Casebook for
TEXTBOOK OF
THERAPEUTICS

Drug and Disease Management

SEVENTH EDITION

Casebook for
TEXTBOOK OF
THERAPEUTICS

Drug and Disease Management

Editors

Greta K. Gourley, Pharm.D., Ph.D.
Associate Professor Pharmacy Practice
 and Pharmacoeconomics
College of Pharmacy
University of Tennessee
Memphis, Tennessee

James M. Holt, Pharm.D., BCPS, CDE
Associate Professor Pharmacy Practice
 and Pharmacoeconomics
College of Pharmacy
University of Tennessee
Memphis, Tennessee

Consulting Editors

Camille W. Thornton / J. Douglas Wurtzbacher / Caroline S. Zeind

Textbook of Therapeutics Editors

Eric T. Herfindal / Dick R. Gourley

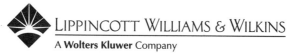

LIPPINCOTT WILLIAMS & WILKINS
A **Wolters Kluwer** Company
Philadelphia • Baltimore • New York • London
Buenos Aires • Hong Kong • Sydney • Tokyo

Editor: Daniel Limmer
Managing Editor: Matthew J. Hauber
Marketing Manager: Anne E. P. Smith
Production Editor: Shannon T. Benner

351 West Camden Street
Baltimore, MD 21201-2436 USA

530 Walnut Street
Philadelphia, PA 19106-3621 USA

Printed in the United States of America

Library of Congress Cataloging-in-Publication Data

Casebook for textbook of therapeutics : textbook of therapeutics / editors, Greta K. Gourley, James M. Holt ; consulting editors, Camile W. Thornton, J. Douglas Wurtzbacher, Caroline S. Zeind.–7th ed.
    p. cm.
  ISBN 0-7817-2415-5
  1. Chemotherapy–Case studies. 2. Therapeutics–Case studies. I. Gourley, Greta K. II. Holt, James M. III. Textbook of therapeutics.

  RM262.C5 2000 Suppl.
  615.5'8–dc21

00-042813

To purchase additional copies of this book, call our customer service department at **(800) 638-3030** or fax orders to **(301) 824-7390.** International customers should call **(301) 714-2324.**

00 01 02 03 04
1 2 3 4 5 6 7 8 9 10

To

My Father
for encouraging my educational endeavors

My Mother
for her attention to detail and steadfast principles

My Husband
for his wonderful devotion to family and the profession of pharmacy

My Child, Kristin
for her commitment to learning and the encouragement of others
and for making everything worthwhile

My Teachers and Colleagues
for sharing their excitement for lifelong learning and
for their abundant support, patience, and understanding

G.K.G.

To

Dick Gourley
for having the confidence in me and giving me the opportunity
to serve as co-editor for the casebook, and most of all for
being a friend and mentor

Greta Gourley
for having the patience to work with me throughout this
project and for being a good friend and colleague

J.M.H.

Preface

The purpose of the *Casebook,* like the previous edition, is to help the student develop skills in therapeutics. While the textbook, *Textbook of Therapeutics: Drug and Disease Management,* Seventh Edition, as well as other sources, provides the facts and knowledge to make therapeutic decisions, students must develop their analytical skills before they attain competence. The *Casebook,* when used with the seventh edition of the *Textbook of Therapeutics: Drug and Disease Management* under the guidance of a clinical educator, will help the student develop skills in therapeutics and make patient-specific decisions.

As with the previous edition, a standard case format is used. The "Introduction" presents the problem-oriented approach to therapy. This approach, used extensively by health care providers, is a comprehensive and organized method for assessing and treating problems.

The cases are organized in sections that correspond to the sections of *Textbook of Therapeutics: Drug and Disease Management,* Seventh Edition. In addition, the cases are presented at three levels of complexity, a feature new to this edition. This use of graded case studies helps the student continually review information from the textbook and coursework, and allows for development of the problem-oriented approach. To enable individual study, the problem lists, SOAP notes, and answers to questions for several cases of varying level of difficulty are contained at the end of the *Casebook* in the "Answers to Selected Cases" section.

The student should not memorize the SOAP notes that are provided, since each is patient-specific and may not apply to other patients. Information in the *Casebook* may become outdated or incorrect as new discoveries are made or new drugs become available. The cases in the *Casebook* do not cover all of the material in the textbook. Based on personal interpretation of the literature or clinical experience, practitioners frequently disagree about the best way to treat a patient, and some may disagree with the approach taken by the consulting editors or contributors. This is expected and is one of the lessons all students must learn; there are often several correct answers to any clinical problem. The student should try to develop the most patient-specific therapeutic plan by carefully weighing the risk versus benefit for the patient.

The *Casebook* includes over 150 cases. This large number of cases allows repetition of the problem-oriented approach to drug therapy. The student can practice on these patients, and no error can result in harm to the patients. Thus, the authors have provided the opportunity for the student to assess current therapy, to recommend new therapy, to monitor therapy, and to provide patient education.

We are pleased to welcome to this edition our three consulting editors, who have provided valuable editorial assistance throughout the editorial process: Drs. Camille W. Thornton, J. Douglas Wurtzbacher, and Caroline S. Zeind. We and the consulting editors would like to thank our other contributors for all their excellent work (see "Contributors"). In addition, we are most grateful to Kelli Beard, our outstanding editorial assistant, who helped us track the progress of the case contributors and consulting editors and the flow of correspondence and revisions necessary to successfully complete this complex undertaking. We would also like to express our appreciation to our colleagues at Lippincott Williams & Wilkins for being responsive to our editorial needs.

We look forward to your feedback on ways to improve the *Casebook* for the next edition.

G.K.G.
J.M.H.

Contributors

Note: Although a number of the cases contained in the *Casebook* were newly authored for this edition, many were adapted from cases originally written for the previous edition; hence, the name listed on the case is the person who either authored the case or adapted it from the original.

Donna L. Baxter, Pharm.D.
Clinical Specialist in Oncology
Department of Pharmacy
University of Arkansas for Medical Sciences
Little Rock, Arkansas

Daphne B. Bernard, Pharm.D.
Assistant Professor
Department of Pharmacy Practice
Howard University College of Pharmacy,
    Nursing, and AHS Division of Pharmacy
Clinical Pharmacist
Howard University Hospital
Washington, D.C.

Michelle Ceresia, Pharm.D.
Assistant Professor
Department of Pharmacy Practice
Massachusetts College of Pharmacy
Boston, Massachusetts

Dawn Chandler-Toufieli, Pharm. D.
Assistant Professor
Department of Pharmacy Practice
Massachusetts College of Pharmacy
Boston, Massachusetts

Stephen Cooke, Pharm.D., BCPP
Assistant Professor
Department of Pharmacy Practice and Pharmacoeconomics
University of Tennessee College of Pharmacy
Memphis, Tennessee

Catherine M. Crill, Pharm.D., BCPS
Assistant Professor
Department of Clinical Pharmacy
University of Tennessee College of Pharmacy
Memphis, Tennessee

Monica Daftary, Pharm.D.
Assistant Professor
Department of Pharmacy Practice
Howard University College of Pharmacy,

Nursing, and AHS Division of Pharmacy
Washington, D.C.

Tammy C. Dawkins, Pharm.D.
Associate Professor
Department of Pharmacy Practice
Howard University College of Pharmacy,
    Nursing, and AHS Division of Pharmacy
Washington, D.C.

Kutay Demirkan, Pharm.D.
Resident
Department of Clinical Pharmacy
University of Tennessee College of Pharmacy
Memphis, Tennessee

Greta K. Gourley, Pharm.D., Ph.D.
Associate Professor
Department of Pharmacy Practice and Pharmacoeconomics
University of Tennessee College of Pharmacy
Memphis, Tennessee

Scott D. Hanes, Pharm.D.
Assistant Professor
Department of Clinical Pharmacy
University of Tennessee College of Pharmacy
Memphis, Tennessee

Valerie W. Hogue, Pharm.D.
Associate Professor
Department of Pharmacy Practice
Howard University College of Pharmacy,
    Nursing, and AHS Division of Pharmacy
Washington, D.C.

James M. Holt, Pharm.D., BCPS, CDE
Associate Professor
Department of Pharmacy Practice and Pharmacoeconomics
University of Tennessee College of Pharmacy
Clinical Pharmacy Specialist
Department of Veteran Affairs
Pharmacy Department
Memphis, Tennessee

Joanna Q. Hudson, Pharm.D., BCPS
Assistant Professor
Department of Clinical Pharmacy
University of Tennessee College of Pharmacy
Memphis, Tennessee

Jeff Hulstein, Pharm.D.
Clinical Specialist
Pharmacy Services
Parkland Health and Hospital System
Dallas, Texas

Lori N. Justice, Pharm.D.
Assistant Professor
Department of Pharmacy Practice and Pharmacoeconomics
University of Tennessee College of Pharmacy
Memphis, Tennessee

Bob Lobo, Pharm.D., BCPS
Assistant Professor
Department of Clinical Pharmacy
University of Tennessee College of Pharmacy
Clinical Pharmacist
Methodist Central Hospital
Memphis, Tennessee

Bill McIntyre, Pharm.D.
Assistant Professor
Department of Pharmacy Practice
University of Arkansas for Medical Sciences
Little Rock, Arkansas

Susan W. Miller, Pharm.D., FASCP, CGP
Professor
Department of Pharmacy Practice
Mercer University Southern School of Pharmacy
Atlanta, Georgia

Nicole G. Parker, Pharm.D.
Fellow, Women's Health
Department of Pharmacy Practice and Pharmacoeconomics
University of Tennessee College of Pharmacy
Memphis, Tennessee

Anne Reaves, Pharm.D., BCPS
Assistant Professor
Department of Clinical Pharmacy
University of Tennessee College of Pharmacy
Ambulatory Care Therapeutics
Methodist Central Hospital
Memphis, Tennessee

Ted L. Rice, M.S., BCPS
Associate Professor
Department of Pharmacy Practice
University of Pittsburgh School of Pharmacy
Pittsburgh, Pennsylvania

Dorthea Rudorf, Pharm.D.
Assistant Professor
Department of Pharmacy Practice
Massachusetts College of Pharmacy
Boston, Massachusetts

R. Michelle Sanders, Pharm.D., BCNSP
Clinical Pharmacy Specialist
Pharmaceutical Department
St. Jude Children's Research Hospital
Memphis, Tennessee

Debbie Scholtz, Pharm.D., BCPS, CDE
Assistant Professor
Department of Pharmacy Practice and
Pharmacoeconomics
University of Tennessee College of Pharmacy
Memphis, Tennessee

Amy Seabrook, Pharm.D.
University of Tennessee College of Pharmacy
Memphis, Tennessee

Kevin M. Sowinski, Pharm.D., BCPS
Assistant Professor
Department of Pharmacy Practice
Purdue University Pharmacy Programs at Indianapolis
Indianapolis, Indiana

Robert C. Stevens, Pharm.D., BCPS
Associate Professor
Department of Clinical Pharmacy
University of Tennessee College of Pharmacy
Memphis, Tennessee

Melanie P. Swims, Pharm.D., BCPS
Assistant Professor
Department of Pharmacy Practice
University of Tennessee College of Pharmacy
Clinical Pharmacy Specialist
Department of Veterans Affairs
Pharmacy Department (119)
Memphis, Tennessee

Simone E. Taylor, Pharm.D., BCPS
Clinical Pharmacy Coordinator
Royal Melbourne Hospital
Melbourne, Australia

Camille W. Thornton, Pharm.D.
Assistant Professor
Department of Pharmacy Practice and Pharmacoeconomics
University of Tennessee College of Pharmacy
Memphis, Tennessee

Donna Topping, Pharm.D., BCOP
Assistant Professor
Department of Clinical Pharmacy
University of Tennessee College of Pharmacy
Clinical Pharmacist
Methodist Hospital-Central
Memphis, Tennessee

Nicole Turcotte, Pharm. D.
Assistant Professor
Department of Pharmacy Practice
Massachusetts College of Pharmacy
Boston, Massachusetts

Jennifer Wiseman, Pharm.D.
University of Tennessee College of Pharmacy
Memphis, Tennessee

G. Christopher Wood, Pharm.D., BCPS
Assistant Professor
Department of Clinical Pharmacy
University of Tennessee College of Pharmacy
Memphis, Tennessee

Lorianne Wright, Pharm. D.
Assistant Professor
Department of Pharmacy Practice
Massachusetts College of Pharmacy and Allied Health Sciences
Boston, Massachusetts

J. Douglas Wurtzbacher, Pharm.D.
Assistant Professor
Department of Pharmacy Practice and Pharmacoeconomics
University of Tennessee College of Pharmacy
Memphis, Tennessee

Caroline S. Zeind, Pharm.D.
Assistant Professor
Department of Pharmacy Practice
Massachusetts College of Pharmacy and Allied Health Sciences
Boston, Massachusetts

Contents

Contents by Topic

GUIDELINES FOR USING CASEBOOK

This casebook was designed to accompany the 7th edition of *Textbook of Therapeutics: Drug and Disease Management;* it is organized in sections that correspond to the sections in the textbook. Specific discussions in the textbook, such as clinical pharmacodynamics, drug interactions, adverse drug reactions, and clinical lab tests and interpretation, are interwoven into the cases. The cases within each section illustrate patients with diseases that are discussed in the textbook. Under the "Educational Materials" heading the textbook chapter is listed, followed in parentheses by the specific discussions within that chapter to which the student should refer for appropriate background material on the case. The cases are realistic and represent those that would likely be encountered in a hospital or clinic.

CASES: THREE TYPES IN EACH SECTION

Cases are categorized as Level 1, 2, or 3 based on their degree of therapeutic difficulty. The three level classification system allows the user to identify the level of knowledge and problem-solving required to design a pharmaceutical care plan as well as answer pertinent questions for each case. The case levels are described below:

Level 1 Cases

a. Involve *simple* therapeutic and disease management problems.
b. Require application of baseline (fundamental) knowledge of therapeutics, pathophysiology, and disease management expected of the *beginner* student.
c. Include development of a pharmaceutical plan of care for such therapeutic-related problems as:
  (1) Epidemiologic considerations and other factors contributing to the condition
  (2) Pharmacokinetic differences
  (3) Physical assessment parameters (including signs and symptoms), laboratory tests, diagnostic tests, serum drug concentrations, and pharmacokinetic abnormalities
  (4) Actual/potential drug interactions
  (5) Adverse drug effects
  (6) Nonoptimal pharmacologic and nonpharmacologic treatment regimens
  (7) Nonadherence to therapy
  (8) Psychosocial problems and/or
  (9) Potential or actual pharmacoeconomic problems
d. Provide for analysis of **2–3 case problems** (e.g., a patient with uncontrolled hypertension on hydrocholorothiazide and experiencing hypokalemia).

e. Require summarization of therapeutic, pathophysiologic, and disease management concepts for a given condition utilizing a key points format.
f. Provide opportunity for *beginning* level application of knowledge for problem-solving.

Level 2 Cases

a. Include *moderately complex* therapeutic and disease management problems.
b. Require application of intermediate (median) knowledge of therapeutics, pathophysiology, and disease management expected of the *intermediate* student.
c. Include development of a pharmaceutical plan of care for such therapeutic-related problems listed under the Level 1 cases with an emphasis on application of a broader knowledge base.
d. Provide for analysis of **4–5 case problems** (e.g., a patient with uncontrolled hypertension, angina, CAD, and type 2 diabetes mellitus who has not been placed on an ACE inhibitor. A patient with type 2 diabetes, angina, CAD, and renal insufficiency (elevated serum creatinine) who should not be put on metformin [Glucophage]).
e. Require summarization of therapeutic, pathophysiologic, and disease management concepts for a given condition utilizing a key points format.
f. Provide opportunity for *intermediate level* application of knowledge for problem-solving.

Level 3 Cases

a. Include *highly complex* therapeutic and disease management problems.
b. Require application of a superior (outstanding) knowledge of therapeutics, pathophysiology, and disease management expected of the *advanced* student.
c. Include development of a pharmaceutical plan of care for such therapeutic-related problems as depicted for level 1 and 2 cases with a greater emphasis on critical thinking.
d. Provide for analysis of **greater than 5 case problems** (e.g., a patient with multiple diagnoses and therapeutic-related problems requiring use of such decision-making tools as treatment algorithms).
e. Require summarization of therapeutic, pathophysiologic, and disease management concepts for a given condition utilizing a key points format.
f. Provide opportunity for *advanced level* application of knowledge for problem-solving and critical thinking.

The ascending level of complexity of the cases in each section provides the student with an opportunity to demonstrate knowledge attainment and acquire increasing problem-solving and critical thinking ability. In addition, it assists the student to develop self-efficacy in many therapeutic areas while building a disease and disease management knowledge base.

Cases are to be fully analyzed using the SOAP method of documentation (discussed later in this introduction). Following the case scenarios, multiple choice questions (with a single correct answer) and open-ended questions are presented. The case questions are developed using the universal set of educational objectives (see below), and the questions correspond to the complexity level of the case. The objectives correspond to the following areas of learning: knowledge acquisition, application, problem-solving, and critical thinking. The educational objective(s) (EO) from the Universal Set of Objectives that correspond to the case questions are in parentheses following each of the questions. This assists the educator who plans to use the cases for a seminar/class by providing both specific evaluation questions and the corresponding objectives. It also helps the student who is doing a self-directed study to determine which educational objectives have been accomplished. Though the case study is generally viewed as a problem-solving, teaching, and learning strategy, the case questions may be written to assess the knowledge attained, the application of knowledge, and problem-solving and critical thinking ability.

All aspects of each disease and every potential therapeutic problem cannot be discussed in the case studies. Therefore, the casebook cannot be used to ensure understanding of all the material in the textbook. However, it is likely that a student who is able to analyze the case, prioritize the problems, document pharmaceutical care utilizing the SOAP note format, and answer the case questions has a good grasp of the material presented in the casebook, as well as the corresponding textbook chapter(s).

To allow students the opportunity to study correct approaches to the cases, the problem lists, SOAP notes, and answers to questions for selected cases are included in the "Answers to Selected Cases" section at the end of the casebook. (These cases are identified under the "Problem List" and "Questions" headings.)

UNIVERSAL SET OF EDUCATIONAL OBJECTIVES (EO)

For the conditions presented, the student should be able to:

1. Describe the etiology and pathophysiology including sequelae.
2. Identify signs and symptoms.
3. Discuss epidemiologic considerations such as incidence, prevalence, demographics (e.g., age, gender, sex, racial and ethnic groups), and other contributing factors.
4. Analyze pharmacokinetic differences as they relate to age, gender, genetic factors (racial and ethnic groups), environment and cultural factors, disease states, alcohol consumption, and smoking.
5. Evaluate pertinent physical assessment parameters, laboratory studies, diagnostic tests, serum drug concentrations and pharmacokinetics for abnormal findings.
6. Apply general principles of clinical pharmacokinetics including calculations as required.
7. Describe the mechanism of action of pharmacologic and nonpharmacologic interventions employed in the treatment.
8. Analyze factors that should be considered when choosing pharmacologic and nonpharmacologic therapy.
9. Identify potential or actual drug interactions (e.g., drug–drug, drug–food, drug–disease, etc.).
10. Recognize common adverse effects of pharmacologic treatments.
11. Evaluate present pharmacologic and nonpharmacologic treatment for problems (e.g., lack of appropriate indication, dose, etc.).
12. Suggest recommendations for optimizing pharmacologic and nonpharmacologic treatment to achieve optimal control of the disease state(s) (e.g., through use of treatment algorithms found in the accompanying 7th edition of Herfindal and Gourley's therapeutics textbook).
13. Use the Problem List and SOAP note format to analyze, synthesize, and prioritize pertinent data in order to develop a pharmaceutical care plan. (This objective will *not* be used to develop case questions. However, it is met in each case through use of the Problem List and SOAP Note.)
14. Develop a detailed education plan for the patient including necessary lifestyle changes, medication counseling information, specific counseling (communication) techniques, and adherence strategies. (This objective may be met in each case through use of the Plan portion of the SOAP Note or by use of specific case questions.)
15. Analyze psychosocial factors that may affect patient adherence with both pharmacologic and nonpharmacologic therapy (e.g., influence of family, significant others, and/or peer group(s); financial resources; perceived susceptibility or severity of long-term consequences; interference with lifestyle).
16. Describe the health care provider's role relative to psychosocial factors.

17. Evaluate the pharmacoeconomic considerations relative to the patient's pharmaceutical plan of care; summarize therapeutic, pathophysiologic, and disease management concepts for a given condition utilizing a key points format.

PROBLEM–ORIENTED APPROACH

In order to use the casebook, it is necessary to become familiar with the Problem–Oriented Medical Record (POMR). In 1964, Lawrence E. Weed published the problem-oriented approach to medical records, patient care, and medical education. The method differs from the earlier method in which health care providers approached the patient from the point of view of their medical specialities. Prior to 1964, a physician would write a note in the chart about one of the patient's diseases. The note usually stated the condition of the patient at that time; if a procedure was performed, the note would describe the procedure and its results. The note usually did not summarize previous data and rarely outlined a thought process about how a diagnosis was made or how a particular treatment was chosen. Many notes were contradictory. The "source method," as this method was called, was cited as a cause of fragmented patient care, and Dr. Weed suggested that this form of record keeping was inappropriate for more sophisticated health care where the medical record was used as a means of communication between health care providers. The problem-oriented method, in addition to being comprehensive due to better communication among all persons contributing to health care, allows auditing of care to assure quality. Today, nearly all health care providers use some form of the problem-oriented method for documentation of patient care in the medical record.

Clinicians should learn the problem-oriented method of health care so that a systematic, disciplined approach to each patient is used and so that no important therapeutic considerations are missed. The approach should always be the same regardless of the simplicity or complexity of the problem.

TWO MAIN COMPONENTS OF THE PROBLEM–ORIENTED METHOD

Problem List

A problem is defined as a patient concern, a health professional concern, or a concern of both. Many problems are diseases that have been fully worked-up and diagnosed, but all problems are not diagnoses. A problem may be a patient complaint (i.e., a symptom), abnormal results from a laboratory test or an abnormal finding from a physical exam (i.e., a sign), a social or financial situation, a psychological concern, or a physical limitation. A problem is identified as generally or as specifically as possible, based on available information. A symptom may result in a sign after a physical examination is completed; this may lead to a diagnosis after the completion of the appropriate diagnostic tests. The diagnosed disease may then be cured by treatment. For example, a patient may complain of cough, fever, and sputum production. A physician hears rales and rhonchi on chest auscultation and orders a sputum culture and chest radiograph, which leads to the diagnosis of pneumococcal pneumonia. Penicillin is administered and the pneumonia is cured. Thus, problems are dynamic: problems are resolved and new problems develop. Patients frequently have some stable and some inactive problems, but they usually have one problem that is the most severe or that demands attention before the others.

The problem list is developed from the data in a medical record, which would typically include the chief complaint, history of the present illness, past medical history, past surgical history, family history, social history, medication and allergy history, physical examination, review of systems, results of laboratory tests, serum drug concentrations, and diagnostic procedures such as electrocardiogram and radiographs. Health care providers gather information to contribute to the data and organize the data to develop the problem list. However, each health care provider may not interpret the data in exactly the same manner, nor will he or she consider each problem in the same rank of importance; ranking will depend upon the perspective of the health care provider. The problem list is the table of contents of the medical record and the framework for patient care.

SOAP Note

The second component of the problem-oriented medical record is the organization of the data into the SOAP (subjective, objective, assessment, and plan) Note. Each entry is recorded in this format. A generally accepted clinical practice is the use of a single SOAP note per patient encounter. **Therefore, a single SOAP note versus a note per problem is to be used to analyze the cases in this casebook.** The subjective and objective data are recorded for the problem(s). Assessments along with their etiologies should be numbered like the problem list in priority order; and the plan(s) should also follow such numbering. A blank SOAP sheet is included with the Introductory Case at the end of Section 1. **Students should make copies of this sheet** for writing each of their SOAP notes. Each component of the SOAP note is discussed next, and a sample case follows the discussion.

SUBJECTIVE (S)

Subjective data record how the patient feels or what can be observed about the patient. Subjective data are descriptive in nature and usually cannot be confirmed by procedures or tests. The primary way to obtain subjective data is to lis-

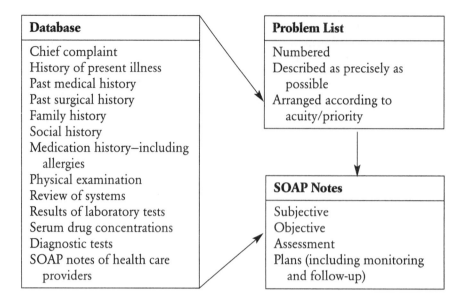

Database	Problem List
Chief complaint History of present illness Past medical history Past surgical history Family history Social history Medication history–including allergies Physical examination Review of systems Results of laboratory tests Serum drug concentrations Diagnostic tests SOAP notes of health care providers	Numbered Described as precisely as possible Arranged according to acuity/priority

SOAP Notes

Subjective
Objective
Assessment
Plans (including monitoring and follow-up)

ten to the patient's descriptions of complaints or symptoms and responses to questions that are asked in a systematic fashion as a review of systems (ROS). Subjective data are also obtained by observing how the patient looks, talks, acts, responds, etc.

OBJECTIVE (O)

Objective data include the history as documented in the medical record and their results of various tests, procedures, and assessments. Objective data may include vital signs, findings on physical examination, results of laboratory tests, and findings for diagnostic procedures such as radiographs, CT scans, and electrocardiograms. Current medications are listed under objective data. This is to remind the clinician what the patient is receiving for each problem. Every medication that the patient is receiving should correspond to a problem. If a patient is receiving medications for an unidentified problem, the problem list is incomplete. Note that some drugs may treat more than one problem.

ASSESSMENT (A)

The clinician uses the subjective and objective data to assess therapy or develop a therapeutic plan. A systematic method for assessing each problem should be developed so that the assessment is complete. There are three components to the assessment of each problem.

1. **Etiology:** The clinician should first assess whether this is a drug-induced problem. Many problems are not diseases but are adverse reactions to drugs. Under etiology, the clinician should also identify any risk factors or predisposing factors for a problem in the

patient. Modification or reduction of these factors may be a part of the treatment plan and may be as important as drug therapy.

2. **Assessment if therapy is indicated:** Problems may be mild, moderate, or severe; they may be acute or chronic; and they may be stable or progressing. Obviously, the need and urgency of treatment varies with each of these. For acute, severe problems, emergency aggressive therapy may be required, while for mild stable problems, a wait-and-watch approach may be more appropriate. Some problems may not be severe enough for drug treatment, and nondrug therapy may be more appropriate for some problems. At times, the diagnosis may not yet be established; more data may be required for diagnosis or an isolated abnormal value may not be a rational basis for drug therapy.

3. **Assessment of current therapy and/or new therapy:** Patients frequently have multiple chronic problems and are therefore already receiving drug therapy. However, this therapy may not be the best possible choice for this patient. New therapy may be initiated for new or old problems. The clinician must systematically evaluate the patient's current therapy as well as the new therapy. The same process applies to both situations. The SOAP note should list all of the reasons for the current assessment. The reasons are important for all health care providers to understand why therapy was changed, for auditing the quality of care, and for helping the health care professional remember the reasons for the changes.

   a. **Optimal therapy (i.e., drug of choice):** The clinician should determine that this is the optimal therapy for this patient. This does not necessarily mean that it is the usual "drug of choice" for this disease. There may be patient-specific reasons why the usual "drug of choice" would be contraindicated or inappropriate for this patient. The drug should be chosen considering the patient's other problems (drug-disease interactions), other drugs (drug-drug interactions), age, renal and hepatic function, allergies (considering cross-sensitivities), risk factors for adverse reactions or side effects, convenience, compliance, and cost.

b. Correct dose: The clinician should determine the correct dose of the drug for this patient considering the patient's age, sex, weight, renal and hepatic function, other drugs that the patient is taking, and any other pertinent factors. The pharmacist on the team should always perform pharmacokinetic calculations based on population parameters or previous drug levels.

c. Correct dosage form: The correct dosage form, route, and schedule of administration should be determined. Patient-specific factors, convenience, compliance, costs, and lifestyle should be considered.

d. Correct duration: The correct duration of therapy should be determined. Patient-specific factors may require that therapy be longer or shorter than what is usually recommended for this problem. Some problems require that therapy be continued for life or until circumstances change, while other problems are cured by a single course of therapy. Unfortunately, patients are frequently started on therapy that is never discontinued, although the problem has resolved. Some patients need to be treated longer because the disease is severe or they have certain predisposing factors. Other patients may need to be treated only during an acute exacerbation of their disease. Thus, the duration of therapy is patient-specific.

e. Drug(s) required: A determination should be made as to whether or not all the drugs that the patient is taking are required. All drugs taken by the patient should be for problems identified on the problem list. The patient should not be taking additional drugs; if there are additional drugs, the problem list is incomplete. Duplication of drugs from the same therapeutic category frequently occurs, and some of these drugs may be discontinued. A higher dose of a single agent may be preferred to two drugs for the same problem. At times, a single drug may be used to treat more than one problem. Some problems do not require drug therapy. Health care professionals should always try to minimize the number of drugs that a patient is taking.

f. Additional monitoring parameters: For current therapy, in addition to the above, the following should be determined.

(1) Response to therapy: If the patient is responding appropriately to therapy. Patient-specific factors should be considered and include the items discussed under goals and monitoring parameters below.

(2) Untoward reactions: If the patient is having any adverse reactions, side effects, or drug interactions. Obviously, the plan will be influenced by the occurrence of any of these.

(3) Compliance issues: If the medications have been taken as prescribed. Drugs that are not taken as prescribed are usually not effective. The plan for treatment of a noncompliant patient is different from the plan for a patient who is compliant but not responding. Serious consequences can occur in a noncompliant patient when therapy is altered based on the assumption of compliance. Questions must be phrased carefully to obtain accurate information about compliance.

PLAN (P)

After the assessment of the subjective and objective data and therapy, a plan is developed.

1. Therapeutic: Current therapy must be either continued or discontinued. The reasons for continuing or discontinuing current therapy should have been stated in the assessment portion of the SOAP note. If new therapy is initiated, the clinician should state the drug, dose, dosage form, route, schedule, duration, and exactly how therapy will be initiated. Therapy may be initiated at full doses or the dose may be titrated, depending on the drug and the patient or problem. If the drug is to be titrated, the size and frequency of the dosage changes should be stated. Precise instructions for drug administration should be included. The reasons for selecting the drug, dose, dosage form, route, schedule, and duration should have been stated in the assessment portion of the SOAP note.

2. Drugs to be avoided: The clinician should list all drugs that could potentially be used to treat this problem but that should be avoided in this patient for patient-specific reasons. If the patient is likely to receive a drug for another problem that would interact with the therapy for this problem, it should be stated that it, too, should be avoided. If these drugs are not documented in the POMR as ones to avoid, other health care providers may inadvertently prescribe them. The clinician should list the reasons why these drugs are being avoided, such as allergies, age, drug-disease interactions, drug-drug interactions, renal or hepatic dysfunction, risk factors for adverse reactions or side effects, convenience, compliance, or cost, if not already stated in the assessment portion of the SOAP note.

3. **Goals:** Each treatment plan should have a long-term goal that should be both problem- and patient-specific. Some problems are cured, while others are controlled or relieved. In some patients, the subjective and objective evidence of the problem will return to normal; in other patients with severe problems the subjective and objective evidence will only return toward normal. Other appropriate goals include preventing acute complications, preventing long-term morbidity and mortality, avoiding adverse drug reactions or drug interactions, improving compliance, improving quality of life, and decreasing health care costs.

4. **Therapeutic and toxicity monitoring parameters:** Each therapeutic plan should be monitored by specific parameters to assess response and to document that no adverse drug reactions or side effects are occurring.

   a. **Therapeutic monitoring parameters:** The clinician must select the appropriate subjective and objective data that will be followed to assess the response to therapy. These parameters should be chosen carefully, considering cost, invasiveness, risks of the procedure, sensitivity, and reliability. Usually the same subjective and objective data that were used to diagnose the disease are used to monitor therapy, except expensive or invasive tests are not always repeated as monitoring parameters. The frequency for monitoring these parameters should be stated. Some critically ill patients should be monitored every 5 minutes, while other tests may be performed only yearly in stable patients. End points should be established for each therapeutic plan. The end points should be patient-, drug-, and problem-specific. Like the goals, the monitoring parameters may return to normal or toward normal, depending upon the patient, drug, or problem. The end point may indicate that therapy is complete or has been inadequate. If the end point shows that therapy is complete, then it should be stated that the drugs will be discontinued. If the end point shows that therapy is inadequate, additional or alternative therapy may be prescribed.

   b. **Toxicity monitoring parameters:** Each therapeutic plan should be monitored for adverse drug reactions, side effects, and drug interactions. The

clinician must select the appropriate subjective and objective data that will be observed for assessment of toxicity. The intervals for monitoring these data should be stated. Any abnormalities that would be revealed by routine screening tests and that would indicate a drug-induced problem should also be identified in the plan along with the frequency of these observations. The plan should include how serious or frequently encountered adverse effects should be handled.

5. **Patient education:** The plan will be useless unless it is implemented correctly. All patients should know the name(s), dose, indication, schedule, storage, precautions, duration, and side effect/adverse reactions of the drugs that they are using. Some plans involve nondrug therapy or lifestyle changes as well as drug therapy. Some dosage forms require more detailed instruction for administration than others. Specific information or techniques to enhance compliance should be discussed and documented in the POMR. Any patient concerns about the medication should be addressed. Any information required for the safe and proper use of the drug should be discussed.

6. **Future plans:** It is likely that the patient will be seen again, so some plans should be made for follow-up. Another clinic visit may be scheduled, additional tests may be required to establish a baseline before treatment is initiated, or contingency plans may be made in case the patient does not respond to therapy or develops a drug-induced problem. The clinician should document what future plans are needed for this patient.

Using the SOAP format is a systematic way to critique or plan pharmacologic and nonpharmacologic therapy for a patient. Because it is a systematic approach if it is employed in a disciplined way for each patient, only patient-specific treatment decisions will be made.

A sample case is analyzed at the end of this section using the SOAP format to illustrate the method that is used in this casebook. The information is obtained from the medical record. For the sake of saving space, all information from the record has been abbreviated and condensed. The laboratory data have been reported in SI units followed by traditional units in parentheses. Abbreviations have been used less frequently than they are used in medical charts, but common abbreviations are used to save space and familiarize the student with these abbreviations.

CONCLUSION

The SOAP format allows a systematic approach to therapy and is widely used in medical education and practice. However, individual practitioners may analyze a case slightly differently. In many cases, the correct therapy for an individual patient will be agreed upon by all who analyze the case, because in these situations there is only one possible therapy based upon the contraindications or other patient variables. In other cases, the correct therapy is not so straightforward, and two or three alternatives may be equally acceptable. In these cases, the choice of therapy frequently rests with the individual practitioner's preference. In other cases, there may be one therapy that would be the best for the patient, but other alternatives may be acceptable because of extenuating circumstances such as a history of noncompliance. Therefore, the student should use the cases in the casebook primarily to learn a method for analyzing cases. The answers given in these cases may not be the only acceptable answers, and other available alternatives would be equally efficacious and safe. In addition, the therapy and information given in these cases may become incorrect as new knowledge is accumulated.

In some cases, the available literature is conflicting or controversial, and two practitioners may have different opinions based on the available information. In all cases, the case analysis and answers to the questions pertain only to the patient involved. The information may or may not be applicable to other patients with the same problem. Therefore, the student is warned against memorizing these cases. This casebook allows the student to practice analyzing cases and making decisions concerning therapeutics in a situation that cannot harm a patient. By this process the student should develop skill in therapeutics. If this casebook is used as intended, the student will make a commitment to a method of analyzing the patient's case. This will be useful in developing the skills that are necessary for performance in a clinical setting. Thus, the student is highly encouraged to write the SOAP notes. A single book cannot be responsible for the development of critical evaluation skills, but this casebook, in conjunction with the seventh edition of *Textbook of Therapeutics: Drug and Disease Management* and with the guidance of faculty in appropriate courses, will aid in preparing students in therapeutics.

INTRODUCTORY CASE

INTRODUCTORY CASE
James M. Holt
Topics: Anemia, Degenerative
Joint Disease, Seizures

Level I

EDUCATIONAL MATERIALS
Chapter 13: Anemias; Chapter 24: Peptic Ulcer
Disease; Chapter 32: Osteoarthritis

SCENARIO

RJ, a 74-year-old male; outpatient clinic

Chief Complaint

Weakness and lethargy

History of Present Illness

Experiencing these symptoms for approximately 2 months

Past Medical History

Seizure disorder since motor vehicle accident 2 years ago
Degenerative joint disease (DJD) in knees and hips

Past Surgical History

Not applicable

Family/Social History

Tobacco–none
Alcohol–heavy since death of wife about 6 months ago

Medication History

Phenytoin, 300 mg PO QHS
Aspirin, 650 mg PO QID and PRN
Reports compliance with medication regimen

Allergies

No known allergies (NKA)

Physical Examination (PE)

GEN (General):	Well-developed, well-nourished (WDWN) male in no acute distress (NAD)
VS (Vital signs):	BP 120/80, RR 20, T 37°C, Wt 62 kg, Ht 180 cm
HEENT (Head, Eyes, Ears, Nose, Throat):	Pale mucous membranes and skin; no nystagmus
COR (Coronary):	Normal S1 and S2, no murmurs, rubs, or gallops
Chest:	Clear to auscultation and percussion
ABD (Abdomen):	Soft, nontender, with no masses or organomegaly
GU (Genitourinary):	Normal male genitalia
RECTAL:	Guaiac-positive stool
EXT (Extremities):	Pale nail beds; tenderness of both knees but no signs of

PROBLEM LIST and SOAP NOTE FOR CASE _____

Problem List:

SUBJECTIVE:

OBJECTIVE:

ASSESSMENT:

PLAN:

Neuro (Neurological): inflammation; limited range of motion of both hips

Alert and oriented × 3 (person, place, and time); cranial nerves intact; normal deep tendon reflexes (DTRs); no seizures in 6 months

Results of Pertinent Laboratory Tests, Serum Drug Concentrations, and Diagnostic Tests

Hct 0.32 (32) [6 month prior–0.38 (38)] Hgb 100 (10) Plts 320 × 10⁹ (320 × 10³) MCV 80 (80) MCHC 280 (28) Serum Fe 6.8 (38) TIBC 91 (510)

Peripheral blood smear: Normocytic red blood cells

The person analyzing this case should first prioritize the problem list for the clinic visit. RJ's complaint today is consistent with the problem of anemia, and this problem should be assigned the highest priority. Other problems that could be contributing to the anemia should be discussed next (e.g., aspirin use for DJD, alcohol abuse). Stable problems (i.e., seizure disorder) should be listed last and given the least priority. The SOAP format should then be utilized to systematically document the patient's problems, as well as recommended interventions.

PROBLEM LIST

1. Anemia
2. DJD–aspirin use
3. Seizure disorder

SOAP NOTE\

S: "I've been weak and lethargic for 2 months. My arthritis has been bothering me, so I've been taking aspirin regularly for relief." Seizure history–none in 6 months; reports compliance with medications. Wife passed away recently–reports increased alcohol use since her death.

O: Vitals–stable
Pertinent findings on physical exam: Pale mucous membranes, guaiac-positive stool, pale nail beds; limited range of motion both hips
Pertinent laboratory: Hct 0.32 (32) [6 month prior–0.38 (38)], Hgb 100 (10), Plts 320 × 10⁹ (320 × 10³), MCV 80 (80), MCHC 280 (28), Serum Fe 6.8 (38), TIBC 91 (510)

A: **Problem 1:** Anemia; guaiac positive. Reports regularly taking aspirin for arthritis relief. Rule out (R/O) possible gastrointestinal bleed from excessive aspirin use.

Problem 2: Degenerative joint disease–needs an agent with less GI toxicity. Recommend acetaminophen 500 mg–2 tablets QID.

Problem 3: Seizure disorder–stable. No change in medications

P: Problem 1: Anemia

- Discuss with patient's provider–would recommend upper GI series to R/O possible ulcer secondary to excessive aspirin usage.
- Iron levels normal–supplementation not recommended
- Recommend H-2 blocker therapy: ranitidine 150 mg BID until UGI results available
- Counsel to monitor bowel movements closely–if black, tarry stools (melena) or worsening of physical symptoms, instruct to report to the emergency room immediately
- Counsel on excessive alcohol use and educate that this, too, can contribute to anemia

Problem 2: DJD

- Recommend stopping aspirin therapy immediately
- Counsel to avoid all OTC products that may contain salicylate
- Recommend scheduled acetaminophen–500 mg–2 tablets QID for arthritis symptoms
- Counsel on the need to avoid excess alcohol while taking acetaminophen because of potential for hepatotoxicity

Problem 3: Seizure disorder

- Stable problem. Recommend continuation of current phenytoin regimen; no recent phenytoin level on record; consider checking at next scheduled follow-up appointment

QUESTIONS

1. The most likely cause of RJ's anemia is: (EO-1 [Educational Objective])
   a. Alcohol abuse
   b. Phenytoin overdose
   c. Aspirin use
   d. Anemia of chronic disease secondary to arthritis

2. Signs and symptoms that RJ is experiencing which might indicate anemia are: (EO-2)
   a. Excessive joint pain
   b. Extreme fatigue
   c. Exacerbation of seizure disorder
   d. High hemoglobin and hematocrit

3. Based on the evaluation of RJ's lab parameters, the health care provider determines his anemia is: (EO-5)

a. Microcytic
b. Macrocytic
c. Normocytic
d. Eosinophilic

4. You recommend acetaminophen as an alternative to aspirin because it: (EO-8)
   a. Is less likely to exacerbate seizures
   b. Is less GI toxic
   c. Can be taken less often than aspirin
   d. Has greater anti-inflammatory properties than aspirin

5. The patient has been drinking alcohol heavily since the death of his wife; a warranted recommendation is: (EO-15)
   a. Alcoholics Anonymous
   b. A support group for grieving spouses
   c. Immediate admission for alcohol detoxification
   d. He limit his alcohol to 3 ounces per day

6. Develop a detailed education plan for this patient. (EO-14)

7. Another provider recommends the patient be placed on celexocib instead of acetaminophen. Discuss pharmacoeconomic implications of this choice. (EO-17)

8. This patient returns 3 months later. He is no longer taking aspirin; however, he continues to drink alcohol heavily. His hematocrit is still low and his MCV is elevated. What type of anemia does this patient probably have? (EO-18)

9. Summarize therapeutic, pathophysiologic, and disease management concepts for anemia and DJD utilizing a key points format. (EO-18)

ANSWERS TO QUESTIONS

1. c: Aspirin use
2. b: Extreme fatigue
3. c: Normocytic
4. b: Is less GI toxic

5. b: A support group for grieving spouses
6. Counsel to take acetaminophen using a scheduled dosage regimen, which should maximize pain relief. Counsel to avoid all over-the-counter agents which may contain salicylate products (e.g., Pepto-Bismol, B.C. powders, etc.). Instruct to let his provider know if he is not getting adequate pain relief with acetaminophen so an alternative therapy can be tried.

7. Celexocib is a COX-2 inhibitor and will require a provider visit to obtain a prescription. While studies show this agent is relatively safe in patients who have a history of GI toxicity from traditional agents, celexocib is much more expensive than OTC acetaminophen and may be cost prohibitive.

8. Based on laboratory parameters and ETOH abuse—a macrocytic anemia probably related to folate deficiency. Fasting B_{12}/folate levels can be obtained to verify this.

9. Key points are:
   - Control of arthritis pain with least toxic agents
   - Education of patients and family about degenerative arthritis and its therapies
   - Acetaminophen is considered first-line therapy and cost-effective treatment for degenerative arthritis
   - Patients with potential ulcer disease should avoid ulcerogenic drugs such as aspirin-containing products
   - Drug therapy for the management of ulcer disease includes:
       H-2 blockers
       Sucralfate, misoprostol
       Detect and eradicate *Helicobacter pylori*
   - Patients with ulcer disease should be counseled to avoid alcohol
   - Patients with a history of alcohol abuse frequently experience macrocytic anemias related to folate deficiency. Cessation of alcohol use and treatment with daily folic acid is recommended.

CASE 1
G. Christopher Wood
Topic: Enteral Nutrition
Level 3
EDUCATIONAL MATERIALS
Chapter 12: Parenteral and Enteral Nutrition in
Adult Patients (nutritional assessment, total protein
and calorie requirements, enteral nutrition);
Chapter 9: Fluid and Electrolyte Therapy and
Acid-Base Balance (phosphorus)

SCENARIO

Patient and Setting
AW, a 37-year-old male; neurotrauma intensive care unit (NICU)

Chief Complaint
Intolerance of enteral feedings

History of Present Illness
Sustained a severe traumatic brain injury (TBI) in a motor vehicle accident (MVA) 5 days ago; other significant injury was 3 broken ribs on right side, generalized tonic-clonic seizure activity was noted at the scene of the accident; an intracranial pressure (ICP) monitor was placed upon admission; on hospital day two, nasogastric enteral feeding was begun with Jevity at 50 mL/hr; however, only a minimal amount of nutrition was able to be administered over the past 4 days (total of 500 mL) due to persistently high gastric residuals (>150 mL) and high blood glucose concentrations; ICP monitor was removed following several days of well-controlled ICPs, however, remains unresponsive to commands and mechanically ventilated; currently being treated empirically for suspected pneumonia

Past Medical History
Type 1 diabetes mellitus (DM) for 26 years

Past Surgical History
Craniotomy, 5 days ago

Family/Social History
Noncontributory

Medication History
Ceftazidime, 2 g IV q8h in 100 mL D5W

Vancomycin, 1.5 g IV q12h in 250 mL D5W

Ranitidine, 150 mg/250 mL NS at 10 mL/hr

Heparin, SC 5000 units q12h

Phenytoin, 150 mg per feeding tube q8h

Morphine, 2–4 mg IV q1h PRN agitation

NS, IV at 75 mL/hr

Accuchecks with sliding scale regular human insulin q6h (if <200 no insulin, 201–250 4 units, 250–300 6 units, >300 8 units and call MD)

Allergies
NKDA

Physical Examination
GEN: Well-developed, well-nourished male in no apparent distress
VS: BP 116/76, HR 85, RR 20, T 38.5°C, Wt 90 kg, Ht 194 cm
HEENT: Craniotomy site healing well, no visible redness, minimal swelling and tenderness
COR: Normal heart sounds
CHEST: Coarse breath sounds bilaterally
ABD: Soft, nontender, nondistended, no masses, hypoactive bowel sounds
GU: WNL
RECTAL: WNL
NEURO: Withdraws to pain, no verbal response (intubated), no eye opening

Results of Pertinent Laboratory Tests, Serum Drug Concentrations, and Diagnostic Tests

Na 142 (142)	Glu 13.3 (240)	AST 0.3 (18)
K 4.5 (4.5)	Ca 2.2 (8.9)	ALT 0.32 (20)
Cl 98 (98)	PO$_4$ 0.30 (0.9)	LDH 1.0 (60)
HCO$_3$ 26 (26)	Mg 0.9 (2.2)	Alb 26 (2.6)
BUN 6.0 (17)	TG 0.96 (85)	T Bili 12 (0.7)
Cr 80 (0.9)	Hct 0.32 (32%)	Hgb 100 (10)
Plts 160 × 10^9	PTT 29	PT 11
(160 × 10^3)	Prealbumin 9	Lkcs 9.0 × 10^9 (9.0 × 10^3)
INR 0.98		

Phenytoin: 8.0 mg/dL (drawn 7 hours after a dose today)

Urine dipstick shows 2+ glucose in urine

Accuchecks yesterday: 13.1 (235), 13.8 (248), 12.2 (219)

Bronchoalveolar lavage (BAL), blood, and urine culture and sensitivity reports pending

PROBLEM LIST

Identify principal problems from the scenario in priority order [completed Problem List and SOAP Note at end of casebook]

SOAP NOTE

To be completed by student

QUESTIONS

[Answers at end of casebook]

1. Why should enteral feedings and phenytoin doses be separated in AW? (EO-6, 9, 12)
   a. Enteral feedings may increase serum phenytoin concentrations if administered to AW concurrently
   b. Enteral feedings may decrease serum phenytoin concentrations if administered to AW concurrently
   c. Phenytoin will precipitate out and clog the feeding tube
   d. Phenytoin will "crack" the enteral feeding emulsion

2. A week after first seeing AW, it is evident that he will not tolerate tube feedings at a rate greater than 115 mL/hr. With regard to antiepileptic therapy, which of the following options should be tried now? (EO-8, 11, 12)
   a. Change to IM phenytoin
   b. Change to IV fosphenytoin
   c. Discontinue phenytoin therapy
   d. Change to IV phenytoin

3. Enteral feedings should not be started until the phosphorus infusion is administered because: (EO-1, 5, 12)
   a. Dextrose from feedings may induce intracellular shift of phosphorus and result in dangerously low serum level
   b. Phosphorus from the feedings plus the IV bolus will cause hyperphosphatemia
   c. IV phosphorus is being used as a prokinetic agent
   d. IV phosphorus will lower blood glucose concentrations

4. AW's acute hyperglycemia while in the ICU may cause all of the following *except:* (EO-1)
   a. Dehydration from osmotic diuresis
   b. Hypokalemia
   c. Diabetic retinopathy and microvascular disease
   d. Increased infection risk

5. AW's 24-hour urine collection results are UUN 900 mg/dL and urine volume 2600 mL. Assume that he received all of his nutrition at the goal rate. What is his approximate nitrogen balance (g/day)? (EO-5)
   a. +5
   b. +1
   c. −5
   d. −10

6. Based on AW's nitrogen balance, what change should be made in his enteral feeding at this time? (EO-11, 12)
   a. Take out protein supplement
   b. Increase protein supplement to 40 g/L
   c. Change to concentrated (2 kcal/mL) formula
   d. No change, nitrogen balance is acceptable for now

7. The neurosurgery resident wants to place a central line and begin total parenteral nutrition. When comparing total parenteral nutrition and enteral nutrition, all of the following are advantages of enteral nutrition *except:* (EO-10, 11)
   a. Decreased risk of aspiration pneumonia
   b. Decreased risk of line sepsis
   c. Decreased risk of pneumothorax
   d. Maintains gastrointestinal mucosal integrity

8. Morphine may complicate enteral nutrition by causing all of the following gastrointestinal side effects *except:* (EO-10)
   a. Aspiration
   b. Constipation
   c. Diarrhea
   d. Vomiting

9. AW develops hyponatremia and his laboratory parameters are consistent with the syndrome of inappropriate antidiuretic hormone secretion (SIADH). What changes, if any, should be made to the EN regimen? (EO-11, 12)

10. Explain the rationale for selecting metoclopramide for prokinetic therapy in AW. (EO-17, 11, 12)

11. Should AW's home insulin regimen (AM: 20 U NPH/10 U regular; PM: 10 U NPH/5 U regular) be restarted when enteral nutrition is initiated in order to maximize control of hyperglycemia? Please provide rationale for answer. (EO-8, 11, 12)

12. In patients requiring home enteral nutrition support, describe issues that should be discussed with the patient prior to discharge. (EO-16)

13. Summarize nutritional assessment, development, and management of a specialized nutrition regimen in AW using a key points format. (EO-18)

CASE 2
G. Christopher Wood
Topic: Fluid and Electrolyte Therapy
 Level 2

EDUCATIONAL MATERIALS
Chapter 9: Fluid and Electrolyte Therapy and Acid-Base Balance (maintenance fluid and electrolyte requirements; disorders of body water and solute; acid-base balance; electrolytes—potassium, calcium, phosphorus); Chapter 10: General Nutrition (population-specific recommendations)

SCENARIO

Patient and Setting

CB, a 36-year-old female; emergency department

Chief Complaint

Weakness, extreme fatigue, and intermittent fevers to 38.5°C

History of Present Illness

Consumed orange juice, ice cream, and antacid for the past 3 days because of nausea and vomiting; also stopped taking all of her medications; co-workers have been recently sick with the flu

Past Medical History

Polycystic kidney disease for 10 years; CB's last clinic visit 6 days ago; at that time, serum creatinine was 270 μmol/L (3 mg/dL), BUN was 17 mmol/L (46 mg/dL), and electrolytes were WNL

Past Surgical History

Noncontributory

Family/Social History

Noncontributory

Medication History

Aluminum hydroxide, 1 cap PO QID

Calcitriol, 100 μg PO QD

Calcium carbonate, 1250 mg PO TID

Aluminum hydroxide/magnesium hydroxide with simethicone, 30 mL PO TID PRN

Allergies

NKDA

Physical Examination

GEN: Thin woman who responds appropriately to questions but is quite lethargic

VS: BP 120/80, HR 100, T 38.2°C, RR 20, Wt 53 kg (usual wt 55 kg), Ht 173 cm

HEENT: Dry, cool skin, parched lips, sunken eyes

COR: Mildly tachycardic

CHEST: Few rales, no rhonchi

ABD: Soft, nontender, nondistended

GU: Deferred

RECT: Deferred

EXT: Cool hands and feet, slightly depressed reflexes, some peripheral muscle wasting

NEURO: Moderate lethargy as above

Results of Pertinent Laboratory Tests, Serum Drug Concentrations, and Diagnostic Tests

Na 128 (128)	BUN 20 (57)	Alb 34 (3.4)
K 5.2 (5.2)	Cr 280 (3.1)	Hct 0.45 (45)
Cl 90 (90)	Ca 2.6 (10.3)	Hgb 8.7 (14)
HCO$_3$ 29 (29)	PO$_4$ 1.8 (5.6)	Lkcs 9.0×10^9 (9.0×10^3)
	Mg 2 (4)	

Lkc differential: Neutrophils 0.85 (85%), lymphocytes 0.08 (8%), no bands

Urinalysis WNL, no bacteria found

Urine and sputum cultures show no growth to date

Urine output 20 mL/hr (normal per history)

PROBLEM LIST

Identify principal problems from the scenario in priority order [completed Problem List and SOAP Note at end of casebook]

SOAP NOTE

To be completed by student

QUESTIONS

[Answers at end of casebook]

1. CB's repeat serum potassium level is 6.5 mmol/L (6.5 mEq/L) but her electrocardiogram remains normal. Which of the following treatments for hyperkalemia is indicated at this time? (EO-5, 8, 12)
   a. Sodium polystyrene sulfonate 30 g IV
   b. Sodium polystyrene sulfonate 30 g PO
   c. Calcium chloride 2 g IV
   d. Insulin 10 units IV plus dextrose 50% 50 mL IV

2. Why is CB taking calcitriol rather than ergocalciferol to regulate calcium utilization? (EO-4, 8, 11)
   a. Calcitriol has a longer half life than ergocalciferol
   b. Calcitriol is much less expensive than ergocalciferol
   c. Patients with renal dysfunction do not absorb ergocalciferol well
   d. Vitamin D is not hydroxylated to its most active form in patients with renal dysfunction

3. Which of the following is the most likely clinical consequence of severe hyperphosphatemia (calcium/phosphorus product >5)? (EO-1, 10)
   a. Calcium phosphate precipitation in soft tissue
   b. Cardiac arrhythmias
   c. Seizures
   d. Respiratory insufficiency

4. If CB's hematocrit drops to 0.25 (25%), which of the following is not a likely contributing cause of anemia in CB? (EO-1, 5)
   a. Decreased red blood cell life span
   b. Iron deficiency
   c. Dehydration
   d. Erythropoietin deficiency

5. After receiving 3 liters of IV NS in the ED, CB's signs and symptoms of dehydration have resolved. Follow-up serum Na is 133 mmol/L. The physician wants to keep CB for observation and begin a maintenance IV fluid infusion. Which regimen should CB receive at this time? (EO-5, 8, 12)
   a. NS + KCl 20 mEq/L at 65 mL/hr
   b. D5W at 65 mL/hr

    c. NS at 65 mL/hr

    d. NS at 35 mL/hr

6. Which of the following is potentially the most serious clinical consequence of long-term aluminum hydroxide therapy in CB? (EO-10)

    a. Worsening renal dysfunction from aluminum toxicity

    b. Bad taste leads to noncompliance

    c. Central nervous system dysfunction from aluminum toxicity

    d. Cardiac arrhythmias from aluminum toxicity

7. All of the following are true regarding sodium polystyrene sulfonate therapy *except:* (EO-10)

    a. It may cause sodium overload in CHF patients

    b. Causes intracellular shift of potassium

    c. Exhibits a slow onset of action compared with insulin/dextrose

    d. Has unpleasant taste and is constipating

8. Which of the following acid-base disorders would be expected in CB? (EO-5)

    a. Contraction metabolic alkalosis

    b. Metabolic lactic acidosis

    c. Respiratory alkalosis

    d. Respiratory acidosis

9. Explain why 3 liters of normal saline IV was chosen as fluid replacement for CB. (EO-5, 8, 11)

10. During dietary counseling, CB is advised to increase her intake of protein. She is afraid her renal function will deteriorate and that she will need hemodialysis due to excessive BUN from the breakdown of more dietary protein. Please provide an appropriate response to her concerns. (EO-12, 15)

11. Determine CB's dietary protein and calorie goals. (EO-5, 12)

12. Compare the cost of crystalloid (NS, Lactated Ringer's) and colloid solutions (albumin, hetastarch, plasma protein fraction). (EO-17)

13. Summarize pathophysiologic, therapeutic, and disease management concepts for fluids and electrolytes utilizing a key points format. (EO-18)

CASE 3
G. Christopher Wood
Topic: Vitamins
 Level 1
EDUCATIONAL MATERIALS
Chapter 11: Vitamins and Minerals
(vitamin c, vitamin a, vitamin stability)

SCENARIO

Patient and Setting

GM, a 35-year-old female; ambulatory care clinic

Chief Complaint

"My right side has been hurting pretty bad for the past couple of days. Also, I've got dry, scaly spots on both of my arms that have been getting worse over the past month or so. I've had some diarrhea lately too."

History of Present Illness

Skin scaling and itching has gotten progressively worse over the last month; right-sided flank pain started yesterday and is moderate to severe; mild diarrhea over the past month; recently (2 months ago) started taking high-dose vitamins in an attempt to prevent the common cold

Past Medical History

Seasonal allergies in the spring and 3–4 common colds/year

Past Surgical History

None

Family/Social History

Noncontributory

Medication History

Ascorbic acid, 3 g PO QD

Multivitamin, 4 tabs PO QD

Kaolin/pectin, 30 mL PO PRN diarrhea

Pseudoephedrine, 60 mg PO q6h PRN sinus congestion

Allergies

NKA

Physical Examination

    GEN: Well-developed, well-nourished female with dermatitis and complaints of being tired

      VS: BP 120/80, HR 74, T 37°C, Wt 59 kg, Ht 167 cm

    ABD: Moderate/severe intermittent right flank pain

    EXT: Mild/moderate areas of dry, scaling skin on upper extremities

All other systems: WNL

Results of Pertinent Laboratory Tests, Serum Drug Concentrations, and Diagnostic Tests

Urinalysis WNL, no bacteria

PROBLEM LIST

Identify principal problems from the scenario in priority order [completed Problem List and SOAP Note at end of casebook]

SOAP NOTE

To be completed by student

QUESTIONS

[Answers at end of casebook]

1. Which of the following have been reported following acute discontinuation of high-dose ascorbic acid therapy? (EO-10)
   a. Bleeding gums
   b. Increased diarrhea
   c. Increased susceptibility to colds
   d. Impaired wound healing

2. Describe the roles of diet and vitamin supplements in average, healthy patients, with regard to obtaining adequate vitamin intake. (EO-16)

3. What other vitamin or mineral supplements may be useful in treating GM's common colds when they occur? (EO-8, 12)
   a. No supplements are useful
   b. Zinc lozenges
   c. Vitamin E
   d. Riboflavin

4. GM wants to switch to vitamins produced from natural sources rather than synthetically produced. What is the primary difference between natural and synthetic vitamins? Natural vitamins are: (EO-17)
   a. More effective
   b. Less effective
   c. More expensive
   d. Less toxic

5. What is the maximum daily dose of vitamin A that may be taken daily without increasing the risk of teratogenicity? (EO-10, 12)
   a. 1000 IU
   b. 5000 IU
   c. 10,000 IU
   d. 50,000 IU

6. Describe the most likely mechanism for the development of kidney stones in GM. (EO-1)
   a. Increased oxalate concentrations as a result of ascorbic acid metabolism
   b. Direct effect of ascorbic acid in the kidney
   c. Vitamin A toxicity
   d. Use of pseudoephedrine PRN

7. Ascorbic acid is required for proper absorption of which mineral? (EO-7)
   a. Calcium
   b. Sodium
   c. Potassium
   d. Iron

8. Which of the following vitamins is most likely to be destroyed during cooking? (EO-8)
   a. Vitamin A
   b. Vitamin C
   c. Vitamin K
   d. Vitamin D

9. Which of the following is required to be prominently displayed on food labels to describe the percent of the daily value for each nutrient that a serving of food provides? (EO-14)
   a. Daily reference value
   b. Dietary reference intake
   c. Daily value
   d. Recommended daily allowance

10. Since GM has unilateral flank pain, should she be evaluated for a possible complicated urinary tract infection? Provide rationale for response. (EO-2, 5, 8, 12)

11. GM wants to continue to take ascorbic acid. Explain the current state of medical knowledge regarding the use of ascorbic acid for prevention of the common cold. (EO-8, 14)

12. Since GM has a history of diarrhea, should she be evaluated for possible *Clostridium difficile* colitis? Provide rationale for response. (EO-2, 5, 8, 12)

13. Summarize pathophysiologic, therapeutic, and disease management concepts for vitamins and minerals utilizing a key points format. (EO-18)

CASE 4
G. Christopher Wood
Topic: Acid-Base Disorders

 Level 2

EDUCATIONAL MATERIALS
Chapter 9: Fluid and Electrolyte Therapy and Acid-Base Balance (maintenance fluid and electrolyte requirements, disorders of body water and solute, metabolic acidosis, potassium, magnesium, calcium); Chapter 11: Vitamins and Minerals (thiamine)

SCENARIO

Patient and Setting
HR, a 56-year-old male; emergency department (ED)

Chief Complaint
None (unconscious)

History of Present Illness
Found unconscious at home; neighbor has arrived at the ED with HR's suicide note and an empty bottle of aspirin

Past Medical History
None

Past Surgical History
None

Family/Social History

Neighbor reports that HR began to drink alcohol heavily after death of his wife from cancer 3 months ago; HR has lost about 18 kg during that time

Medication History

None

Allergies

Unknown

Physical Examination

GEN: Thin, well-developed man who opens eyes and moans when stimulated, but otherwise nonresponsive

VS: BP 130/70, HR 90, T 37.1°C, RR 25, Wt 60 kg, HT 188 cm

HEENT: Dry mucus membranes, sunken eyes, well-healed craniotomy scar

COR: Mild tachycardia

CHEST: WNL

ABD: WNL

GU: Urine output 15 mL/hr

RECT: WNL

EXT: Cool fingers and toes, dry skin, decreased skin turgor without tenting

NEURO: Localizes to pain, unintelligible speech

Results of Pertinent Laboratory Tests, Serum Drug Concentrations, and Diagnostic Tests

Na 145 (145)	Cr 120 (1.3)	Alb 36 (3.6)
K 4.0 (4.0)	Hct 0.53 (53)	Glu 5 (90)
Cl 107 (107)	Hgb 160 (16)	Ca Total 2.5 (10)
HCO_3 15 (15)	AST 0.3 (18)	PO_4 1.3 (4)
BUN 10 (27)	ALT 0.3 (17)	Mg 1 (2)
	Alk Phos 1 (60)	

ABG: pH 7.25, pO_2 98, pCO_2 35

Urinalysis: WNL

ECG: WNL

EEG: WNL

Stool: Guaiac-negative

Toxicology screen: Salicylate 0.45 g/L (45 mg/dL); ethanol 2.5 g/L (0.25%)

PROBLEM LIST

Identify principal problems from the scenario in priority order

SOAP NOTE

To be completed by student

QUESTIONS

1. What is HR's serum potassium level (mmol/L) when "corrected" for acidosis? (EO-5)
   a. 4.0
   b. 3.1
   c. 4.9
   d. 3.7

2. Why does acidosis affect serum potassium concentrations? (EO-1)

3. How should HR's potassium level be treated? (EO-5, 8, 11, 12)
   a. 60 mmol K acetate IV over 6 hours
   b. 60 mmol K acetate IV over 2 hours
   c. 30 mmol KCL IV over 3 hours
   d. 30 mmol KCL via nasogastric tube

4. After administration of charcoal and sorbitol, which of the following should be done next to treat HR's metabolic acidosis? (EO-5, 8, 11, 12)
   a. Hemodialysis to remove salicylate ions
   b. IV sodium bicarbonate infusion
   c. Fluid and electrolyte replacement
   d. IV sodium bicarbonate PRN pH <7.30

5. What is HR's calcium level (mmol/L) when corrected for acidosis? (EO-5)
   a. 2.5
   b. 3.2
   c. 1.8
   d. 3.8

6. Twenty-four hours after admission, HR remains unresponsive despite undetectable salicylate and ethanol levels, normal EEG, and pH 7.4. The total serum calcium level is now 2.8 mmol/L (11.2 mg/dL) and albumin is 31 (3.1). Which treatment for hypercalcemia should be administered now? (EO-5, 8, 11, 12)
   a. Subcutaneous calcitonin
   b. Intranasal calcitonin
   c. IV glucocorticoids
   d. IV etidronate

7. Why should HR receive thiamine in the ER? (EO-1)
   a. Prevent pellagra
   b. Prevent beri-beri
   c. Thiamine lowers calcium levels acutely
   d. Prevent Wernicke-Korsakoff syndrome

8. The ER physician wants to give magnesium replacement therapy via the nasogastric tube. Which of the following is the most likely adverse effect of oral magnesium replacement? (EO-10)
   a. Constipation
   b. Hypermagnesemia
   c. Diarrhea
   d. Cardiac arrhythmias

9. Which acid-base disorder would HR be at risk of developing if his nasogastric tube was placed to continuous suction for an extended period of time? Why would this happen? (EO-1)

10. Which of the following should be HR's initial protein and calorie goals? (EO-5, 9, 12)
    a. 1800–2000 kcal/day, 125 g protein/day
    b. 2400–2600 kcal/day, 125 g protein/day

c. 2400–2600 kcal/day, 75 g protein/day

d. 1800–2000 kcal/day, 75 g protein/day

11. Twenty-four hours after admission, HR's serum Alb level has decreased to 31 g/L (3.1 g/dL). Does this alter your initial nutritional goal? (EO-5, 8, 11, 12)

12. Describe psychosocial interventions that may benefit HR. (EO-15)

13. Describe why hemodialysis is not indicated for removal of salicylate ions in HR. (EO-10, 17)

14. Summarize pathophysiologic, therapeutic, and disease management concepts for acid-base disorders utilizing a key points format. (EO-18)

CASE 5
G. Christopher Wood
Topic: General Nutrition
Level 1
EDUCATIONAL MATERIALS

Chapter 10: General Nutrition (calcium supplements and osteoporosis); Chapter 12: Parenteral and Enteral Nutrition in Adult Patients (nutritional assessment, total calorie and protein requirements, enteral nutrition)

SCENARIO

Patient and Setting

CM, a 61-year-old female; ambulatory care clinic

Chief Complaint

Loss of appetite, pain upon swallowing, and significant weight loss

History of Present Illness

Progressive weight loss (10 kg in 6 months), with increasing difficulty in swallowing food or liquids over the past 6 months

Past Medical History

Currently being treated for prevention of osteoporosis; chooses not to take estrogen

Past Surgical History

None

Family/Social History

Tobacco—40 pack/year history

Medication History

Alendronate, 10 mg PO QD × 9 months

Calcium carbonate, 650 mg 3 tablets PO QD × 9 months

Oral supplement, 1 can (240 mL) PO TID × 6 months

Allergies

NKDA

Physical Examination

GEN: Malnourished female in no apparent distress

VS: BP 135/85, HR 60, T 37.0°C, RR 12, Wt 47 kg (57 kg 6 months ago), Ht 165 cm

HEENT: Hoarseness, difficulty swallowing

COR: WNL

CHEST: WNL

ABD: Soft, nontender, no masses or organomegaly, nausea and vomiting with eating, esophageal pain on swallowing

GU: WNL

RECT: Guaiac-negative

EXT: Normal skin turgor

NEURO: Oriented to time, place, and person; normal deep tendon reflexes

Results of Pertinent Laboratory Tests, Serum Drug Concentrations, and Diagnostic Tests

Na 139 (139)	Cr 100 (1.1)	Alk Phos 1 (60)
K 3.7 (3.7)	Glu 5 (90)	Alb 28 (2.8)
Cl 100 (100)	Ca Total 2.2 (8.8)	PO_4 1.3 (4)
HCO_3 26 (26)	AST 0.66 (40)	Mg 1 (2)
BUN 6.5 (18)	ALT 0.76 (45)	

Bone density scan shows mild osteopenia in lumbar spine

Endoscopy shows moderate to severe erosive esophagitis

PROBLEM LIST

Identify principal problems from the scenario in priority order [completed Problem List and SOAP Note at end of casebook]

SOAP NOTE

To be completed by student

QUESTIONS

[Answers at end of casebook]

1. CM has had poor oral intake and continued weight loss over the past 2 weeks and is admitted to the hospital for gastrostomy placement. Enteral nutrition with a standard formula (1 kcal/mL, 38 g protein/L, no dietary fiber) will be needed at which of the following rates to provide approximately 30 kcal/kg/day: (EO-5, 8, 12)

a. 120 mL/hr

b. 100 mL/hr

c. 80 mL/hr

d. 60 mL/hr

2. Two days after beginning enteral feedings, CM develops mild diarrhea. Which of the following should be done to treat the diarrhea? (EO-8, 11, 12)
   a. Switch to a fiber-containing enteral feeding
   b. Evaluate for *Clostridium difficile* colitis
   c. Discontinue feeds until diarrhea resolves
   d. Discontinue feeds and begin TPN

3. CM "doesn't want to be hooked up to the nutrition pump all day" at home, and needs to be transitioned to an overnight feeding regimen. Which of the following will provide the same amount of nutrition CM is receiving in the hospital? (EO-12)
   a. 75 mL/hr from 10 PM to 10 AM
   b. 100 mL/hr from 8 PM to 10 AM
   c. 125 mL/hr from 8 PM to 10 AM
   d. 100 mL/hr from 10 PM to 8 AM

4. After 2 months of acid suppression therapy, CM's esophagitis has healed. She desires to start drinking oral supplements and discontinue gastrostomy feedings. Her current weight is 50 kg. Choose the most appropriate regimen to deliver CM's protein and calorie requirements with an oral supplement (1 kcal/mL, 35 g protein/L). (EO-8, 12)
   a. 3 cans QD
   b. 3 cans BID
   c. 2 cans TID
   d. 1 can q4h

5. How much calcium carbonate should CM take daily for prevention of osteoporosis? (EO-12)
   a. 1500 mg
   b. 3750 mg
   c. 600 mg
   d. 2000 mg

6. Which of the following is correct regarding administration of alendronate? (EO-14)
   a. Take with semi-viscous liquid such as orange juice
   b. Take with over-the-counter histamine-2 antagonists
   c. Take with food first thing in the morning
   d. Take with a full glass of plain water and remain in an upright position for 30 min.

7. Which of the following will dramatically decrease bioavailability of alendronate? (EO-9)
   a. Administration on an empty stomach
   b. Administration with breakfast
   c. Administration with plain water
   d. Administration at least 30 min. prior to breakfast

8. Which of the following is true regarding calcium and magnesium intake and hypertension? (EO-3)
   a. Lower calcium and magnesium intake seems to be associated with a higher prevalence of hypertension
   b. JNC VI recommends the use of calcium and magnesium supplements in the treatment of hypertension
   c. Higher calcium and magnesium intake seems to be associated with a higher prevalence of hypertension
   d. Higher calcium and magnesium intake may be associated with a lower prevalence of hypertension

9. What potential complications may CM experience due to enteral feedings? (EO-10)

10. CM's albumin is 28 (2.8). Discuss the use of parenteral albumin therapy in CM at this time. (EO-5, 8, 17)

11. CM is moderately malnourished. Upon starting enteral nutrition, what syndrome may occur? Describe the mechanism of this syndrome and appropriate management. (EO-1, 10, 12)

12. Describe common psychosocial impediments to good nutrition. (EO-16)

13. Summarize disease management concepts of malnourished patients using the key points format. (EO-18)

CASE 6
G. Christopher Wood
Topic: Minerals
 Level 2

EDUCATIONAL MATERIALS
Chapter 11: Vitamins and Minerals (minerals); Chapter 10: General Nutrition (patients with high blood pressure, chromium)

SCENARIO

Patient and Setting
RB, a 16-year-old female; ambulatory care clinic

Chief Complaint
Loss of taste and smell, dysuria

History of Present Illness
Progressive loss of taste and smell over the past 2–3 months; 2-day history of increasing dysuria; added chromium to existing insulin regimen for the past month after reading about its use in a women's magazine; RB claims to have good control of her diabetes but has not seen a health care provider in 6 months; began oral contraceptives 6 months ago

Past Medical History
Type 1 diabetes mellitus (DM) for 12 years

Past Surgical History
None

Family/Social History
Moderate/heavy alcohol use for 12 months

Lives at home with single mother who "works all the time" and with 19-year-old sister

Medication History

Human insulin 70/30, 28 units SC AC breakfast, 18 units AC supper

Oral contraceptive (20 μg ethinyl estradiol, 1 mg norethindrone acetate), 1 tablet PO QD

Chromium picolinate, 1 mg PO QD

Generic multivitamins, 2 tablets PO QD

Calcium carbonate, 650 mg PO QD

Allergies

Sulfa drugs, penicillin, melons (all three cause rash/hives)

Physical Examination

GEN: Well-developed, well-nourished female in no apparent distress

VS: BP 110/59, HR 69, RR 16, T 37°C, Wt 50 Kg, Ht 160 cm

HEENT: WNL

GU: Pain upon urination

All other systems: WNL

Results of Pertinent Laboratory Tests, Serum Drug Concentrations, and Diagnostic Tests

Accucheck in clinic 11.3 (203)   Accucheck 2 days ago 10.4 (187) HbA_{1C} 8.4 (8.0 2 months ago)

UA: glucose positive; bacteria 3+; Lkcs 10

PROBLEM LIST

Identify principal problems from the scenario in priority order [completed Problem List and SOAP Note at end of casebook]

SOAP NOTE

To be completed by student

QUESTIONS

[Answers at end of casebook]

1. Chromium supplements have been reported to cause all of the following *except:* (EO-10)
   a. Renal dysfunction
   b. Dermatitis
   c. Thrombocytopenia
   d. Toxic hepatitis

2. It has been estimated that what percent of Americans' diets are deficient in chromium? (EO-3)
   a. 1%
   b. 10%
   c. 50%
   d. 90%

3. Describe to RB the current state of knowledge regarding the use of chromium supplements to help treat diabetes. (EO-11)

4. Which of the following is a side effect of zinc sulfate therapy that RB should be told about? (EO-10)
   a. Gastrointestinal irritation
   b. Rash/hives
   c. Drowsiness
   d. Hyperglycemia

5. RB has been taking calcium since her mother was recently diagnosed with mild osteoporosis. Approximately how much calcium carbonate will RB have to take daily to receive 1500 mg of elemental calcium? (EO-12)
   a. 1500 mg
   b. 3500 mg
   c. 5000 mg
   d. 7000 mg

6. Which form of calcium will be absorbed best in a patient taking lansoprazole? (EO-8, 9, 12)
   a. Calcium carbonate
   b. Calcium citrate
   c. Calcium acetate
   d. Calcium chloride

7. RB complains because her mother has cut back on the family's salt use to "keep from getting high blood pressure." What is the recommended daily sodium intake? (EO-14)
   a. 50 mmol (0.9 g)
   b. 200 mmol (3.6 g)
   c. 150 mmol (2.4 g)
   d. 100 mmol (1.8 g)

8. RB is at risk for iron deficiency. All of the following are high-risk groups for iron deficiency *except:* (EO-3)
   a. Children
   b. Women of child-bearing age
   c. Frequent blood donors
   d. Vegetarians

9. Alcohol impairs the absorption of which of the following? (EO-9)
   a. Magnesium
   b. Copper
   c. Iron
   d. Phosphorus

10. How should RB be counseled to take her new drug therapy (ciprofloxacin 250 mg PO q12h, zinc sulfate 220 mg PO TID)? (EO-9,11,12)

11. RB has been reading a lot about organic vitamins and supplements and wants to take a "more natural" calcium supplement made from bone meal. Provide an appropriate recommendation. (EO-12, 15, 17)

12. Describe how friends/family should be informed to recognize and treat hypoglycemia due to drinking alcohol without eating food. (EO-16)

13. Summarize disease management concepts for minerals utilizing a key points format. (EO-18)

CASE 7
G. Christopher Wood
Topic: Parenteral Nutrition
Level 3

EDUCATIONAL MATERIALS
Chapter 12: Parenteral and Enteral Nutrition in Adult Patients (total calorie and protein requirements, parenteral nutrition)

SCENARIO

Patient and Setting
SD, a 53-year-old female; hospital–general surgery ward

Chief Complaint
Postoperative ileus; presumed catheter sepsis

History of Present Illness
Surgery for lysis of adhesions and breakup of mechanical obstruction of small intestine 7 days ago; developed postoperative ileus; cannot tolerate enteral nutrition; the hospital's standard total parenteral nutrition (TPN) formula was started via central line 4 days ago; surgery service has consulted the clinical pharmacist to manage TPN; also with presumed catheter sepsis; febrile × 48 hours with erythema around central catheter site; vancomycin and gentamicin started yesterday empirically

Past Medical History
Moderate to heavy alcohol use × 30 years

Past Surgical History
Tubal ligation 25 years ago

Family/Social History
None

Medication History
Vancomycin, 1 g IV q12h in 250 mL D5W

Gentamicin, 300 mg IV QD in 150 mL D5W

Acetaminophen suppository, 650 mg PR q6h PRN
    T >38.3°C

Parenteral nutrition solution at 75 mL/hr with the following:
    Dextrose, 450 g/day (250 g/L)
    Aminosyn II amino acid formula, 90 g/day (50 g/L)

Sodium chloride, 54 mEq/day (30 mEq/L)

Sodium phosphate, 27 mmol/day (15 mmol/L)

Potassium acetate, 72 mEq/day (40 mEq/L)

Calcium gluconate, 9 mEq/day (5 mEq/L)

Magnesium sulfate, 22 mEq/day (12 mEq/L)

Multivitamins, 10 mL/day

Trace elements, 3 mL/day

Ranitidine, 150 mg/day

Allergies
NKDA

Physical Examination
GEN: Well-developed female in mild distress, complaining of chills

VS: BP 104/70, HR 110, RR 10, T 39.4°C, Wt 60 kg, HT 163 cm

HEENT: WNL

COR: Tachycardic, otherwise normal

CHEST: Clear to auscultation and percussion, central line site has redness, without swelling or tenderness

ABD: Distended and tender, no bowel sounds, surgical wound site healing well without redness, swelling, or tenderness; NG tube in place to suction with 2500 mL out over past 24 hours

GU: Deferred

RECT: Guaiac negative

EXT: WNL

NEURO: Oriented to time, place, and person

Results of Pertinent Laboratory Tests, Serum Drug Concentrations, and Diagnostic Tests

Na 130 (130)	Lkcs 17.0×10^9 (17.0×10^3)	Prealbumin 11
K 3.3 (3.3)	Cr 90 (1.0)	AST 1.5 (90)
Cl 94 (94)	PO_4 0.78 (2.4)	ALT 1.7 (100)
HCO_3 25 (25)	Mg 0.62 (1.5)	LDH 1.66 (100)
BUN 8.9 (25)	Ca 2.14 (8.6)	Alb 30 (3.0)
T Bili 22 (1.3)	Glu 12.5 (225)	

Lkc differential: Neutrophils 0.89 (89%), bands 0.02 (2%)

Blood: Gram-positive cocci on Gram-stain, culture and sensitivity pending

Urine: Culture negative

Total in/out over past 4 days is approximately negative 7000 mL

Urine output (UOP): Approximately 15 mL/hr

CT of abdomen: No intraabdominal abscess

PROBLEM LIST

Identify principal problems from the scenario in priority order

SOAP NOTE

To be completed by student

QUESTIONS

1. When deciding to add a drug to a parenteral nutrition (PN) formulation, all of the following must exist *except:* (EO-8, 9, 12)
   a. No dosage changes anticipated
   b. A distinct cost advantage
   c. Pharmacodynamics consistent with continuous infusion
   d. Physical compatibility

2. Due to incompatibility, which of the following should not be added to total nutrient admixtures? (EO-8, 9, 12)
   a. Heparin
   b. Insulin
   c. Cimetidine
   d. Iron dextran

3. In order to avoid hyperglycemia and associated complications, glucose administration should not exceed: (EO-10)
   a. 5 kcal/kg/day
   b. 15 kcal/kg/day
   c. 20 kcal/kg/day
   d. 25 kcal/kg/day

4. Which of the following trace elements should be removed from the PN formula if SD develops liver failure? (EO-4, 5, 8,12)
   a. Copper, manganese
   b. Zinc, selenium
   c. Chromium, manganese
   d. Copper, zinc

5. Due to high gastrointestinal losses, SD may have higher requirements of which of the following trace elements: (EO-8)
   a. Zinc
   b. Selenium
   c. Chromium
   d. Manganese

6. The culture and sensitivity results from the catheter tip and blood show *Staphylococcus aureus* sensitive to vancomycin, gentamicin, oxacillin, tetracycline, clindamycin, and ciprofloxacin. Which of the following should be used as definitive treatment of SD's catheter sepsis? (EO-5, 8, 11, 12)
   a. Vancomycin and gentamicin
   b. Vancomycin
   c. Gentamicin
   d. Nafcillin

7. Which of the following vitamins is not included in intravenous multivitamin formulations? (EO-11)
   a. Vitamin K
   b. Thiamine
   c. Folic acid
   d. Vitamin C

8. All of the following are advantages of total nutrient admixtures (three-in-one solutions) *except:* (EO-9, 11)
   a. Decreased pharmacy and nursing preparation time
   b. Inability to visually detect particulates
   c. Decreased risk of infection from fewer central line manipulations
   d. Less potential for immunosuppression due to slow, continuous administration of lipids

9. Because of SD's alcohol history and elevated liver function tests, should HepatAmine be used as the amino acid source in SD to prevent hepatic encephalopathy? Please provide rationale for response. (EO-8, 12, 17)

10. The surgery service asks if peripheral parenteral nutrition should be started in SD, since the first catheter became infected. Please provide rationale for response. (EO-8, 12)

11. Describe what SD's protein requirements would be if she developed renal failure and required intermittent hemodialysis, continuous hemodialysis, peritoneal dialysis, and no dialysis. Also, what type of specialized amino acid formula should be used in renal failure? (EO-5, 8, 12)

12. In patients requiring home parenteral nutrition support, describe issues that should be discussed with the patient prior to discharge. (EO-16)

13. Summarize disease management concepts for parenteral nutrition utilizing a key points format. (EO-18)

CASE 8
Anne Reaves
Topic: Iron Deficiency Anemia
Level 2
EDUCATIONAL MATERIALS
Chapter 13: Iron Deficiency and Megaloblastic Anemias (clinical findings and manifestations, diagnosis of iron deficiency, treatment of iron deficiency anemia, monitoring iron therapy)

SCENARIO

Patient and Setting

AM, a 22-year-old female; emergency department

Chief Complaint

Bloody diarrhea (approximately nine/day) with severe abdominal pain, arthritic pain in both knees, increased fatigue, and decreased appetite

History of Present Illness

Diagnosed 1½ months ago with ulcerative colitis (UC) by sigmoidoscopy; extent of disease at diagnosis was 22 cm; symptoms included increased fatigue, moderate abdominal pain, and approximately six bloody stools/day; started on sulfasalazine 2 g/day and titrated up to 6 g/day due to persistent symptoms; began to experience increased headaches, intermittent nausea and vomiting, malaise, and anorexia; over the past 3 weeks, experienced weight loss of approximately 3.6 kg (8 pounds); began menstruating heavily 4 days prior to admission

Past Medical History

Depression

Past Surgical History

None

Family/Social History

Family History: Noncontributory
Social History: Patient denies tobacco smoking, but admits occasional binge alcohol drinking

Medication History

Diphenoxylate/atropine 2 tabs PO QID PRN for diarrhea
Sulfasalazine 1500 mg PO QID
Fluoxetine 40 mg PO QID
Calcium carbonate 500 mg PO QID

Allergies

PCN–rash

Physical Examination

GEN: Thin, pale female in moderate-to-severe distress
VS: BP 120/84, HR 104, RR 18, T 99.8°F, Wt 43 kg, Ht 156 cm
HEENT: WNL
COR: Tachycardic
CHEST: Lungs clear to auscultation and percussion
ABD: Soft, lower abdomen tender to palpation
GU: WNL, menstruating
RECT: Bloody, watery diarrhea
EXT: Tenderness and warmth of both knees
NEURO: WNL

Results of Pertinent Laboratory Tests, Serum Drug Concentrations, and Diagnostic Tests

Na 137 (137)	Hct 0.28 (28)	T Bili 13.68 (0.8)
K 3.3 (3.3)	Hgb 87 (8.7)	Alb 41 (4.1)
HCO$_3$ 24 (24)	Plts 240 × 10^9	Uric Acid 120 (20)
BUN 5.4 (16)	(240 × 10^3)	Ca 2.45 (9.8)
Cr 68.63 (0.9)	MCV 60 (60)	Mg 1.0 (2.0)
Cl 96 (96)	Alk Phos 3.0 (180)	S Ferr 11 (11)
Glu 5.0 (90)	AST 0.75 (45)	Trans Sat 14 (14)
WBC 16 × 10^9	ALT 0.58 (35)	ESR 60 (60)
(16 × 10^3)		

Urinalysis, chest radiography, ECG: All WNL

Stool examination: Numerous WBC, RBC

Stool culture: Negative

Repeat sigmoidoscopy: Edematous and friable mucosa, extent of disease 23 cm

PROBLEM LIST

Identify principal problems from the scenario in priority order [completed Problem List and SOAP Note at end of casebook]

SOAP NOTE

To be completed by student

QUESTIONS

[Answers at end of casebook]

1. All of the following factors presented in AM's history could contribute to the development of iron deficiency anemia *except:* (EO-1)
   a. Ulcerative colitis
   b. Anorexia/malnutrition
   c. Increased fatigue
   d. Heavy menstruation

2. AM presented with all the following signs and symptoms of anemia *except:* (EO-2)
   a. Tachycardia (HR 104)
   b. T 99.8°F
   c. Increased fatigue
   d. Pallor

3. AM reports increased GI upset (nausea, vomiting, anorexia). This is most likely due to which medication? (EO-10)
   a. Diphenoxylate/atropine
   b. Sulfasalazine
   c. Fluoxetine
   d. Calcium carbonate

4. All the following findings are consistent with an ulcerative colitis exacerbation in AM *except:* (EO-2,5)
   a. Heavy menstruation
   b. Increased number of bloody stools
   c. Stool with numerous WBCs and RBCs
   d. Sigmoidoscopy: edematous and friable mucosa

5. Describe the mechanisms of action of the pharmacologic and nonpharmacologic interventions in AM. (EO-7)

6. List the pharmacologic treatment problem(s) present in AM's treatment plan. (EO-11)

7. Calculate the total dose of iron in milligrams necessary to replete stores in AM. (EO-6)

8. What is the uncommon, but severe adverse reaction seen with parenteral iron that warrants a test dose prior to therapy? (EO-10)
   a. Stevens-Johnson syndrome
   b. Severe hypoglycemia
   c. Anaphylaxis
   d. Bradycardia

9. Total dose infusion of iron dextran offers all the following advantages over IM or bolus IV dosing *except:* (EO-10, 15)
   a. Lower total dose required, so less expensive
   b. Fewer office visits
   c. Less needle sticks (so less patient discomfort and more convenient)
   d. Less local side effects

10. All of the following could result in reduced absorption of oral iron in AM *except:* (EO-10)
    a. Use of calcium carbonate
    b. Chronic diarrhea
    c. Acute inflammation
    d. Anorexia

11. Discuss possible lifestyle changes and medication counseling that will be required for AM for ferrous sulfate therapy. (EO-14)

12. What psychosocial factors may affect AM's adherence to pharmacologic and nonpharmacologic therapy? (EO-15)

13. Summarize pathophysiologic, therapeutic, and disease management concepts for iron deficiency anemia utilizing a key points format. (EO-18)

CASE 9
Anne Reaves
Topic: Megaloblastic Anemia

EDUCATIONAL MATERIALS
Chapter 13: Iron Deficiency and Megaloblastic Anemias (folate deficiency, diagnosis and management of folate deficiency, monitoring therapy)

SCENARIO

Patient and Setting
KL, a 62-year-old male; emergency medical clinic

Chief Complaint
Stomach pains, weakness, and dizziness

History of Present Illness
Complains of stomach pain for 2 weeks; food relieves pain, but poor appetite; self-medicating with antacids for a few weeks, but pain relief only temporary; also feeling depressed lately due to receiving a second DUI; desires to quit drinking alcohol and "willing to do anything" to stop so life can return to normal

Past Medical History
None

Past Surgical History
None

Family/Social History
Family History: Father died age 65 liver disease

Social History: Tobacco: 1 PPD; alcohol: drinks 5 martinis after work daily and an occasional "pick me up" in the morning

Medication History
Ibuprofen 600–800 mg QID PRN for headaches

Magnesium/aluminum antacid PRN for stomach pain

Allergies

NKDA

Physical Examination

GEN: Pale, elderly-appearing male in moderate distress
VS: BP 120/75, HR 80, RR 12, T 37.5°C, Wt 55 kg
HEENT: WNL
COR: RRR
CHEST: Clear to auscultation and percussion
ABD: Soft, slightly tender, no hepatosplenomegaly
GU: Exam deferred
RECT: Guaiac positive stool
EXT: Pale nail beds, bruising on upper arms and thighs
NEURO: Oriented to person, place, and time

Results of Pertinent Laboratory Tests, Serum Drug Concentrations, and Diagnostic Tests

Na 138 (138)
K 4.0 (4.0)
Cl 99 (99)
HCO_3 22 (22)
BUN 3.6 (12)
Cr 80 (0.9)

Hct 0.25 (25)
Hgb 100 (10)
Plts 150×10^9 (150×10^3)
WBC 3.8×10^9 (3.8×10^3)

MCV 104 (104)
RBC 4.0 (4.0)
Serum Vit B_{12} 225 (300)
Serum folate 2 (1.2)

Endoscopy: 0.5-cm ulcer in the duodenum, no active bleeding

PROBLEM LIST

Identify principal problems from the scenario in priority order [completed Problem List and SOAP Note at end of casebook]

SOAP NOTE

To be completed by student

QUESTIONS

[Answers at end of casebook]

1. All of the following are common causes of folate deficiency *except:* (EO-1)
   a. Inadequate diet
   b. Pregnancy
   c. Alcoholism
   d. GI blood loss

2. In addition to ethanol, all the following drugs can reduce folate absorption and result in folate deficiency *except:* (EO-9)
   a. Digoxin
   b. Sulfasalazine
   c. Cholestyramine
   d. Oral contraceptives

3. Factors contributing to the development of peptic ulcer disease in KL include all the following *except:* (EO-1)
   a. Ethanol abuse
   b. Cigarette smoking
   c. Depression
   d. NSAID use

4. A physical assessment finding apparent in KL that is consistent with anemia includes: (EO-5)
   a. Pale nail beds
   b. BP 120/75
   c. Soft, tender abdomen
   d. HR 80 with RRR

5. Describe the mechanism of action of pharmacologic and nonpharmacologic interventions used in KL. (EO-7)

6. Parenteral administration of folate should be considered in which of the following: (EO-4, 8, 9)
   a. Achlorhydria
   b. Intrinsic factor deficiency
   c. *H. pylori* infections
   d. Post gastric resection

7. Discuss the possible classes of pharmacologic agents that could be used to treat KL's duodenal ulcer and any advantages or disadvantages they possess. (EO-7, 8)

8. KL has completed 8 weeks of appropriate H2 blocker therapy. He states that he has abstained from ethanol and NSAID use during this time. KL still complains of abdominal pain. Follow-up endoscopy reveals a new duodenal ulcer. Which of the following would be the best action to consider at this time? (EO-1)
   a. Evaluation for *H. pylori*
   b. Switching to a different H2 blocker
   c. Adding antacids to H2 blocker therapy
   d. Checking a gastrin level

9. KL decides to try disulfiram therapy. Develop an education plan for him (including necessary lifestyle changes and medication counseling). (EO-14)

10. What psychosocial factors may affect KL's adherence to both pharmacologic and nonpharmacologic therapy? (EO-15)

11. Evaluate the pharmacoeconomic considerations relative to KL's plan of care. (EO-17)

12. Summarize pathophysiologic, therapeutic, and disease management concepts for megaloblastic anemias utilizing a key points format. (EO-18)

CASE 10
Anne Reaves
Topic: Megaloblastic Anemia

Level 3

EDUCATIONAL MATERIALS

Chapter 13: Iron Deficiency and Megaloblastic Anemias (pernicious anemia, clinical manifestations and diagnosis of B_{12} deficiency, management and monitoring of B_{12} deficiency)

SCENARIO

Patient and Setting

DR, a 64-year-old female; internal medicine clinic

Chief Complaint

Numbness and tingling in hands and feet, sore tongue, constipation, new rash

History of Present Illness

Reports numbness and tingling in lower extremities for approximately 2 months, diagnosed as peripheral neuropathy due to diabetes; started amitriptyline 50 mg daily; amitriptyline induced constipation requiring laxatives 3–4 times a week; has noted numbness/tingling in hands × 1 month and recently developed soreness in tongue making it difficult to eat; seen by podiatrist 1 week ago, given griseofulvin for onychomycosis; 3 days after starting therapy, broke out in diffuse rash on trunk and abdomen

Past Medical History

Diabetes mellitus type 2 for 4 years, controlled on oral hypoglycemic agent; hypertension (HTN) for 9 years

Past Surgical History

None

Family/Social History

Family History: Diabetes mellitus—mother and sister; mother died age 60 of MI; father died age 64 of CVA

Social History: Negative for tobacco or illicit drug use; positive for occasional alcohol use

Medication History

Triamterene/hydrochlorothiazide 37.5/25 mg 1 tablet PO q AM

Glipizide, 5 mg BID

Amitriptyline, 50 mg QHS

Griseofulvin, 500 mg BID

Allergies

Penicillin—rash

Physical Examination

GEN: Well-developed, slightly overweight female
VS: BP 170/100, HR 84, RR 14, T 37.5°C, Wt 73 kg, Ht 165 cm

HEENT: Glossitis
COR: RRR
CHEST: Clear to auscultation and percussion
ABD: Slightly distended, slight tenderness to palpation, decreased bowel sounds; pale, diffuse, maculopapular rash
GU: Deferred
RECT: Guaiac negative stool
EXT: Warm extremities, normal pulses, decreased sensation to touch, onychomycotic toenails on left foot
NEURO: Alert, O × 4

Results of Pertinent Laboratory Tests, Serum Drug Concentrations, and Diagnostic Tests

Na 138 (138)	Hgb 120 (12)	Ca 2.2 (8.8)
K 4.0 (4.0)	Plts 300 × 10^9	PO$_4$ 0.92 (3.0)
Cl 96 (96)	(300 × 10^3)	Mg 1.2 (2.5)
HCO$_3$ 24 (24)	MCV 109 (109)	HbA$_{1C}$ 0.07 (7%)
BUN 5.7 (16)	MCH 1.9 (30)	Serum B$_{12}$ 98.7 (123)
Cr 88.4 (1.0)	RDW 16 (16)	Serum Folate 18 (8)
Hct 0.32 (32)	Glu 6.1 (110)	

Peripheral blood smear: Normochromic, macrocytic RBCs

Urinalysis: 1+ protein

Schilling test: Stage I abnormal
Stage II normal

PROBLEM LIST

Identify principal problems from the scenario in priority order

SOAP NOTE

To be completed by student

QUESTIONS

1. What is the prevalence of pernicious anemia in the general population? (EO-3)
   a. 20%
   b. 10%
   c. 5%
   d. 1%

2. What is the cause of DR's pernicious anemia? (EO-1)
   a. Loss of intrinsic factor secretion
   b. Malabsorption due to diabetes mellitus
   c. Drug-induced
   d. Postmenopausal bleeding

3. Other causes of vitamin B$_{12}$ deficiency include all the following *except*: (EO-1)

a. Inadequate dietary intake
b. Bacterial overgrowth
c. GI blood loss
d. Transcobalamin II deficiency

4. DR presented with which of the following signs and symptoms of vitamin B_{12} deficiency: (EO-2)
   a. Rash
   b. Constipation
   c. Proteinuria
   d. Peripheral neuropathy

5. In the United States, vitamin B_{12} deficiency is most commonly seen in which of the following patient populations: (EO-3)
   a. Elderly (>65 years of age)
   b. Adolescents
   c. Menstruating females
   d. Pregnant/lactating females

6. Describe the mechanism of action of the pharmacologic and nonpharmacologic interventions in this case. (EO-7)

7. List the pharmacologic and nonpharmacologic treatment problems present in DR's treatment plan on presentation. (EO-11)

8. Which of the following medications used in the treatment of diabetes mellitus has been associated with drug-induced vitamin B_{12} deficiency? (EO-10)
   a. Glipizide
   b. Metformin
   c. Acarbose
   d. Troglitazone

9. DR presents with several risk factors for developing coronary artery disease. This includes all the following *except:* (EO-1, 3)
   a. Diabetes mellitus
   b. Hypertension
   c. Pernicious anemia
   d. Family history of premature CAD

10. DR develops an intolerable dry cough on lisinopril, which recurs upon rechallenge. Which of the following medications would be the most appropriate second-line choice for management of her hypertension and proteinuria? (EO-8, 12)
    a. Losartan
    b. Atenolol
    c. Prazosin
    d. HCTZ

11. What psychosocial factors may affect DR's adherence to both pharmacologic and nonpharmacologic therapy? (EO-15)

12. Describe the health care provider's role relative to the proposed psychosocial factors identified. (EO-16)

13. Evaluate the pharmacoeconomic considerations relative to DR's plan of care. (EO-17)

14. Summarize pathophysiologic, therapeutic, and disease management concepts for megaloblastic anemia utilizing a key points format. (EO-18)

CASE 11
Anne Reaves
Topic: Other Anemias

EDUCATIONAL MATERIALS
Chapter 14: Other Anemias (hemolytic anemia)

SCENARIO

Patient and Setting
RB, a 67-year-old male; adult cardiology clinic

Chief Complaint
Recent onset of fatigue and shortness of breath; also reports a pink discoloration in his urine

History of Present Illness
Diagnosed 3 months prior with new-onset atrial fibrillation (A. fib.) accompanied by mild shortness of breath and dizziness; ventricular response rate at that time was 110 beats/min; started digoxin for rate control and anticoagulated with warfarin for 1 month; procainamide initiated; chemically converted to normal sinus rhythm with resolution of symptoms 2 days later; warfarin discontinued 2 weeks later; procainamide and digoxin continued for 3 additional months to prevent recurrence of arrhythmia; over the next 4–6 weeks, experienced increasing fatigue and difficulty catching breath; current symptoms different than those experienced with A. fib.; 5 days prior to presentation returned to his cardiologist due to pink discoloration of urine; ECG showed normal sinus rhythm; referred to clinic for further evaluation and treatment

Past Medical History
New-onset A. fib. (resolved); osteoarthritis (5-year history); chronic sinusitis

Past Surgical History
Tonsillectomy at age 6

Family/Social History
Family History: Noncontributory

Social History: No history of tobacco, ethanol, or illicit drug use

Medication History
Procainamide sustained-release, 500 mg PO q6h

Digoxin, 0.25 mg PO QD

Naproxen, 250 mg BID with food

Pseudoephedrine, 60 mg q4h PRN

Antacids, PRN

Allergies

Aspirin, most NSAIDs—dyspepsia

Physical Examination

GEN: Well-developed, well-nourished male appearing somewhat anxious about his current state of health

VS: BP 130/80, HR 64, RR 22, afebrile; Wt 82 kg, Ht 183 cm

HEENT: Pale conjunctiva, icteric sclera, rhinorrhea, swollen nasal mucous membranes

COR: Normal S1 and S2, no murmurs, rubs, or gallop

CHEST: Clear to auscultation and percussion

ABD: Soft, nontender, no masses, mild splenomegaly

GU: WNL

RECT: Guaiac negative, enlarged prostate gland

EXT: Nail beds and palms of hands slightly pale, both knees swollen and mildly tender, limited range of motion in both knees and right hip

NEURO: Alert, O × 4

Results of Pertinent Laboratory Tests, Serum Drug Concentrations, and Diagnostic Tests

Na 139 (139)	MCHC 350 (35)	Haptoglobin 0.13
K 4.3 (4.3)	Retic 0.15 (15)	(13)
BUN 5.0 (14)	Corrected 0.1 (10)	Direct Coombs 2+
Cr 99.5 (1.1)	LDH 5.1 (300)	Procain 14.4 (3.4)
Hct 0.25 (25%)	T Bili 41 (2.4)	NAPA 31 (7.3)
Hgb 79 (7.9)	D Bili 5 (0.3)	Digoxin 1.1 (0.9)
MCV 82 (82)	Ind Bili 36 (2.1)	

Peripheral blood smear: Normochromic, normocytic RBCs

ECG (12-lead): Normal sinus rhythm

Urinalysis: Hemoglobin present

PROBLEM LIST

Identify principal problems from the scenario in priority order

SOAP NOTE

To be completed by student

QUESTIONS

1. RB appears to have drug-induced hemolytic anemia. This is most likely due to which of his medications? (EO-1, 10)
   a. Procainamide
   b. Naproxen
   c. Digoxin
   d. Pseudoephedrine

2. Physical findings apparent in RB that are consistent with hemolytic anemia include all of the following *except:* (EO-5)
   a. Hemoglobinuria
   b. Icteric sclera
   c. Enlarged prostate gland
   d. Splenomegaly

3. Describe the mechanisms of action of the pharmacologic interventions in this case. (EO-7)

4. The cardiologist would like to start another antiarrhythmic agent for RB. Which of the following would not be a good choice due to a risk of causing drug-induced hemolytic anemia? (EO-8, 10)
   a. Propafenone
   b. Quinidine
   c. Amiodarone
   d. Sotalol

5. List the pharmacologic and nonpharmacologic treatment problems present in RB's treatment plan. (EO-11)

6. RB complains of dyspepsia with aspirin and most NSAIDs. Which of the following alternative agents has been demonstrated to be effective in the treatment of osteoarthritis, and void of GI side effects and ulceration? (EO-4, 8, 10, 12)
   a. Celecoxib
   b. Acetaminophen
   c. Tramadol
   d. Meperidine

7. RB's hemolytic anemia does not respond to corticosteroid therapy and requires him to have a splenectomy. RB should have all the following vaccinations prior to surgery *except:* (EO-7)
   a. Pneumococcal vaccine
   b. Meningococcal vaccine
   c. *H. influenzae* vaccine
   d. Varicella zoster vaccine

8. Which of the following is a long-term risk associated with chronic atrial fibrillation? (EO-1, 2)
   a. Cardioembolic stroke
   b. Congestive heart failure
   c. Renal insufficiency
   d. Peripheral vascular disease

9. RB converts back to atrial fibrillation. Warfarin and digoxin are both restarted. Which of the following medications that RB is taking has a significant interaction with warfarin that he must be counseled on? (EO-9)
   a. Fluticasone
   b. Misoprostol
   c. Pseudoephedrine
   d. Naproxen

10. What is the role of digoxin therapy in the management of atrial fibrillation? (EO-7)
    a. Antiarrhythmic (to convert to NSR)
    b. Stroke prevention
    c. Ventricular rate control
    d. Blood pressure management

11. What psychosocial factors may affect RB's adherence to both pharmacologic and nonpharmacologic therapy? (EO-15)

12. Describe the health care provider's role relative to the proposed psychosocial factors identified. (EO-16)

13. Summarize pathophysiologic, therapeutic, and disease management concepts for hemolytic anemias utilizing a key points format. (EO-18)

CASE 12
Anne Reaves
Topic: Other Anemias
Level 3
EDUCATIONAL MATERIALS
Chapter 14: Other Anemias (sickle cell anemia)

SCENARIO

Patient and Setting

AB, a 25-year-old black female; internal medicine service

Chief Complaint

Diffuse pain affecting abdomen, arms, and legs, typical of previous painful crises; pain is unrelieved by oral hydro-morphone

History of Present Illness

Sickle cell anemia; reports malaise, fevers to 38.9°C, and diarrhea over the past 3–4 days and dizziness upon standing since previous day; unable to eat or drink much and reports recent contact with the flu; denies melena, BRBPR, cough, SOB, headache, or dysuria

Past Medical History

Sickle cell anemia; multiple admissions for sickle cell crises; narcotic dependence; pneumococcal pneumonia, unsure if pneumococcal vaccine ever received

Past Surgical History

Splenectomy

Family/Social History

Family History: Mother, father, and 23-year-old brother have sickle cell trait, and 20-year-old brother has sickle cell anemia; older sister died last year (at 27 years) of complications of sickle cell anemia

Social History: No tobacco or ethanol use; history of narcotic abuse

Medication History

Hydromorphone 8 mg PO q4h PRN (usually 32 mg/day)
Folic acid 1 mg PO QD

Allergies

NKDA

Physical Examination

GEN: Black female appearing younger than stated age, in acute distress
VS: BP 100/60, HR 104, RR 18, T 38.0°C, Wt 46 kg, Ht 160 cm (usual weight 48 kg)
HEENT: Mildly icteric sclera, pupils equal and reactive, no sinus tenderness, pale and dry mucous membranes
COR: Nl S1 and S2; II/VI systolic ejection murmur
CHEST: Clear to auscultation and percussion
ABD: Hyperactive bowel sounds; + diffuse, non-localized tenderness; no hepatomegaly
GU: Deferred
RECT: Guaiac negative
EXT: Dry skin; + clubbing; tenderness to palpation: legs & arms; pale nail beds; no cyanosis or edema
NEURO: Alert and oriented × 4; CN II-XII intact; motor grossly intact

Results of Pertinent Laboratory Tests, Serum Drug Concentrations, and Diagnostic Tests

Na 140 (140)	Hct 0.243 (24.3)	Lkcs 13.6 × 10⁹
K 4.1 (4.1)	Hgb 81 (8.1)	(13.6 × 10³)
BUN 5.0 (14)	MCV 90.2 (90.2)	Iron 16 (88)
Cr 70 (0.8)	MCH 30.2 (30.2)	TIBC 68 (380)

Peripheral blood smear: Widespread sickled cells and few schistocytes; normochromic, normocytic RBCs

Chest radiography: No infiltrates or effusions, enlarged cardiac shadow

ECG: Normal sinus rhythm with rate of 100 beats/min, left ventricular hypertrophy

PROBLEM LIST

Identify principal problems from the scenario in priority order [completed Problem List and SOAP Note at end of casebook]

SOAP NOTE

To be completed by student

QUESTIONS

[Answers at end of casebook]

1. Sickle cell disease is seen predominantly in all the following countries with the *exception* of: (EO-3)
   a. United States
   b. Africa
   c. Saudi Arabia
   d. India

2. All of the following factors probably contributed to the development of the pain crisis in AB *except:* (EO-1)
   a. Decreased oral intake
   b. Viral gastroenteritis
   c. Diarrhea
   d. Malaise

3. Which of the following physical assessment findings in AB is a complication associated with sickle cell disease? (EO-5)
   a. Hyperactive bowel sounds
   b. Dry mucous membranes
   c. Systolic ejection murmur
   d. HR 104

4. Which of the following findings is indicative of a painful crisis in AB? (EO-2)
   a. Dry skin with clubbing in the extremities
   b. S1 and S2 heart sounds
   c. Tenderness to palpation in legs and arms
   d. Hyperactive bowel sounds

5. AB is receiving chronic folic acid supplementation in order to reduce which of the following risks associated with folate deficiency: (EO-1, 8)
   a. Infection
   b. Aplastic crisis
   c. Vaso-occlusive crisis
   d. Autosplenectomy

6. Describe the mechanisms of action of the pharmacologic and nonpharmacologic interventions in this case. (EO-7)

7. Patients who have had splenectomies are at increased risk for infections by encapsulated bacteria. This includes all the following *except:* (EO-18)
   a. Pneumococcus
   b. Meningococcus
   c. *H. influenzae*
   d. *C. difficile*

8. Which of the following would *not* be an appropriate medication to discharge AB home on for pain relief? (EO-6, 10)
   a. Morphine
   b. Hydromorphone
   c. Meperidine
   d. Naproxen sodium

9. What is the mechanism by which hydroxyurea decreases the incidence of painful crises? (EO-7)
   a. Increases production of hemoglobin F
   b. Decreases amount of hemoglobin S
   c. Increases splenic clearance of sickled cells
   d. Causes dilatation of capillaries, thus preventing vaso-occlusion

10. AB will be discharged home on the following medications: folic acid, ibuprofen, hydromorphone, and hydroxyurea. Please provide appropriate discharge counseling, including common adverse effects, for these medications. (EO-10, 14)

11. What psychosocial factors may affect AB's adherence to both pharmacologic and nonpharmacologic therapy? (EO-15)

12. Describe the health care provider's role relative to the proposed psychosocial factors identified. (EO-16)

13. Evaluate the pharmacoeconomic considerations relative to AB's plan of care. (EO-17)

14. Summarize pathophysiologic, therapeutic, and disease management concepts for sickle cell anemia utilizing a key points format. (EO-18)

CASE 13
James M. Holt, Amy Seabrook
Topic: Thrombocytopenia
 Level 1
EDUCATIONAL MATERIALS
Chapter 15: Coagulation Disorders (thrombocytopenia, treatment goals, drug-induced platelet disorders)

SCENARIO
Patient and Setting
PA, a 30-year-old white male; primary care clinic

Chief Complaint
4-day history of epistaxis

History of Present Illness
Has had intermittent epistaxis for 4 days; has handled epistaxis by leaning head back and using tissues to collect blood; also noticed the appearance of a few flat dark-red spots on arms about this same time; reports that the unpredictable epistaxis has recently made him very frustrated and upset

Past Medical History
Rheumatoid arthritis for 2 years

Past Surgical History
None

Family/Social History

Family History: Noncontributory

Social History: Smokes ½ PPD × 9 years, drinks 2–3 beers per week, no illicit drug use

Medication History

Indomethacin 25 mg PO TID

Multivitamin 1 tablet PO QD

Diphenhydramine 25 mg PO QHS

Allergies

None

Physical Examination

GEN: Agitated, upset, and concerned male

VS: BP 142/88, RR 22, HR 116, T 39°C, Wt 90 kg, Ht 6'1" (185 cm)

HEENT: Irritated and reddened skin near nasal areas, PERRLA

COR: Tachycardic, normal S1, S2

CHEST: No rales or rhonchi

ABD: (+) BS

GU: WNL

RECT: Deferred

EXT: Mild petechiae, purpura on upper arms; swelling and mild tenderness bilaterally knees

NEURO: WNL

Results of Pertinent Laboratory Tests, Serum Drug Concentrations, and Diagnostic Tests

Na 140 (140)
Ca 2.3 (9.2)
Hgb 115 (11.5)

K 4.1 (4.1)
PO_4 1.2 (3.8)
WBC 9.2 × 10^9

Cl 101 (101)
Mg 1.2 (2.9)
(9.2 × 10^3)

HCO_3 26 (26)
Plts 55 × 10^9
ALT 0.48 (29)

BUN 4.3 (12)
(55 × 10^3)
AST 0.47 (28)

Cr 88.4 (1.0)
MCV 87 (87)
Alb 49 (4.9)

Glu 6.0 (108)
Hct 0.29 (29)

WBC with differential: PMNs 0.61 (61%), monocytes 0.06 (6%), lymphs 0.33 (33%)

PROBLEM LIST

Identify principal problems from the scenario in priority order [completed Problem List and SOAP Note at end of casebook]

SOAP NOTE

To be completed by student

QUESTIONS

[Answers at end of casebook]

1. All of the following are mechanisms of drug interference found in drug-induced platelet disorders *except:* (EO-1)
   a. Platelet membranes or membrane receptor sites
   b. Phosphodiesterase activity
   c. Acetylcholine activity
   d. Prostaglandin biosynthetic pathways

2. All of the following can be found in a clinical presentation of drug-induced thrombocytopenia *except:* (EO-2)
   a. Vomiting
   b. Mucous membrane bleeding
   c. Petechiae
   d. Purpura

3. Which of the following drugs would be a good choice in a situation of drug-induced thrombocytopenia? (EO-8, 9)
   a. Piroxicam
   b. Aspirin
   c. Fenoprofen
   d. Celecoxib

4. What is the mechanism of action of indomethacin and other NSAIDs? (EO-1, 7)
   a. Interferes with hepatic synthesis of vitamin K dependent coagulation factors
   b. Prevents thromboxane A_2 generation by inhibiting cyclooxygenase
   c. Prevents conversion of fibrinogen to fibrin
   d. Blocks adenosine diphosphate receptors

5. All of the following could be considered for management of patients with platelet function disorders *except:* (EO-8, 12)
   a. Avoidance of high risk bleeding situations
   b. Correction with platelet transfusions for all patients
   c. Avoidance of medications that alter platelet function
   d. Correction of the underlying disorder when possible

6. Thrombocytopenia may be caused by all of the following *except:* (EO-1)
   a. Increased destruction of platelets
   b. Altered distribution (sequestration) of platelets
   c. Increased production of white blood cells
   d. Decreased production of platelets

7. Which of the following platelet counts defines "moderate thrombocytopenia?" (EO-5)
   a. 0–20,000
   b. >100,000
   c. 50,000–100,000
   d. 20,000–50,000

8. Drug-induced immune thrombocytopenia has all of the following characteristics *except:* (EO-1, 3)
   a. Dose-related
   b. Associated with antibody persistence for many years
   c. Rapid sustained recovery after drug is terminated
   d. More common in adults

9. Explain the rationale for using salsalate in PA at this time. (EO-8, 12)

10. Describe the pharmacoeconomic considerations relative to PA's plan of care. (EO-17)

11. Describe psychosocial aspects involved in PA's plan of care. (EO-15)

12. Summarize pathophysiologic, therapeutic, and disease management concepts for this case utilizing a key points format. (EO-18)

CASE 14
James M. Holt, Jennifer Wiseman
Topic: Protein C Deficiency
Level 2
EDUCATIONAL MATERIALS
Chapter 15: Coagulation Disorders (protein C deficiency, clinical presentation and diagnosis, treatment, long-term management)

SCENARIO

Patient and Setting
JD, a 27-year-old male; local emergency room

Chief Complaint
Pain and swelling of LLE × 2 days; sudden SOB, cough, dyspnea, chest pain × 20 minutes

History of Present Illness
Presented to ER 4 days ago with deep vein thrombosis (DVT) in RLE; was given warfarin 10 mg, then started on warfarin 5 mg PO QD and scheduled to clinic in 5 days to check INR; presents again to ER with new symptoms as above

Past Medical History
Significant only for HTN × 2 years

Past Surgical History
None

Family/Social History
Family History: Father died age 51 after massive CVA; had protein C deficiency; brother with history of DVT

Social History: Smokes 1½ PPD × 9 years; denies alcohol or illicit drug use

Medication History
Hydrochlorothiazide (HCTZ) 25 mg PO QD
Warfarin 5 mg PO QD
Multivitamin PO QD

Allergies
Codeine—rash and hives

Physical Examination
GEN: Obese, anxious male in mild respiratory distress
VS: BP 132/68, HR 110, RR 30, O_2 sat 88%, T 38°C, Wt 240 lb (109 kg), Ht 5'9" (175 cm)
HEENT: Unremarkable
CV: Regular rhythm, tachycardic
CHEST: CTA, coarse breath sounds throughout, tachypneic
ABD: Benign
EXT: LLE—erythematous w/ 2+ pitting edema, + calf tenderness, + Homans' sign; RLE—mild edema
NEURO: No focal deficit

Results of Pertinent Laboratory Tests, Serum Drug Concentrations, and Diagnostic Tests

Na 137 (137)	Hgb 130 (13.0)	CK 0 (0)
K 4.6 (4.6)	WBC 8 × 10⁹	LDH 83 (83)
Cl 103 (103)	(8 × 10³)	Fibrinogen 6.3 (0.2)
HCO₃ 22 (22)	Plts 200 × 10⁹	ATIII 92%
BUN 6.0 (16.8)	(200 × 10³)	Protein C 13%
Cr 65 (0.7)	Alb 50 (5.0)	ABG: pH 7.38 (7.38)
AST 16 (16)	aPTT 32 (32)	pO₂ 9.2 (69)
ALT 22 (22)	INR 1.7	pCO₂ 4.0 (30)
Hct 0.4 (40%)		

Doppler ultrasound: Consistent with bilateral DVT
V/Q scan: High probability of pulmonary embolism (PE)
ECG: NSR; tachycardia; no signs of ischemia

PROBLEM LIST
Identify principal problems from the scenario in priority order [completed Problem List and SOAP Note at end of casebook]

SOAP NOTE
To be completed by student

QUESTIONS
[Answers at end of casebook]

1. Based on JD's age of thrombosis onset, clinical symptoms, and protein C level, which of the following types of protein C deficiency does he most likely have? (EO-1)
   a. Autosomal-recessive, heterozygous
   b. Autosomal-recessive, homozygous
   c. Autosomal-dominant, heterozygous
   d. Autosomal-dominant, homozygous

2. In individuals *without* protein C deficiency, the normal range for protein C is: (EO-5)
   a. 15–40%
   b. 40–65%
   c. 65–130%
   d. 130–180%

3. Symptomatic patients with the autosomal-dominant form of protein C deficiency most frequently present with: (EO-2)
   a. DVT and/or PE
   b. Neonatal purpura fulminans
   c. Myocardial infarction
   d. Ischemic stroke

4. Protein C levels are: (EO-8)
   a. Affected by heparin
   b. Affected by warfarin
   c. Not measurable
   d. Affected by enoxaparin

5. Heparin should be overlapped with warfarin for treatment of DVT in protein C-deficient patients: (EO-6)
   a. For 3–5 days
   b. Until therapeutic INR is achieved
   c. Until symptoms resolve
   d. Indefinitely

6. The goal INR in JD's case is: (EO-6)
   a. 2.0–3.0
   b. 3.0–4.0
   c. 3.5–4.5
   d. 4.5–5.5

7. Which of the following warfarin adverse effects occurs in higher frequency in protein C-deficient patients vs. the general population? (EO-10)
   a. Confusion
   b. Hemorrhage
   c. Alopecia
   d. Skin necrosis

8. Warfarin works to treat recurrent DVT in protein C-deficient patients by: (EO-7)
   a. Dissolving fibrin clots
   b. Inhibiting hepatic synthesis of vitamin K-dependent clotting factors
   c. Increasing activity of functional protein C
   d. Stopping the coagulation cascade

9. Which of the following would be the next best option in JD for long-term treatment if he developed warfarin-induced skin necrosis? (EO-12, 17)
   a. Protein C concentrate
   b. Unfractionated heparin
   c. Low molecular weight heparin
   d. Fresh frozen plasma

10. How should JD's first DVT have been managed, knowing that he has protein C deficiency? (EO-11)

11. From a pharmacoeconomic standpoint, what might be a better option for immediate anticoagulation in JD? (EO-17)

12. List the symptoms, laboratory values, patient factors, and details of history in JD that are consistent with protein C deficiency. (EO-2, 5)

13. List two options (other than anticoagulation) for DVT prevention in high-risk situations. (EO-12)

14. Summarize pathophysiologic, therapeutic, and disease management concepts for this case utilizing a key points format. (EO-18)

CASE 15
Debbie Scholtz
Topics: Type 2 DM, Community-Acquired Pneumonia
Level 1
EDUCATIONAL MATERIALS
Chapter 19: Diabetes; Chapter 67: Pneumonia

SCENARIO

Patient and Setting

JG, a 52-year-old female; primary care clinic

Chief Complaint

3-day history of fever, chills, pleuritic chest pain, productive cough, extreme fatigue

History of Present Illness

Returned 3 days ago from a stressful 5-day business trip; since then developed the symptoms described above; for 1 week has felt restless, anxious, and has been unable to sleep soundly; frequent cough, fever, and increased nocturia are interfering with her sleep; noticed increased numbness in her toes and burning leg pain at night for the past 2 months that was not adequately controlled by her current medications

Past Medical History

Type 2 DM for 8 years

Past Surgical History

None

Family/Social History

Smokes 2 PPD × 15 years

Drinks 2–3 glasses of wine per week

Drinks 3 cups of coffee per day (more on business trips)

Not following diabetic diet consistently

Medication History

Pseudoephedrine, 60 mg PO QID for the past 5 days

Glipizide, 10 mg PO BID

Acetaminophen with codeine, PO q6h PRN pain

Allergies

None

Physical Examination

GEN: Tired, obese, agitated female in moderate respiratory distress

VS: BP 140/90, RR 28, HR 125, T 39.5°C, Wt 73 kg, Ht 5′4″

HEENT: "Bags under the eyes," yellow purulent sputum for 3 days

COR: Normal S1, S2, no murmur, tachycardic

CHEST: LLL dullness

ABD: WNL

GU: WNL

RECT: Deferred

EXT: Numbness to toes bilaterally

NEURO: Decreased DTR lower extremities

Results of Pertinent Laboratory Tests, Serum Drug Concentrations, and Diagnostic Tests

Na 135 (135)	Hct 0.35 (35%)	ALT 0.52 (31)
K 4.5 (4.5)	Hgb 119 (11.9)	Ca 2.2 (8.8)
Cl 105 (105)	WBC 14 × 10⁹	PO$_4$ 0.66 (2.0)
HCO$_3$ 25 (25)	(14 × 10³)	Mg 1.15 (2.8)
BUN 7.1 (20)	Plts 2.1 × 10⁹	Alb 37 (3.7)
Cr 126 (1.2)	(210 × 10³)	Fast Glu 12.2 (220)
HbA$_{1C}$ .12 (12%)	MCV 90 (90)	AST 0.42 (25)

WBC with differential: PMN 0.85 (85%), bands 0.12 (12%), lymphs 0.03 (3%)

Sputum: Gram stain shows many pleomorphic gram (−) coccobacilli, few gram (+) cocci in pairs, chains, and clusters, 30 neutrophils, <10 epithelial cells per low-power field; culture pending

Blood: Smear negative; culture × 2 pending

Urine: 1+ protein, 1+ glucose, (−) ketone; culture pending

Chest radiography: LLL consolidation, no pleural effusion

Doppler: Negative

PROBLEM LIST

Identify principal problems from the scenario in priority order [completed Problem List and SOAP Note at end of casebook]

SOAP NOTE

To be completed by student

QUESTIONS

[Answers at end of casebook]

1. What is the *most* common pathogen associated with community-acquired pneumonia? (EO-1)
   a. *Staphylococcus aureus*
   b. *Streptococcus pneumoniae*
   c. *Haemophilus influenzae*
   d. *Streptococcus pyogenes*

2. All of the following signs or symptoms present in JG are frequently associated with community-acquired pneumonia *except:* (EO-2)
   a. Fever
   b. Increased respirations
   c. Nocturia
   d. Fatigue

3. Which of the following antibiotics would *not* be an appropriate choice for this patient? (EO-8)
   a. Cephalexin
   b. Cefuroxime axetil
   c. Cefpodoxime proxetil
   d. Amoxicillin/clavulanate

4. Which of the following findings is an indication that JG is developing long-term complications from her diabetes? (EO-5)
   a. Tachycardia
   b. Glucosuria
   c. Leukocytosis
   d. Proteinuria

5. What is the primary mechanism of action of metformin? (EO-7)
   a. Decreased hepatic glucose production
   b. Increased secretion of insulin from pancreatic beta cells
   c. Inhibition of alpha glucosidase enzymes
   d. Increased glucose disposal in muscle tissues

6. Which of the following statements regarding self-monitoring of blood glucose is true? (EO-8)
   a. All diabetics should monitor blood glucose four times a day
   b. Frequency of testing is dependent on patient variables
   c. All monitors utilize inexpensive strips
   d. Only patients using insulin need to monitor blood glucose routinely

7. JG should be monitored for factors that would predispose her to lactic acidosis due to metformin. Which of the following may increase her risk for this problem? (EO-4, 6, 8)
   a. Serum potassium <3.5 mmol/L
   b. Cigarette smoking
   c. HgA$_{1C}$ >12%
   d. Serum creatinine >124 (1.4)

8. JG returns in 1 month with slightly improved blood glucose and improved adherence with diet, yet with a new complaint of frequent diarrhea. What approach would be the *most* appropriate at this time? (EO-8, 10, 12)
   a. Stop the amitriptyline
   b. Decrease the metformin
   c. Increase the metformin
   d. Add metoclopramide

9. In light of JG's proteinuria, what class of drugs may be used to prevent progression of diabetic nephropathy? (EO-12)
   a. Beta-blockers
   b. Thiazolidinediones
   c. ACE inhibitors
   d. Tricyclic antidepressants

10. Explain the rationale for using metformin in this patient at this time. (EO-8, 12)

11. Describe the general nutritional principles JG should follow to manage her diabetes. (EO-8, 14)

12. List methods a health care provider may use to assist JG in adhering to a "diabetic" diet. (EO-14, 16)

13. Discuss the pharmacoeconomic considerations relative to JG's plan of care. (EO-17)

14. Describe how an exercise program may benefit JG. (EO-7, 14)

15. Summarize pathophysiologic, therapeutic, and disease management concepts for this case utilizing a key points format. (EO-18)

CASE 16
Debbie Scholtz
Topic: Diabetes
Level 2
EDUCATIONAL MATERIALS
Chapter 19: Diabetes; Chapter 39: Hypertension

SCENARIO

Patient and Setting

AH, a 57-year-old black man; primary care clinic

Chief Complaint

Several episodes of sweating, tremors, and nervousness in the past several weeks; also has felt more fatigued in the past 2 months

History of Present Illness

Reports three episodes, all occurring between 10:30 AM and 12:00 PM; checked blood glucose on one occasion and reported it was 3.0 mmol/L (55 mg/dL); drinking soda relieved all episodes; does not check blood glucose regularly; when checked runs "between 55 and 180"

Past Medical History

DM Type 2 × 7 years, HTN × 10 years

Past Surgical History

Appendectomy 1981

Family/Social History

Family History: Positive for hypertension, diabetes, and MI (father, age 64)

Social History: Works as contractor and has an unpredictable schedule from day to day; often skips breakfast and eats fast food on the run; nonsmoker; drinks beer frequently

Medication History

Glyburide, 20 mg q AM

HCTZ, 50 mg q AM

KCl, 40 mEq q AM

Allergies

NKA

Physical Examination

GEN: Obese male in no apparent distress

VS: 154/94 (previous BPs range from 150/92–160/96), HR 88 reg, RR 14, Wt 90 kg (increased 3 kg), Ht 173 cm

HEENT: EOM intact, PERRLA

COR: NSR

CHEST: Without rales or rhonchi

ABD: Normal, positive bowel sounds, no guarding, no organomegaly

EXT: No peripheral edema

NEURO: DTR intact, without signs of diabetic neuropathy

Results of Pertinent Laboratory Tests, Serum Drug Concentrations, and Diagnostic Tests

Na 140 (140)	Hct 0.32 (32)	Glu (random)
K 4.5 (4.5)	Hgb 100 (10)	10 (189)
Cl 98	Lkcs 6.8×10^9	Chol 6.4 (250)
HCO$_3$ 21 (21)	(6.8×10^3)	TG 2.68 (238)
BUN 10 (28)	MCV 91 (91)	HbA$_{1C}$ 7.9%
Cr 150 (1.7)	MCH 24 (24)	AST 0.33 (20)
Cr one year ago	MCHC 310 (31)	ALT 0.36 (22)
115 (1.3)		

Folate: 4.5 nmol/L (2 μg/dL)

Fe: 14.7 μmol/L (82 μg/dL)

Vitamin B$_{12}$: 162 pmol/L (220 ng/dL)

UA: (+) glucose, (−) ketone, (+) protein

PROBLEM LIST

Identify principal problems from the scenario in priority order

SOAP NOTES

To be completed by student

QUESTIONS

1. What sulfonylurea has been associated with the highest incidence of hypoglycemia? (EO-10)
   a. Tolazamide
   b. Glyburide
   c. Chlorpropamide
   d. Glimepiride

2. Sulfonylureas lower blood glucose primarily by: (EO-7)
   a. Decreasing hepatic glucose production
   b. Increasing insulin secretion by pancreatic beta cells
   c. Decreasing intestinal absorption of carbohydrates
   d. Increasing glucose disposal in muscle tissue

3. Metformin would *not* be an option for this patient because: (EO-5, 10)
   a. He has folate deficiency anemia
   b. He has impaired renal function
   c. His hypertension is poorly controlled
   d. He has Type 2 diabetes

4. Which of the following medications can cause hypoglycemia when used as monotherapy? (EO-10)
   a. Troglitazone
   b. Metformin
   c. Acarbose
   d. Glyburide

5. Which of the following is *not* a reason for AH's fatigue? (EO-1, 2, 5)
   a. Poorly controlled hypertension
   b. Poorly controlled diabetes
   c. Folate deficiency anemia
   d. Poor and irregular diet

6. Thiazide diuretics have been associated with which adverse metabolic effect? (EO-10)
   a. Hyperkalemia
   b. Hypokalemia
   c. Hypoglycemia
   d. Hypocalcemia

7. If the change in glyburide dose is insufficient in achieving good diabetes control in this patient, what combination with glyburide would be the next best option? (EO-8, 12)
   a. A thiazolidinedione
   b. Metformin
   c. Repaglinide
   d. Regular insulin sliding scale

8. What other preventive measure should be considered for AH? (EO-12)
   a. Vitamin E
   b. Clopidogrel
   c. Atorvastatin
   d. Low-dose aspirin

9. What factors have contributed to AH's increased risk for hypoglycemia? (EO-10, 15)

10. Why are beta-blockers relatively contraindicated in this patient? (EO-8, 9, 10)

11. List psychosocial factors that may affect LH's ability to adhere to the treatment plan. (EO-15)

12. Describe methods health care providers may utilize to address the identified psychosocial factors in question 11. (EO-16)

13. Summarize pathophysiologic, therapeutic, and disease management concepts for this case utilizing a key points format. (EO-18)

CASE 17
Debbie Scholtz
Topic: Hyperlipidemia
Level 2

EDUCATIONAL MATERIALS
Chapter 19: Diabetes; Chapter 20: Hyperlipidemia;
Chapter 39: Hypertension

SCENARIO

Patient and Setting

TT, a 52-year-old female; general medicine clinic

Chief Complaint

Ran out of several medicines 3 days ago; now has heartburn and painful feet

History of Present Illness

Frequent difficulty getting refills on time due to financial and transportation difficulties; reports running out of benazepril, amitriptyline, and ranitidine 3 days ago and mentions heartburn symptoms and a burning pain in feet have returned; checks blood glucose twice a day before breakfast and dinner and reports a range of 122–161 mg/dL.

Past Medical History

DM Type 1 × 24 years, with diabetic neuropathy × 4 years; hypertension × 7 years; hyperlipidemia × 5 years; gastroesophageal reflux disease × 3 years

Past Surgical History

Total abdominal hysterectomy with bilateral salpingoophorectomy 1986

Family/Social History

Mother also had diabetes and died of renal failure; father died of a stroke at age 68; does not drink alcohol or smoke; follows an ADA diet and walks three times a week.

Medication History

Insulin regular, 10 U SC q AM, 8 U SC q PM

Insulin NPH, 20 U SC q AM, 16 U SC q PM

Simvastatin, 10 mg q PM

Benazepril, 10 mg BID

Amitriptyline, 25 mg QHS

Ranitidine, 150 mg BID

Conjugated estrogens, 0.625 mg q AM

Allergies

NKA

Physical Examination

GEN: WDWN female in no apparent distress
VS: BP 164/100, HR 85, RR 14, T 37.5°C, Wt 68 kg, Ht 160 cm
HEENT: PERRLA
COR: Normal S1 and S2
CHEST: Clear to auscultation and percussion
ABD: Soft, nontender, no hepatosplenomegaly
RECT: Guaiac negative
EXT: No clubbing, cyanosis, or edema
NEURO: Oriented to time, place, and person, cranial nerves intact, decreased deep tendon reflexes

Results of Pertinent Laboratory Tests, Serum Drug Concentrations, and Diagnostic Tests

Na 140 (140)	Lkcs 10 × 10⁹	Alb 55 (5.5)
K 4.0 (4.0)	(10 × 10³)	T Bili 10.3 (0.6)
Cl 136 (136)	Plts 170 × 10⁹	HbA₁C 8.2%
HCO₃ 25 (25)	(170 × 10³)	TG 2.1 (186)
BUN 7.1 (20)	MCV 85 (85)	LDH 1.34 (80)
Cr 132.6 (1.5)	Glucose 13.3 (240)	Ca 2.4 (9.6)
Uric Acid 333 (5.6)	Chol 6.2 (240)	PO₄ 0.9 (2.8)
Hct 0.40 (40)	ALT 0.33 (20)	Mg 0.98 (2.4)
Hgb 130 (13)	AST 0.58 (35)	HDL 1.34 (52)
	Alk Phos 0.83 (50)	LDL 3.9 (151)

Urinalysis: 2+protein, 2+glucose, no organisms seen, clear, pH 7.5, SG 1.020, no RBC/leuk/casts

ECG: Left ventricular hypertrophy

PROBLEM LIST

Identify principal problems from the scenario in priority order [completed Problem List and SOAP Note at end of casebook]

SOAP NOTES

To be completed by student

QUESTIONS

[Answers at end of casebook]

1. How many risk factors for coronary heart disease does TT have? (EO-3)
   a. One
   b. Two
   c. Three
   d. Four

2. Which factor present in this case significantly increases risk for coronary heart disease more than the others? (EO-3)
   a. Hypertension
   b. Father's history of stroke at age 68
   c. Diabetes
   d. HDL cholesterol <60 mg/dL

3. What impact may oral estrogen replacement therapy be expected to have on TT's lipid profile? (EO-5, 7)
   a. Increase HDL, increase triglycerides
   b. Increase HDL, increase LDL
   c. Increase HDL, decrease triglycerides
   d. Decrease LDL, decrease triglycerides

4. Which lipid-lowering agent may potentially worsen TT's diabetic control? EO-10)
   a. Gemfibrozil
   b. Cholestyramine
   c. Simvastatin
   d. Niacin

5. Which of the following is *not* a contraindication to lipid-lowering therapy with statin-type drugs? (EO-8, 9)
   a. Renal impairment
   b. Pregnancy
   c. Active liver disease
   d. Unexplained elevations in liver enzymes

6. Drug therapy with statins is clearly cost-effective in which groups of patients? (EO-3, 17)
   a. Primary prevention in premenopausal women
   b. All patients over 70 years old
   c. Secondary prevention in those with established CHD
   d. All patients with diabetes and hypertension

7. TT should be advised to take her simvastatin in the evening because: (EO-12, 14)
   a. Simvastatin may cause sedation
   b. Most people have the highest cholesterol intake with the evening meal
   c. Absorption is decreased when taken with food
   d. Cholesterol synthesis peaks at night

8. What other laboratory monitoring besides liver function tests should be performed routinely to monitor for toxicity from statin drugs? (EO-5, 10)
   a. Creatine kinase
   b. No other routine tests are necessary
   c. Serum creatinine
   d. Hemoglobin and hematocrit

9. Besides lowering her blood pressure, what other advantage may benazepril provide TT? (EO-8)
   a. Delayed progression of neuropathy
   b. Decreased LDL cholesterol
   c. Delayed progression of nephropathy
   d. Increased esophageal sphincter tone

10. Which of the following screening tests would *not* be necessary for TT at this time? (EO-1)
    a. Echocardiography
    b. Mammogram
    c. Dilated eye exam
    d. Foot exam

11. Describe the principles of the NCEP-ATPII Step I diet for hypercholesterolemia. (EO-8, 14)

12. What factors may be involved in interfering with TT's ability to adhere to the treatment plan? (EO-15)

13. What assistance may the health care provider give in helping TT to improve her adherence? (EO-16)

14. List advantages and disadvantages of using niacin therapy for hyperlipidemia. (EO-7, 8, 9, 10)

15. Summarize pathophysiologic, therapeutic, and disease management concepts for this case utilizing a key points format. (EO-18)

CASE 18
Debbie Scholtz
Topic: Diabetes

EDUCATIONAL MATERIALS
Chapter 19: Diabetes

SCENARIO

Patient and Setting

BK, a 23-year-old male; emergency room

Chief Complaint

Nausea, vomiting, myalgias, polydipsia, and polyuria × 2 days

History of Present Illness

Has Type 1 diabetes; 3 days ago at a party drank an excessive amount of alcohol and woke up the next day "sick to his stomach"; has vomited six times since then, and is unable to keep any food or drink down; stopped taking insulin; currently has a headache; denies chest pain, cough, fever, upper respiratory symptoms, and abdominal pain

Past Medical History

DM Type 1 × 11 years (3 hospitalizations for DKA); depression × 2 years; allergic rhinitis × 5 years

Past Surgical History

None

Family/Social History

Family History: No family history of diabetes; mother committed suicide

Social History: Smokes approximately ½ pack per day, drinks socially; denies IV drug abuse; works for father; does not follow diabetic diet

Medication History

Human 70/30 insulin, 30 U q AM

Sertraline, 100 mg q PM

Fluticazone nasal spray, 2 sprays each nostril PRN

Loratidine, 10 mg QD

Acetaminophen, 500 mg PRN

Allergies

Amoxicillin—causes rash

Physical Examination

GEN: Well-developed, well-nourished pale 23-year-old male in mild distress

VS: Breathing is deep and labored with a fruity odor; BP 100/84, HR 120 (supine); BP 98/60, HR 140 (sitting); RR 34; T 37.0°C; Wt 68 kg (decreased 4 kg); Ht 178 cm

HEENT: Dry tongue and mucous membranes

CHEST: Clear to auscultation and percussion, no rales, wheezing, or rhonchi

COR: Tachycardia, regular rhythm

EXT: Poor skin turgor

NEURO: Alert and oriented × 3

ABD: Voluntary guarding secondary to nervousness, mildly tender, positive bowel sounds

Results of Pertinent Laboratory Tests, Serum Drug Concentrations, and Diagnostic Tests

Na 130 (130)	Cr 141 (1.6)	Glu 30 (541)
K 6.0 (6.0)	Hct 0.457 (45.7)	PO_4 1.5 (4.8)
Cl 96 (96)	Hgb 152 (15.2)	ABG: pH 7.2
HCO_3 14 (14)	Lkcs 14 × 10⁹	PCO_2 26
BUN 14.2 (40)	(14 × 10³)	

Urinalysis: Trace protein, 4+ glucose, +ketones, −nitrites

Chest radiography: No infiltrates

ECG: Within normal limits

Blood cultures × 2: Pending

Urine cultures: Pending

Problem List

Identify principal problems from the scenario in priority order [completed Problem List and SOAP Note at end of casebook]

SOAP NOTES

To be completed by student

QUESTIONS

[Answers at end of casebook]

1. What is the most probable cause of BK's DKA? (EO-1)
   a. Viral gastroenteritis
   b. Lack of insulin
   c. Urinary tract infection
   d. Stress from depression

2. Which one of the following findings in BK is *not* a common sign or symptom of DKA? (EO-2)
   a. Tachycardia
   b. Fruity breath
   c. Rapid respiration
   d. Headache

3. BK's hyperventilation is probably due to: (EO-1, 2)
   a. Compensation for metabolic acidosis
   b. Respiratory acidosis
   c. Stress and anxiety
   d. Cigarette smoking

4. When should bicarbonate replacement be considered for BK? (EO-8, 12)
   a. It should be given now, since his pH is <7.2
   b. It should be given if his CO_2 decreases to <12
   c. It should be given if his pH is <7.0
   d. It should never be given because it would cause hypokalemia

5. If BK's blood glucose does not decrease by at least 2.8 (50 mg/dL) in the first 2 hours, what should be done? (EO-5, 6, 12)
   a. Double the insulin infusion rate
   b. Give an insulin bolus dose of 2 U/kg
   c. Increase the insulin infusion to 0.5 U/kg/hr
   d. Check blood glucose again in 2 hours

6. The DCCT study is important in a case such as BK's because it showed: (EO-1, 8)
   a. Lowering blood glucose to <11.1 (200 mg/dL) within the first 24 hours shortens length of hospital stay
   b. Intensive control of Type 1 diabetes will decrease risk of long-term complications
   c. Patients with uncontrolled diabetes for >10 years will develop diabetic neuropathy
   d. Utilizing insulin infusions results in quicker resolution of DKA

7. What should BK be told about the use of alcohol in diabetics? (EO-11, 14)
   a. He should never drink alcoholic beverages
   b. Mixed drinks would be less likely to affect his blood sugar vs. light beer
   c. In people using insulin, alcohol is likely to cause significant hyperglycemia
   d. Use of alcohol should be kept to a minimum and be taken with food

8. BK is switched back to his usual dose of insulin, 30 U of 70/30 insulin once a day, when he is discharged from the

hospital. Three weeks later, he returns with the following blood glucose records:

AM	noon	PM	hs
186	105	118	138
154	99	115	144
168	111	130	129
141	94	104	124
147	118	108	142

What would be the most reasonable adjustment in his insulin dose? (EO-6, 12)
a. Increase dose to 35 U 70/30 every morning
b. Add 5 U of regular insulin at bedtime
c. Change insulin to 20 U NPH and 15 U regular each morning
d. Add 3 U 70/30 insulin at suppertime

9. One year later, BK is on the following insulin regimen: 28 U NPH + 14 U Humalog before breakfast and 15 U NPH + 15 U Humalog before supper. What is the difference between regular insulin and Humalog? (EO-7)
a. Regular insulin has a quicker onset of action and shorter duration
b. Only Humalog insulin can be given either intravenously or subcutaneously
c. Humalog has a quicker onset of action and shorter duration
d. Humalog is made through recombinant DNA technology

10. BK's blood sugars are as follows:

AM	noon	PM	hs	3 AM
165	92	103	85	
172	106	110	94	88
144	88	90	102	
150	101	105	92	98
147	75	87	98	

What would be the most reasonable adjustment in his insulin dose? (EO-6, 12)
a. For the Somoygi effect, his evening NPH dose should be decreased
b. His supper NPH dose should be moved to bedtime
c. For the dawn phenomenon, his morning regular dose should be increased
d. No changes are necessary; overall control is good

11. Describe what patients should be taught about sick-day management. (EO-14)

12. Explain why dextrose is added to BK's intravenous fluids while he is still hyperglycemic. (EO-8, 10)

13. As BK is being readied for discharge from the hospital, what specific educational topics are most important to address at this time? (EO-17)

14. What psychosocial factors may affect BK's ability to adhere to the treatment plan? (EO-15)

15. How can health care providers address the psychosocial factors that may affect BK's ability to adhere to the treatment plan? (EO-16)

16. What direct and indirect costs are involved in BK's case? (EO-17)

17. Summarize pathophysiologic, therapeutic, and disease management concepts for this case utilizing a key points format. (EO-18)

CASE 19
Debbie Scholtz
Topic: Acute Adrenal Insufficiency

EDUCATIONAL MATERIALS
Chapter 16: Adrenocortical Dysfunction and Clinical Use of Steroids; Chapter 9: Fluid and Electrolyte Therapy and Acid-Base Balance; Chapter 31: Rheumatoid Arthritis

---

SCENARIO

Patient and Setting
EM, a 65-year-old female; emergency department

Chief Complaint
Acute change in mental status

History of Present Illness
Brought to ER by husband who states has become progressively confused over the past 24–48 hours; now only semiconscious; also experiencing weakness, dizziness, diarrhea, and severe vomiting prior to the onset of confusion; just returned from vacation during which ran out of prednisone.

Past Medical History
Rheumatoid arthritis × 5 years (on prednisone × 1 year), GERD × 6 months, hypertension × 14 years, osteoporosis × 2 years, postmenopausal

Past Surgical History
Hysterectomy 12 years prior

Family/Social History
Family History: Noncontributory

Social History: Married × 37 years, retired teacher, nonsmoker, nondrinker

Medication History
Prednisone, 20 mg QD, ran out 1 week ago
Ibuprofen, 400 mg TID since prednisone ran out
Famotidine, 20 mg QHS
Atenolol, 50 mg QD

Magnesium hydroxide/aluminum hydroxide suspension
  PRN heartburn

Allergies

None

Physical Examination

    GEN: Pale, semiconscious, elderly female
     VS: BP 100/52, P 112, RR 28, T 37.3°C, Wt 65 kg
          (72 kg 1 month ago)
  HEENT: Moon facies, pale gums
  CHEST: WNL
    COR: Normal S_1, S_2, no S_3 or S_4; rapid heart rate;
          mild mitral valve murmur suggestive of mitral
          valve prolapse
    ABD: Obese; diffuse abdominal tenderness; normal
          bowel sounds
    EXT: Thin, cool extremities; proximal muscle
          weakness, 1–2+ pulses throughout; pale nail
          beds
   SKIN: Dry, +tenting, +striae on abdomen

Results of Pertinent Laboratory Tests, Serum Drug Concentrations, and Diagnostic Tests

Na 119 (119)	PO$_4$ 1.2 (3.8)	Plts 170 × 10^9
K 5.8 (5.8)	Mg 0.9 (1.8)	(170 × 10^3)
Cl 92 (92)	Uric Acid 238 (4)	MCV 80 (80)
HCO$_3$ 26 (26)	T Bili 14 (0.8)	MCHC 320 (32)
BUN 17.8 (50)	Hct 0.38 (38)	MCH 27 (27)
Cr 150 (1.7)	Hgb 110 (11)	ALT 0.37 (22)
Glu 2.8 (50)	Lkcs 6.5 × 10^9	LDH 1.43 (86)
Ca 5 (10)	(6.5 × 10^3)	Alk Phos 1.3 (78)
		Alb 30 (3.0)

Stool: Guaiac positive
UA: SG 1.025
ECG: Tachycardia, regular rhythm

PROBLEM LIST

*Identify principal problems from the scenario in priority order
[completed Problem List and SOAP Note at end of casebook]*

SOAP NOTE

To be completed by student

QUESTIONS

[Answers at end of casebook]

1. Which of the following signs or symptoms exhibited by EM
   is *not* characteristic of acute adrenal insufficiency? (EO-2)
   a. Hypotension
   b. Confusion
   c. Moon facies
   d. Hyperkalemia

2. Intravenous treatment with hydrocortisone may cause which
   of the following: (EO-10)
   a. Hyperglycemia
   b. Renal insufficiency
   c. Hyperkalemia
   d. Leukopenia

3. The minimum dose at which prednisone may cause HPA axis
   suppression if used for longer than 2–3 weeks is: (EO-3, 10)
   a. 5.0 mg/day
   b. 7.5 mg/day
   c. 10.0 mg/day
   d. 15.0 mg/day

4. EM exhibits several markers of chronic corticosteroid excess.
   Which of the following findings is *not* characteristic of this?
   (EO-10)
   a. Proximal muscle weakness
   b. Striae on abdomen
   c. Moon facies
   d. Mitral valve prolapse

5. The type of hyponatremia EM exhibits is called: (EO-5)
   a. Hypotonic
   b. Isotonic
   c. Hypertonic
   d. Hypervolemic

6. What are the consequences of replacing EM's sodium
   deficits too quickly? (EO-7, 8, 10)
   a. Congestive heart failure
   b. Osmotic brain injury
   c. Hypertension
   d. Renal failure

7. Which of the following would *not* be necessary to monitor
   during the tapering of EM's intravenous hydrocortisone
   regimen? (EO-5)
   a. Blood pressure
   b. Serum sodium
   c. Weight
   d. Serum glucose

8. At what point would hyperkalemia be treated in a patient
   such as EM? (EO-1, 8)
   a. Serum potassium remains elevated after 6 hours
   b. Serum potassium exceeds 6 mmol/L
   c. She complains of muscle cramping
   d. ECG changes occur

9. What analgesic *may* be a safe and effective option for EM if
   her anemia is due to gastritis from prednisone and ibuprofen
   use? (EO-11, 12)
   a. Acetaminophen
   b. Misoprostil
   c. Sulindac
   d. Celecoxib

10. EM does not need to be on progesterone replacement with
    her estrogen because: (EO-8)
    a. She is not at risk for uterine cancer

b. She is not experiencing hot flashes

c. Progesterone replacement negates the estrogen effect on bone

d. She is not experiencing irregular bleeding

11. If, after discharge, EM continues to complain of heartburn on famotidine 20 mg QHS and her tapering dose of prednisone, what should be done? (EO-11)

a. Test for *Helicobacter pylori*

b. Increase famotidine to 20 mg twice a day

c. Add lansoprazole 15 mg every day

d. Increase famotidine to 40 mg at bedtime

12. If EM had developed acute gastrointestinal bleeding during her first day of hospitalization, what complications could this cause and how would it be treated? (EO-1, 8)

13. What patient education should EM receive regarding her prednisone use? (EO-14)

14. List 10 long-term complications from using supraphysiologic doses of corticosteroids chronically. (EO-10)

15. Why or why not might alternate-day therapy with prednisone be an option for EM? (EO-1, 6, 8)

16. Summarize pathophysiologic, therapeutic, and disease management concepts for this case utilizing a key points format. (EO-18)

CASE 20
Debbie Scholtz
Topic: Cushing's Syndrome
Level 2
EDUCATIONAL MATERIALS
Chapter 16: Adrenocortical Dysfunction and Clinical
Use of Steroids

SCENARIO

Patient and Setting

RM, a 56-year-old male; hospital

Chief Complaint

Extreme weakness in arms and legs, headache, and increased thirst

History of Present Illness

States hasn't felt well for the previous 1–2 months; notes a 15-pound weight gain; had to quit working recently due to extreme fatigue and weakness; wife states his mood has been more irritable and depressed; progressively weaker in the past several days

Past Medical History

Tuberculosis diagnosed 5 months ago, hypertension × 15 years, depression × 2 years

Past Surgical History

Appendectomy 32 years prior

Family/Social History

Family History: Positive for prostate cancer and hypertension in father, positive for diabetes in mother

Social History: Positive tobacco history (1 pack per day × 40 years), history of alcohol abuse

Medication History

Isoniazid, 300 mg QD × 5 months

Rifampin, 600 mg QD × 5 months

Pyridoxine, 50 mg QD × 5 months

Nifedipine XL, 90 mg QD

Fosinopril, 10 mg QD

Imipramine, 75 mg QHS

Acetaminophen, 650 mg PRN headache

Allergies

Penicillin—rash

Physical Examination

GEN: Obese male appearing very anxious

VS: BP 140/104, HR 84, RR 20, T 36.9°C, Wt 94 kg

HEENT: Rounded face, ruddy skin color, no hemorrhages or exudates

CHEST: Normal breath sounds

COR: Normal S_1, S_2, $+S_4$

ABD: Protuberant abdomen, +striae, normal bowel sounds

EXT: Thin wasted appearance; bilateral proximal muscle weakness of arms and legs; unhealed bruise on left lower leg; 2+ pitting edema of lower extremities

SKIN: Hyperpigmented

Results of Pertinent Laboratory Tests, Serum Drug Concentrations, and Diagnostic Tests

Na 140 (140)	PO$_4$ 1.3 (4.0)	MCV 92 (92)
K 3.9 (3.9)	Mg 1.0 (2.0)	AST 0.58 (35)
Cl 100 (100)	Uric Acid 321 (5.4)	ALT 0.55 (33)
HCO$_3$ 22 (22)	Hct 0.36 (36)	LDH 1.8 (110)
BUN 6.4 (18)	Hgb 120 (12)	Alk Phos 1.7 (105)
Cr 106 (1.2)	Lkcs 8 × 10^9	Alb 36 (3.6)
Glu Fasting 10.8 (195)	(8 × 10^3)	T Bili 15.4 (0.9)
Ca 4.6 (9.2)	Plts 313 × 10^9	
	(313 × 10^3)	

Serum cortisol: 1048 nmol/L (38 μg/dL)

Serum ACTH: 0.8 pmol/L (3.3 pg/mL)

UA: 3+ glucose, no ketones, SG 1.022

Urine free cortisol (24 hr): 827 nmol/day (300 μg/24 hr)

ECG: WNL

PROBLEM LIST

Identify principal problems from the scenario in priority order

SOAP NOTE

To be completed by student

QUESTIONS

1. An additional test which may be used to establish hypercortisolism in a patient such as RM is the: (EO-5)
   a. High-dose dexamethasone suppression test
   b. Low-dose dexamethasone suppression test
   c. CRH stimulation test
   d. Magnetic resonance imaging (MRI)

2. Tests which help differentiate between adrenal and non-adrenal causes of Cushing's syndrome include all of the following *except:* (EO-5)
   a. Basal plasma ACTH
   b. Metyrapone test
   c. CRH stimulation test
   d. 24-hour urinary free cortisol test

3. Which of RM's current medications may interfere with the dexamethasone suppression test? (EO-9)
   a. Rifampin
   b. Imipramine
   c. Nifedipine
   d. Isoniazid

4. All of the following signs or symptoms exhibited by RM are indicative of Cushing's syndrome *except:* (EO-2)
   a. Weight gain
   b. Proximal muscle weakness
   c. Serum potassium of 3.9 mmol/L
   d. Fasting glucose of 10.8 mmol/L

5. A CT scan of RM's adrenal glands and further testing reveals an adrenal adenoma, and a unilateral adrenalectomy is scheduled. What medication should RM receive pre- and postoperatively? (EO-8, 12)
   a. Prednisone
   b. Ketoconazole
   c. Hydrocortisone
   d. Mitotane

6. Four days after his operation, RM develops acute nausea and vomiting, confusion, hyperkalemia, and hypoglycemia. What is the most likely cause of these symptoms? (EO-11, 12)
   a. Continuing hypercortisolism
   b. Acute adrenal insufficiency
   c. Wound infection
   d. Diabetic ketoacidosis

7. How should RM's acute nausea, vomiting, confusion, hyperkalemia, and hypoglycemia be managed? (EO-8)

   a. Increase the hydrocortisone dose
   b. Decrease the hydrocortisone dose
   c. Start antibiotic therapy
   d. Increase the insulin dose

8. If RM's surgery had to be delayed for several months, what purpose would adding ketoconazole serve in this situation? (EO-7)
   a. Provides prophylaxis for fungal infections
   b. Blocks glucocorticoid receptors
   c. Suppresses growth of adrenal tumors
   d. Blocks formation of pregnenolone and steroid precursors

9. What information should be provided to RM's physician regarding the use of ketoconazole in RM? (EO-7, 8, 9)
   a. Most patients respond to a dose of 200 mg every day
   b. Ketoconazole may decrease response to nifedipine
   c. Rifampin significantly lowers ketoconazole levels
   d. Renal function should be monitored closely while taking ketoconazole

10. If RM's hypertension remains uncontrolled despite a reduction in his hypercortisolism and fluid retention, what would be the most reasonable next step? (EO-11, 12)
    a. Increase nifedipine XL to 120 mg every day
    b. Increase fosinopril to 20 mg every day
    c. Increase furosemide to 80 mg every day
    d. Add atenolol 50 mg every day

11. Give three examples of alternative drug therapies to ketoconazole and describe their mechanisms of action and common side effects. (EO-7, 10)

12. Describe psychological complications RM may experience as a result of his Cushing's syndrome. (EO-15)

13. List ways a health care provider may address psychological problems RM may experience as a result of his Cushing's syndrome. (EO-16)

14. After RM's surgery, he is to be discharged on hydrocortisone and fludrocortisone. Why is fludrocortisone necessary? (EO-8)

15. What should RM be counseled on regarding the use of hydrocortisone and fludrocortisone? (EO-14)

16. Summarize pathophysiologic, therapeutic, and disease management concepts for this case utilizing a key points format. (EO-18)

CASE 21
Debbie Scholtz
Topic: Hyperlipidemia

Level 1

EDUCATIONAL MATERIALS
Chapter 20: Hyperlipidemia

SCENARIO

Patient and Setting

MG, a 53-year-old male; family medicine clinic

Chief Complaint

Patient reports an elevated cholesterol at a health fair screening 2 weeks ago

History of Present Illness

Told at health fair screening to notify his physician about his elevated cholesterol

Past Medical History

Type 2 diabetes mellitus for 5 years
Hypothyroidism for 20 years

Past Surgical History

None

Family/Social History

Family History: Father died of myocardial infarction at age 53; brother had a myocardial infarction at age 44

Social History: Works as a salesman; travels frequently; golfs on weekends; otherwise no exercise; follows a good diabetic diet; does not smoke; drinks 3–4 glasses of wine with evening meal and at frequent social occasions

Medications

Levothyroxine, 0.15 mg QD
Glyburide, 10 mg BID

Allergies

NKA

Physical Examination

GEN: Healthy appearing male in no apparent distress
VS: BP 138/88, HR 85 regular, RR 18, Wt 83 kg, Ht 180 cm
HEENT: Normal
COR: Normal
ABD: Positive bowel sounds
EXT: Skin normal with good turgor
NEURO: Tendon reflexes normal

Results of Pertinent Laboratory Tests, Serum Drug Concentrations, and Diagnostic Tests (fasting)

Total Cholesterol 6.03 (233)	LDLC 4.14 (160)	Glucose 7.5 (135)
	Triglycerides 2.3 (201)	HbA$_{1C}$ 7.0%
HDLC 0.83 (32)	TSH 4.2 mU/L (4.2 μU/mL)	UA normal, -glucose, -protein

PROBLEM LIST

Identify principal problems from the scenario in priority order [completed Problem List and SOAP Note at end of casebook]

SOAP NOTE

To be completed by student

QUESTIONS

[Answers at end of casebook]

1. How many risk factors for coronary heart disease does MG have? (EO-3)
   a. Two
   b. Three
   c. Four
   d. Five

2. Treatment of MG's hyperlipidemia may decrease the risk of all of the following events *except:* (EO-1, 3)
   a. Myocardial infarction
   b. Congestive heart failure
   c. Unstable angina
   d. Angioplasty

3. All of the following could be secondary causes of MG's hyperlipidemia *except:* (EO-5, 8)
   a. Elevated blood pressure
   b. Diabetes
   c. Hypothyroidism
   d. Excessive alcohol use

4. MG has a healthy 22-year-old son. How often should the son have his cholesterol level checked? (EO-3)
   a. Not until he is 45 years old
   b. Not until he has a risk factor for coronary heart disease
   c. Every year starting now
   d. Every 5 years starting now

5. All of the following may improve HDL cholesterol levels *except:* (EO-4, 12)
   a. Smoking cessation
   b. Exercise
   c. Moderate alcohol use
   d. High consumption of fish

6. For what reason would bile acid resins *not* be an ideal first choice for MG? (EO-8, 9)
   a. May interfere with absorption of levothyroxine
   b. May cause hyperglycemia
   c. May further decrease HDL cholesterol
   d. He is unlikely to be compliant with the regimen

7. Atorvastatin lowers LDL cholesterol by which primary mechanism? (EO-7)
   a. Decreases production of hepatic LDL cholesterol receptors
   b. Decreases cholesterol production and upregulates LDL receptors
   c. Decreases enterohepatic recycling of cholesterol
   d. Decreases production of VLDL particles

8. Which "statin" type drug would be unlikely to achieve MG's LDL goal of <2.6 (<100)? (EO-12)
   a. All statins should be effective
   b. Fluvastatin 40 mg every day
   c. Lovastatin 80 mg every day
   d. Simvastatin 40 mg every day

9. What advice should MG be given regarding his use of alcohol? (EO-4, 14)

10. What difficulties may MG encounter with the diet and drug treatment of his hyperlipidemia? (EO-15)

11. How might a health care provider address the problems MG may encounter with his treatment? (EO-16)

12. What pharmacoeconomic considerations are relevant to MG's plan of care? (EO-17)

13. Summarize pathophysiologic, therapeutic, and disease management concepts for this patient utilizing a key points format. (EO-18)

CASE 22
Debbie Scholtz
Topic: Hypothyroidism
Level 1

EDUCATIONAL MATERIALS
Chapter 17: Thyroid Disorders

SCENARIO

Patient and Setting

PJ, a 38-year-old woman; general medicine clinic

Chief Complaint

Reports increasing fatigue and concern about a "lump" in her throat

History of Present Illness

Has gained 5 kg over the past 6 months and has experienced decreased energy and ability to concentrate; frequently feels cold; menstrual periods have been unusually heavy and painful; constipated; describes the lump in throat as one that interferes with swallowing but does not experience any choking or respiratory difficulties; headaches ~3 times/month

Past Medical History

Iron deficiency anemia × 4 months

Family/Social History

Family History: Mother with Graves' disease, father with hypertension, grandmother with diabetes

Social History: No tobacco; drinks 2–3 glasses of wine daily

Medications

Ferrous sulfate, 325 mg TID (not taking due to stomach upset and constipation)

Ibuprofen, 200 mg, 2 tablets PRN menstrual cramps or headaches

Kelp tablets daily (from health food store)

Ethinyl estradiol and norgestrel daily

Allergies

NKA

Physical Examination

GEN: Lethargic female in no apparent distress
VS: BP 138/82, HR 78, RR 10, T 37.8°C, Wt 60 kg, Ht 157 cm
HEENT: Flaky dry scalp, pale mucous membranes and gums, diffusely enlarged goiter with no palpable nodules
COR: Normal, regular rate and rhythm
CHEST: Clear to auscultation
ABD: Soft, nontender
GU: WNL
RECT: WNL, guaiac negative
EXT: + pretibial myxedema, dry scaly skin, pale nailbeds
NEURO: Delayed deep tendon reflexes

Results of Pertinent Laboratory Tests, Serum Drug Concentrations, and Diagnostic Tests

Na 144 (144)	TT_4 84 (6.5)	Hgb 120 (12)
K 4.2 (4.2)	TSH 20	Lkcs 7.5 × 10⁹
Cl 100 (100)	MCV 78 (78)	(7.5 × 10³)
HCO₃ 30 (30)	MCHC 260 (26)	Plts 180 × 10⁹
BUN 5.4 (15)	Ferritin 9 (9)	(180 × 10³)
Cr 88 (1.0)	TIBC 75 (418)	FT_4I 4.5
Glu 5.4 (98)	Hct 0.30 (30)	Thyroid antibodies (+)
Chol 6.7 (258)		

ECG: WNL

PROBLEM LIST

Identify principal problems from the scenario in priority order [completed Problem List and SOAP Note at end of casebook]

SOAP NOTE

To be completed by student

QUESTIONS

[Answers at end of casebook]

1. All of the following signs or symptoms exhibited by PJ are characteristic of hypothyroidism *except:* (EO-2)
   a. Headaches
   b. Cold intolerance
   c. Fatigue
   d. Heavy menses

2. What effect does the use of Lo-Ovral in PJ have on the results of her thyroid function tests? (EO-5)
   a. Low-dose oral contraceptives are unlikely to affect her test results
   b. Estrogen may falsely increase TSH due to alterations in TSH secretion
   c. Estrogen may falsely decrease FT_4I due to alterations in TBG
   d. Estrogen may falsely elevate total T_4 levels due to alterations in TBG

3. Why should PJ discontinue the use of the kelp tablets? (EO-5, 9)
   a. Kelp tablets may be worsening her constipation
   b. Iodide in kelp causes an inability to escape the Wolff-Chaikoff block in this patient
   c. Kelp tablets may block the absorption of levothyroxine
   d. Iodide in kelp may cause a false elevation in TSH

4. Women are more likely to develop hypothyroidism than men. What other factor in PJ's case has increased her risk of developing hypothyroidism? (EO-3)
   a. Her age
   b. Her family history of thyroid disease
   c. Her use of oral contraceptives
   d. Her daily alcohol use

5. What is the most common cause of hypothyroidism in the United States? (EO-1, 3)
   a. Iatrogenic hypothyroidism
   b. Graves' disease
   c. Hashimoto's thyroiditis
   d. Postpartum thyroiditis

6. How should PJ's elevated cholesterol be addressed? (EO-8, 11)
   a. Start a Step 1 diet to lower cholesterol
   b. Start lipid-lowering therapy to lower cholesterol to <200 mg/dL
   c. Discontinue use of oral contraceptives, which may be adversely affecting her lipids
   d. Correct hypothyroidism first before implementing lipid-lowering treatment

7. PJ returns in 6 weeks for follow up. She has taken her levothyroxine faithfully but reports she still feels tired and cold frequently. Her difficulty swallowing has improved. Her TSH level drawn that day was 12. What would be the most reasonable action to take at this time? (EO-6, 11)
   a. Continue same dose of levothyroxine; not yet at steady state
   b. Increase levothyroxine to 0.112 mg every day
   c. Switch her to the branded levothyroxine product
   d. Increase levothyroxine to 0.15 mg every day

8. If PJ should become pregnant, how might her levothyroxine replacement be affected? (EO-4)
   a. She may require a 20 to 30% increase in dose
   b. She may require a 20 to 30% decrease in dose
   c. She will probably not require any changes in dose
   d. TT_4 levels should also be monitored because of changes in TBG

9. What other medication that PJ is taking may interfere with her levothyroxine therapy? (EO-9)
   a. Ethinyl estradiol and norgestrel
   b. Ibuprofen
   c. Ferrous sulfate
   d. There are no significant drug interactions present

10. Describe what patient education points should be covered regarding PJ's levothyroxine therapy. (EO-14)

11. List reasons why desiccated thyroid products are no longer recommended for thyroid replacement. (EO4, EO8)

12. Describe how the approach to thyroid replacement changes in patients with cardiac disease. (EO-8)

13. List pharmacoeconomic considerations relevant to PJ's plan of care. (EO-17)

14. Summarize pathophysiologic, therapeutic, and disease management concepts for this case utilizing a key points format. (EO-18)

CASE 23
Debbie Scholtz
Topic: Hyperthyroidism
 Level 3
EDUCATIONAL MATERIALS
Chapter 17: Thyroid Disorders

SCENARIO

Patient and Setting

JK, a 30-year-old female; hospital Family Practice service

Chief Complaint

Complains of generalized weakness, the "shakes," feelings of "burning up," palpitations, intermittent chest pains, shortness of breath, and swelling in feet

History of Present Illness

Symptoms have worsened lately; has been anxious, forgetful, and confused; has frequent diarrhea; numbness and tingling in feet and hands; no period in 4 months; has lost 7 kg over the past few months despite a "ravenous" appetite; feels that eyes are protruding and frequently has tearing, pain, double vision, and light sensitivity; takes propylthiouracil only once or twice a day because forgets to take it and thinks it causes diarrhea and an itchy rash all over; denies any joint pain or sore throat

Past Medical History

Diagnosed with Graves' disease 2 years ago, which was complicated by ophthalmopathy, pretibial myxedema, and pernicious anemia; was started on PTU 200 g q6h and vitamin B_{12} injections; nine months ago was hospitalized with thyroid storm secondary to nonadherence with therapy; symptoms were controlled and PTU and vitamin B_{12} injections were restarted; lost to follow-up until now; also treated for anxiety in the past

Past Surgical History

Tonsillectomy at 10 years of age

Family/Social History

Family History: Grandmother with Graves' disease and ophthalmopathy

Social History: Nonsmoker; drinks 2–4 beers intermittently when anxious; lives with boyfriend

Medication History

Propylthiouracil, 200 mg PO q6h (takes sporadically)
Vitamin B_{12}, 100 μg IM q month (none $\times$ 8 months)
Pseudoephedrine, 60 mg PRN nasal congestion
Diphenhydramine, 25 mg, 2 at bedtime PRN insomnia
Ethinyl estradiol and norethindrone, 1 tablet daily

Allergies

Cephalexin–rash

Physical Examination

GEN: Thin, tremulous, anxious, and restless female in apparent respiratory distress, intermittently stuporous

VS: BP 180/100, HR 130 irreg, RR 28, T 40.0°C, Wt 52 kg, Ht 170 cm

HEENT: Thin, fine hair with patches of baldness; bilateral proptosis R>L; (+) lid lag; (+) stare; (+) chemosis and conjunctivitis; (+) painful tongue; diffusely enlarged goiter 5 times normal size; (+) bruit in right thyroid lobe; (+) JVD

COR: Rapid irregular rhythm; (+) S_3 (+) S_4; displaced PMI

CHEST: Bilateral rales and crackles

ABD: Soft; (−) masses; (+) abdominal tenderness; hepatomegaly; hyperdynamic bowel sounds

GU: WNL

RECT: Guaiac negative

EXT: 2+ pitting edema bilaterally; (+) pretibial myxedema; hot flushed skin with fine,

maculopapular rash; (+) palmar erythema; nail onycholysis

NEURO: Rapid DTRs with mild clonus; decreased pinprick and vibratory sensation in lower legs; weakness of large muscle groups; (+) coarse tremor

Results of Pertinent Laboratory Tests, Serum Drug Concentrations, and Diagnostic Tests

Na 130 (130)	Plts 150 $\times$ 10^9 (150 $\times$ 10^3)	TT$_4$ 257 nmol/L (20 μg/dL)
K 3.2 (3.2)	MCV 120 (120)	TT$_3$ 12.7 nmol/L
Cl 90 (90)	AST 2.5 (150)	(830 ng/dL)
HCO$_3$ 26 (26)	ALT 2.42 (145)	FT$_4$I 121 mmol/L (9.4)
BUN 12.5 (35)	LDH 4.67 (280)	TSH <0.05 mU/L
Cr 133 (1.5)	Alk Phos 5.8 (350)	ATgA (+)
Hct 0.23 (23)	Alb 33 (3.3)	Vit B$_{12}$ 59 pmol/L (80
Hgb 80 (8)	T Bili 60 (3.5)	pg/mL)
Lkcs 14.3 $\times$ 10^9	Glu 6.7 (121)	
(14.3 $\times$ 10^3)	PT/INR 15.0/1.2	

Urinalysis: WNL

Chest radiograph: Cardiomegaly, pulmonary edema

ECG: HR 130–150, atrial fibrillation, (+) LVH

PROBLEM LIST

Identify principal problems from the scenario in priority order

SOAP NOTE

To be completed by student

QUESTIONS

1. All of the following signs or symptoms exhibited by JK are characteristic of Graves' disease *except:* (EO-2)
   a. Diarrhea
   b. Thinning hair
   c. Painful tongue
   d. Increased systolic pressure

2. Why should JK receive PTU instead of methimazole for treatment of thyroid storm? (EO-7, 8)
   a. Less expensive
   b. Available for intravenous use
   c. Better tolerated than methimazole
   d. Inhibits the peripheral conversion of T_4 to T_3

3. All of the following would be appropriate reasons to measure thyroid receptor antibodies (Trab) *except:* (EO-5)
   a. Pregnant woman with a history of Graves' disease
   b. Patient with classic signs of Graves' disease
   c. Patient with an atypical presentation and clinical euthyroidism
   d. Patient for which the potential for relapse or remission might be helpful to determine treatment

4. The most common cause of hyperthyroidism in the U.S. is: (EO-1)
   a. Toxic multinodular goiter
   b. Graves' disease
   c. Postpartum thyroiditis
   d. Drug-induced hyperthyroidism

5. What information should be provided to JK regarding the treatment of her ophthalmopathy? (EO-12)
   a. Optimal treatment for prevention of progression is still unknown
   b. It will resolve when she becomes euthyroid
   c. Only radioactive iodine therapy will reverse ophthalmopathy
   d. Only thyroidectomy will reverse ophthalmopathy

6. All of the following are reasons why hydrocortisone is ordered for JK *except:* (EO-7, 8)
   a. Helps reduce T_3 levels
   b. Helps relieve itchy rash from PTU
   c. Helps relieve symptoms of hyperthyroidism
   d. Treats underlying adrenal insufficiency if present

7. Because of JK's thyrotoxicosis-induced high-output congestive heart failure, she may require higher doses of: (EO-6)
   a. Propylthiouracil
   b. Hydrocortisone
   c. Vitamin B_{12}
   d. Digoxin

8. The mechanism of action for iodide therapy in this case is to: (EO-7)
   a. Enhance uptake of PTU into the thyroid gland
   b. Rapidly reduce release of thyroid hormone
   c. Decrease peripheral conversion of T_3 to T_4
   d. Prepare JK for future radioactive iodine therapy

9. Anticoagulation with warfarin could be affected by all of the following *except:* (EO-3, 4, 5)
   a. Elevated BUN and creatinine
   b. History of poor adherence
   c. History of alcohol use
   d. Current hepatomegaly and elevated liver enzymes

10. Diltiazem was used in place of propranolol in JK because: (EO-8, 10)
    a. Diltiazem has a quicker onset of action
    b. Propranolol may exacerbate her CHF
    c. Diltiazem is more effective in reducing symptoms
    d. Propranolol may worsen her anxiety

11. If JK were to undergo RAI in the future, which medication would need to be stopped several months before treatment? (EO-8, 12)
    a. Propylthiouracil
    b. Diltiazem
    c. Prednisone
    d. Iodides (Lugol's solution)

12. If JK should become pregnant before she receives RAI, how should she be managed? (EO-3, 8)

13. List the most common or serious adverse effects from thioamide therapy. (EO-10)

14. List advantages of methimazole therapy over PTU. (EO-8)

15. What psychosocial factors may interfere with JK's ability to adhere to the treatment plan? (EO-15)

16. How can health care providers address psychosocial factors that may affect JK's adherence? (EO-16)

17. Summarize pathophysiologic, therapeutic, and disease management concepts for this case utilizing a key points format. (EO-18)

CASE 24
Debbie Scholtz
Topic: Diabetes with End-Stage Renal Disease

EDUCATIONAL MATERIALS
Chapter 19: Diabetes; Chapter 23: Dialytic and Pharmacotherapy for End-Stage Renal Disease

SCENARIO

Patient and Setting
KJ, a 29-year-old male; diabetes clinic

Chief Complaint
Decreased energy, feeling more tired, and occasionally short of breath

History of Present Illness
In the past few months tires more easily; on several occasions felt short of breath with exertion; complains of impotence; reports no change in mood; follows a diabetic diet; checks blood glucose four times a day

Past Medical History
DM Type 1 × 15 years, Graves' disease treated 10 years ago with thyroidectomy, hypothyroidism × 8 years, end-stage renal disease (ESRD) on hemodialysis 3 ×/week

Past Surgical History
Thyroidectomy 10 years ago

Family/Social History
Family History: Noncontributory

Social History: Nonsmoker, nondrinker; following low-protein diabetic diet

Medications
Human insulin, 20 U NPH/8 U R q AM, 12 U NPH/5 U R q PM

Levothyroxine, 0.15 mg every day

B-complex vitamins every day

Vitamin C, 500 mg BID

Calcium carbonate, 500 mg TID

1,25-Dihydroxy vitamin D, 0.25 μg every day

Folic acid, 1 mg every day

Ferrous sulfate, 325 mg every day

Ranitidine, 75 mg PRN heartburn

Allergies

Codeine–rash

Physical Examination

GEN: Well-developed male in no apparent distress
VS: BP 124/84, HR 84, RR 12, T 37.9°C, Wt 75 kg, Ht 178 cm
HEENT: PERRLA, EOM intact
COR: NSR
CHEST: Without rales or rhonchi
ABD: No organomegaly
GU: Normal
RECT: Guaiac negative
EXT: AV fistula–left arm
NEURO: Within normal limits

Results of Pertinent Laboratory Tests, Serum Drug Concentrations, and Diagnostic Tests

Na 138 (138)
K 3.9 (3.9)
Cl 103 (103)
HCO_3 28 (28)
BUN 14 (39) stable
Cr 318 (3.6) stable
Glucose 7.5 (135)

Ca 2.24 (9.0)
PO_4 1.38 (4.3)
Alb 38 (3.8)
HbA_{1C} 9.2%
Hct 0.28 (28)
Hgb 90 (9)
Lkcs 5.7 × 10⁹ (5.7 × 10³)

Plts 238 × 10⁹ (238 × 10³)
MCV 88 (88)
Serum Fe 13.4 (75)
Ferritin 160 (160)
TIBC 300 (300)
Transferrin Saturation 25%
Mg 1.0 (2.0)

TSH <0.4 μU/L

UA: (−)glucose, (−)ketone, (+) protein

Results of home blood glucose monitoring (averages)

AM: 6.4 (115)

Noon: 6.7 (120)

5 PM: 10.8 (195)

11 PM: 6.6 (118)

PROBLEM LIST

Identify principal problems from the scenario in priority order [completed Problem List and SOAP Note at end of casebook]

SOAP NOTE

To be completed by student

QUESTIONS

[Answers at end of casebook]

1. KJ needs to take folic acid and B vitamins to: (EO-7)
   a. Improve his energy
   b. Replace lost nutrients from hemodialysis
   c. Treat his anemia
   d. Supplement his insufficient diabetic diet

2. Another approach to decreasing KJ's 5-PM hyperglycemia would be to: (EO-12)
   a. Increase his morning regular insulin dose
   b. Decrease his caloric intake at dinner
   c. Decrease his caloric intake at breakfast
   d. Decrease his caloric intake at lunch

3. All of the following vaccinations should be considered for KJ *except:* (EO-8, 11)
   a. Varicella
   b. Influenza
   c. Pneumococcus
   d. Hepatitis B

4. KJ's HbA_{1C} of 9.2% roughly correlates to an average blood glucose of: (EO-5)
   a. 8.3 (150)
   b. 11.6 (210)
   c. 10.0 (180)
   d. 13.3 (240)

5. Another test which may be used to monitor KJ's glycemic control and response to therapy would be the: (EO-5)
   a. Urine microalbumin
   b. Urine glucose
   c. Serum fructosamine
   d. Serum aldose reductase

6. All of the following statements about mixing NPH and regular insulins are true *except:* (EO-6)
   a. The injection must be taken within 10 minutes of mixing
   b. Regular insulin is drawn up before the NPH dose
   c. Mixtures of NPH and regular insulin are stable in any ratio
   d. Mixing insulins allows greater flexibility versus 70/30 insulin

7. KJ is most likely receiving calcium carbonate for the purpose of: (EO-5, 7, 8)
   a. Treating heartburn
   b. Preventing osteoporosis
   c. Binding phosphate in the GI tract
   d. Improving absorption of ferrous sulfate

8. In patients with Type 1 DM with an irregular lifestyle in terms of erratic meal and work/school schedules, what approach may work best with their insulin regimen? (EO-8, 12)
   a. Long-acting insulin once a day
   b. Advising the patient to make the daily routine more consistent

c. Mixed insulin (NPH/regular) before each meal

d. Quick-acting insulin before meals with long-acting insulin once or twice a day

9. Why should patients on insulin be advised to rotate their sites for insulin injection? (EO-10)

a. This recommendation is no longer necessary with the use of human insulin

b. Reduces the risk of infection

c. Reduces the risk of lipoatrophy

d. Reduces the risk of lipohypertrophy

10. Explain how glucagon works and how it should be administered. (EO-7)

11. Give an example of a sliding scale insulin regimen and how it might be used for KJ. (EO-12)

12. What should KJ be counselled about regarding his oral medications? (EO-14)

13. Describe how KJ's medical conditions may affect his psychological health. (EO-15)

14. Summarize pathophysiologic, therapeutic, and disease management concepts for this case utilizing a key points format. (EO-18)

CASE 25
Debbie Scholtz
Topic: Hyperparathyroidism

EDUCATIONAL MATERIALS
Chapter 18: Parathyroid Disorders

SCENARIO

Patient and Setting

EE, a 46-year-old commercial fisherman; hospital medicine service

Chief Complaint

Dehydration secondary to sun exposure, nausea and vomiting; increased confusion and memory loss

History of Present Illness

Diagnosed with primary hyperparathyroidism 10 years ago and refused surgery; serum calcium ranged 2.62–2.82 mmol/L (10.5–11.3 mg/dL) and an intact PTH level ranged 60–70; has passed 2 kidney stones in the past few years; recently has felt dizzy, fatigued, thirsty; frequent urination without burning or pain; constipated with bowel movements every 4–5 days; Senokot has helped some; bones and joints have been aching more; unable to work recently; increasingly concerned about forgetfulness, especially about taking his medications

Past Medical History

Primary hyperparathyroidism × 10 years, hypertension × 4 years, hyperlipidemia × 2 years

Past Surgical History

None

Family/Social History

Family History: Uncle with Type 1 DM; father with HTN, gout, and angioplasty at age 52

Social History: Divorced, smokes 2 PPD × 25 years, drinks alcohol with binges on weekends

Medications

Hydrochlorothiazide 50 mg/triamterene 75 mg every day

Verapamil, 80 mg TID

Gemfibrozil, 600 mg BID

Senna, 2 BID–TID for previous 3 weeks

Aluminum sodium carbonate PRN abdominal pain

Allergies

NKA

Physical Examination

GEN: Ill-appearing male in moderate distress

VS: BP 170/100, HR 96 (sitting); BP 130/60, HR 120 (standing); RR 22, T 37.0°C, Wt 85 kg, Ht 183 cm

HEENT: PERRLA, (+) arteriolar narrowing, dry and pale mucous membranes and gums

COR: Normal S_1 and S_2, sinus tachycardia

CHEST: Clear to auscultation and percussion

ABD: Positive bowel sounds; lower quadrant tenderness

GU: WNL

RECT: Guaiac negative; (+) impacted stool

EXT: (+) bone tenderness; poor skin turgor

NEURO: 3+ DTRs; (+) ataxia; unable to do "serial 7's"

Results of Pertinent Laboratory Tests, Serum Drug Concentrations, and Diagnostic Tests

Na 150 (150)	PO₄ 0.58 (1.8)	Plts 300 × 10⁹
K 3.6 (3.6)	Uric Acid 714 (12)	(300 × 10³)
Cl 110 (110)	TG 3.6 (316)	MCV 100 (100)
HCO₃ 19 (19)	LDL 3.8 (146)	AST 1.08 (65)
BUN 23.2 (65)	Hct 0.43 (43)	ALT 0.92 (55)
Cr 221 (2.5)	Hgb 160 (16)	Alk Phos 3.3 (200)
Glu 20.3 (365)	Lkcs 13 × 10⁹	Alb 3.6 (3.6)
Ca 3.99 (16)	(13 × 10³)	Chol 6.3 (245)
		HDL 0.93 (36)

PTH: 95 pg/mL

Lkcs differential: No left shift

UA: SG 1.002, (+) glucose, (−)ketones, (−)protein, (−) nitrates, 0–2 RBC

Ultrasound of neck: (+) parathyroid mass

ECG: Sinus rate 120, shortened QT interval

PROBLEM LIST

Identify principal problems from the scenario in priority order [completed Problem List and SOAP Note at end of casebook]

SOAP NOTE

To be completed by student

QUESTIONS

[Answers at end of casebook]

1. All of the following signs or symptoms exhibited by EE are characteristic of hyperparathyroidism *except:* (EO-2)
   a. Memory loss
   b. Hypophosphatemia
   c. Polyuria
   d. Hyperuricemia

2. The etiology of EE's hyperparathyroidism is most likely: (EO-1)
   a. Hyperplastic parathyroid gland
   b. Parathyroid adenoma
   c. Multiple endocrine neoplasia syndrome
   d. Drug-induced

3. Ionized calcium levels should be drawn in patients with: (EO-5)
   a. Concurrent lithium use
   b. Low serum albumin
   c. Low serum potassium
   d. High serum creatinine

4. Hydrochlorothiazide was discontinued in EE primarily because thiazide diuretics: (EO-9, 11)
   a. Lose effectiveness with decreased renal function
   b. Cause an increase in calcium excretion
   c. Cause a decrease in calcium excretion
   d. Frequently cause hypokalemia

5. All of the following are advantages of using pamidronate instead of etidronate *except:* (EO-8, 12)
   a. Can often be given orally
   b. Is less likely to affect bone mineralization
   c. Reduces serum calcium to a greater extent
   d. Is less expensive

6. Calcitonin is advantageous over other calcium-lowering therapies because it: (EO-8, 12)
   a. Lowers calcium to the greatest extent
   b. Is less expensive
   c. Has a longer duration of action
   d. Has the most rapid onset of action

7. Parathyroid surgery is indicated at this time for EE for all of the following reasons *except:* (EO-3, 12)
   a. He is <50 years old
   b. His hypertension may be exacerbated by hypercalcemia
   c. He is likely to progress to malignancy
   d. He has renal involvement

8. Both benazepril and verapamil may effectively lower EE's blood pressure. What additional advantage may the ACE inhibitor provide? (EO-8)
   a. Available in once-daily dosing regimens
   b. More data to support their use for delaying nephropathy
   c. Less expensive than verapamil
   d. Better tolerated than verapamil

9. Why was glipizide a more appropriate choice than glyburide to treat EE's diabetes? (EO-8)
   a. Less likely to cause hypoglycemia with renal impairment
   b. Longer duration of action
   c. Less expensive
   d. Less potential for drug interactions

10. EE returns in 2 months for review of his fasting lipid panel and diabetes. His blood sugars have been controlled on glipizide 10 mg XL every day. His labs reveal the following:

    Glucose 7.8 (141)

    Cholesterol 6.0 (231)

    Triglycerides 2.7 (240)

    HDL 1.0 (39)

    LDL 3.7 (144)

    What would be the most appropriate action at this time? (EO-11, 12)
    a. Change to pravastatin 20 mg every evening
    b. Continue gemfibrozil 600 mg twice a day
    c. Increase gemfibrozil to 1200 mg twice a day
    d. Add cholestyramine 5 g three times a day

11. Describe how EE's serum calcium levels should be managed postsurgery. (EO-8, 12)

12. List the ways in which PTH prevents hypocalcemia. (EO-1)

13. Describe the mechanism of action for plicamycin and when it would be used. (EO-7)

14. Describe the pharmacoeconomic considerations of the agents used to treat hypercalcemia. (EO-17)

15. Summarize pathophysiologic, therapeutic, and disease management concepts for this case utilizing a key points format. (EO-18)

CASE 26
Joanna Q. Hudson
Topic: Acute Renal Failure

EDUCATIONAL MATERIALS
Chapter 21: Acute Renal Disease (definition, pathophysiology, prerenal azotemia, ARF from therapeutic agents, clinical evaluation of renal function in ARF)

SCENARIO

Patient and Setting

CL, a 37-year-old African-American female; Emergency Department

Chief Complaint

"Lately I've been nauseous and vomiting and I can't seem to keep anything down. I also have had a fever and chills and sometimes feel very dizzy when I stand up."

History of Present Illness

5-day history of nausea, vomiting, fever, and chills; began taking ibuprofen for generalized aches 3 days ago; recent blood sugar readings unavailable–normally checks blood glucose once weekly but reports running out of test strips

Past Medical History

Diabetes mellitus (DM), Type 1 × 21 years
One previous episode of diabetic ketoacidosis 4 months ago
Peripheral neuropathy

Past Surgical History

No prior surgery

Family/Social History

Family History: Father–Hypertension (HTN) and died of acute MI age 65
Social History: Social use of alcohol, nonsmoker; lives with older sister, works as a sales clerk in department store

Medication History

Insulin NPH, 20 units q AM and 40 units q PM
Ibuprofen, 400 mg PO q6h (for past 3 days)
Amitriptyline, 150 mg PO QHS

Allergies

NKDA

Physical Examination

GEN: Thin, ill-appearing, lethargic female in acute distress
VS: BP 103/56 (sitting), HR 125, RR 18, Wt 50 kg, Ht 152 cm, T 39.5°C
HEENT: PERRLA
COR: Tachycardic, otherwise WNL
CHEST: Clear to auscultation and percussion
ABD: Soft and nontender
GU: WNL
RECT: Guaiac negative
EXT: Dry mucous membranes, dry skin
NEURO: A & O × 3, cranial nerves intact

Results of Pertinent Laboratory Tests, Serum Drug Concentrations, and Diagnostic Tests

Na 138 (138)	Cr 212 (2.4)	Glu 8.9 (160)
K 4.1 (4.1)	Hct 0.47 (47)	HbA_{1C} 0.082 (8.2)
Cl 105 (105)	Hgb 150 (15)	WBC 15,000
HCO_3 22 (22)	Plts 150 × 10⁹	
BUN 17.5 (49)	(150 × 10³)	

Urinalysis & Urine Chemistries: 1+ proteinuria, glucose (−), pH 6.8, SG 1.035, WBC (−), RBC (−), no bacteria or casts, Na 10 (10), FE_{Na} 0.6% osmolality 480 mmol/kg, volume 350 mL in 24 hr

PROBLEM LIST

Identify principal problems from the scenario in priority order [completed Problem List and SOAP Note at end of casebook]

SOAP NOTE

To be completed by student

QUESTIONS

[Answers at end of casebook]

1. Objective data supporting the development of acute renal failure in CL include all of the following *except:* (EO-5)

a. Serum creatinine
b. Serum BUN
c. Hematocrit
d. Urine Output

2. Which of the following would be consistent with acute renal failure in CL if her renal function further deteriorates despite fluid replacement? (EO-2, 5)
   a. Prolonged fever
   b. Hyponatremia
   c. Hypokalemia
   d. Fluid overload

3. All of the following are potential contributors to CL's acute decline in renal function *except:* (EO-1, 9)
   a. Decreased fluid intake
   b. Vomiting
   c. Fever
   d. Ibuprofen use

4. A complication of acute renal failure frequently observed is: (EO-1)
   a. Hypercalcemia
   b. Dehydration
   c. Hyperkalemia
   d. Metabolic alkalosis

5. Based on CL's urine output, her ARF would be classified as: (EO-2, 5)
   a. Anuric
   b. Oliguric
   c. Nonoliguric
   d. Excessive

6. All of the following are used to differentiate between prerenal and intrinsic causes of acute renal failure *except:* (EO-5)
   a. Urine pH
   b. Fractional excretion of sodium (FE_{Na})
   c. Urine Sodium
   d. Urine Osmolality

7. Which of the following agents may further precipitate acute renal failure in CL? (EO-9)
   a. Furosemide
   b. Acetaminophen
   c. Amitriptyline
   d. Insulin

8. During states of renal hypoperfusion the kidney compensates to increase intraglomerular pressure through vasoconstriction of which of the following: (EO-1)
   a. Renal artery
   b. Glomerulus
   c. Afferent arteriole
   d. Efferent arteriole

9. The best initial treatment strategy for CL is to: (EO-12)
   a. Send her home with oral antibiotics
   b. Increase the NPH insulin dose
   c. Provide IV fluid replacement
   d. Administer pressor agents to increase blood pressure

10. Identify three factors that put CL at high risk of developing acute renal failure and describe the basis of each. (EO-1, 3)

11. Describe the mechanisms of action of each of the pharmacologic and nonpharmacologic interventions in this case. (EO-7)

12. Develop a detailed educational plan for the patient including necessary lifestyle changes, medication counseling information, specific counseling (communication) techniques, and adherence strategies. (EO-14)

13. What psychosocial factors may affect CL's adherence to both pharmacologic and nonpharmacologic therapy? (EO-15)

14. Identify goals of treatment for CL. (EO-12, 13)

15. Evaluate the pharmacoeconomic considerations relative to CL's plan of care. (EO-17)

16. Summarize pathophysiologic, therapeutic, and disease management concepts for acute renal failure from prerenal causes utilizing a key points format. (EO-18)

CASE 27
Joanna Q. Hudson
Topic: Acute Renal Failure
Level 2
EDUCATIONAL MATERIALS
Chapter 21: Acute Renal Disease (pathophysiology of acute renal failure, ARF from therapeutic agents, clinical evaluation of renal function in ARF, pharmacological agents, indications for initiating RRT, drug-dosing issues)

SCENARIO

Patient and Setting
JW, a 47-year-old white male; emergency department

Chief Complaint
Nausea/vomiting and dizziness over the past 2 days

History of Present Illness
2-day history of nausea, vomiting, and dizziness following discharge from hospital for prosthetic mitral valve replacement for valvular endocarditis. Symptoms worse with procainamide use (reports taking two 1-g tablets every 6 hours).

Past Medical History
Rheumatic heart disease (RHD) at age 2

Partial complex seizures after possible embolic event in 1988 (well-controlled with phenytoin)

Prosthetic mitral valve replaced 2 weeks ago for valvular endocarditis (*Staphylococcus epidermidis*—received a 2-week course of gentamicin & vancomycin during hospital admission)

Atrial fibrillation (developed during admission for mitral valve replacement–prescribed procainamide)

Past Surgical History

Mitral valve placement–1989

Mitral valve replacement (MVR)–2 weeks ago

Family/Social History

Family History: Father–Type 2 Diabetes Mellitus

Social History: Tobacco–30 pack-year history; alcohol–occasional use; lives with spouse; works as a plant manager in textile mill

Medication History

Procainamide SR, 1 g PO q6h

Rifampin, 300 mg PO BID

Warfarin, 5 mg PO QD

Phenytoin, 300 mg PO BID (increased on last admission from 300 mg QHS)

Vancomycin, 750 mg IV q12h (home IV therapy)

Allergies

Penicillin (rash)

Physical Examination

GEN: Well-developed, well-nourished male in acute distress

VS: BP 120/74 (sitting), 128/70 (standing); HR 74 (sitting), 70 (standing); RR 20; T 36.9°C, Wt 70 kg (68 kg on last admission), Ht 178 cm

HEENT: Nystagmus

COR: JV pulse 8 cm, quick S_1, normal S_2, 2/6 systolic ejection murmur, 2/6 early diastolic murmur

CHEST: Clear to auscultation and percussion

ABD: WNL

GU: WNL

RECT: WNL

EXT: WNL

NEURO: Ataxia

Abdominal sonography: No urinary obstruction

Results of Pertinent Laboratory Tests, Serum Drug Concentrations, and Diagnostic Tests

Na 132 (132)	Hgb 104 g/L (10.4)	Alb 28 (2.8)
K 3.5 (3.5)	Lkcs 6.7 × 10⁹	T Bili 10.3 (0.6)
Cl 98 (98)	(6.7 × 10³)	Ca 2.2 (8.9)
HCO₃ 26 (26)	Plts 390 × 10⁹	PO₄ 1.4 (4.5)
BUN 8.8 (24)	(390 × 10³)	Mg 0.62 (1.5)
Cr 283 (3.2)	ALT 0.28 (17)	
Hct 0.31 (31.1)	Alk Phos 2.6 (154)	

Urine electrolytes: Cl 86 (86), Cr 40 mg/dL, Na 74 (74), K 33 (33), osmolality 335 (mmol/kg), SG 1.010

Urine output: 1500 mL/24 hr (24-hr urine collection)

Antinuclear antibodies (ANA): < 40 (titer)

Sedimentation rate: 62 (mm/hr)

Phenytoin: 103.1 μmol/L (26)

Procainamide: 113 μmol/L (26.6)

N-Acetyl procainamide: 60.6 μmol/L (16.8)

Chest radiography: Mild increase in heart size, no signs of CHF

ECG: First-degree AV block

Last vancomycin concentrations: Peak 35 mg/L, trough 9 mg/L (assessed 3 days ago prior to hospital discharge)

PROBLEM LIST

Identify principal problem(s) from the scenario in priority order

SOAP NOTE

To be completed by student

QUESTIONS

1. Which of the following is least likely to be associated with development of acute renal failure in JW? (EO-1)
   a. Recent surgery
   b. Aminoglycoside therapy
   c. Volume depletion from vomiting
   d. Increase in phenytoin dose

2. Characteristic features of aminoglycoside (AG)-induced renal failure include an increase in SCr_____ after the start of therapy with _____. (EO-10, 12)
   a. 5–7 days; normal electrolytes
   b. 5–7 days; hypomagnesemia & hypokalemia
   c. Immediately, normal electrolytes
   d. Immediately, hypomagnesemia & hypokalemia

3. JW's renal failure is most likely classified as: (EO-1, 5)
   a. Prerenal, nonoliguric
   b. Prerenal, oliguric
   c. Intrinsic, nonoliguric
   d. Intrinsic, oliguric

4. Calculate JW's creatinine clearance using the 24-hour urine data along with serum data. (EO-5, 6)

5. A decrease in which of the following is most likely to occur in the presence of renal impairment to account for the increase in total phenytoin concentration observed in JW: (EO-5, 6)
   a. Hepatic metabolism
   b. Protein binding
   c. Volume of distribution
   d. Renal elimination

6. All of the following should be avoided in JW due to their nephrotoxic potential *except:* (EO-10)
   a. Ranitidine
   b. Radiocontrast media
   c. Captopril
   d. Ibuprofen

7. Identify the abnormal findings from the urine data that support the classification of JW's acute renal failure and provide an interpretation for each finding. (EO-5)

8. Identify risk factors for the development of nephrotoxicity from aminoglycoside use. Indicate those specific to JW. (EO-3, 4)

9. The best strategy for management of JW's acute renal failure is to: (EO-11, 12)
   a. Monitor renal function for signs of reversal
   b. Discontinue vancomycin due to potential nephrotoxicity
   c. Administer furosemide to increase urine flow rate
   d. Administer renal dose dopamine to increase GFR

10. All of the following are correct regarding acute renal failure *except:* (EO-1, 3)
    a. Prerenal causes are the most common etiologies
    b. ARF is commonly a hospital-acquired illness
    c. Mortality rates are lower with intrinsic vs. prerenal causes
    d. ARF may persist for days to weeks

11. JW is most likely in which phase of acute renal failure? (EO-1, EO-2)
    a. Initiation of injury
    b. Maintenance
    c. Diuretic
    d. Recovery

12. Describe the mechanism of action of furosemide, mannitol, and dopamine when used in the treatment of acute renal failure. (EO-7)

13. Which of the following conditions is an indication for initiation of dialysis therapy in a patient with renal insufficiency? (EO-8)
    a. Metabolic alkalosis
    b. Hyperphosphatemia
    c. Oliguria
    d. Hyperkalemia

14. What psychosocial factors may influence JM's disease state management? (EO-15)

15. Identify pharmacoeconomic considerations related to JM's case. (EO-17)

16. Summarize pathophysiologic, therapeutic, and disease management concepts for acute renal failure from nephrotoxic agents utilizing a key points format. (EO-18)

CASE 28
Joanna Q. Hudson
Topic: Chronic Renal Failure

EDUCATIONAL MATERIALS

Chapter 22: Chronic Renal Disease (treatment goals, pathogenesis and mechanisms of CRD progression, metabolic and systemic consequences of CRD, therapeutic plan, pharmacotherapeutic management of CRD, pharmacokinetic considerations and drug-dosing)

SCENARIO

Patient and Setting

HP, a 58-year-old widowed female; diabetes clinic

Chief Complaint

Episodes of restlessness and anxiety over the last week; weight has increased by approximately 2 kg (5 lb) since last appointment

History of Present Illness

Scheduled for outpatient follow-up every 3 months; has missed the last 2 regular appointments; last evaluation 9 months ago (fasting blood glucose 150 mg/dL, Cr 1.8 mg/dL, BP 138/82, UA 100 mg protein in 24 hours)—glipizide dose was increased from 35 mg/day to 40 mg/day; reports blood sugars at home 130–180 mg/dL; medication adherence verified by daughter

Past Medical History

Type 2 diabetes mellitus × 10 years; migraine headaches – 1 episode every 2–3 months (last episode 6 months ago)

Past Surgical History

Hysterectomy 5 years ago

Family/Social History

Family History: Mother–Type 2 DM; father–died age 53 of MI

Social History: Smoker–25 pack-year history; no alcohol use

Medication History

Glipizide, 20 mg PO BID (2 years, current dose × 9 months)

Sumatriptan, 1 injection SC PRN migraine

Conjugated estrogens, 0.625 mg PO QD (5 years)

Allergies

Sulfa, unknown reaction

Physical Examination

GEN: Well-developed, well-nourished female in no acute distress

VS: BP 148/84 (sitting), HR 92, RR 15, T 37.1°C, Wt 70.3 kg (68 kg at last visit), Ht 163 cm

HEENT: Retinal edema, punctate hemorrhages

COR: WNL

CHEST: WNL

ABD: WNL

GU: WNL

RECT: WNL

EXT: WNL

NEURO: WNL

Results of Pertinent Laboratory Tests, Serum Drug Concentrations, and Diagnostic Tests

Na 143 (143)   Hct 0.38 (38)   Alb 29 (2.9)
K 4.7 (4.7)   Hgb 127 (12.7)   T Bili 13.7 (0.8)
Cl 102 (102)   Plts 230 × 10⁹   Ca 2.1 (8.3)
HCO₃ 23 (23)   (230 × 10³)   PO₄ 1.6 (5.0)
BUN 14 (38)   ALT 0.47 (28)   Mg 1.0 (2.5)
Cr 176 (2.0)   Alk Phos 1.9 (112)   HbA₁C 0.084 (8.4)
Glu 10 (180)

UA: Protein 260 mg in 24 hrs, (1+) glucose

PROBLEM LIST

Identify principal problem(s) from the scenario in priority order [completed Problem List and SOAP Note at end of casebook]

SOAP NOTE

To be completed by student

QUESTIONS

[Answers at end of casebook]

1. Which of the following is the most appropriate assessment of HP's current condition? (EO-1)
   a. Acute renal failure secondary to diabetes mellitus
   b. Acute renal failure secondary to proteinuria
   c. Chronic renal insufficiency secondary to diabetes mellitus
   d. Chronic renal insufficiency secondary to proteinuria

2. The best option to improve glycemic control in HP is to: (EO-12)
   a. Increase the glipizide dose
   b. Continue glipizide and add NPH insulin
   c. Switch from glipizide to metformin
   d. Switch from glipizide to chlorpropamide

3. All of the following can be used to monitor the progression of renal disease *except:* (EO-5)
   a. Calculation of 1/serum creatinine
   b. Serum creatinine
   c. Urine protein
   d. Urine glucose

4. The agent most clearly indicated for HP to slow/delay the progression of renal insufficiency is: (EO-8, 12)
   a. Furosemide
   b. Enalapril
   c. Nifedipine
   d. Labetalol

5. Calculate HP's estimated creatinine clearance using the Cockroft-Gault method; comment on the degree of renal impairment. (EO-2, 5)

6. Without intervention, HP will likely develop end-stage renal disease (GFR ≤ 10) in approximately: (EO-6)
   a. <5 years
   b. 5–<10 years
   c. 10–<15 years
   d. 15–<20 years

7. HP is at greatest risk of developing which of the following complications as renal function declines: (EO-1)
   a. Metabolic alkalosis
   b. Hypokalemia
   c. Hypotension
   d. Anemia

8. Which of the following calcium (Ca) and phosphorus (P) profiles is most likely to be observed in HP as chronic renal disease progresses (assume no treatment intervention)? (EO-5)
   a. Ca 7.8 mg/dL, P 1.5 mg/dL
   b. Ca 7.8 mg/dL, P 7.2 mg/dL
   c. Ca 11.5 mg/dL, P 1.5 mg/dL
   d. Ca 11.5 mg/dL, P 7.2 mg/dL

9. Describe the mechanisms of action of the pharmacologic and nonpharmacologic interventions selected for HP. (EO-7)

10. If HP requires additional pharmacological treatment for migraine headaches, which of the following agents would be the best choice given the concomitant factors present? (EO-4, 6)
    a. Codeine
    b. Morphine
    c. Acetaminophen
    d. Meperidine

11. Patients receiving insulin therapy generally require which of the following interventions with progression to end-stage renal disease: (EO-4, 6)
    a. Decrease in total insulin dose
    b. Increase in total insulin dose
    c. Increase in frequency of insulin administration
    d. No change in insulin regimen

12. Discuss psychosocial factors that may affect patient adherence in this case with both pharmacologic and nonpharmacologic therapy. (EO-15)

13. Describe the health care provider's role with consideration of these psychosocial factors. (EO-16)

14. Identify pharmacoeconomic issues to consider in HP. (EO-17)

15. Summarize therapeutic, pathophysiologic, and disease management concepts for progression of chronic renal disease in the diabetic population using a key points format. (EO-18)

CASE 29
Joanna Q. Hudson
Topic: Chronic Renal Failure
Level 3
EDUCATIONAL MATERIALS
Chapter 22: Chronic Renal Disease (epidemiology; hypertension; metabolic and systemic consequences of CRD; pharmacotherapeutic management of CRD; cardiovascular disease: antihypertensives; pharmacokinetic considerations and drug-dosing; nonpharmacologic therapy)

SCENARIO

Patient and Setting
HJ, a 67-year-old African-American male; clinic

Chief Complaint
Chronic fatigue and weakness, unchanged from his last visit 1 month ago; occasional nausea/vomiting, decreased appetite, and "funny" heart beat

History of Present Illness
Nausea/vomiting started 2 weeks ago, antacids (magnesium hydroxide/aluminum hydroxide) used without relief; denies shortness of breath, edema, or weight gain; reports compliance with medication and diet regimen

Past Medical History
Chronic renal insufficiency × 2 years secondary to analgesic abuse for chronic pain — baseline Cr (3.3–3.5); congestive heart failure (CHF) × 5 years — New York Heart Association Class II; hypertension (HTN) × 20 years

Past Surgical History
No prior surgery

Family/Social History
Family History: Father HTN (died age 72)

Social History: Smokes 1 cigar per week, no alcohol intake

Medication History
Digoxin, 0.25 mg PO QD

Lisinopril, 30 mg PO QD

Triamterene/HCTZ, 37.5/25 mg 1 PO QD

Acetaminophen, 650 mg PO q4h PRN pain

Allergies
No known medication allergies

Physical Examination
GEN: Well-developed, well-nourished male in no acute distress
VS: BP 135/80, HR 54, RR 20, T 37.1°C, Wt 73 kg, Ht 173 cm
HEENT: Pale mucous membranes and skin
COR: Normal S1 and S2, early S3
CHEST: Few rales and dullness over bases of lungs
ABD: WNL
GU: No flank pain
RECT: WNL
EXT: Pale nail beds
NEURO: WNL

Results of Pertinent Laboratory Tests, Serum Drug Concentrations, and Diagnostic Tests

Na 133 (133)	Hct 0.28 (28.0)	Alk Phos 2.0 (122)
K 5.5 (5.5)	Hgb 93 (9.3)	Alb 31 (3.1)
Cl 105 (105)	Plts 3.75 × 10⁹ (375)	T Bili 13.7 (0.8)
HCO₃ 17 (17)	Lkcs 5.4 × 10⁹	Ca 2.2 (8.9)
BUN 20 (56)	(5.4 × 10³)	PO₄ 1.97 (6.1)
Cr 309.4 (3.5)	MCV 85 fL	Mg 1.15 (2.8)
Glu 5.27 (95)	ALT 47 (28)	

Peripheral smear: Normochromic, normocytic

Chest radiography: Enlarged heart

ECG: Prolonged P-R interval with occasional PVCs

Digoxin level: 2.8 ng/mL

PROBLEM LIST
Identify principal problem(s) from the scenario in priority order [completed Problem List and SOAP Note at end of casebook]

SOAP NOTE
To be completed by student

QUESTIONS
[Answers at end of casebook]

1. In addition to decreased renal elimination, which of the following are most likely to contribute to the elevated digoxin concentration observed in HJ? (EO-4)
   a. Decreased digoxin tissue binding
   b. Decreased plasma protein binding
   c. Increased gut absorption
   d. Increased liver metabolism

2. The best strategy to address digoxin toxicity in HJ is to: (EO-12)
   a. Administer digoxin antibodies to rapidly bind digoxin
   b. Discontinue digoxin since contraindicated in renal failure
   c. Hold digoxin until level in therapeutic range
   d. Initiate hemodialysis to remove digoxin

3. Elevated potassium levels in HJ may be attributed to all of the following agents *except:* (EO-10)
   a. Mg/Al Antacid
   b. Lisinopril
   c. Triamterene/HCTZ
   d. Digoxin

4. Describe factors that put HJ at risk for developing acute renal failure. (EO-1)

5. Identify problems related to HJ's current pharmacologic and nonpharmacologic regimen. (EO-11)

6. If HJ develops end-stage renal disease, he is at greatest risk of mortality from which of the following conditions: (EO-1, 3)
   a. Anemia
   b. Metabolic Acidosis
   c. Congestive Heart Failure
   d. Renal Osteodystrophy

7. Which of the following phosphate binding agents should be prescribed for initial management of hyperphosphatemia in HJ? (EO-12)
   a. Sevelamer Hydrochloride
   b. Aluminum Hydroxide
   c. Magnesium Hydroxide
   d. Calcium Carbonate

8. HJ should be instructed to take his phosphate binder: (EO-9, 14)
   a. With meals to promote phosphorus elimination
   b. With meals to enhance calcium and phosphorus absorption
   c. Between meals to minimize GI side effects
   d. With vitamin C to enhance absorption

9. Assuming iron indices are above target levels, the most appropriate regimen for maintaining adequate iron in HP is: (EO-8, 12)
   a. Ferrous sulfate 1 g PO QD
   b. Ferrous sulfate 300 mg PO TID
   c. Iron dextran 1 g IV × 1 dose
   d. Iron dextran 50 mg IV q week

10. Therapy with erythropoietin may lead to which of the following: (EO-10)
    a. Thrombocytopenia
    b. Hypokalemia
    c. Neuropathy
    d. Hypertension

11. HJ may benefit from dietary restriction of all of the following *except:* (EO-12)
    a. Potassium
    b. Vitamin D
    c. Phosphorus
    d. Protein

12. Discuss factors to consider when choosing agents for pain management in HJ. (EO-8)

13. Describe the secondary complications expected at each stage of renal disease. (EO-1)

14. Identify psychosocial factors that may influence HJ and management of his disease processes. (EO-15)

15. Which of the following assessments should be completed for all patients with chronic renal failure to optimize pharmacoeconomic outcomes of erythropoietin therapy? (EO-17)
    a. Determine need for folate supplementation
    b. Determine need for iron supplementation
    c. Assess renal function
    d. Assess liver function

16. Summarize pharmacokinetic considerations in chronic renal disease using a key points format. (EO-18)

CASE 30
Joanna Q. Hudson
Topic: Dialysis Therapy

 Level 3

EDUCATIONAL MATERIALS
Chapter 23: Dialytic and Pharmacotherapy for End-Stage Renal Disease (principles of dialysis, indications for dialysis, principles of hemodialysis, adequacy of hemodialysis, complications of hemodialysis, pharmacotherapeutic considerations for dialysis patients, drug dosing considerations in dialysis patients)

SCENARIO

Patient and Setting
TR, a 42-year-old African-American female; admitted to the hospital

Chief Complaint
Shortness of breath, decreased appetite, nausea & vomiting, fatigue, weakness & itching

History of Present Illness
Seen regularly in predialysis clinic for the past year for evaluation of progressive renal failure and secondary complications; arteriovenous fistula placed 2 weeks ago in preparation for hemodialysis anticipated to begin in approximately 1–2 months; new onset (last 2–3 days) of shortness of breath, nausea & vomiting, itching

Past Medical History

Chronic renal disease–secondary to lupus erythematosus and hypertension; systemic lupus erythematosus (SLE) × 9 years–last active flare 6 months ago; hypertension (HTN) × 12 years

Past Surgical History

No prior surgery

Family/Social History

Family History: Mother with SLE–died age 58; father with coronary artery disease (age 67)

Social History: Tobacco negative, alcohol negative

Medication History

Calcium carbonate, 1000 mg PO TID with meals

Felodipine, 10 mg PO QD

Furosemide, 80 mg PO BID

Prednisone, 5 mg PO QD

Erythropoietin, 4000 U SC twice weekly for 8 weeks

Ferrous sulfate, 300 mg PO TID

Sodium bicarbonate, 325 mg tablet–2 tabs PO TID

Calcium carbonate antacid, 1 tab (500 mg) PRN indigestion

ALLERGIES

NKDA

Physical Examination

GEN: Pale, thin, anxious-appearing female

VS: BP 160/ 90, HR 110, RR 22, T 37.0°C, Wt 53 kg (last weight: 49 kg 2 weeks ago), Ht 165 cm

HEENT: Scarring on R cheek from prior discoid lesion

COR: Normal S1 and S2, no murmurs

CHEST: Bibasilar rales

ABD: WNL

GU: WNL

RECT: Guaiac negative

EXT: 2+ pitting ankle edema

NEURO: Alert and oriented × 3

Results of Pertinent Laboratory Tests, Serum Drug Concentrations, and Diagnostic Tests

Na 142 (142)

K 5.9 (5.9)

Cl 107 (107)

HCO_3 16 (16)

BUN 31.8 (89)

Cr 672 (7.6)

Hgb 85 (8.5)

Hct 0.26 (26)

Plts 180 × 10⁹ (180 × 10³)

Lkcs 6.0 × 10⁹ (6.0 × 10³)

Glu 8.32 (150)

Ca 2.2 (8.8)

PO_4 2.1 (8.5)

Mg 1.15 (2.8)

Alb 28 (2.8)

AST 0.47 (28)

ALT 0.53 (32)

T Bili 17.1 (1.0)

LDH 1.2 (70)

Alk Phos 1.2 (70)

MCV 75 (75)

MCH 1.7 (28)

Iron 6.3 (35)

B_{12} 295 (400)

TIBC 86 (480)

Folate 34 (15)

Ferritin 10 (10)

Aluminum 72.1 (2)

ECG: WNL

ANA titer: 1:225 with rim fluorescent pattern (normal < 1:160)

Serum complement: WNL

PROBLEM LIST

Identify principal problem(s) from the scenario in priority order

SOAP NOTE

To be completed by student

QUESTIONS

1. Which of the following is *not* an indication for dialytic therapy in TR? (EO-8)
   a. Fluid overload
   b. Anemia
   c. Metabolic acidosis
   d. Hyperkalemia

2. The minimum target Kt/V for TR is: (EO-12)
   a. 0.2
   b. 0.8
   c. 1.2
   d. 2.0

3. Describe pharmacologic and nonpharmacologic aspects to consider for optimization of blood pressure in TR. (EO-12)

4. Summarize the principles of hemodialysis including the hemodialysis system (components) and factors incorporated in the hemodialysis prescription. (EO-7)

5. Identify short-term and long-term complications that may occur in TR with initiation of hemodialysis. (EO-10, 11)

6. An option other than hemodialysis to acutely treat hyperkalemia in TR is to: (EO-12)
   a. Increase sodium bicarbonate dose to correct acidosis
   b. Restrict dietary potassium to 1 mEq/kg/day
   c. Administer furosemide IV to promote potassium excretion
   d. Administer sodium polystyrene sulfonate

7. The most appropriate phosphate binder to prescribe for TR is: (EO-10, 12)
   a. Aluminum hydroxide
   b. Magnesium hydroxide
   c. Calcium carbonate
   d. Calcium acetate

8. Laboratory data in TR most suggestive of resistance as a potential cause of an inappropriate response to erythropoietin include: (EO-11)
   a. Glucose
   b. Urea
   c. Ferritin
   d. Aluminum

9. Which of the following regimens are most appropriate to replete iron in TR? (EO-8, 12)

a. Continue ferrous sulfate 300 mg PO TID

b. Increase ferrous sulfate to 600 mg PO TID

c. IV iron dextran 25-mg test dose, then 100 mg Q dialysis × 10 doses

d. IV iron dextran 25-mg test dose, then 1 g administered over 1 hour

10. Evaluate TR's current nutritional status based on subjective and objective findings. (EO-2, 5)

11. TR's current therapy with prednisone put her at increased risk for which of the following: (EO-10)

a. Lupus flares

b. Bone disease

c. Acidosis

d. Anemia

12. Assuming TR is dialyzed using high-flux hemodialysis, a drug with which of the following characteristics is most likely to be removed during the procedure: (EO-6, 11)

a. Protein binding 12%, V_D 0.7 L/kg

b. Protein binding 94%, V_D 0.7 L/kg

c. Protein binding 12%, V_D 7 L/kg

d. Protein binding 94%, V_D 7.0 L/kg

13. What psychosocial and pharmacoeconomic factors may affect TR's adherence with pharmacologic and nonpharmacologic therapy? (EO-15, 17)

14. Describe the health care provider's role relative to the psychosocial factors identified. (EO-16)

15. Summarize pathophysiologic, therapeutic, and disease management concepts for end-stage renal disease using a key points format. (EO-18)

CASE 31
Joanna Q. Hudson
Topic: Dialysis Therapy
Level 2

EDUCATIONAL MATERIALS
Chapter 23: Dialytic and Pharmacotherapy for End-Stage Renal Disease (peritoneal dialysis, adequacy of peritoneal dialysis, complications of peritoneal dialysis, drug dosing in CAPD)

SCENARIO

Patient and Setting
FK, a 52-year-old white male; outpatient peritoneal dialysis clinic

Chief Complaint
Painful continuous ambulatory peritoneal dialysis (CAPD) exchanges, "hazy" dialysate fluid, fatigued, feverish, decreased appetite; "I cannot do all my exchanges—I feel too bad."

History of Present Illness
4-day history of painful sensation during exchanges, cloudy effluent drained from peritoneal cavity; fatigued, feverish × 2 days, swollen ankles; brought effluent and residual urine for assessment of dialysis adequacy and residual renal function; dextrose content increased from 2.5 to 4.25% 2 weeks ago per verbal instructions by nephrologist; has become less motivated to do exchanges in last 6 months per spouse

Past Medical History
End-stage renal disease secondary to Type 2 diabetes; CAPD × 5 years; peritonitis—approximately 2 episodes per year; Type 2 diabetes mellitus × 14 years

Past Surgical History
Amputation of R middle digit 2 years ago

Family/Social History
Family History: Father—MI age 53

Social History: Nonsmoker; denies alcohol use

Medication History
Erythropoietin, 4000 units SC BIW (Monday, Thursday)

Ferrous sulfate, 325 mg PO TID

Folic acid, 1 mg PO QD

NPH insulin, 8 units SC q AM

Metoclopramide, 5 mg PO AC & HS

4.25% dextrose solution, 2 L IP (8 AM, 1 PM, 6 PM, 11 PM)

Aluminum hydroxide, 30 mL PO with meals & HS

Allergies
NKDA

Physical Examination
GEN: Well-developed male in no acute distress

VS: BP 138/88, HR 75, RR 14, T 38°C, Wt 84 kg (normal weight: 80 kg), Ht 172 cm

HEENT: WNL

COR: WNL

CHEST: Few rales in lower third of lung fields

ABD: Abdominal tenderness and guarding

GU: WNL

RECT: WNL

EXT: 1+ edema in ankles

NEURO: WNL

Results of Pertinent Laboratory Tests, Serum Drug Concentrations, and Diagnostic Tests

Na 142 (142)	Plts 230×10^9	Mg 0.91 (2.2)
K 5.2 (5.2)	(230×10^3)	Alb 36 (3.6)
Cl 104 (104)	Lkcs 9.7×10^9	Aluminum 2783 (75)
HCO$_3$ 22 (22)	(9.7×10^3)	PTH (4 times normal)
BUN 35 (98)	Glu 10.6 (190)	Total Cholesterol 6.2 (240)
Cr 601 (6.8)	HbA$_{1C}$ 0.062 (6.2)	LDL Cholesterol 4.8 (184)
Hgb 114 (11.4)	Ca 2.45 (9.8)	HDL Cholesterol 0.72 (28)
Hct 0.34 (34.2)	PO$_4$ 1.73 (6.9)	Trig 1.6 (140)

Dialysate effluent: WBC 200/mm^3, neutrophils 110/mm^3 (Gram stain and culture pending)

Measured Kt/V = 1.1

Weekly creatinine clearance = 45 L/1.73 m^2

Urine volume in 24 hr = 300 mL

PROBLEM LIST

Identify principal problem(s) from the scenario in priority order [completed Problem List and SOAP Note at end of casebook]

SOAP NOTE

To be completed by student

QUESTIONS

[Answers at end of casebook]

1. Identify subjective and objective findings in FK consistent with peritonitis. (EO-2, 5)

2. The best antibiotic selection for empiric treatment of peritonitis in FK is: (EO-12)
   a. Cefazolin + gentamicin
   b. Vancomycin + gentamicin
   c. Cefazolin alone
   d. Gentamicin alone

3. Compared to intravenous administration, intraperitoneal (IP) administration of antibiotics for treatment of CAPD peritonitis: (EO-7, EO-8)
   a. Requires a longer time for resolution of infection
   b. Results in minimal systemic drug concentrations
   c. Places patients at increased risk for systemic toxicity
   d. Is the preferred method of administration

4. Which of the following would be the appropriate antibiotic selection if FK's culture reveals *Pseudomonas?* (EO-12)
   a. Gentamicin alone
   b. Vancomycin alone
   c. Ceftazidime + gentamicin
   d. Fluconazole + gentamicin

5. Discuss possible options for prevention of CAPD infections in FK. (EO-7, 12)

6. Inadequate dialysis for FK is supported by all of the following measurements *except:* (EO-11)
   a. Measured Kt/V
   b. Urine output
   c. Weekly creatinine clearance
   d. Urea concentration

7. The most likely cause of hyperglycemia in FK is: (EO-1)
   a. Decreased response to insulin therapy
   b. Decreased renal elimination of glucose
   c. Increased removal of insulin during PD exchanges
   d. Increased glucose absorption from the dialysate solution

8. FK's target LDL level, based on the 2000 American Diabetes Association guidelines, is: (EO-8)
   a. <100 mg/dL
   b. <130 mg/dL
   c. <160 mg/dL
   d. <190 mg/dL

9. Which of the following is the most appropriate option to prevent renal bone disease in FK? (EO-8, 10)
   a. Change the phosphate binder to sevelamer
   b. Change the phosphate binder to calcium acetate
   c. Increase the aluminum hydroxide dose
   d. Add oral 1,25-dihydroxyvitamin D$_3$ (calcitriol)

10. Which of the following is most likely to influence the potential for drug removal during CAPD? (EO-6)
    a. Dialysate flow rate
    b. Molecular weight
    c. Protein binding
    d. Volume of distribution

11. Evaluate FK's current regimen for management of the anemia of chronic renal failure. (EO-11)

12. What pharmacoeconomic factors should be considered in FK's situation? (EO-17)

13. Identify psychosocial factors that may influence FK's adherence with his PD exchanges. (EO-15)

14. Summarize therapeutic, pathophysiologic, and disease management concepts for peritonitis using a key points format. (EO-18)

CASE 32
Monica Daftary
Topic: Peptic Ulcer Disease

Level 2

EDUCATIONAL MATERIALS

Chapter 24: Peptic Ulcer Disease (duodenal ulcer, clinical presentation of PUD, diagnosis, therapeutic plan, and pharmacoeconomics)

SCENARIO

Patient and Setting

AJ, a 35-year-old female; clinic

Chief Complaint

Abdominal pain

History of Present Illness

Abdominal pain for the past 3 weeks, pain awakens her at night and is relieved by food and antacids

Past Medical History

Diagnosed with Graves' disease 2 months ago (symptoms of hyperthyroidism [tachycardia]); chronic renal dysfunction due to polycystic kidney disease; irritable bowel syndrome (IBS) with complaints of diarrhea and constipation (increasing episodes of diarrhea over past 2 months); iron deficiency anemia

Past Surgical History

None

Family/Social History

Family History: Married; 2 children

Social History: Cigarette smoker ½ PPD; alcohol 2 glasses of wine per day with dinner; coffee 2–6 cups per day

Medication History

Propylthiouracil, 200 mg PO q6h for 2 months

Magnesium hydroxide, 300 mg/5 mL, aluminum hydroxide 600 mg/5 mL–15 mL PO PRN

Propranolol, 20 mg PO QID

Allergies

NKDA

Physical Examination

GEN: Well-developed, thin female in mild distress
VS: BP 140/88, HR 84, RR 18, T 37.0°C, Wt 55 kg, Ht 165 cm
HEENT: Small, symmetric goiter, much smaller than 2 months ago
COR: NL S1 and S2; no murmurs, rubs, or gallops
CHEST: WNL
ABD: Intermittent, crampy, lower abdominal pain relieved by passage of flatus; point tenderness between the xiphoid and umbilicus
GU: WNL
RECT: Guaiac positive
EXT: Pruritic pretibial myxedema
NEURO: WNL

Results of Pertinent Laboratory Tests, Serum Drug Concentrations, and Diagnostic Tests

Na 128 (128)	Plts 120 × 10⁹	Ca 2.1 (8.6)
K 4.8 (4.8)	(120 × 10³)	PO₄ 1.6 (4.8)
Cl 102 (102)	MCV 68 (68)	Mg 1.35 (2.7)
HCO₃ 20 (20)	AST 0.42 (25)	Uric Acid 535 (9)
BUN 28.6 (80)	ALT 0.45 (27)	TT₄ 100 (7.8)
Cr 283 (3.2)	LDH 1.1 (65)	RT₃U 0.3 (30%)
Hct 0.29 (29%)	Alk Phos 1.1 (65)	FT₄I 34 (2.6)
Hgb 100 (10)	Alb 35 (3.5)	TSH 5 (5)
Lkcs 5 × 10⁹	T Bili 15.4 (0.9)	Fe 9.8 (55)
(5 × 10³)	Glu 4.7 (84)	

Na 128 (128) — Ca 2.1 (8.6)
$Na\ 128\ (128)$

Lkc differential: WNL

Urinalysis: Hematuria, proteinuria

Chest radiography: WNL

ECG: WNL

Endoscopy: Two small duodenal ulcers

Peripheral blood smear: Microcytic anemia

PROBLEM LIST

Identify principal problems from the scenario in priority order [completed Problem List and SOAP Note at end of casebook]

SOAP NOTE

To be completed by student

QUESTIONS

[Answers at end of casebook]

1. AJ should be counseled on all of the following to avoid complications of PUD *except:* (EO-4)
   a. Smoking cessation
   b. Discontinue alcohol intake
   c. Eat after the evening meal to prevent acid secretion during the night
   d. Avoid caffeine intake

2. AJ presents with signs and symptoms consistent with the findings of a duodenal ulcer: (EO-2)
   a. Pain over midepigastrium, worsened by food
   b. Abdominal pain, relieved by food and antacids
   c. Anorexia
   d. Vomiting

3. AJ's calculated creatinine clearance: (EO-6, 8)
   a. 30 mL/min
   b. 21 mL/min
   c. 42 mL/min
   d. 15 mL/min

4. Based on AJ's calculated creatinine clearance, the appropriate recommended dose of ranitidine for treatment of duodenal ulcers is: (EO-6)
   a. 300 mg PO QHS
   b. 150 mg PO BID
   c. 450 mg PO QHS
   d. 150 mg PO QHS

5. If famotidine, rather than ranitidine, were the H$_2$-antagonist on formulary at AJ's HMO Pharmacy, what would be an equivalent treatment dose of famotidine for her duodenal ulcers? (EO-6, 8)
   a. 40 mg PO BID
   b. 20 mg PO QHS
   c. 20 mg PO BID
   d. 40 mg PO TID

6. AJ has experienced increasing episodes of diarrhea over the past 2 months. Which of the following drug(s) is most likely contributing to this problem? (EO-10)
   a. PTU and magnesium hydroxide
   b. Propranolol
   c. Aluminum hydroxide
   d. Alcohol

7. Physical assessment and laboratory findings apparent in AJ that support the diagnosis of PUD include all of the following *except:* (EO-5)
   a. Small, symmetric goiter
   b. Guaiac-positive stools
   c. Endoscopy: 2 small duodenal ulcers
   d. Point tenderness between the xiphoid and umbilicus

8. AJ is placed on ferrous sulfate 325 mg PO TID for her iron deficiency anemia. AJ should be instructed that this medication is best absorbed: (EO-10, 14)
   a. With antacids
   b. On an empty stomach
   c. With food
   d. With propylthiouracil

9. AJ's propranolol can be considered for tapering because: (EO-8, 12)
   a. The hemoglobin and hematocrit have normalized
   b. The duodenal ulcer has healed
   c. The patient is no longer tachycardic because of Graves' disease
   d. The patient had episodes of constipation from the ferrous sulfate

10. All of the following are aggressive factors that influenced the development of PUD in AJ *except:* (EO-1)
    a. Rapid gastric epithelial cell turnover
    b. Nicotine use
    c. Ethanol use
    d. Caffeine use

11. List the pharmacologic and nonpharmacologic treatment problem(s) present in AJ's treatment plan. (EO-11)

12. Evaluate the pharmacoeconomic considerations relative to AJ's treatment plan for duodenal ulcer. (EO-17)

13. What psychosocial factors affect AJ's adherence to both pharmacologic and nonpharmacologic therapy? (EO-15)

14. Summarize pathophysiologic, therapeutic, and disease management concepts for duodenal ulcers utilizing a key points format. (EO-18)

CASE 33
Monica Daftary
Topic: Peptic Ulcer Disease
Level 2
EDUCATIONAL MATERIALS
Chapter 24: Peptic Ulcer Disease (duodenal ulcer, clinical presentation of PUD, diagnosis of *H. pylori*, treatment of *H. pylori*)

SCENARIO

Patient and Setting
NK, a 62-year-old male; clinic

Chief Complaint
Heartburn and gnawing feeling which increases in between meals

History of Present Illness
Increasing heartburn over past 2 weeks which increases in between meals; taking magaldrate with no relief

Past Medical History
Type 2 diabetes × 20 years; hypertension (HTN) × 15 years; 1 myocardial infarction (MI); hyperlipidemia; peptic ulcer disease (PUD); diabetic nephropathy

Past Surgical History

1 angioplasty (PTCA)

Family/Social History

Family History: Father died at age 65 from MI

Social History: No alcohol or tobacco use

Medication History

Magaldrate, 540 mg 1 tsp PO q3h PRN heartburn

Metformin, 500 mg PO BID

Amlodipine, 5 mg PO QD

Atorvastatin, 10 mg PO QHS

Allergies

NKDA

Physical Examination

GEN: Well-developed, obese male in moderate pain
VS: BP 150/92, HR 80, RR 20, T 37.0°C, Wt 101 kg, HT 180 cm
HEENT: WNL
COR: NSR
CHEST: WNL
ABD: Abdominal pain
GU: Deferred
RECT: WNL
EXT: 1+edema bilat LE
NEURO: WNL

Results of Pertinent Laboratory Tests, Serum Drug Concentrations, and Diagnostic Tests

Na 137 (137)
K 4.2 (4.2)
Cl 100 (100)
HCO_3 27 (27)
BUN 7 (20)
Cr 123 (1.4)
Hct 0.40 (40)
Hgb 150 (15)
Lkcs 9.0 × 10⁹
  (9.0 × 10³)

Plts 150 × 10⁹
  (150 × 10³)
MCV 78 (78)
AST 0.58 (35)
ALT 0.58 (35)
LDH 2.66 (150)
Alk Phos 2.0 (120)
Alb 30 (3.0)
T Bili 2 (0.1)
Glu 9.9 (180)

Ca 2.58 (10.3)
PO_4 0.80 (2.5)
Mg 0.80 (1.6)
UA 120 (2.0)
TC 5.2 (200)
LDL 3.7 (140)
HDL 1.6 (60)
Trig 1.8 (160)
HbA_{1C} 10%

Urinalysis: 1+ protein

Endoscopy: 3 duodenal ulcers

Biopsy with culture: Consistent with *H. pylori*

PROBLEM LIST

Identify principal problem(s) from the scenario in priority order

SOAP NOTE

To be completed by student

QUESTIONS

1. The probable cause of NK's heartburn is: (EO-1)
   a. Use of magaldrate
   b. Obesity
   c. Hypertension
   d. *H. pylori* infection

2. NK presents with all of the signs and symptoms of PUD *except:* (EO-2)
   a. Proteinuria
   b. Heartburn
   c. Abdominal pain
   d. Gnawing feeling

3. NK appears to have drug-induced pedal edema. This may be due to which one of his medications: (EO-10)
   a. Atorvastatin
   b. Amlodipine
   c. Metformin
   d. Magaldrate

4. NK should be monitored for lactic acidosis while receiving metformin therapy. Which of the following may increase the risk for this adverse effect? (EO-4, 6, 8)
   a. Hypoglycemia
   b. Serum creatinine >1.5
   c. Hyperglycemia
   d. Proteinuria

5. All of the following are acceptable regimens for the eradication of *H. pylori except:* (EO-12)
   a. Omeprazole 40 mg PO QD for 28 days + clarithromycin 500 mg PO TID for 14 days
   b. Omeprazole 20 mg PO BID + metronidazole 250 mg PO BID + amoxicillin 1 g PO QD for 7–14 days
   c. Omeprazole 20 mg PO BID + clarithromycin 500 mg PO BID + amoxicillin 1 g PO QD for 7 days
   d. Omeprazole 80 mg PO BID + clarithromycin 1 g PO TID + amoxicillin 2 g PO QD for 14 days

6. NK is placed on metronidazole 500 mg PO BID as a part of his treatment for *H. pylori*. NK should be instructed: (EO-10, 14)
   a. To take the medication with antacids
   b. Of possibility of darkening of the urine
   c. Of possibility of darkening of the feces
   d. To take the medication with alcohol

7. Physical assessment and laboratory findings apparent in NK that point to PUD include all of the following *except:* (EO-5)
   a. Endoscopy: 3 duodenal ulcers
   b. 1+ edema bilat LE
   c. Biopsy with culture: consistent with *H. pylori*
   d. Abdominal pain

8. Invasive diagnostic measures for the detection of *H. pylori* include all of the following *except:* (EO-5)
   a. Serological tests for IgG antibodies to *H. pylori*
   b. Endoscopy with gastric biopsy

c. Histologic demonstration of organisms

d. Biopsy with culture of the *H. pylori* organism

9. List the pharmacologic and nonpharmacologic treatment problem(s) present in NK's treatment plan. (EO-11)

10. Name four factors that should be considered when choosing therapy for NK in the management of PUD to make the decision pharmacologically sound. (EO-17)

11. What psychosocial factors may affect NK's adherence to both pharmacologic and nonpharmacologic therapy? (EO-15)

12. Summarize the pathophysiologic, therapeutic, and disease management concepts for *H. pylori*-associated duodenal ulcers utilizing a key points format. (EO-18)

CASE 34
Tammy C. Dawkins
Topic: Gastroesophageal Reflux Disease
Level 2
EDUCATIONAL MATERIALS
Chapter 24: Peptic Ulcer Disease
(gastroesophageal reflux disease)

SCENARIO

Patient and Setting

TM, a 42-year-old female; clinic

Chief Complaint

Severe heartburn, morning hoarseness, laryngitis, and fatigue

History of Present Illness

Experiencing intense episodes of heartburn for past 3 days, despite increased antacid use

Past Medical History

Gastroesophageal reflux disease (GERD) × 3 years, occasional heartburn, usually responds to antacids; hypertension (HTN) × 5 years (controlled with verapamil and propranolol); deep venous thrombosis (DVT) diagnosed 3 weeks ago (on warfarin therapy); motion sickness problems for past month (scopolamine transdermal system initiated 1 week ago)

Past Surgical History

Cesarean section for twins 20 years ago

Family/Social History

Family History: Mother living with emphysema; father deceased at 62 with myocardial infarction (MI)

Social History: Smokes 1 PPD × past 20 years; drinks 2–3 glasses of wine per day

Medication History

Antacid containing aluminum hydroxide, magnesium carbonate, alginic acid, and sodium bicarbonate, 2 tablets PO q2h PRN heartburn

Verapamil sustained release, 120 mg PO QD

Propranolol, 40 mg PO BID

Warfarin, 5 mg PO QD

Scopolamine transdermal system, 1 topically q 3 days × 1 week

Allergies

NKDA

Physical Examination

GEN: Well-developed, obese female in moderate pain

VS: BP 130/85, HR 80, RR 16, T 37°C, Wt 90 kg, HT 157 cm

HEENT: Dysphagia

COR: NL S_1 and S_2; no murmurs, rubs, or gallops

CHEST: Clear to auscultation

ABD: Nontender, no masses

GU: Deferred

RECT: Guaiac negative

EXT: Few small healing bruises, right thigh slightly larger than left

NEURO: Alert, O × 3

Results of Pertinent Laboratory Tests, Serum Drug Concentrations, and Diagnostic Tests

Na 140 (140)	Lkcs 5.3 × 10⁹	Alk Phos 1.1 (65)
K 3.8 (3.8)	(5.3 × 10³)	Alb 40 (4.0)
Cl 102 (102)	Plts 160 × 10⁹	T Bili 15.4 (0.9)
HCO₃ 24 (24)	(160 × 10³)	Glu 4.4 (80)
BUN 3.2 (9)	MCV 68 (68)	Ca 2.2 (9)
Cr 80 (0.9)	AST 0.42 (25)	PO₄ 0.87 (2.7)
Hct 0.35 (35%)	ALT 0.45 (27)	Mg 0.85 (1.7)
Hgb 130 (13)	LDH 1.1 (65)	Uric Acid 557 (9)

INR 2.4

Lkc differential: WNL

Urinalysis: Normal PT: 15.9/10.6 (control)

ECG: WNL

Esophagoscopy: Moderate esophagitis, friable mucosa

PROBLEM LIST

Identify principal problems from the scenario in priority order [completed Problem List and SOAP Note at end of casebook]

SOAP NOTE

To be completed by student

QUESTIONS

[Answers at end of casebook]

1. A common clinical manifestation of GERD present in TM: (EO-2)
   a. Dizziness
   b. Constipation
   c. Heartburn
   d. Headache

2. The consequences of an ineffective or incompetent lower esophageal sphincter (LES) in GERD: (EO-1)
   a. Allows retrograde flow of gastric contents into esophagus
   b. Increases retrograde flow of gastric contents into stomach
   c. Causes peptic ulcer disease
   d. Allows retrograde flow of gastric contents into duodenum

3. A drug-induced cause of GERD in TM: (EO-1, 8, 10)
   a. Anticoagulant activity of warfarin
   b. Anticholinergic activity of scopolamine transdermal system
   c. Beta-blocking action of propranolol
   d. Neutralizing capacity of antacid

4. All of the following factors listed in TM's medical history can reduce the LES pressure *except:* (EO-1, 3, 4)
   a. Motion sickness
   b. Calcium channel blockers
   c. Nicotine use
   d. Ethanol consumption

5. Use of the esophagoscopy in TM allows for: (EO-5)
   a. Nonsurgical visualization of esophagus
   b. Visualization of colon and rectum
   c. Measurement of gastric pH
   d. Direct delivery of enteral feedings to stomach

6. Describe the mechanism of action of the pharmacologic and nonpharmacologic interventions for this case. (EO-7)

7. TM should be monitored for factors that will alter the elimination of medications. Which of the following warrants a dosage adjustment in TM's ranitidine therapy? (EO-4, 5, 6, 8)
   a. AST 0.35 (35)
   b. ALT 0.40 (40)
   c. CrCl <75 mL/min
   d. CrCl <50 mL/min

8. Select the best description for an interaction between warfarin and ranitidine: (EO-9)
   a. Significant increase in warfarin absorption
   b. Minimal increase in warfarin absorption
   c. Significant reduction in warfarin clearance
   d. Minimal reduction in warfarin clearance

9. Describe the pharmacologic and nonpharmacologic problems in TM's treatment plan. (EO-11)

10. Omeprazole would be indicated when which of the following occurs in TM: (EO-4, 5, 6, 8, 12)
    a. Creatinine clearance >40 mL/min
    b. Hemodialysis is required
    c. Severe, erosive esophagitis occurs
    d. Patient no longer has GERD symptoms

11. What psychosocial factors may affect TM's adherence to pharmacologic and nonpharmacologic therapy? (EO-15)

12. Describe the health care provider's role relative to the identified psychosocial factors. (EO-16)

13. Evaluate the pharmacoeconomic considerations relative to TM's pharmaceutical plan of care. (EO-17)

14. Summarize the therapeutic, pathophysiologic, and disease management concepts for moderate GERD utilizing a key points format. (EO-18)

CASE 35
Tammy C. Dawkins
Topic: Gastroesophageal Reflux Disease

EDUCATIONAL MATERIALS
Chapter 24: Peptic Ulcer Disease
(gastroesophageal reflux disease)

SCENARIO

Patient and Setting

PR, a 48-year-old male; urgent care center

Chief Complaint

Occasional heartburn after meals, and a bitter taste in mouth

History of Present Illness

Heartburn started 1 month ago while on camping trip; reluctantly started antacid 3 days ago with some relief

Past Medical History

Gallstones 4 years ago; gout diagnosed 3 years ago; gout attacks respond to colchicine; last attack 1 year ago

Past Surgical History

Gallstones removed

Family/Social History

Family History: Mother good health; father Parkinson's disease

Social History: Camp director; drinks 1 six pack each weekend; nonsmoker

Medication History

Antacid suspension, 400 mg aluminum hydroxide, 2 tsp
  PO BID

Colchicine, 0.6 mg PO PRN at first sign of gout attack

Allergies

Aspirin—difficulty breathing, rash

Physical Examination

    GEN: Well-developed, overweight male in some
         discomfort
     VS: BP 105/80, HR 68, RR 18, T 37.5°C, Wt 80 kg,
         Ht 175 cm
  HEENT: Bitter taste in mouth; otherwise normal
    COR: Regular heart rate and rhythm
  CHEST: Clear to auscultation
    ABD: WNL
     GU: Deferred
   RECT: Hard stool present, guaiac negative
    EXT: No edema or pain
  NEURO: Alert O × 3

Results of Pertinent Laboratory Tests, Serum Drug Concentrations, and Diagnostic Tests

Na 137 (137)   Lkcs 6.2 × 10⁹   Alk Phos 50 (50)
K 4.2 (4.2)   (6.2 × 10³)   Alb 38 (3.8)
Cl 100 (100)   Plts 175 × 10⁹   T Bili 8.55 (0.5)
CO_2 21 (21)   (175 × 10³)   Glu 5.1 (92)
BUN 3.5 (10)   MCV 81 (81)   Ca 3.5 (7)
Cr 88.4 (1.0)   AST 0.55 (33) PO_4 0.48 (1.5)
Hct 0.38 (38%)   ALT 0.47 (28)   Mg 0.9 (2.2)
Hgb 126 (12.6)   LDH 0.75 (75)   Uric Acid 588 (9.5)

PROBLEM LIST

Identify principal problems from the scenario in priority order [completed Problem List and SOAP Note at end of casebook]

SOAP NOTE

To be completed by student

QUESTIONS

[Answers at end of casebook]

1. The probable cause for PR's GERD: (EO-1)
   a. High-fat, spicy meals eaten late at night
   b. Aluminum hydroxide antacid use
   c. Prior use of colchicine
   d. History of gallstones

2. Which of the following is a common symptom of GERD? (EO-2)
   a. Bitter taste in mouth
   b. Swollen big toe
   c. Constipation
   d. Heartburn

3. A factor that can worsen GERD in PR: (EO-1, 3)
   a. History of gout
   b. Male gender
   c. Ethanol use
   d. Age group

4. Which best describes the mechanism for the symptoms of GERD in PR? (EO-1)
   a. Backward flow of gastric contents into esophagus
   b. An impaired esophagus
   c. An ulcer in the stomach
   d. Reduced acid secretion in the esophagus

5. PR will be taking famotidine, a drug renally eliminated. Which of the following would represent a decrease in renal function for PR? (EO-4, 5, 6, 8)
   a. Serum creatinine 3.5 mg/dL
   b. Uric acid 7.0 mg/dL
   c. Creatinine clearance 98 mL/min
   d. Serum creatinine 0.5 mg/dL

6. Describe the mechanism of action of pharmacologic and nonpharmacologic interventions used in this case. (EO-7)

7. PR has developed constipation. Which of the following may have contributed to constipation? (EO-10)
   a. Untreated GERD
   b. Aluminum content of antacid
   c. Ethanol use
   d. Prior colchicine therapy

8. List the pharmacologic and nonpharmacologic treatment problem(s) present in PR's treatment plan. (EO-11)

9. Which medication(s) can treat symptomatic, severe GERD? (EO-12)
   a. Hydroxymagnesium aluminate antacid
   b. Low-dose, over-the-counter ranitidine or famotidine
   c. Omeprazole
   d. Sodium chloride tablets

10. PR's disease progresses and lansoprazole is prescribed. The mechanism of lansoprazole: (EO-12)
    a. Reduces gastric acid secretion
    b. Increases gastric acid secretion
    c. Binds to lining of esophagus
    d. Binds to stomach ulcer

11. What psychosocial factors may affect PR's adherence to the pharmacologic and nonpharmacologic interventions? (EO-15)

12. Describe the health care provider's role relative to the proposed psychosocial factors identified. (EO-16)

13. Evaluate the pharmacoeconomic considerations relative to the plan of care. (EO-17)

14. Summarize the pathophysiologic, therapeutic, and disease management concepts for GERD utilizing a key points format. (EO-18)

CASE 36
Daphne Bernard
Topic: Crohn's Disease
Level 3
EDUCATIONAL MATERIALS
Chapter 25: Inflammatory Bowel Disease

SCENARIO

Patient and Setting

GK, a 32-year-old male; surgery department

Chief Complaint

Severe abdominal pain, crampy diarrhea, recent 10-lb weight loss; postoperative nausea and vomiting secondary to narcotic medication

History of Present Illness

Resection of terminal ilium performed due to unresponsiveness to a 72-hour course of intravenous steroid therapy (methylprednisolone 20 mg PO q6h)

Past Medical History

Severe recurrent Crohn's disease (CD), first diagnosed at age 18, with involvement of the terminal ileum and colon and "cobblestoned" appearing mucosa (uncontrolled with sulfasalazine and oral steroid therapy); arthritis in both knees for several years with pain onset associated with exacerbation of intestinal disease (relieved by NSAIDs); NSAID-induced peptic ulcer disease (PUD) 1 year ago (relieved by famotidine)

Past Surgical History

Small bowel resection 3 years ago; postsurgical relapse treated with one course of azathioprine 1.5 mg/kg (discontinued after 8 weeks due to leukopenia)

Family/Social History

Unremarkable

Medication History

Prednisone, 30 mg PO q AM and 20 mg PO q PM for 3 years

Sulfasalazine, 1 g PO QID for 3 years

Ibuprofen, 600 mg PO q4–6h PRN arthritic and muscle pain (average of 2400 mg/day for the past 2 weeks)

Oxycodone/aspirin 1–2 tabs PO q4–6h PRN abdominal pain (4 tabs/day for the past 2 weeks)

Allergies

NKDA

Physical Examination

GEN: Ill-appearing thin male, febrile, and in acute distress
VS: BP 145/85, HR 95, T 38.0°C, RR 14, Wt 61.4 kg, HT 173 cm
HEENT: WNL
CHEST: WNL
ABD: Abdominal tenderness and guarding
RECT: Guaiac positive
EXT: Reduced reflexes, swollen knees, mild lower extremity edema, dry skin, ecchymosis

Results of Pertinent Laboratory Tests, Serum Drug Concentrations, and Diagnostic Tests

Na 135 (135)
K 3.5 (3.5)
Cl 98 (98)
CO_2 22 (22)
BUN 11.4 (32)
T Bili 13.7 (0.8)
Hct 0.37 (37)
Hgb 130 (13)

Lkcs 1.4×10^9 (1.4×10^3)
Plts 260×10^9 (260×10^3)
Alb 23 (2.3)
AST 0.65 (39)
ALT 0.53 (32)
LDH 3.2 (190)

Alk Phos 1.5 (90)
Uric Acid 357 (6)
Glu 10 (180)
Ca 2.3 (9.2)
PO_4 1.4 (4.3)
Mg 1.2 (2.4)
Cr 115 (1.3)

PROBLEM LIST

Identify principal problem(s) from the scenario in priority order

SOAP NOTE

To be completed by student

QUESTIONS

1. GK presents with all the following signs and symptoms of severe CD exacerbation *except:* (EO-2)
   a. Abdominal pain
   b. Diarrhea
   c. Perianal disease
   d. Malnutrition

2. A probable cause for GK's CD exacerbation is: (EO-1)
   a. Smoking
   b. NSAID use
   c. Mesalamine sensitivity
   d. Genetic influence

3. All of the following statements are true *except:* (EO-9)
   a. Sulfasalazine and azathioprine may cause leukocytosis
   b. NSAIDs may precipitate IBD
   c. Sulfasalazine may increase digoxin's bioavailability and increase digoxin serum concentrations
   d. Sulfasalazine may enhance the effect of warfarin

4. Physical assessment findings apparent in GK, which point to CD, include all of the following *except:* (EO-5)
   a. Mucosa with cobblestone appearance
   b. Low-grade fever
   c. Rectal guaiac-positive
   d. Chest pain

5. What are the indications for surgery in this case? (EO-8)

6. Which epidemiologic factors for CD should be considered in regards to GK? (EO-3)
   a. Age of onset 15–25 years
   b. More common in Blacks than Caucasians
   c. More common in males than females
   d. More common in tobacco smokers

7. Which drug is recognized as a probable cause for GK's previous development of leukopenia? (EO-10)
   a. Prednisone
   b. Azathioprine
   c. Sulfasalazine
   d. Ibuprofen

8. Provide an appropriate steroid-tapering regimen when converting intravenous methylprednisolone (current dose is 60 mg q6h IV) to oral prednisone for GK. (EO-6, 8)

9. Tapering of long-term corticosteroid therapy is indicated when which of the following occurs: (EO-4, 6, 8, 12)
   a. Glu 10 (180) (fasting)
   b. BP 130/84
   c. Cl 98
   d. K 3.5

10. Evaluate pharmacoeconomic considerations relative to GK's plan of care. (EO-17)

11. GK has been recommended to receive a single intravenous dose of Infliximab. During the patient counseling session, he should be instructed to monitor for signs of: (EO-10, 14)
    a. Bradycardia
    b. Infections
    c. Rebound hypertension
    d. Heat intolerance

12. What psychosocial factors may affect GK's adherence to both pharmacologic and nonpharmacologic therapy? (EO-15)

13. Summarize the pathophysiologic, therapeutic, and disease management concepts for CD utilizing a key points format. (EO-18)

CASE 37
Daphne Bernard
Topic: Ulcerative Colitis
Level 1
EDUCATIONAL MATERIALS
Chapter 25: Inflammatory Bowel Disease

SCENARIO

Patient and Setting

DD, a 35-year-old female; internal medicine department

Chief Complaint

Increasing fatigue, increased frequency of bowel movements, rectal bleeding, and abdominal cramping

History of Present Illness

Made appointment to see gastroenterologist for recurrent ulcerative colitis (UC); increased frequency of bowel movements, rectal bleeding, and abdominal cramping (that is usually relieved upon defecation) since 2 weeks ago; has 6–7 bloody bowel movements per day; increased fatigue for the past month

Past Medical History

Proctosigmoiditis diagnosed 3 years ago; initially treated with sulfasalazine 2–4 g/day (discontinued by physician after 6 weeks of treatment due to occurrence of severe headache, increased fatigue, malaise, upset stomach with nausea, and an itchy rash); hydrocortisone enemas begun, and remission of UC achieved in 1 month

Past Surgical History

None

Family History/Social History

Family History: Unremarkable

Social History: Increased work-related stress, alcohol consumption, and poor nutrition during this past month, nonsmoker

Medication History

Hydrocortisone enema, 100 mg/60 mL PR QHS for 1 month

Sulfasalazine, 2–4 g/day PO for 6 weeks

Multivitamin with minerals, 1 PO q AM

Calcium carbonate, 1250 mg PO q AM

Loperamide, PRN diarrhea (Rx—with onset of diarrhea take 4 mg followed by 2 mg q4–6h until diarrhea resolves)

Allergies

Sulfasalazine

Physical Examination

GEN: Thin female in mild-to-moderate distress
VS: BP 128/80, HR 85, T 37.5°C, Wt 45.5 kg, Ht 157 cm
HEENT: WNL
CHEST: WNL

ABD: Mild tenderness, hyperactive bowel sounds

RECT: Bloody, watery diarrhea

Results of Pertinent Laboratory Tests, Serum Drug Concentrations, and Diagnostic Tests

Na 135 (135)

K 3.9 (3.9)

Cl 95 (95)

CO_2 27 (27)

BUN 8.9 (25)

T PROT 59 (5.9)

Hct 0.32 (32)

Hgb 102 (10.2)

Lkcs 1.2×10^9

(1.2×10^3)

Plts 270×10^9

(270×10^3)

Alb 30 (3)

AST 0.45 (27)

ALT 0.5 (30)

LDH 2.0 (120)

Alk Phos 1.6 (95)

Uric Acid 297 (5)

Glu 3.9 (70)

Ca 2.2 (8.9)

PO_4 1.4 (4.2)

Mg 1.3 (2.5)

Cr 97 (1.1)

Sigmoidoscopy report: Mucosal surface irregular and granular in appearance; mucosa friable with spontaneous bleeding

PROBLEM LIST

Identify principal problems from the scenario in priority order [completed Problem List and SOAP Note at end of casebook]

SOAP NOTE

To be completed by student

QUESTIONS

[Answers at end of casebook]

1. The probable cause for DD's UC exacerbation: (EO-1)
   a. Viral infection
   b. Diet
   c. Stress
   d. Discontinuation of maintenance therapy

2. DD presents with the following signs and symptoms of UC exacerbation *except:* (EO-2)
   a. Absent bowel sounds
   b. Leukocytosis
   c. Fever
   d. Rectal bleeding

3. DD has clinical symptoms that include an increase in frequency of bowel movements, rectal bleeding, and abdominal cramping that is usually relieved upon defecation. This stage of UC would be classified as: (EO-1, 2, 5, 8, 12)
   a. Mild
   b. Moderate
   c. Severe
   d. Complex

4. Develop a detailed education plan for DD including necessary lifestyle changes, and medication counseling information. (EO-9, 11, 14)

5. Which epidemiologic factor is likely to have predisposed DD to develop UC? (EO-3)
   a. Age of onset 15–25 years
   b. More prevalent in females than males
   c. More common in tobacco smokers
   d. More common in Hispanics

6. What psychosocial factors may affect DD's adherence to both pharmacological and nonpharmacological therapy? (EO-15)

7. Evaluate pharmacoeconomic considerations relative to DD's pharmaceutical care plan. (EO-17)

8. If DD plans to get pregnant, which drug would be safe to use during pregnancy? (EO- 4, 8, 10)
   a. Mesalamine
   b. Methotrexate
   c. Metronidazole
   d. Cyclosporine

9. Physical assessment findings apparent in DD that point to UC include all of the following *except:* (EO-5)
   a. Lkcs 1.2×10^9 (1.2×10^3)
   b. Wt 45.5 kg
   c. Plts 270×10^9 (270×10^3)
   d. T 37.5°C

10. The presence of DD's rectal bleeding increases the risk of developing anemia. What is the most common hematological complication of UC? (EO-1, 2)
    a. Folic acid-deficiency anemia
    b. B_{12}-deficiency anemia
    c. Hemolytic anemia
    d. Iron deficiency anemia

11. Which of the following is true concerning topical treatment of UC? (EO-6, 8)
    a. More than 25% of a rectally administered 5-ASA dose is absorbed.
    b. Rectal 5-ASA suppositories are indicated for distal ulcerative proctitis.
    c. Patients refractory to oral sulfasalazine usually get no benefit from the use of rectal aminosalicylates.
    d. In patients with mild to moderate active UC, the 5-ASA enema is not as effective as a GCS enema.

12. Summarize therapeutic, pathophysiologic, and disease management concepts for UC utilizing a key points format. (EO-18)

CASE 38

Valerie W. Hogue

Topic: Traveler's Diarrhea

 Level 2

EDUCATIONAL MATERIALS

Chapter 27: Constipation and Diarrhea (definition and epidemiology, clinical presentation and diagnosis, prevention, treatment, acute nonspecific diarrhea)

SCENARIO

Patient and Setting

KT, a 39-year-old American male; hospital in Guatemala

Chief Complaint

Abdominal cramps, diarrhea, vomiting, fatigue, polydipsia, and blurred vision

History of Present Illness

Decreased oral intake for 2 days (only ice cubes)

Past Medical History

Type 2 diabetes mellitus (controlled) for 4 years; hyperlipidemia for 1 year; deep venous thrombosis (DVT) (hospitalized 2 months ago)

Past Surgical History

None

Family/Social History

Family History: Father (age 69) has angina
Social History: Smokes 1 PPD

Medication History

Warfarin, 5 mg PO QD (for 5 weeks)
Glimepiride, 2 mg PO QD
Atorvastatin, 20 mg PO QD

Allergies

NKDA

Physical Examination

GEN: Obese male with decreased skin turgor
VS: BP 116/72, HR 100 (lying); 100/66, 110 (sitting); T 37.9°C; RR 18, Wt 84 kg (usual Wt 88 kg); Ht 175 cm
HEENT: Dry mucous membranes
COR: Tachycardia
CHEST: WNL
ABD: Soft, hyperactive bowel sounds; pain on palpation
GU: WNL
RECT: Guaiac negative
EXT: (−) edema; (−) pain
NEURO: WNL

Results of Pertinent Laboratory Tests, Serum Drug Concentrations, and Diagnostic Tests

Na 132 (132)	Hgb 150 (15)	LDH 0.82 (50)
K 2.7 (2.7)	Lkcs 7.1 × 10⁹	Alk Phos 0.80 (48)
Cl 100 (100)	(7.1 × 10³)	Alb 42 (4.2)
CO₂ 20 (20)	Plts 350 × 10⁹	T Bili 3.6 (0.21)
BUN 13.2 (37)	(350 × 10³)	Glu 16.8 (303)
Cr 114 (1.3)	MCV 90 (90)	Ca 2.3 (9.2)
Uric Acid 178.4 (3.0)	AST 0.50 (30)	PO₄ 0.80 (2.5)
Hct 0.45 (45)	ALT 0.40 (24)	Mg 0.90 (1.8)

PT (control) 12.0

PT 16.2

INR 2.3

Total plasma cholesterol: 4.1 mmol/L (160 mg/dL)

Fasting plasma triglyceride: 1.58 mmol/L (140 mg/dL)

High-density lipoprotein cholesterol: 1.03 mmol/L (40 mg/dL)

Low-density lipoprotein cholesterol: 3.2 mmol/L (125 mg/dL)

Stool culture: Pending

PROBLEM LIST

Identify principal problem(s) from the scenario in priority order

SOAP NOTE

To be completed by student

QUESTIONS

1. The primary cause of KT's episode of TD: (EO-1)
   a. Lack of vitamin K in diet
   b. Oral intake of contaminated food and water
   c. Age
   d. Dehydration/hypovolemia
2. Physical assessment findings that suggest dehydration secondary to TD include all of the following *except:* (EO-5)
   a. Stool guaiac negative
   b. Dry mucous membranes
   c. Tachycardia
   d. Weight loss
3. KT's stool culture is pending. What organism is most likely the cause of KT's TD? (EO-1)
   a. *Clostridium difficile*
   b. Enterotoxigenic *E. coli*
   c. *Pseudomonas aeruginosa*
   d. *Giardia lamblia*
4. KT has a history of type 2 diabetes mellitus. Which problem in this case predisposed him to loss of glucose control? (EO-1)
   a. DVT
   b. Hyperlipidemia

   c. Family history of CAD

   d. Dehydration/hypovolemia

5. All of the following are correct regarding loperamide *except:* (EO-7)

   a. Decreases gastrointestinal motility

   b. Synthetic congener of meperidine

   c. Affects circular and longitudinal intestinal muscles

   d. Reduction of gastric acid secretions

6. All of the following are risk factors in KT's history that predispose him to atherosclerosis *except:* (EO-4)

   a. Tachycardia

   b. Male

   c. Diabetes

   d. Tobacco use

7. Which of the following is *not* an appropriate option for KT in the treatment of TD? (EO-8)

   a. Bismuth subsalicylate

   b. Loperamide

   c. Vancomycin (oral)

   d. Trimethoprim/sulfamethoxazole

8. Side effects of loperamide include all of the following *except:* (EO-10)

   a. Drowsiness

   b. Constipation

   c. Dry mouth

   d. Mild tinnitus

9. KT's diarrhea persisted after loperamide therapy. What considerations should be made when selecting pharmacological intervention for KT? (EO-8)

10. KT is planning a business trip to Asia 1 month after returning from Guatemala. His primary care provider suggested that he take bismuth subsalicylate 2 tablets PO QID for 1 week prior to the trip. What problems can be identified with this regimen? (EO-9)

11. What drug-drug interactions may occur while KT is taking bismuth subsalicylate? (EO-11)

12. What psychosocial factors may affect KT's adherence with both pharmacologic and nonpharmacologic therapy? (EO-15)

13. Evaluate the pharmacoeconomic considerations relative to KT's plan of care. (EO-17)

14. Summarize pathophysiologic, therapeutic, and disease management concepts for TD utilizing a key points format. (EO-18)

CASE 39
Valerie W. Hogue
Topic: Constipation

Level 3

EDUCATIONAL MATERIALS
Chapter 27: Constipation and Diarrhea (clinical presentation and diagnosis, bulk-forming agents, hyperosmotic agents, stool softeners, saline laxatives)

SCENARIO

Patient and Setting
DH, a 55-year-old male; walk-in clinic

Chief Complaint
Fatigue, weakness, and abdominal discomfort

History of Present Illness
Over the past 3 weeks experienced the passage of hard stools with straining; decreased bowel movements (2 × week); laxative use without relief of symptoms; antihypertensive medications recently changed

Past Medical History
Hypertension (HTN)

Chronic renal failure (CRF) on hemodialysis

Parkinson's disease

Benign prostatic hyperplasia (BPH)

Past Surgical History
None

Family/Social History
Family History: Mother, age 75 with HTN and CRF

Social History: Sedentary lifestyle; smokes 1/2 PPD

Medication History
Verapamil sustained release, 240 mg PO q AM

Furosemide, 40 mg PO BID

Levodopa/carbidopa 25 mg/100 mg sustained release, 1 tablet PO BID

Benztropine, 2 mg PO QHS

Aluminum hydroxide suspension, 2 tbsp PO TID

Sodium bicarbonate, 650 mg PO TID

Calcitriol, 0.5 μg PO QD

Magnesium sulfate salt, 1 tsp dissolved in 1/2 glass water PO PRN for constipation

Allergies
NKDA

Physical Examination
GEN: Pale male; appearing listless; with complaints of gastrointestinal discomfort

VS: BP 130/82, HR 62, T 37.6°C, RR 22, Wt 71 kg, Ht 177.8 cm

HEENT: Dry mucous membranes
  COR: WNL
CHEST: Clear to auscultation
  ABD: Tender, decreased bowel sounds
   GU: Soft, enlarged asymmetrical prostate gland
 RECT: Guaiac negative
  EXT: No edema
NEURO: Cranial nerves II-XII WNL, strength 5/5 bilaterally upper extremities, 5/5 lower extremities, gait with small steps and reduced arm swing, (+) slow, resting hand tremor, sensory intact, alert × 3

Results of Pertinent Laboratory Tests, Serum Drug Concentrations, and Diagnostic Tests

Na 142 (142)	Plts 180 × 10^9	T Bili 2.6 (0.15)
K 4.5 (4.5)	(180 × 10^3)	Glu 6.1 (110)
Cl 105 (105)	MCV 75 (75)	Ca 2.32 (9.3)
HCO$_3$ 24 (24)	MCH 24 (24)	PO$_4$ 122 (3.8)
BUN 17.1 (48)	MCHC 300 (30)	Mg 1.2 (2.4)
Cr 274 (3.1)	Retic 0.0005 (0.5)	Uric Acid 297 (5.0)
Hct 0.24 (24)	AST 0.47 (28)	Fe 7 (40)
Hgb 83 (8.3)	ALT 0.53 (32)	TIBC 81 (450)
Lkcs 4.5 × 10^9	LDH 1.2 (70)	Ferritin 9.0 (9.0)
(4.5 × 10^3)	Alk Phos 0.95 (57)	Folate 11 (5)
	Alb 45 (4.5)	B$_{12}$ 443 (600)

Diagnostic test: Barium enema, no obstruction

PROBLEM LIST

Identify principal problems from the scenario in priority order [completed Problem List and SOAP Note at end of casebook]

SOAP NOTE

To be completed by student

QUESTIONS

[Answers at end of casebook]

1. The primary cause of DH's episode of acute constipation: (EO-1)
   a. Age
   b. Change in antihypertensive medication to verapamil
   c. Use of magnesium sulfate salt
   d. Sedentary lifestyle

2. Which of the following diseases listed in DH's medical history probably contributed to the development of chronic constipation? (EO-1)
   a. Hypertension
   b. Chronic renal failure
   c. Parkinson's disease
   d. Benign prostatic hypertrophy

3. Saline laxatives would be appropriate for DH to use if he experiences: (EO-8)
   a. Hard, pellet-like stools
   b. Diarrhea
   c. Chronic constipation
   d. Fecal impaction

4. All of the following tests are important in the diagnosis of constipation *except:* (EO-5)
   a. Barium enema
   b. Stool guaiac
   c. Blood chemistry
   d. Abdominal examination

5. List pertinent information to discuss with DH regarding nonpharmacologic treatment of constipation. (EO-14)

6. It is important for DH to follow a dose of bulk-forming laxative with a glass of liquid to prevent: (EO-10)
   a. Aspiration of the psyllium husks
   b. Intestinal and esophageal obstruction
   c. Electrolyte imbalances in a patient with renal disease
   d. Rectal irritation and burning

7. DH should anticipate the laxative effects of the glycerin suppository to occur within: (EO-8)
   a. 15–30 minutes
   b. 24–48 hours
   c. 12–24 hours
   d. 2–3 days

8. All of the following are factors to consider when selecting laxative therapy for DH *except:* (EO-8)
   a. Description of symptoms
   b. Length of time DH experienced symptoms
   c. DH's normal bowel habits
   d. Gender

9. After 2 weeks of the current treatment, DH occasionally experienced constipation. He began taking bisacodyl 10 mg 1 tablet PO QHS for 2 weeks and subsequently noticed very loose stools. How should DH be advised on the use of this laxative? (EO-10, 14)

10. DH has been self-medicating with magnesium sulfate salt for the relief of constipation. What factor may predispose him to magnesium toxicity? (EO-4, 6, 8)
    a. Iron deficiency anemia
    b. Decreased bowel sounds
    c. Sodium bicarbonate
    d. Chronic renal failure

11. Describe the mechanism of action of recombinant erythropoietin therapy in DH for anemia of chronic renal failure. (EO-7)

12. What psychosocial issues may influence DH's ability to adhere to the nonpharmacologic and pharmacologic interventions for constipation? (EO-15)

13. What pharmacoeconomic issues should be considered regarding DH's plan of care? (EO-17)

14. Utilizing a key points format, summarize the definition, therapeutic, and disease management concepts for constipation. (EO-18)

CASE 40
Camille W. Thornton
Topic: Hepatitis: Drug-Induced
Level 3
EDUCATIONAL MATERIALS
Chapters 28: Hepatitis, Viral and Drug-Induced;
Chapter 2: Adverse Drug Reactions and
Drug-Induced Diseases

SCENARIO

Patient and Setting

SR, a 41-year-old male; emergency department

Chief Complaint

Semicomatose

History of Present Illness

Per report of wife, patient had an episode of hematemesis about 24 hours prior to admission and has remained asleep and unresponsive since that time; began taking wife's prescribed valproic acid 2 months ago secondary to recurring migraine headaches; has had no medications for the last 24 hours

Past Medical History

Type 2 Diabetes
Migraine headaches

Past Surgical History

None

Family/Social History

Family History: Unremarkable
Social History: Nonsmoker, nondrinker

Medication History

NPH insulin (human), 30 units SC QD

Valproic acid PO (dose not known)

Amitriptyline, 25 mg PO QHS (stopped taking due to no change in migraine frequency 2 months ago and began wife's valproic acid for prophylaxis of migraine headache)

Asprin, 650–1300 mg PO PRN

Allergies

NKDA

Physical Examination

GEN: Thin male with jaundice, semicomatose, responding only to noxious stimuli
VS: BP 110/60, HR 92, T 38.0°C, RR 16, Wt 59 kg, Ht 177.5 cm
HEENT: Semicomatose, pupils unequal, icterus in the sclera, dried blood around mouth and in throat
COR: Tachycardic, no S3 or S4, no murmurs
CHEST: WNL
ABD: Slightly rotund, responds to RUQ pressure, liver enlarged, + JVD
GU: Deferred
RECT: Guaiac negative
EXT: Reflexes equal but exaggerated, poor skin turgor, dry skin, + liver flap, pale nail beds
NEURO: Semicomatose, responds to pain

Results of Pertinent Laboratory Tests, Serum Drug Concentrations, and Diagnostic Tests

Na 142 (142)	RBC 4.3 × 10¹²	Alk Phos 1.8 (108)
K 4.6 (4.6)	(4.3 × 10⁶)	Alb 26 (2.6)
Cl 109 (109)	Lkcs 18 × 10⁹	T Bili 70.1 (4.1)
HCO₃ 22 (22)	(18 × 10³)	Glu 14 (252)
BUN 6.5 (18)	Plts 94 × 10⁹ (94 × 10³)	Ca 2.2 (4.4)
Cr 97 (1.1)	MCV 76 (76)	PO₄ 1.36 (4.2)
Ammonia 106	AST 7.1 (426)	PT 33.1
Hct 0.24 (24)	ALT 5.6 (336)	PTT 90
Hgb 98 (9.8)	LDH 3.8 (229)	INR 1.6

Lkc differential: segs 0.37, lymph 0.19, mono 0.3, eos 0.7

Toxicology screen: Negative for 27 drugs, including cocaine

Alcohol screen: Negative

Valproic acid: 305 μmol/liter (44 μg/mL)

Blood, urine, CSF cultures pending

Hepatitis screen: HBsAg (−), HBsAb (−), anti-HCV (−), HAV (−), anti-HAV (−)

Coffee ground-appearing material recovered via gastric suction

PROBLEM LIST

Identify principal problems from the scenario in priority order

SOAP NOTE

To be completed by student

QUESTIONS

1. Explain why this patient should or should not be fed orally. (EO-8)

2. What considerations are there for deciding the specific TPN formulation? (EO-8)

3. What was the purpose of thiamine and folic acid in this patient? (EO-7)

4. How could SR's compliance with insulin therapy be assessed? (EO-12)

5. The patient has a slightly rounded abdomen, which could have been ascites. If ascites were present, what treatment should be recommended? (EO-18)
   a. Furosemide 40 mg IV QD
   b. Hydrochlorothiazide 25 mg PO via NG tube QD
   c. Spironolactone 50 mg PO via NG tube QD
   d. Hydralazine 50 mg IV QD

6. All of the following are goals of treatment of drug-induced hepatitis *except:* (EO-12)
   a. Give immune suppressive drugs to slow hepatic damage
   b. Avoid agents known to cause hepatitis
   c. To detect drug-induced hepatitis early and discontinue the offending agent
   d. To avoid significant liver damage

7. Which of the following is *NOT* a sign or symptom of SR's hepatotoxicity? (EO-2)
   a. Jaundice
   b. Elevated liver enzymes
   c. Hepatotoxicity
   d. Rash

8. Which laboratory monitoring parameters would be most important to assess to evaluate SR's liver function from valproic acid-induced hepatotoxicity? (EO-5)
   a. INR, PT, Alk Phos, AST
   b. AST, ALT, INR, bilirubin
   c. AST, LDH, INR, Alk Phos
   d. AST, ALT, Alk Phos, bilirubin

9. Which of the following medications is effective for the prophylaxis of migraine headaches? (EO-5)
   a. Atenolol
   b. Tramadol
   c. Sumatriptan
   d. Ketorolac

10. SR is released from the hospital and comes to the family medicine clinic for follow-up. At the time he is noted to have hemoglobin A_{1C} of 11.2. Which of the following would *not* be an appropriate intervention? (EO-11)
    a. Educate on proper diet and exercise and reevaluate at next visit.
    b. Change regimen to NPH 15 units SC and regular 5 units SC q AM and NPH 15 units SC and regular 3 units SC q PM and reevaluate at next visit. Provide hypoglycemic counseling.

    c. Continue current therapy; it is too soon after his acute drug-induced hepatitis to make an evaluation.
    d. Instruct on blood glucose monitoring, encourage keeping a journal, and instruct to bring the journal to clinic appointments.

11. SR most likely has which type of drug induced hepatitis? (EO-1)
    a. Nonspecific hepatitis, characterized by focal hepatocellular necrosis with a mononuclear infiltrate and variable amounts of portal inflammation.
    b. Viral-like hepatitis, characterized by an inflammatory infiltrate, variable amounts of hepatocyte necrosis, bile stasis, and lobular disarray.
    c. Granulomatous hepatitis, characterized by aggregates of epithelioid histiocytes with variable types and amounts of inflammatory cells.
    d. Autoimmune-like hepatitis characterized by a hepatitis with positive antinuclear antibodies.

12. This patient should be educated concerning all of the following pertinent items concerning his current medical history *except:* (EO-14)
    a. How to dose insulin on sick days
    b. To discard all medications that are not currently a part of the patient's drug therapy
    c. The importance of only taking medications that are prescribed to you
    d. To report any signs and symptoms of chest pain

13. Summarize pathophysiologic, therapeutic, and disease-management concepts for drug-induced hepatitis utilizing a key points format. (EO-18)

CASE 41
Camille W. Thornton
Topic: Cirrhosis
 Level 2
EDUCATIONAL MATERIALS
Chapter 29: Cirrhosis

SCENARIO

Patient and Setting

ST, a 52-year-old female; emergency department

Chief Complaint

2 episodes of vomiting bright red blood this morning and has experienced mental status changes throughout the day

History of Present Illness

Has been complaining of increased nausea and abdominal pain over the past 2 weeks per report of husband; has also had 4 bloody stools during the past 2 weeks; began exhibiting mental confusion early this morning after vomiting bright red blood; mental confusion has gotten progressively worse

Past Medical History

Cirrhosis (diagnosed 5 years ago)

Ascites

Alcoholic (drank for 30 years, stopped drinking 5 years ago)

Family/Social History

Family History: Mother has Type 2 diabetes, father died of MI at age 42

Social History: Stopped drinking 5 years ago, nonsmoker

Medication History

Spironolactone, 50 mg PO QD

Conjugated estrogen, 0.625 mg PO QD

Medroxyprogesterone, 2.5 mg PO QD

Allergies

NKDA

Physical Examination

GEN: Semi-comatose female, slightly protuberant abdomen, thin extremities

VS: BP 124/80 supine, 108/60 sitting, HR 88 supine, 110 sitting, + tilt test, T 37.0°C, RR 20, Wt 61 kg, Ht 163 cm

HEENT: Nystagmus, foul breath with possible fetor hepaticus

COR: RRR, no gallops, no rubs

CHEST: Clear to auscultation and percussion

ABD: Slightly increased girth, + hepatomegaly, + fluid wave, spider angiomas

RECT: Heme +

EXT: Muscle wasting in arms and legs, + nail clubbing, + palmar erythema, little to no hair on extremities, no peripheral edema

NEURO: Liver flap in both hands (asterixis), oriented to person only

Results of Pertinent Laboratory Tests, Serum Drug Concentrations, and Diagnostic Tests

Na 132 (132)	Hgb 90 (9)	Alk Phos 2.0 (120)
K 5.2 (5.2)	Lkcs 9.8 × 10⁹	T Bili 87 (5.1)
Cl 100 (100)	(9.8 × 10³)	Protein 54 (5.4)
HCO₃ 23 (23)	Plts 50 × 10⁹	Ca 2.24 (9.0)
BUN 2.9 (8)	(50 × 10³)	Alb 24 (2.4)
Cr 71 (0.8)	MCV 90 (90)	PO₄ 1.4 (4.3)
Glu 6.6 (120)	AST 3.2 (189)	Mg 0.7 (1.4)
Hct 0.27 (27)	ALT 0.55 (33)	

Ammonia 88 (150)

INR 1.4, PT 18 seconds (control 11 seconds)

WBC differential: WNL

Urinalysis: WNL

Chest radiography: Heart and lungs normal

Endoscopy: Shows actively bleeding esophageal varices

PROBLEM LIST

Identify principal problems from the scenario in priority order [completed Problem List and SOAP Note at end of casebook

SOAP NOTE

To be completed by student

QUESTIONS

[*Answers at end of casebook*]

1. ST presents with all of the following signs and symptoms of hepatic encephalopathy *except:* (EO-2)
   a. Asterixis
   b. Mental confusion
   c. Fetor hepaticus
   d. Vomiting

2. The probable cause of ST's hepatic encephalopathy is: (EO-5)
   a. Bleeding into the GI tract
   b. Ascites
   c. NSAID use
   d. Malnutrition

3. Explain the ammonia and branched chain amino acids theory in relation to the pathogenesis of hepatic encephalopathy. (EO-1)

4. After 48 hours, ST remains in a semiconscious state. Her ammonia levels are falling but it appears it will be another 4–5 days before she will be able to be fed orally. What type of nutrition should be given and how much should ST receive? How should she be monitored? (EO-5, 6, 8)

5. Which of the following is not a sign or symptom of cirrhosis exhibited by ST? (EO-2)
   a. Fetor hepaticus
   b. Palmar erythema
   c. Chest pain
   d. Spider angiomas

6. Three months later, ST presents with fever, chills, vomiting, abdominal pain, and tenderness. A paracentesis is performed, and the culture reveals PMN cell counts of 300/mm³. A diagnosis of spontaneous bacterial peritonitis (SBP) is made. What is the most likely pathogen? (EO-5)
   a. Anaerobes
   b. Gram-negative bacilli
   c. *Pseudomonas aeruginosa*
   d. *Staphylococcus aureus*

7. ST is treated with a 5-day course of cefotaxime 2 mg IV q8h.

It is decided to start a prophylactic agent. Of the following, which would be the best choice? (EO-8)
   a. Ciprofloxacin 750 mg PO every Monday
   b. Erythromycin 500 mg PO BID
   c. Azithromycin 1 g PO every Monday
   d. Doxycycline 100 mg PO BID

8. Describe the mechanisms of action of the pharmacologic and nonpharmacologic interventions used in this case. (EO-11)

9. List interventions (pharmacologic and nonpharmacologic) that, if complied with, can be expected to decrease hospital admissions and increase survival in patients with cirrhosis. (EO-14, 15)

10. All of the following are true about spironolactone *except:* (EO-10)
   a. It is a gentle, slow-acting diuretic allowing a slow diuresis
   b. It antagonizes the effects of hyperaldosteronism that exist in many of these patients
   c. It can increase potassium levels
   d. It should be dosed BID to TID

11. Vasopressin, a natural hormone also known as antidiuretic hormone, is sometimes used before sclerotherapy of bleeding varices. Which of the following is not true concerning vasopressin? (EO-10)
   a. It significantly decreases portal blood flow and pressure by constricting portal and other splanchnic arterioles. This slows or stops bleeding long enough to allow thrombus formation at the site of the bleeding.
   b. The intense vasoconstrictor action decreases cardiac output and may cause coronary ischemia.
   c. Tachycardia due to inhibition of the vagus nerve is the most commonly observed side effect.
   d. Bradycardia due to stimulation of the vagus nerve is the most commonly observed side effect.

12. An alternative to lactulose for the treatment of hepatic encephalopathy is neomycin. All of the following are true concerning neomycin *except:* (EO-10)
   a. Diarrhea is uncommon with neomycin
   b. It destroys colonic bacteria, slowing the degradation of protein to ammonia
   c. Ototoxicity has been reported in patients on chronic oral neomycin therapy
   d. Neomycin has been implicated in development of hepatorenal syndrome

13. What psychosocial factors should be considered when managing an alcoholic patient? (EO-15)

14. Summarize pathophysiologic, therapeutic, and disease-management concepts for cirrhosis utilizing a key points format. (EO-18)

CASE 42
Camille W. Thornton
Topic: Hepatitis: Viral
Level 1
EDUCATIONAL MATERIALS
Chapter 28: Hepatitis, Viral and Drug-Induced

SCENARIO

Patient and Setting
CB, a 42-year-old female; office visit

Chief Complaint
Right upper quadrant pain, fatigue, anorexia, N/V

History of Present Illness
Feeling progressively worse for about a year; only mentioned this to physician 1 month ago; full hepatitis panel done; found to be positive for anti-HCV by ELISA-2 and RIBA confirmatory tests; has lost 9 kg (20 lb) over the last year.

Past Medical History
Depression
Hypertension

Family/Social History
Family History: Unknown
Social History: IV drug use for 15 years (has been drug free for the past 10 years); alcohol use for 20 years (has not drunk for the past 5 years); nonsmoker and lives with her husband of 20 years and 2 teenage children

Medication History
Sertraline, 50 mg PO QD
HCTZ, 25 mg PO QD

Allergies
Penicillin

Physical Examination
   GEN: Well-developed, slightly underweight female
     VS: BP 132/82, HR 72, T 37°C, RR 21, Wt 50 kg, HT 160 cm
   HEENT: WNL
     COR: WNL
   CHEST: WNL
     ABD: Right upper quadrant pain,–JVD,–ascites,
     GU: No assessment
   RECT: Deferred
     EXT: Unremarkable
   NEURO: Alert and oriented × 4

Results of Pertinent Laboratory Tests, Serum Drug Concentrations, and Diagnostic Tests

Na 140 (140)
K 4.0 (4.0)
Cl 99 (99)
HCO_3 26 (26)
BUN 5.7 (16)
Cr 88.4 (1.0)
Glu 5.5 (100)
Uric Acid 190 (3.2)
Hct 0.35 (35)
Hgb 160 (16)

Lkcs 6.1×10^9
   (6.1×10^3)
Plts 250×10^9
   (250×10^3)
MCV 84 (84)
AST 1.63 (98)
ALT 1.87 (112)
LDH 1.7 (100)
Alk Phos 1.9 (118)
Alb 40 (4.0)

T Bili 15.4 (0.9)
PT 12 (12)
INR 1.1 (1.1)
Ca 1.15 (4.6)
PO_4 1.29 (4.0)
Mg 1.0 (2.0)
TSH 4.2 (4.2)
FT_4 20.6 (1.6)

HCV RNA: 585,000 copies/mL

Hepatitis C genotype: 1

ANA negative

Pregnancy test: negative

Lkc differential: WNL

HIV: negative

HBsAg: negative

Alpha-fetoprotein: 10 (10)

Liver biopsy: bridging fibrosis and moderate degrees of inflammation and necrosis

PROBLEM LIST

Identify principal problem(s) from the scenario in priority order [completed Problem List and SOAP Note at end of casebook]

SOAP NOTE

To be completed by student

QUESTIONS

[Answers at end of casebook]

1. List 6 side effects of interferon. (EO-10)

2. Which of the following is a side effect of ribavirin that requires monitoring at every patient visit? (EO-10)
   a. Anemia (hemolysis)
   b. Hypertension
   c. Depression
   d. Pulmonary fibrosis

3. Discuss the assessment required for determining the response to therapy. (EO-5)

4. Discuss thyroid disorder and depression in relation to treatment with interferon. (EO-4)

5. Which of the following is not a predictor of response to combination therapy? (EO-4)
   a. Absence of decompensated liver disease
   b. Hepatitis C genotype 2 or 3
   c. High iron in liver
   d. Low serum HCV RNA levels (<100,000 copies/mL)

6. Which of the following is not a treatment goal for viral hepatitis? (EO-14)
   a. Improve or normalize serum aminotransferases
   b. Prevent progression of hepatic disease
   c. Clear the virus as measured by polymerase chain reaction
   d. Restore lost hepatic function

7. Hepatitis A is mainly transmitted through: (EO-1)
   a. The parenteral route
   b. The fecal/oral route
   c. Sexual contact
   d. Insect vectors

8. All of the following are true concerning hepatitis B *except:* (EO-1)
   a. Anti-HBe positive is the lab test that confirms the presence of hepatitis B
   b. It is a DNA virus
   c. It is transmitted mainly through parenteral and sexual exposure
   d. 5–10% of infected adult individuals will become chronically infected with hepatitis B

9. What psychosocial issues pertain to patients with chronic hepatitis B and C? (EO-15)

10. All of the following are acceptable treatments for hepatitis B *except:* (EO-11)
    a. Interferon alfa-2b 5 million IU SC QD for 4 months
    b. Interferon alfa-2b 10 million IU SC 3/week for 4 months
    c. Interferon alfa-2b 5 million IU SC QD and 100 mg PO BID for 4 months
    d. Lamivudine 100 mg PO QD for 1 year

11. During the third month of treatment, CB experiences a decrease in leukocytes to 1.4×10^9 (1.4×10^3) and platelets to 50×10^9 (50×10^3). Which of the following is the most reasonable action? (EO-11)
    a. Advise to continue therapy. Tell patient to report any fevers or infection immediately. Check again in 2 weeks.
    b. Decrease ribavirin to 300 mg PO BID, and decrease interferon to 1.5 million units SC 3 times a week. Tell patient to report any fevers or infection immediately. Check again at next month's appointment.
    c. Just decrease the interferon, it is the most likely cause of this decrease in leukocytes and platelets.
    d. Hold both medications until lab values increase to baseline levels.

12. All of the following are true about hepatitis C *except:* (EO-1)
    a. A vaccine is available
    b. It is a RNA virus
    c. 85% of patients become chronically infected
    d. It is mainly transmitted through the parenteral route

13. Summarize pathophysiologic, therapeutic, and disease-management concepts for viral hepatitis utilizing a key points format. (EO-18)

CASE 43
Camille W. Thornton
Topic: Pancreatitis
Level 2
EDUCATIONAL MATERIALS
Chapter 30: Pancreatitis

SCENARIO

Patient and Setting

JG, a 59-year-old male; emergency department

Chief Complaint

Abdominal pain, radiating to the back; nausea and vomiting; gets some relief by sitting and leaning forward

History of Present Illness

Alcoholic binge beginning 2 days ago because of problems at work; awoke this morning with the above complaints that have continued throughout the day; for the last 6 months has had intermittent abdominal pain and diarrhea which is worse after eating

Past Medical History

Type 1 diabetes (10 years)

Chronic pancreatitis (10 years)

Chronic diarrhea and abdominal pain that worsens with meals

9.1 kg (20 lb) weight loss in the last 6 months

Alcohol abuse

Family/Social History

Family History: Unknown

Social History: Alcohol: 1–2 quarts of beer daily and occasional binges with scotch

Medication History

NPH insulin, 15 units SC 8 AM and 6 PM

Regular insulin, 5 units SC 8 AM and 6 PM

Pancrelipase, 2 tabs PO TID AC

Cimetidine, 400 mg PO BID

Allergies

NKDA

Physical Examination

GEN: Disheveled, thin-appearing male
VS: BP 110/70, HR 116-regular, T 38.0°C, RR 20, Wt 80 kg (89 kg 6 months ago), Ht 182 cm
HEENT: Anicteric sclera, poor dentition
COR: RRR
CHEST: Clear to auscultation and percussion
ABD: Midepigastric pain radiating to the back, (−) bowel sounds
RECT: Guaiac negative
EXT: Ulcer L foot
NEURO: Uncooperative

Results of Pertinent Laboratory Tests, Serum Drug Concentrations, and Diagnostic Tests

Na 133 (133)	Lkcs 10 × 10⁹	Alk Phos 3.67 (220)
K 3.4 (3.4)	(10 × 10³)	Alb 19 (1.9)
Cl 104 (104)	Plts 250 × 10⁹	T Bili 25.65 (1.5)
HCO₃ 20 (20)	(250 × 10³)	Trig 3.23 (286)
BUN 6.5 (18)	MCV 91 (91)	Mg 0.86 (2.1)
Cr 132 (1.5)	Amylase 6.52 (370)	Ca 1.62 (6.5)
Glu 15 (270)	Lipase 166.7 (10,000)	PO₄ 1.13 (3.5)
Hct 0.36 (36)	AST 3.17 (190)	
Hgb 108 (10.8)	ALT 0.58 (35)	

Lkc differential: WNL

Abdominal x-ray: Nonspecific air fluid levels in large and small bowel suggestive of an ileus; calcifications in pancreas also noted

PROBLEM LIST

Identify principal problems from the scenario in priority order

SOAP NOTE

To be completed by student

QUESTIONS

1. JG's serum calcium level is below normal. What ionized (free) level does his calcium level represent? Is the ionized level normal or abnormal? (EO-6)

2. Three days after admission, JG has a serum potassium level of 6.5 mmol/L (6.5 mEq/L) with peaked T waves on ECG. What treatment would you recommend for his condition? (EO-5)

3. Following discharge, JG still complains of diarrhea and foul-smelling, oily stools. His abdominal pain continues to worsen with food. How would you adjust JG's therapy for chronic pancreatitis to lessen his symptoms? (EO-12)

4. What is the theoretical reason meperidine might be the opioid of choice for pain in the setting of acute pancreatitis? (EO-8)

5. Which of the following is not a common cause of chronic pancreatitis? (EO-1)
   a. Alcohol
   b. Hypertriglyceridemia
   c. Cystic fibrosis
   d. Graves' disease

6. Which drug is associated with acute pancreatitis? (EO-1)
   a. Theophylline
   b. Didanosine
   c. Amphotericin B
   d. Digoxin

7. JG exhibited all of the following complications of acute pancreatitis *except:* (EO-2)
   a. Renal failure
   b. Hypocalcemia
   c. Hyperglycemia
   d. Ileus

8. Cimetidine was most likely included in this patient's medication regimen to: (EO-6)
   a. Treat the PUD
   b. Increase absorption of oral pancreatic enzymes
   c. Treat the GERD
   d. Treat the chronic abdominal pain

9. A majority of patients (80%) who develop acute pancreatitis will have interstitial pancreatitis as opposed to necrotizing pancreatitis. All of the following statements are true concerning interstitial pancreatitis *except:* (EO-1, 2)
   a. Mortality associated with interstitial pancreatitis is less than 2%
   b. It is characterized by interstitial edema with or without mild peripancreatic fat necrosis
   c. Interstitial pancreatitis may be associated with serious systemic toxicity, but its clinical course is usually mild with minimal organ dysfunction
   d. No treatment or monitoring is generally needed with interstitial pancreatitis

10. Which of the following is not a reason for JG to be a candidate for TPN? (EO-11)
    a. Severe preexisting malnutrition
    b. JG is an alcoholic
    c. Extended need for NPO status for bowel rest
    d. No bowel sounds and the presence of an ileus

11. Which of the following is not a treatment goal in acute pancreatitis? (EO-8)
    a. Pancreatic enzyme replacement
    b. Correction of intravascular volume and electrolyte loss with aggressive fluid resuscitation
    c. Relief of pain with parenteral analgesia
    d. Nutritional support when oral intake is suspended for an extended time to minimize pancreatic exocrine secretion

12. Which of the following is not an exocrine function of the pancreas? (EO-1)
    a. Secretion of digestive enzymes
    b. Secretion of sodium and potassium
    c. Pancreatic enzyme replacement
    d. Secretion of bicarbonate and chloride

13. Summarize pathophysiologic, therapeutic, and disease-management concepts for pancreatitis utilizing a key points format. (EO-18)

CASE 44
Lori N. Justice
Topic: Rheumatoid Arthritis
Level 2
EDUCATIONAL MATERIALS
Chapter 31: Rheumatoid Arthritis (etiology, anatomy and physiology, pathogenesis; diagnosis and clinical findings, treatment)

SCENARIO

Patient and Setting

BN, 62-year-old female; hospital, internal medicine floor

Chief Complaint

Acute pain in the low back and left hip region

History of Present Illness

Acute lower back and left hip pain began after falling from a standing position 2 days ago

Past Medical History

Osteoporosis × 2 years; rheumatoid arthritis (RA) for 5 years (Class II functional class, steroid dependent × 3 years, no previous treatment with DMARDS); carpal tunnel syndrome of right upper extremity; history of peptic ulcer disease (PUD); chronic active hepatitis B detected 3 months PTA; menopause at age 55

Family/Social History

Family History: Breast cancer in mother and one sister
Social History: Drinks 2 cups of coffee each morning

Medication History

Acetaminophen, 2 × 500 mg PO QID PRN arthritis pain (previous therapy with full-dose aspirin, ibuprofen, and piroxicam discontinued due to GI upset; naproxen discontinued after guaiac-positive stool; indomethacin SR discontinued due to dizziness and confusion)

Cimetidine, 400 mg PO BID for several years (adherence related to GI symptoms)

Prednisone, up to 40 mg/day; 10 mg PO BID for past 6 months (makes her "feel better")

Calcium carbonate chewable tablets, 500 mg 1 BID

Allergies

NKDA

Physical Examination

GEN: Pale woman of Scandinavian descent with truncal obesity, appearing tired
VS: BP 128/84, HR 70, RR 20, T 37.2°C, Wt 61 kg, Ht 5′3″
HEENT: Pale mucous membranes; moon facies
COR: RRR
CHEST: Clear to auscultation and percussion
ABD: Right upper quadrant (RUQ) pain; liver nonpalpable; striae
GU: Atrophy of urogenital area
RECT: WNL; guaiac negative
EXT: Ecchymoses on both arms; MCP and PIP tender and swollen
NEURO: MS WNL; proximal muscle weakness in both legs

Results of Pertinent Laboratory Tests, Serum Drug Concentrations, and Diagnostic Tests

Na 139 (139)	LDH 6.00 (360)	Plts 240 × 10^9 (240 × 10^3)
K 3.2 (3.2)	Mg 0.74 (1.8)	Glu 6.1 (110)
Cl 101 (101)	MCV 76 (76)	Ca 2.10 (8.4)
Alk Phos 1.0 (60)	AST 8.00 (480)	HCO$_3$ 25 (25)
BUN 5.4 (15)	ALT 8.66 (520)	Uric Acid 178 (3.0)
Lkcs 14.1 × 10^9	PO$_4$ 1.61 (5.0)	T Bili 8.6 (0.5)
(14.1 × 10^3)	Alb 3.1 (3.1)	PT 11.6 (11.6)
Hct 0.35 (35)	Cr 71 (0.8)	INR 1.2 (1.2)
Hgb 140 (14.0)		

Lkc differential: PMN 72, lymph 15, mono 9, eos 0, baso 1, bands 3

HBsAg-positive

Rheumatoid factor titer of 1:65

ECG: NSR

X-ray films: L2-L4 anterior wedge compression fractures; simple fracture of left femoral neck; decreased opacity suggestive of osteoporosis

Muscle biopsy of vastus lateralis: Selective atrophy of type II muscle fibers

PROBLEM LIST

Identify principal problems from the scenario in priority order

SOAP NOTE

To be completed by student

QUESTIONS

1. BN presents with all of the following criteria for rheumatoid arthritis *except:* (EO-2)
   a. Positive rheumatoid factor
   b. Soft tissue swelling in the hand joints
   c. Rheumatoid nodules
   d. Symmetric arthritis in PIP and MCP

2. BN's rheumatoid arthritis is described as Functional Class II. Which of the following best describes this functional class? (EO-2)
   a. Unable to perform self-care
   b. Moderate restrictions but able to do normal activities
   c. Ability to perform daily living activities without restriction
   d. Major restriction in performing self-care activities

3. BN's laboratory analysis revealed a rheumatoid factor titer at 1:650. At what titer is rheumatoid factor generally considered positive? (EO-5)
   a. ≥1:22
   b. ≥1:32
   c. ≥1:52
   d. ≥1:62

4. Which of the following extra-articular features of rheumatoid arthritis is present in BN? (EO-2, 5)
   a. Vasculitis
   b. Rheumatoid nodules
   c. Keratoconjunctivitis
   d. Carpal tunnel syndrome

5. What are the goals of therapy for BN's rheumatoid arthritis? (EO-8)

6. First-line nonpharmacologic therapy for treatment of RA in BN should include all of the following *except:* (EO-8)
   a. Rest
   b. Exercise
   c. Appropriate diet
   d. Surgical intervention

7. List the factors that contributed to the development of osteoporosis in BN. (EO-8, 10, 11)

8. Which of the following laboratory abnormalities is a result of BN's prednisone therapy? (EO-10)
   a. Hypokalemia
   b. Positive rheumatoid factor
   c. Hypoglycemia
   d. Positive HBsAg

9. Which of the following best describes the rationale behind using misoprostol in combination with an NSAID for treating RA in BN? (EO-7, 12)
   a. Prevention of *Helicobacter pylori* infection
   b. Protection against gastric duodenal ulceration with chronic NSAID use
   c. Prevention of gastrointestinal cramping and diarrhea associated with NSAID use
   d. Provision of convenient drug administration method

10. Which of the following antirheumatic agents may be a good choice for BN, considering its lack of hepatotoxic effects? (EO-12)

    a. Methotrexate
    b. Hydroxychloroquine
    c. Leflunomide
    d. Azathioprine

11. What psychosocial factors might negatively affect BN's perception relative to her RA? (EO-15)

12. Evaluate the pharmacoeconomic considerations associated with BN's plan of care. (EO-17)

13. Summarize pathophysiologic, therapeutic, and disease management concepts for rheumatoid arthritis utilizing a key points format. (EO-18)

CASE 45
Lori N. Justice
Topic: Rheumatoid Arthritis (RA)

EDUCATIONAL MATERIALS
Chapter 31: Rheumatic Arthritis (etiology, pathogenesis, diagnosis and clinical findings, treatment)

SCENARIO

Patient and Setting

CJ, 70-year-old female; follow-up at outpatient clinic

Chief Complaint

Fatigue, diarrhea, dry mouth, early morning stiffness, swelling of hands, elbows, and knees, nightly heartburn

History of Present Illness

Experiencing 3–4 bowel movements daily, baseline change which occurred shortly after increase in RA therapy from 6 mg/day to 9 mg/day 2 weeks ago; fatigue, early morning stiffness, and swelling of hands, elbows, and knees worsened over past 2–3 months

Past Medical History

RA for 10 years; admitted to hospital with diagnosis of deep vein thrombosis (DVT) 2 months ago; gastroesophageal reflux disease (GERD) for past 5 years; hypothyroidism for 12 years; menopause at age 50

Past Surgical History

No major surgeries

Family/Social History

Family History: Widowed, lives with sister who assists her with activities of daily living

Social History: Drinks 1–2 glasses of wine almost every day; smokes 1 PPD × 50 years

Medication History

Auranofin, 9 mg PO QD, increased from 6 mg/day 2 weeks ago after 3 months of treatment (previous therapy with injectable gold salts resulted in some permanent decrease in disease, but stopped by patient choice 3 years ago; trials with penicillamine and hydroxychloroquine stopped due to adverse effects)

Piroxicam, 10 mg PO QD (previous treatment failures with aspirin, ibuprofen, and naproxen at maximum doses)

Warfarin, 5 mg PO QD

Levothyroxine, 0.1 mg PO QD

Antacid containing magnesium hydroxide 200 mg/aluminum hydroxide 225 mg PO PRN heartburn

Allergies

NKDA

Physical Examination

GEN: Obese, elderly woman appearing pale and tired
VS: BP 110/70 (supine), 90/60 (sitting), HR 84 (supine), 112 (sitting), RR 16, T 37.0°C, Wt 80 kg (Wt 2 months ago: 79 kg), Ht 150 cm
HEENT: PERRLA, EOMI
COR: RRR
CHEST: Normal breath sounds throughout
ABD: Obese, soft; without guarding or pain
GU: Deferred
RECT: Guaiac negative
EXT: Swelling and tenderness in joints of the hands and elbows, with tenderness in the knees; major restriction in performing work or self-care activities
NEURO: No abnormalities in deep tendon reflexes (DTRs) or cranial nerves

Results of Pertinent Laboratory Tests, Serum Drug Concentrations, and Diagnostic Tests

Na 142 (142)	Lkcs 8.2 × 10⁹	Alk Phos 1.5 (87)
K 4.1 (4.1)	(8.2 × 10³)	Alb 40 (4.0)
Cl 104 (104)	Plts 440 × 10⁹	T Bili 15 (0.9)
HCO₃ 23 (23)	(440 × 10³)	INR 2.3
BUN 8.9 (25)	MCV 84 (84)	Ca 2.2 (8.9)
AST 0.35 (21)	Glu 6.2 (111)	PO₄ 0.9 (2.8)
Hct 0.30 (30)	ALT 0.20 (12)	Mg 1.0 (2.0)
Hgb 120 (12.0)	LDH 2.0 (120)	Urate 120 (2.0)
		Cr 115 (1.3)

WBC differential: PMN 72, lymph 26, mono 1, eos 1, FE 4.5 (25), TIBC 43 (240), ferritin 205

Peripheral blood smear: RBC morphology: normochromic

Urinalysis: pH 7.2, specific gravity 1.031, RBCs 0–2/hpf, dip negative

Chest x-ray films: Not performed

ECG: Not performed

PROBLEM LIST

Identify principal problems from the scenario in priority order [completed Problem List and SOAP Note at end of casebook]

SOAP NOTE

To be completed by student

QUESTIONS

[Answers at end of casebook]

1. Which of the following factors has been shown to be at increased levels in the blood, synovial fluid, and synovial tissue in patients with rheumatoid arthritis and may correlate with disease activity? (EO-1)
   a. Substance P
   b. TNF-alpha
   c. PGE₂
   d. IFN-gamma

2. All of the following signs or symptoms of rheumatoid arthritis are present in CJ *except:* (EO-2)
   a. Morning stiffness
   b. Fatigue
   c. Ulnar deviation
   d. Swollen joints

3. Which of the following symptoms of dehydration might also occur if CJ developed the extra-articular manifestation of secondary Sjogren's syndrome? (EO-2)
   a. Dry mouth
   b. Hypotension
   c. Tachycardia
   d. Diarrhea

4. Which of the following functional classes best describes CJ's ability to perform daily living activities? (EO-2, 5)
   a. Class I
   b. Class II
   c. Class III
   d. Class IV

5. Which of the following laboratory abnormalities represents ongoing inflammation in CJ's case? (EO-5)
   a. Elevated platelet count
   b. BUN:Cr ratio
   c. Elevated serum sodium
   d. Normal MCV

6. Which of the following is true regarding nutrition in rheumatoid arthritis patients such as CJ? (EO-7, 8)
   a. Protein intake should be minimized to avoid enhancement of muscle mass
   b. Alpha-linoleic acid supplementation, a precursor of omega-3 fatty acids found in flaxseed oil, provides sufficient relief in RA to discontinue other therapy
   c. Vitamin E supplementation provides a small amount of pain relief in RA that is additive to anti-inflammatory drug effects
   d. Altering the fatty acid precursors of prostanoids and leukotrienes through vegetarian and elemental diets have shown no benefits at all

7. All of the following psychological manifestations are common in patients with RA *except:* (EO-8, 15)
   a. Anxiety
   b. Depression
   c. Insomnia
   d. Schizophrenia

8. CJ was treated with auranofin for over 3 months. All of the following should have been monitored in CJ every 2–4 weeks during therapy to avoid/detect adverse effects *except:* (EO-10)
   a. Complete blood count
   b. Urinalysis
   c. Mucous membranes
   d. Symptoms of constipation

9. If methotrexate therapy (5 mg PO 1 × week) is initiated in CJ, what baseline laboratory assessments should be performed? (EO-8, 10)

10. Which factors present in CJ's case may increase her risk for methotrexate-induced pulmonary toxicity? (EO-8, 10)

11. What signs and symptoms might indicate methotrexate-induced lung toxicity? (EO-8, 10)

12. CJ's primary care physician inquires about a potential drug-drug interaction between NSAIDs and methotrexate. Should CJ's NSAID be discontinued? Explain. (EO-9)

13. Evaluate the pharmacoeconomic considerations relative to CJ's plan of care. (EO-17)

14. Summarize the pathophysiologic, therapeutic, and disease management concepts for rheumatoid arthritis utilizing a key points format. (EO-18)

CASE 46
Lori N. Justice
Topic: Osteoarthritis (OA)

EDUCATIONAL MATERIALS
Chapter 32: Osteoarthritis (treatment goals, predisposing factors, clinical presentation and diagnosis, psychosocial, therapeutic plan, treatment, pharmacoeconomics)

SCENARIO

Patient and Setting
VB, 72-year-old female; general medicine clinic

Chief Complaint
Nausea, right upper quadrant abdominal pain, and aching pain in left knee

History of Present Illness
Intermittent relief of osteoarthritis (OA) with PRN acetaminophen, ibuprofen; orthopedic surgeon prescribed 7-day supply of propoxyphene napsylate/acetaminophen (100/650 mg) for recent increase in pain level 6 weeks ago; VB did not return for reevaluation as directed and obtained additional courses of propoxyphene napsylate/acetaminophen from internist, dentist, outpatient emergency center over past few weeks; recent increase in activity (weekly bowling, ballroom dance lessons), takes extra propoxyphene napsylate/acetaminophen after activities; new-onset joint swelling in past week; difficulty sleeping, increased irritability ("snapping" at family members often) for 6 weeks

Past Medical History
OA/degenerative joint disease (DJD) for 20 years; difficulty falling asleep for approximately 3 years (time of husband's death)

Past Surgical History
Right knee replacement 1 year ago (left knee replacement recommended, VB reluctant)

Social History
Family History: Lives alone, performs weight bearing tasks regularly; refuses family assistance with chores; eats "fast food" 4–5 times/week

Social History: No tobacco use; drinks caffeinated tea daily and 2 glasses sherry/night to fall asleep

Medication History
Acetaminophen, 325 mg PO q6h PRN pain × 15 years

Ibuprofen, 200 mg PO q6h PRN pain, occasionally × 2 years

Acetaminophen 650 mg/propoxyphene napsylate 100 mg, 1 tab PO q4h PRN pain (per physician order) and 2 tabs PO PRN severe pain (self-initiated); 6 to 8 tablets daily × 6 weeks

Triazolam, 0.0625 to 0.125 mg PO QHS PRN for sleep × 3 years

Allergies

NKDA

Physical Examination

GEN: Elderly, fairly obese woman in moderate distress

VS: BP 140/80, HR 85, RR 20, T 37.0°C, Wt 60 kg, Ht 153 cm

HEENT: WNL

COR: WNL

CHEST: WNL

ABD: RUQ tenderness; mild guarding; moderately obese

GU: Deferred

RECT: Deferred

EXT: Limited range of motion of left knee with mild swelling, tenderness, warmth

NEURO: Alert, O × 3

Results of Pertinent Laboratory Tests, Serum Drug Concentrations, and Diagnostic Tests

Na 140 (140)	WBC 8.5 × 10⁹	Alk Phos 3 (200)
K 3.9 (3.9)	(8.5 × 10³)	Alb 33 (3.3)
Cl 103 (103)	Plts 180 × 10⁹	T Bili 17.1 (1.0)
HCO₃ 27 (27)	(180 × 10³)	Glu 7.8 (140)
BUN 10.4 (29)	MCV 91 (91)	Ca 2.2 (8.9)
ESR 15 (15)	Cr 88.4 (1.0)	PO₄ 1.19 (3.7)
Hct 0.36 (36)	AST 6 (360)	Mg 1.0 (2.0)
Hgb 120 (12)	ALT 4.7 (180)	PT/PTT 11.2 (28.7)

X-ray: Joint-space narrowing, left knee

PROBLEM LIST

Identify principal problems from the scenario in priority order

SOAP NOTE

To be completed by student

QUESTIONS

1. The most likely cause for VB's worsening pain associated with osteoarthritis: (EO-1)
   a. Use of propoxyphene/acetaminophen for pain
   b. Frequent heavy, weight-bearing activities such as mowing the lawn, bowling, and vacuuming
   c. Use of ibuprofen PRN
   d. Elevated liver function tests

2. VB presents with many signs and symptoms of osteoarthritis. Which of the following is *not* present? (EO-2)
   a. Joint stiffness
   b. Crepitus
   c. Joint deformity
   d. Joint space narrowing on radiograph

3. List potential causes for VB's chronic insomnia. (EO-1)

4. What psychosocial factors may adversely influence VB's perception of the pain and disability associated with osteoarthritis? (EO-15)

5. VB is experiencing right upper quadrant abdominal pain. Results of VB's laboratory tests indicate elevated levels of AST, ALT, and alkaline phosphatase. This may be due to which of her medications? (EO-10)
   a. Triazolam
   b. Ibuprofen
   c. Acetaminophen
   d. Propoxyphene

6. Which of the following factors present in VB's history may make her more susceptible to drug-induced liver toxicity? (EO-4, 6, 8)
   a. Alcohol consumption
   b. Caffeine consumption
   c. Preexisting liver impairment
   d. Allergy to aspirin

7. Describe the mechanisms of action of the pharmacologic and nonpharmacologic interventions in this case. (EO-7)

8. Principles of appropriate NSAID use in VB would include all of the following *except:* (EO-8)
   a. Use of minimum effective dose
   b. Assessment of benefit after 1 month
   c. Patient education regarding appropriate use
   d. Use of more than one NSAID simultaneously

9. Which of the following pharmacologic treatment problems is present in VB's existing treatment plan? (EO-11)
   a. Inadequate trial of triazolam for insomnia
   b. Daily acetaminophen therapy exceeds recommended dose
   c. Propoxyphene dose inadequate for pain control
   d. Acetaminophen therapy is inadequate in the treatment of osteoarthritis

10. What risk factor does VB have that may predispose her to NSAID-induced peptic ulcer disease (PUD)? (EO-4, 6, 8, 10)
    a. History of upper GI bleed
    b. Concomitant use of corticosteroids
    c. Age
    d. High NSAID dose

11. After 1 month of therapy with ibuprofen, 400 mg PO QID, and topical capsaicin, VB's response is inadequate and signs of effusion and increased inflammation are present in her left knee. Which of the following treatment modalities would be an appropriate option? (EO-8, 12)
    a. Prednisone 2 mg/kg PO QD
    b. Acetaminophen 1000 mg PO QID, with additional doses PRN
    c. Ibuprofen 1000 mg PO QID
    d. Triamcinolone acetonide 40 mg intra-articular injection

12. Evaluate the pharmacoeconomic considerations associated with VB's plan of care. (EO-17)

13. Summarize pathophysiologic, therapeutic, and disease management concepts for osteoarthritis utilizing a key points format. (EO-18)

CASE 47
Lori N. Justice
Topic: Osteoarthritis
Level 3
EDUCATIONAL MATERIALS
Chapter 32: Osteoarthritis (treatment goals, clinical presentation and diagnosis, treatment, pharmacoeconomics)

SCENARIO

Patient and Setting

MJ, a 46-year-old female; outpatient clinic

Chief Complaint

Worsening pain and joint stiffness in both knees; new-onset pain in hands, wrists, feet; lack of energy, abdominal cramping, and constipation with intermittent watery diarrhea, usually in the morning

History of Present Illness

Knee osteoarthritis (OA) currently treated with aspirin PRN (reports taking 650 mg 3 times/week); experiencing irritable bowel symptoms for 2 weeks; fatigue, lethargy, malaise, arthritic pain in hands, wrists, and feet for 5 days

Past Medical History

OA in both knees × 10 years (morning stiffness of 10 minutes duration, joint cracking, and pain with daily activities); irritable bowel syndrome (IBS) × 4 years (propantheline 15 mg PO TID unsuccessful); diagnosis of premature ventricular contractions (graded 2 on scale of 5) 2 years ago after complaints of "heart jumping out of chest," currently without symptoms on procainamide; irregular menstrual cycle × 1 year (diagnosed as perimenopausal)

Family/Social History

Family History: Professional soccer player until age 30; currently coaches girls' soccer team at local high school (admits to overexertion); divorced for 3 years, 20-year-old daughter away at college

Social History: Drinks 8–10 cups of coffee per day; smokes 30 packs/year

Medication History

Aspirin, 650 mg PO PRN

Procainamide SR, 500 mg TID

Milk of magnesia, 2 tablespoonfuls PRN for dyspepsia

Allergies

NKDA

Physical Examination

GEN: Slightly anxious, mildly obese female in moderate distress
VS: BP 130/80, HR 120, RR 18, T 38.2°C, Wt. 63 kg, Ht 165 cm
HEENT: Dry tongue, mucous membranes
COR: Tachycardia
CHEST: WNL
ABD: RUQ soft, tender, painful
GU: Deferred
RECT: Guaiac negative; small, hardened stool present
EXT: Tenderness and swelling, decreased range of motion of both knees; mild tenderness on both hands, wrists, and feet; poor skin turgor
NEURO: Alert, O × 3

Results of Pertinent Laboratory Tests, Serum Drug Concentrations, and Diagnostic Tests

Na 146 (146)	Cl 105 (105)	WBC 3.5 × 10⁹
K 4.8 (4.8)	BUN 14.6 (41)	(3.5 × 10³)
HCO₃ 27 (27)	Sed Rate 80 (80)	AST 0.25 (15)
T₄ 112 (8.7)	ALT 0.43 (26)	Hgb 152 (15.2)
Cr 97.2 (1.1)	Hct 0.457 (45.7)	TSH 0.45 (0.45)

ANA (+) LE (+)

Rheum Factor (−) VDRL (+)

Procainamide concentration: 25.5 μmol/L (6 mg/L)

Sigmoidoscopy: WNL

Stool: Negative for ova and parasites

X-ray films of knees: Bilateral joint-space narrowing consistent with OA

PROBLEM LIST

Identify principal problem(s) from the scenario in priority order

SOAP NOTE

To be completed by student

QUESTIONS

1. Which of the following factors may have increased MJ's risk for developing knee osteoarthritis? (EO-1, 3)
   a. Age
   b. Family history
   c. Sedentary lifestyle
   d. Athletic activities

2. MJ presents with all of the following signs and symptoms of osteoarthritis *except:* (EO-2)
   a. Worsening pain and joint stiffness in both knees
   b. Morning stiffness of 10 minutes duration
   c. Decreased range of motion of both knees
   d. Limps as result of compensation of surrounding muscle due to atrophy

3. In MJ, analysis of synovial fluid might indicate which of the following: (EO-5)
   a. Mild thrombocytopenia
   b. Increased IL-1 and TNF-alpha
   c. Mild leukocytosis
   d. Increased GM-CSF

4. MJ presents with all of the following clinical features of drug-related lupus *except:* (EO-5)
   a. Fever
   b. Skin rash
   c. Malaise
   d. Arthralgia

5. Which of the following agents most likely caused drug-related lupus in MJ? (EO-10)
   a. Aspirin
   b. Milk of magnesia
   c. Procainamide
   d. Propantheline

6. Describe the mechanism of action of pharmacologic and nonpharmacologic interventions employed in MJ's treatment plan. (EO-7)

7. Describe the goals of therapy for MJ's osteoarthritis. (EO-8)

8. On her next visit to outpatient clinic, MJ states that she saw an advertisement for a natural "miracle cure" for osteoarthritis and heard that the product is available at local pharmacies, but she can't remember its name. As her pharmacist, you explain that the ingredient(s) in the product, _____, is(are) used by some patients, but is not FDA-approved or recognized by the Arthritis Foundation as a treatment for osteoarthritis. (EO-8)
   a. St. John's Wort
   b. Glucosamine/chondroitin
   c. Ginseng
   d. Kava kava

9. Which of the following agents approved for the treatment of pain in knee OA is thought to restore the composition of synovial fluid such that normal tissue regeneration and function may occur? (EO-7)
   a. Aspirin
   b. Triamcinolone
   c. Glucosamine
   d. Hyaluronic acid

10. MJ has been taking acetaminophen 500 mg QID for a few months with intermittent relief and inquires about increasing the daily dose of this medication. Which of the following is the recommended maximum daily dose for this agent? (EO-11)
    a. 2 grams
    b. 3 grams
    c. 4 grams
    d. 6 grams

11. What psychosocial factors may affect MJ's adherence to both pharmacologic and nonpharmacologic therapy? (EO-15)

12. Describe the health care provider's role relative to the proposed psychosocial factors identified in Question 11. (EO-16)

13. Evaluate the pharmacoeconomic considerations associated with MJ's plan of care. (EO-17)

14. Summarize pathophysiologic, therapeutic, and disease management concepts for osteoarthritis utilizing a key points format (EO-18)

CASE 48
Lori N. Justice
Topics: Gout and Hyperuricemia

EDUCATIONAL MATERIALS
Chapter 33: Gout and Hyperuricemia (etiology, pathogenesis, diagnosis and clinical findings, treatment)

SCENARIO

Patient and Setting
DW, a 38-year-old male; primary care center

Chief Complaint
Excruciating pain and swelling in left big toe

History of Present Illness
Awakened about 5:00 this morning by intense pain in toe followed by redness, heat, and swelling of the skin a few hours later; several previous episodes of less intense pain in same toe over past year

Past Medical History
Hypertension × 5 years (controlled by diet and exercise modifications until 1 year ago)

Family/Social History
Family History: Nonapplicable

Social History: Drinks 2 cups of decaffeinated coffee each morning; moderate alcohol consumption (3 drinks per week); quit smoking 4 years ago

Medication History
Hydrochlorothiazide, 50 mg PO QD

Vitamin C, 1000 mg PO QD

Allergies

Aspirin (rash, bronchospasm, and facial swelling)

Physical Examination

GEN: Moderately obese, Caucasian male in moderate distress from the painful experience in his toe early this morning

VS: BP 150/99 (152/102, 1 month ago), HR 70, RR 20, T 38.8°C, Wt. 98 kg, Ht 180 cm

HEENT: WNL

COR: Normal S1 and S2

CHEST: Clear to auscultation and percussion

ABD: Soft, nontender, no distention

GU: WNL

RECT: Deferred

EXT: Redness, heat, and swelling of left first metatarsophalangeal joint

NEURO: Alert, O × 3

Results of Pertinent Laboratory Tests, Serum Drug Concentrations, and Diagnostic Tests

Na 138 (138)   Cl 99 (99)   Plts 150 × 10⁹
Glu 5.55 (100)   Hgb 115 (11.5)   (150 × 10³)
Cr 97 (1.1)   BUN 3.9 (11)   HCO₃ 22 (22)
Lkcs 12.0 × 10⁹   K 3.2 (3.2)   Sed Rate 55 (55)
   (12.0 × 10³)   Hct 0.45 (45)

Uric Acid (colorimetric method) 530 (8.9)

Synovial fluid aspirate (left metatarsophalangeal joint): Cloudy, protein WNL, glucose WNL, Gram stain (−), leukocyte count 19.5 × 10⁹/L (predominance of PMNs), needle-shaped crystals (approximately 5 μm in length)

24-hour urine collection in progress (uric acid clearance pending)

PROBLEM LIST

Identify principal problem(s) from the scenario in priority order [completed Problem List and SOAP Note at end of casebook]

SOAP NOTE

To be completed by student

QUESTIONS

[Answers at end of casebook]

1. Which of the following factors most likely contributed to DW's hyperuricemia? (EO-1)
   a. Hypertension
   b. Hydrochlorothiazide therapy
   c. Decaffeinated coffee
   d. Vitamin C intake

2. What signs and symptoms of acute gout are present in DW? (EO-2)

3. Crystals were noted in the synovial fluid aspirate obtained on DW's arrival to the primary care center. What type of crystals are associated with acute attacks of gout? (EO-5)
   a. Potassium citrate
   b. Calcium oxalate
   c. Monosodium urate
   d. Sodium chloride

4. DW presents with all of the following American Rheumatism Association diagnostic criteria suggestive for acute gout *except:* (EO-2)
   a. Hyperuricemia
   b. Redness over joint
   c. Painful first metatarsophalangeal joint
   d. Tophus

5. A 24-hour urine collection from DW while on a diet with rigid purine restriction revealed uric acid excretion of 5960 mmol per 24 hours. This indicates: (EO-1, 5)
   a. Underexcretion
   b. Overproduction
   c. Normal excretion
   d. Normal production

6. Which of the following factors could contribute to a false elevation in serum urate concentration in DW? (EO-5)
   a. Vitamin C intake
   b. Decaffeinated coffee
   c. Hypertension
   d. Ethanol consumption

7. All of the following statements regarding colchicine are true *except:* (EO-7)
   a. Colchicine is most effective within the first 12–36 hours of an acute gout attack
   b. Colchicine possesses anti-inflammatory activity
   c. Colchicine possesses analgesic activity
   d. Colchicine may be used to establish the diagnosis of gout

8. What side effects may be associated with colchicine therapy in MJ? (EO-10)

9. Would indomethacin have been an appropriate choice for treating DW's acute gout attack? Explain. (EO-8, 9, 10)

10. Based on the 24-hour uric acid excretion data in question 5, which of the following agents would be most appropriate if long-term therapy to control gout attacks is necessary in DW? (EO-8, 12)
    a. Indomethacin
    b. Sulfinpyrazone
    c. Probenecid
    d. Allopurinol

11. Which of the following adverse effects has been most frequently associated with the agent from question 10? (EO-10)
    a. Pruritic maculopapular rash
    b. Gastrointestinal effects
    c. Precipitation of uric acid stones
    d. Acute interstitial nephritis

12. Evaluate the pharmacoeconomic considerations associated with DW's plan of care. (EO-17)

13. Summarize the pathophysiologic, therapeutic, and disease management concepts for gout utilizing a key points format. (EO-18)

CASE 49
Lori N. Justice
Topic: Systemic Lupus Erythematosus
Level 2
EDUCATIONAL MATERIALS
Chapter 34: Systemic Lupus Erythematosus (treatment goals; epidemiology; pathogenesis; clinical features; prognosis; treatment; pregnancy, estrogen, and lupus)

SCENARIO

Patient and Setting

PS, a 38-year-old female; emergency department

Chief Complaint

Fever, fatigue, joint tenderness and swelling, chest pain with mild dyspnea, and dry mouth

History of Present Illness

Low-grade fever for 48 hours with increasing fatigue, joint tenderness and swelling; pleuritic chest pain with some dyspnea in the past 12 hours; currently depressed; often unable to sleep at night

Past Medical History

Systemic lupus erythematosus (SLE) × 3 years (first diagnosed when rash appeared over her cheeks and nose); multiple problems from SLE with periods of remissions and exacerbations; flares consist of joint pain, fatigue, worsening facial rash, increasing serum creatinine levels with proteinuria, fever, and pleurisy; feels weak and has lost 15 pounds since diagnosis; depression

Family/Social History

Family History: Father and mother alive and well; two sisters with no significant medical history

Social History: Elementary school teacher; married with one child (4 years of age); no tobacco or alcohol use

Medication History

Sulindac, 200 mg PO BID

Hydroxychloroquine, 200 mg PO QD × 28 months

Amitriptyline, 100 mg PO QHS (increased from 50 mg QHS 4 weeks ago after 6 months of treatment)

Allergies

NKDA

Physical Examination

GEN: Thin Hispanic woman with mild SOB
VS: BP 150/90, HR 60, RR 20, T 38.2°C, Wt 64 kg, Ht 170 cm
HEENT: Butterfly-shaped erythema covering the cheeks and bridge of nose
COR: Normal S_1 and S_2
CHEST: Clear to auscultation and percussion
ABD: Soft, nontender, no distention
GU: WNL
RECT: Guaiac negative
EXT: Joint swelling and tenderness at ankles, knees, and wrists; warm to touch
NEURO: Alert, O × 3

Results of Pertinent Laboratory Tests, Serum Drug Concentrations, and Diagnostic Tests

Na 135 (135)	Lkcs 3.0 × 10⁹	Alb 32 (3.2)
K 4.8 (4.8)	(3.0 × 10³)	MCV 76 (76)
Cl 98 (98)	Plts 145 × 10⁹	Sed Rate 50 (50)
HCO₃ 22 (22)	(145 × 10³)	AST .47 (28)
Uric Acid 446.1 (7.5)	BUN 12 (35)	PO₄ 1.78 (5.5)
T Bili 13.7 (0.8)	Cr 221 (2.5)	Mg 1.20 (2.4)
Hct 0.33 (33)	ALT 0.58 (35)	Glu 5.55 (100)
Hgb 120 (12.0)	LDH 1.7 (101)	Ca 1.95 (7.8)
	Alk Phos 1.08 (65)	

Urine output over the past 6 hours is 300 mL

Urinalysis: 3+ proteinuria, granular casts, WBC 1+, RBC 2+, nitrates (−), esterase (−)

CXR: NL

ANA titer: 1:480 with a rim fluorescent pattern

Positive LE cell test

Positive anti-DNA antibodies

Positive anti-Sm

Serum complement (C3,C4) decreased

PROBLEM LIST

Identify principal problem(s) from the scenario in priority order [completed Problem List and SOAP Note at end of casebook]

SOAP NOTE

To be completed by student

QUESTIONS

[Answers at end of casebook]

1. Which of the following immune abnormalities present in PS is found exclusively in patients with SLE? (EO-1, 5)
   a. Anti-Sm antibodies
   b. U_1RNP antibodies
   c. Anti-La antibodies
   d. Anti-Ro antibodies

2. Most of the disease manifestations observed in PS and other patients with SLE are related to the key immune pathology, which is _____. (EO-1)
   a. Inflammation
   b. Decreased antibody production
   c. Bacterial infection
   d. Increased testosterone production

3. PS presents with all of the following criteria for classification of SLE *except:* (EO-2)
   a. Immunologic disorder
   b. Malar rash
   c. Oral ulcers
   d. Hematologic disorder

4. Which of the following classifications describes PS's dermatologic manifestations of SLE at the time of her diagnosis? (EO-2)
   a. Acute cutaneous lupus erythematosus (ACLE)
   b. Subacute cutaneous lupus erythematosus (SCLE)
   c. Discoid lupus erythematosus (DLE)
   d. Drug-related lupus (DRL)

5. Which of the following clinical features typically occurs in patients with drug-related lupus (DRL) but not idiopathic SLE? (EO-2)
   a. Fever
   b. CNS disease
   c. Hepatomegaly
   d. Abrupt onset of symptoms

6. Which of the following demographic characteristics associated with SLE is *not* observed in PS? (EO-3)
   a. First-degree relative with SLE
   b. Female sex
   c. Hispanic race
   d. Age <40

7. Describe the clinical, laboratory, and pathological findings of lupus nephritis and chronic renal failure present in PS. (EO-5, 6)

8. For which of the following manifestations of SLE seen in PS would hydroxychloroquine be indicated? (EO-7)
   a. Thrombocytopenia
   b. Depression
   c. Rash
   d. Nephritis

9. List adverse effects that may occur while PS is taking an antimalarial medication. (EO-10)

10. Which of the following agents should be considered in patients with lupus nephritis refractory to high-dose steroid therapy? (EO-8)

a. Methotrexate
b. Cyclophosphamide
c. Ibuprofen
d. Chloroquine

11. List the goals of treatment for PS's SLE. (EO-8, 12)

12. Outline an appropriate prednisone taper schedule to utilize once PS's SLE is controlled and has been maintained at 20 mg PO QD to avoid problems associated with adrenal insufficiency due to hypothalamic-pituitary-adrenal suppression. (EO-10, 12)

13. PS reports to outpatient clinic 6 months after the flare, her SLE now controlled and no longer feeling sad and withdrawn. Her current medications include prednisone 20 mg PO QD and hydroxychloroquine 200 mg PO QD. PS states that she would like to become pregnant. Describe issues that should be addressed with PS related to SLE and pregnancy. (EO-8, 9, 11)

14. What psychosocial factors may affect PS's adherence to both pharmacologic and nonpharmacologic therapy? (EO-15)

15. Describe the health care provider's role relative to PS's proposed plan of care. (EO-16)

16. Evaluate the pharmacoeconomic considerations relative to PS's plan of care. (EO-17)

17. Summarize the pathophysiologic, therapeutic, and disease management concepts for SLE using a key points format. (EO-18)

CASE 50
Lori N. Justice
Topics: Osteoporosis and Osteomalacia

EDUCATIONAL MATERIALS
Chapter 35: Osteoporosis and Osteomalacia (definition, physiology, pathogenesis, signs and symptoms of osteoporosis, diagnosis and clinical findings, prevention and treatment of osteoporosis, benefits other than prevention of osteoporosis, patient education)

SCENARIO

Patient and Setting

TF, a 66-year-old female; outpatient clinic

Chief Complaint

New-onset back pain, joint and stomach pain

History of Present Illness

Back pain of 2 days duration; joint pain and stomach pain not relieved by antacids

Past Medical History

Rheumatoid arthritis for 10 years treated with prednisone after failed therapy with NSAIDs; history of NSAID-induced peptic ulcer disease (PUD) and chronic alcoholism; postmenopausal for 4 years; hip fracture after fall in bathtub 1 year ago

Family/Social History

Family History: Husband died 3 years ago; since then, lives with daughter who is married with two children

Social History: Tobacco (+) 22 pack/year history; alcohol (+) 4 to 6 drinks per day in past; denies use presently, but daughter reports began drinking again when husband died 3 years ago

Medication History

Prednisone, 5 mg PO QD

Ranitidine, 150 mg PO QHS

Aluminum hydroxide 200 mg/magnesium 200 mg suspension, PO as needed

Allergies

NKDA

Physical Examination

GEN: Thin, elderly appearing Caucasian woman in no acute distress

VS: BP 140/85, HR 70, RR 14, Wt 55 kg, Ht 160 cm (Ht at last visit 6 months ago: 160 cm)

HEENT: WNL

COR: Normal S_1 and S_2

CHEST: Clear to auscultation and percussion

ABD: Soft, nontender; liver palpable; hepatomegaly

GU: WNL

RECT: Guaiac negative

EXT: Muscle atrophy in dorsal musculature and joint swelling of both hands

NEURO: Alert, O × 3

Results of Pertinent Laboratory Tests, Serum Drug Concentrations, and Diagnostic Tests:

Na 138 (138)	Alb 25 (2.5)	Cr 106 (1.2)
Glu 5.55 (100)	LDH 1.7 (101)	Plts 100×10^9 (100×10^3)
T Bili 18 (1.0)	Folate 9.064 (4)	HCO$_3$ 22 (22)
AST .58 (35)	Lkcs 3.0×10^9 (3.0×10^3)	Hct 0.25 (25)
PO$_4$ 1.07 (3.3)	K 4.2 (4.2)	ALT .58 (35)
Vit B$_{12}$ 177.1 (240)	Hgb 100 (10)	Mg 1 (2)
Cl 98 (98)	Alk Phos 2.0 (120)	BUN 3.6 (10)
MCV 105 (105)	Ca 2.2 (8.8)	

H. pylori (−)

PROBLEM LIST

Identify principal problem(s) from the scenario in priority order [completed Problem List and SOAP Note at end of casebook]

SOAP NOTE

To be completed by student

QUESTIONS

[Answers at end of casebook]

1. All of following risk factors may have contributed to TF's development of osteoporosis *except:* (EO-1, 3)
   a. Menopause
   b. Glucocorticoid therapy
   c. Alcohol consumption
   d. Ranitidine therapy

2. Which of the following signs/symptoms of osteoporosis are present in TF? (EO-2)
   a. Kyphosis
   b. Wrist fracture
   c. Back pain
   d. Loss in height

3. What percentage range of spinal bone loss must occur in TF for detection of osteoporosis by a routine spinal radiograph? (EO-5)
   a. <5%
   b. 10–15%
   c. 20–50%
   d. 60–90%

4. Describe the mechanism of action of the pharmacologic and nonpharmacologic interventions employed in the treatment of osteoporosis in this case. (EO-7)

5. According to the National Institutes of Health, which of the following is the recommended daily calcium intake for TF? (EO-8)
   a. 800 mg
   b. 1000 mg
   c. 1200 mg
   d. 1500 mg

6. Which of the following calcium salts would provide TF with the highest percentage of elemental calcium? (EO-8)
   a. Calcium carbonate
   b. Calcium citrate
   c. Calcium lactate
   d. Calcium gluconate

7. Which of the following therapeutic options might be useful in TF for its analgesic effect on back pain associated with osteoporotic vertebral fractures? (EO-8, 12)
   a. Calcium carbonate
   b. Calcitonin
   c. Alendronate
   d. Raloxifene

8. Estrogen therapy may increase the effects of which of TF's medications/supplements? (EO-9)

a. Calcium
b. Vitamin D
c. Prednisone
d. Ranitidine

9. Which of the following risks of hormone replacement therapy (estrogen with progestin) should be discussed with TF? (EO-10)
   a. Thromboembolism
   b. Endometrial cancer
   c. Weight loss
   d. Skin irritation

10. Describe benefits of estrogen therapy other than prevention of osteoporosis that should be discussed with TF. (EO-8, 14)

11. During her past three visits to outpatient clinic, TF's blood pressure has measured 140/85, 142/90, and 148/90, respectively. Which of the following would be an appropriate choice for treatment of hypertension in a patient with osteoporosis? (EO-12)
    a. Furosemide
    b. Hydrochlorothiazide
    c. Torsemide
    d. Spironolactone

12. Due to the increased effectiveness of the combination in women with osteoporosis, alendronate may be used in combination with estrogen therapy. Describe appropriate patient counseling points to address with a patient receiving this agent. (EO-14)

13. Evaluate the pharmacoeconomic considerations related to TF's plan of care. (EO-17)

14. Summarize the pathophysiologic, therapeutic, and disease management concepts for osteoporosis using a key points format. (EO-18)

CASE 51
Kutay Demirkan
Topic: Steroid-Dependent Asthma
[Level 1]
EDUCATIONAL MATERIALS
Chapter 36: Asthma (clinical presentations and diagnosis, psychosocial issues, treatment, pharmacoeconomics)

SCENARIO

Patient and Setting

BJ, a 54-year-old female; emergency department

Chief Complaint

Shortness of breath (SOB), flu-like symptoms (nausea, vomiting, and fatigue), palpitations, insomnia, and irritability

History of Present Illness

Abruptly discontinued prednisone 2 days ago; increasing SOB; increased use of inhalers; nausea, vomiting, fatigue, palpitations, insomnia, and irritability; cimetidine started 1 week ago for gastroesophageal reflux disease (GERD)

Past Medical History

Chronic steroid-dependent asthma; two hospital admissions for acute exacerbation of asthma over the past year; GERD diagnosed 3 weeks prior to admission; degenerative joint disease (DJD) controlled with indomethacin

Past Surgical History

None

Family/Social History

Family history: Noncontributory

Social History: Quit smoking 5 years ago ($\frac{1}{2}$ package/day × 18 years); no alcohol intake

Medication History

Theophylline SR tablets, 400 mg PO BID

Cimetidine tablets, 400 mg PO BID (started 1 week ago)

Indomethacin capsules, 50 mg PO TID

Prednisone tablets, 20 mg PO QD (stopped 3 days ago)

Albuterol inhaler, 2 puffs PRN

Cromolyn inhaler, 1 puff PRN

Beclomethasone inhaler, 2 puffs PRN

Erythromycin tablets, 500 mg PO QD (started 1 year ago)

Allergies

NKDA

Physical Examination

GEN: Cushingoid appearance; in obvious respiratory distress

VS: BP 100/60 (sitting), BP 90/50 (standing), RR 27, HR 130, T 37.5°C, Wt 65 kg

HEENT: Moon facies, hirsutism

COR: No murmurs, NL S1, S2

CHEST: Decreased breath sounds bilaterally, inspiratory/expiratory wheezing and rhonchi

ABD: Truncal obesity

GU: Unremarkable

RECT: Unremarkable

EXT: Pale skin with tenting, bruising

NEURO: Oriented × 2, alert but confused

Results of Pertinent Laboratory Tests, Serum Drug Concentrations, and Diagnostic Tests

Na 125 (125)	Hct 0.41 (41)	AST 0.3 (22)
K 5.9 (5.9)	Hgb 140 (14)	Alb 41 (4.1)
Cl 94 (94)	Lkcs 9.0 × 10⁹	T Bili 5.1 (0.3)
HCO$_3$ 33 (33)	(9.0 × 10³)	Ca 2.4 (9.8)
BUN 10.7 (30)	Plts 250 × 10⁹	PO$_4$ 1.45 (4.5)
SCr 212 (2.4)	(250 × 10³)	Mg 0.78 (1.9)

Theophylline: 94.4 μmol/L (17 mg/L) (clinic visit 2 months prior to admission); 138.7 μmol/L (25 mg/L) (admission)

Pulmonary function tests: FEV$_1$/FVC: 55% (before β$_2$-agonist dose); FEV$_1$/FVC: 70% (after β$_2$-agonist dose)

ECG: Atrial fibrillation and occasional premature ventricular contractions

PROBLEM LIST

Identify principal problems from the scenario in priority order [completed Problem List and SOAP Note at end of casebook]

SOAP NOTE

To be completed by student

QUESTIONS

[Answers at end of casebook]

1. Considering the time of onset, the most probable cause of BJ's theophylline toxicity is: (EO-4, 5, 8, 9)
   a. Erythromycin drug interaction
   b. Cimetidine drug interaction
   c. Abrupt discontinuance of prednisone
   d. History of smoking cessation

2. Explain the necessity of tapering steroids in this case. (EO-8, 11)

3. BJ presented with all of the following signs and symptoms of asthma exacerbation *except:* (EO-2)
   a. Dyspnea
   b. Increasing shortness of breath
   c. Cough
   d. Inspiratory and expiratory wheezing

4. The reason that excessive use of β_2-agonist therapy should be avoided in BJ is: (EO-8, 10)
   a. Patient unable to use MDI properly
   b. No additional benefit with high-dose β_2-agonist
   c. To minimize cost
   d. To reduce risk of side effects

5. List the steps for proper technique for metered dose inhalers. (EO-14)

6. BJ presents with flu-like symptoms (nausea, vomiting, and excessive fatigue) that are sign and symptoms of: (EO-2)
   a. Gastroesophageal reflux disease
   b. Theophylline toxicity
   c. Adrenal insufficiency
   d. Indomethacin side effects

7. Factors that would predispose for theophylline toxicity and, therefore, should be monitored include all of the following *except:* (EO-4)
   a. Hyperthyroidism
   b. Prolonged fever
   c. Congestive heart failure
   d. Age <1 year or >60 years old

8. Evaluate the pharmacoeconomic considerations relative to BJ's asthma management. (EO-17)

9. Which of the following MDI regimen is NOT appropriate for BJ after acute symptoms resolve? (EO-8, 12)
   a. Albuterol MDI, 2 puffs QID PRN
   b. Salmeterol MDI, 2 puffs BID PRN
   c. Beclomethasone MDI, 4 puffs QID
   d. Metaproterenol MDI, 2 puffs QID PRN

10. If BJ was discharged with inhaled corticosteroid, which of the following would be appropriate educational efforts? (EO-14)
    a. Corticosteroid inhaler should be used after meals
    b. Spacer devices are not recommended with corticosteroid inhalers
    c. Corticosteroid inhaler should be used PRN, if shortness of breath is not relieved with albuterol inhaler
    d. After inhalation of corticosteroids, rinse mouth with water or mouthwash and expel contents

11. What psychosocial factors may affect BJ's adherence to both pharmacologic and nonpharmacologic therapy? (EO-16)

12. BJ presents with several symptoms of steroid excess *except:* (EO-4)
    a. Hirsutism
    b. Respiratory distress
    c. Moon facies
    d. Bruising

13. Summarize pathophysiologic, therapeutic, and disease management concepts for steroid-dependent asthma utilizing a key points format. (EO-18)

CASE 52
Kutay Demirkan
Topic: Chronic Obstructive Pulmonary Disease (COPD)

EDUCATIONAL MATERIALS
Chapter 37: Chronic Obstructive Pulmonary Disease (clinical presentation and diagnosis, specific therapy)

SCENARIO

Patient and Setting

SB, a 65-year-old male; general medicine clinic

Chief Complaint

Nausea, agitation, tremors, and an increased number of anginal attacks associated with palpitations

History of Present Illness

Underwent treatment for smoking cessation; quit smoking 2 months ago; treated for acute gout with colchicine 1 week ago; chest pain upon exertion; 1 week history of nausea, agitation, and tremors; an increased number of anginal attacks associated with palpitations

Past Medical History

Angina × 5 years; hypertension × 10 years, controlled with hydrochlorothiazide; chronic obstructive pulmonary disease (COPD) × 3 years, stabilized with theophylline and albuterol inhaler PRN

Past Surgical History

None

Family/Social History

Family History: Mother has COPD; father has coronary artery disease and gout

Social History: Prior cigarette smoker 1 PPD × 30 years (discontinued 2 months ago); occasional alcohol use

Medication History

Hydrochlorothiazide tablets, 50 mg PO QD

KCl tablets, 20 mEq PO QD

Isosorbide dinitrate tablets, 30 mg PO TID

Theophylline SR capsules, 300 mg PO BID

Albuterol inhaler, 2 puffs q4h PRN

Nitroglycerin sublingual tablets, 4 mg sublingual (SL) PRN chest pain

Enteric-coated aspirin tablets, 325 mg PO QD

Colchicine tablets, 0.6 mg PO BID (1 week prior)

Allergies

NKDA

Physical Examination

GEN: Well-developed man in mild distress

VS: BP 155/95, HR 100, RR 16, T 37.5°C, Wt 70 kg, Ht 177.8 cm

HEENT: Mild AV nicking

COR: S1, S2, no S3, sinus tachycardia

CHEST: Barrel chest, increased accessory muscle use

ABD: Soft, nontender

GU: WNL

RECT: Unremarkable

EXT: Metatarsophalangeal of left toe is erythematous, tender, warm to touch (1 week ago), now WNL

NEURO: A & O × 3

Results of Pertinent Laboratory Tests, Serum Drug Concentrations, and Diagnostic Tests

Na 139 (139)	Hgb 135 (13.5)	Uric Acid 582 (9.8)
K 4.6 (4.6)	ALT 0.38 (23)	T Bili 17 (1)
Cl 96 (96)	Alk Phos 0.92 (55)	Ca 2.02 (8.1)
HCO_3 27 (27)	WBC 9.5 × 10⁹	PO_4 1.03 (3.2)
Glu 6.1 (110)	(9.5 × 10³)	Mg 0.95 (1.9)
LDH 1.42 (85)	Plts 253 × 10⁹	MCV 90 (90)
BUN 6.78 (19)	(253 × 10³)	
SCr 106 (1.2)	AST 0.467 (28)	
Hct 0.40 (40)	Alb 43 (4.3)	

WBC differential: WNL

Theophylline: 21 mg/L

Urinalysis: WNL

$FEV_1/FVC = 35\%$

Chest x-ray: clear

FEV_1: 700 mL (before bronchodilator); 900 ml (after bronchodilator)

ECG: Sinus tachycardia, occasional PVCs

PROBLEM LIST

Identify principal problems from the scenario in priority order [completed Problem List and SOAP Note at end of casebook]

SOAP NOTE

To be completed by student

QUESTIONS

[Answers at end of casebook]

1. Which of the following therapies is step one for long-term management of COPD? (EO-8, 12)
   a. Albuterol
   b. Theophylline
   c. Beclomethasone
   d. Ipratropium

2. Influenza vaccine: (EO-11, 12)
   a. Has shown no benefit in COPD patients
   b. Is recommended every fall for COPD patients
   c. Is recommended in asthma but not COPD
   d. Should generally be avoided in severe COPD due to a compromised immune system

3. SB's COPD is strongly associated with: (EO-1, 3)
   a. Mother had COPD
   b. Environmental factors
   c. History of smoking
   d. Gender and increasing age

4. List the effects of theophylline on the cardiac and respiratory systems. (EO-7)

5. List the goals of therapy for SB's COPD. (EO-11, 12)

6. Which of the following is *not* a factor that can precipitate SB's acute gouty attack? (EO-4, 8)
   a. Isosorbide dinitrate
   b. Hydrochlorothiazide
   c. Aspirin
   d. Alcohol intake

7. Which of the following is *not* true for proper use of sublingual nitroglycerin? (EO-14)
   a. Place 1 tablet under the tongue at the onset of chest pain
   b. May repeat the dose every 5 minutes for a maximum of three doses as needed
   c. Keep nitroglycerin tablets in the original container and store in a cool dry place
   d. Once open, the tablets have an expiration date of 1 month

8. If SB experiences more than 3 gouty attacks per year, which of the following statements regarding SB's therapy is correct? (EO-8, 11, 12)

a. Allopurinol should be started if SB has underproduction of uric acid

b. Probenecid should be started if SB has overexcretion of uric acid

c. Pharmacologic therapy with an appropriate agent is indicated

d. It is not necessary to know the etiology of hyperuricemia to provide optimal care

9. All of the following would predispose a patient to theophylline toxicity, *except:* (EO-4)

a. Congestive heart failure (CHF)

b. Smoking

c. Hyperthyroidism

d. Cystic fibrosis

10. What psychosocial factors may affect SB's adherence to both pharmacologic and nonpharmacologic therapy? (EO-15)

11. Evaluate the pharmacoeconomic considerations relative to SB's plan of care. (EO-17)

12. Summarize pathophysiologic, therapeutic, and disease management concepts for a given condition utilizing a key points format. (EO-18)

CASE 53
Kutay Demirkan
Topic: Cystic Fibrosis
Level 2

EDUCATIONAL MATERIALS
Chapter 38: Cystic Fibrosis (pathogenesis and pathophysiology, clinical presentation, treatment)

SCENARIO

Patient and Setting
YM, a 30-year-old female; clinic

Chief Complaint
Mild cough, slight fever, dyspnea on exertion, occasional wheezes, decreased appetite, "sleeping a lot," and crying spells approximately 3–4 times a week for the past month

History of Present Illness
History of multiple pulmonary bacterial infections; emergency room visit 2 days before this clinic visit (cultures taken); empirically started on sulfamethoxazole/trimethoprim (SMX-TMP) DS BID which has not helped her symptoms much; seen regularly for nutritional support

Past Medical History
Cystic fibrosis was diagnosed at 5 years of age; multiple hospitalizations for pulmonary infections; chronic renal insufficiency for approximately 2 years

Past Surgical History
None

Family/Social History
Family History: Father had cystic fibrosis

Social History: Occasional alcohol use; nonsmoker

Medication History
Sulfamethoxazole/trimethoprim (SMX-TMP) DS, 1 tablet PO BID

Pancrelipase capsule, 3 capsules PO TID with each meal

Albuterol inhaler, 2 puffs QID PRN for shortness of breath

Hydrochlorothiazide tablet, 25 mg PO QD

Vitamin A tablet, 5000 Units PO QD

Vitamin E tablet, 400 Units PO QD

Vitamin D tablet, 800 Units PO QD

Allergies
NKDA

Physical Examination
GEN: Disheveled, depressed-looking woman in no acute distress

VS: BP 136/82, HR 70, RR 12, T 38.7°C, Wt 55 kg, Ht 165 cm

HEENT: PERRLA

COR: Normal S_1 and S_2

CHEST: Mild rales at base

ABD: Soft, nontender, no hepatosplenomegaly

GU: Unremarkable

RECT: Unremarkable

EXT: Slight bruising on upper thighs

NEURO: Oriented to time, place, and person

Results of Pertinent Laboratory Tests, Serum Drug Concentrations, and Diagnostic Tests

Na 140 (140)	BUN 8.5 (24)	Vit E 14 (0.6)
K 4.0 (4.0)	Cr 178 (2.0)	WBC 12 (12)
HCO_3 24 (24)	AST 0.58 (35)	INR 1.4 (1.4)
Cl 100 (100)	ALT 4.6 (21)	Vit A 0.28 (8)

Culture (sputum): *Pseudomonas aeruginosa*

Culture (blood): (−)

Chest x-ray: bronchovascular markings

O_2 saturation = 92%

PROBLEM LIST

Identify principal problems from the scenario in priority order

SOAP NOTE

To be completed by student

QUESTIONS

1. Which of the following is *not* an alternative to ciprofloxacin to treat YM's *Pseudomonas* infection? (EO-5, 8, 12)
   a. Tobramycin
   b. Ceftazidime
   c. Ampicillin/sulbactam
   d. Imipenem

2. YM presents with all the following signs and symptoms of upper respiratory tract infection *except:* (EO-2)
   a. Increased WBC count
   b. Chest x-ray with positive bronchovascular markings
   c. Slight fever
   d. Positive sputum culture

3. List the pharmacologic and nonpharmacologic treatment problem(s) in YM's treatment plan. (EO-11)

4. YM's estimated CrCl is: (EO-6)
   a. 42 mL/min
   b. 36 mL/min
   c. 27 mL/min
   d. 49 mL/min

5. In the absence of culture and sensitivity, empiric therapy should be directed toward all of the following organisms, *except:* (EO-1)
   a. *H. influenzae*
   b. *S. aureus*
   c. *P. aeruginosa*
   d. *S. pneumonia*

6. Which of the following statement is *false* about YM's antibiotic therapy? (EO-4, 8, 11)
   a. YM has a higher clearance of some antibiotics secondary to cystic fibrosis
   b. YM should receive aggressive antibiotic doses
   c. Inhaled tobramycin is not indicated to treat YM's acute infection
   d. Antibiotic therapy should be continued for 7 days

7. Develop a nutritional support plan for YM. (EO-12)

8. Cystic fibrosis affects all of the following systems *except:* (EO-1)
   a. Reproductive organs
   b. Cardiovascular system
   c. Sweat glands
   d. Gastrointestinal system

9. What psychosocial factors may affect YM's adherence to both pharmacologic and nonpharmacologic therapy? (EO-15)

10. It may be necessary to change YM's hydrochlorothiazide to a loop diuretic if CrCl is less than: (EO-4, 6, 8, 12)
    a. 80 mL/min
    b. 50 mL/min
    c. 25 mL/min
    d. 10 mL/min

11. Evaluate the pharmacoeconomic considerations relative to YM's plan of care. (EO-17)

12. Summarize pathophysiologic, therapeutic, and disease management concepts for cystic fibrosis utilizing a key points format. (EO-18)

CASE 54
Kutay Demirkan
Topic: Asthma

EDUCATIONAL MATERIALS
Chapter 36: Asthma (clinical presentations and diagnosis, psychosocial issues, treatment, pharmacoeconomics)

SCENARIO

Patient and Setting

RP, a 52-year-old female; emergency department

Chief Complaint

Severe wheezing, shortness of breath, and coughing

History of Present Illness

Frequent asthma attacks for the past 2 months; serious motor vehicle accident 10 weeks ago; posttraumatic seizure 2 weeks after the accident; anticonvulsant therapy with phenytoin started; no seizure activity since initiation of anticonvulsant therapy

Past Medical History

History of periodic asthma attacks since early 20s; mild congestive heart failure (CHF) diagnosed 3 years ago; placed on a sodium-restricted diet and hydrochlorothiazide; last year, placed on enalapril due to worsening CHF; symptoms well controlled for the past year

Past Surgical History

None

Family/Social History

Family History: Father died age 59 of kidney failure secondary to hypertension; mother died age 62 of CHF

Social History: Nonsmoker; no alcohol intake; caffeine use: 4 cups of coffee and 4 diet colas per day

Medication History

Theophylline SR capsules, 300 mg PO BID

Albuterol inhaler, PRN

Phenytoin SR capsules, 300 mg PO QHS

Hydrochlorothiazide tablets, 50 mg PO BID

Enalapril tablets, 5 mg PO BID

Allergies

NKDA

Physical Examination

GEN: Pale, well-developed, anxious-appearing woman

VS: Emergency department admission: BP 171/94, HR 122, RR 31, T 38.5°C, Wt 61 kg, Ht 161 cm; Current: BP 142/79, HR 80, RR 18, T 38.3°C

HEENT: PERRLA, oral cavity without lesions, TM without signs of inflammation; no nystagmus noted, positive for AV nicking

COR: RRR, normal S_1 and S_2

CHEST: Bilateral expiratory wheezes

ABD: Nontender, nondistended, no masses

GU: Unremarkable

RECT: Guaiac negative

EXT: 1+ ankle edema on right, no bruising, normal pulses

NEURO: Oriented to time, place, and person; cranial nerves intact

Results of Pertinent Laboratory Tests, Serum Drug Concentrations, and Diagnostic Tests

Na 134 (134)	Cr 106.1 (1.2)	LDH 2.5 (150)
K 4.9 (4.9)	Glu 6.1 (110)	WBC 5.2 × 10⁹
HCO_3 30 (30)	PT 12 sec	(5.2 × 10³)
Mg 0.65 (1.3)	INR 1.0	Hct 0.37 (37)
PO_4 0.872 (2.7)	AST 0.45 (27)	Hgb 8.1 (13)
Ca 2.23 (8.9)	ALT 0.4 (24)	Plts 201 × 10⁹ (201 × 10³)
Cl 100 (100)	Alb 38 (3.8)	Alk Phos 1.32 (79)
BUN 7.5 (21)	T Bili 3.4 (0.2)	

Theophylline: 6.2 μg/mL

Phenytoin: 17 μg/mL

Chest x-ray results: Blunting of the right and left costophrenic angles

ECG: Voltage changes consistent with left ventricular hypertrophy (LVH)

Initial peak flow: 75/min; second reading taken 1 hour after beginning treatment with aerosolized albuterol and oxygen: 102/min

On admission: FEV_1 1.8 L; FVC 3.0 L; FEV_1/FVC 60%

PROBLEM LIST

Identify principal problems from the scenario in priority order

SOAP NOTE

To be completed by student

QUESTIONS

1. The probable cause for RP's recent subtherapeutic theophylline level: (EO-4, 9)
   a. Low theophylline dose
   b. Effect of CHF on theophylline clearance
   c. Noncompliance
   d. Phenytoin interaction

2. All of the following are advantages of using a spacer device, *except:* (EO-8)
   a. Can use 2 puffs at a time
   b. Reduces the amount of hand-lung coordination required for proper use of MDIs
   c. Improves pulmonary drug deposition
   d. Reduces the risks for adverse effects from inhaled medications

3. Describe the mechanisms of actions of the pharmacologic and nonpharmacologic interventions in this case. (EO-7)

4. Educate RP regarding peak flow meter zones. (EO-14)

5. Which of the following statements about administration route of $β_2$-agonists is *false*? (EO-8)
   a. $β_2$-Agonists may be administered orally, subcutaneously, or inhaled
   b. When given orally, much smaller doses must be used compared with the inhaled route
   c. Inhaled route provides more rapid onset of action and fewer systemic adverse effects
   d. Potentially life-threatening adverse effects limit the safety of intravenous administration

6. Which of the following is *not* associated with phenytoin toxicity? (EO-10)
   a. Nystagmus
   b. Dyspnea
   c. Ataxia
   d. Lethargy

7. How long should RP continue to take her antiseizure medication? (EO-12)
   a. Total of 2 years
   b. Life-long
   c. Antiseizure therapy should be maintained for 1–2 years free from seizures
   d. Antiseizure therapy should be maintained for 6 months free from seizures

8. If the physician decided to continue theophylline therapy, which of the following would be the best recommendation? (EO-4, 6, 8)
   a. Continue current dose and educate the patient regarding importance of compliance
   b. Start intravenous aminophylline
   c. Increase maintenance theophylline dose
   d. Give partial loading dose and increase maintenance theophylline dose

9. RP admitted to the emergency department with all of the following signs and symptoms of acute asthma attack *except:* (EO-2)
   a. Severe wheezing and shortness of breath
   b. Unable to speak more than a few words without taking a breath
   c. Decreased FEV_1, FVC, and peak flow
   d. Cardiac dilatation

10. What psychosocial factors may affect RP's adherence to both pharmacologic and nonpharmacologic therapy? (EO-15)

11. The probable cause for RP's asthma exacerbation: (EO-1)
    a. Noncompliance
    b. Exposure to asthma stimulants
    c. Increased theophylline clearance secondary to phenytoin along with improper dose of β_2-agonist
    d. Unable to use MDI with proper technique

12. Evaluate the pharmacoeconomic considerations relative to RP's plan of care. (EO-17)

13. Summarize pathophysiologic, therapeutic, and disease management concepts for a given condition utilizing a key points format. (EO-18)

CASE 55
Kutay Demirkan
Topic: Chronic Obstructive Pulmonary Disease (COPD)
Level 3
EDUCATIONAL MATERIALS
Chapter 37: Chronic Obstructive Pulmonary Disease (clinical presentation and diagnosis, specific therapy)

SCENARIO

Patient and Setting
MM, a 64-year-old male; unscheduled clinic visit

Chief Complaint
"Racing heart beat," increased shortness of breath, wheezing, chest tightness, productive cough, and fever

History of Present Illness
Admitted for COPD exacerbation 6 months ago; current complaints present for 3 days

Past Medical History
Hypertension for 6 years; congestive heart failure (CHF)

Past Surgical History
None

Family/Social History
Family History: Both parents died in MVA in their mid-30s

Social History: Smokes 1 PPD × 28 years; occasional alcohol use

Medication History
Hydrochlorothiazide tablets, 50 mg PO q AM

Nadolol tablets, 80 mg PO q AM

Theophylline SR capsules, 300 mg PO QD

Albuterol inhaler, 2 puffs q4h PRN

Digoxin tablets, 0.125 mg PO QD

Aspirin, 325 mg; heat-treated sodium bicarbonate, 1700 mg; citric acid, 1000 mg tablet effervescent PRN for GI upset

Allergies
NKDA

Physical Examination
GEN: Confused and pale elderly male in acute respiratory distress, complaining of chest pain and palpitations
VS: BP 145/94, HR 140, RR 26, T 39.9°C, Wt 65 kg, Ht 178 cm
HEENT: PERRLA
COR: Jugular venous distention (JVD)
CHEST: Inspiratory and expiratory wheezing, rales, and rhonchi
ABD: Hepatojugular reflux, hepatomegaly
GU: WNL
RECT: Guaiac negative
EXT: 2+ pedal edema
NEURO: Oriented × 1, confused

Results of Pertinent Laboratory Tests, Serum Drug Concentrations, and Diagnostic Tests

Na 134 (134)	Hct 0.35 (35)	AST 0.33 (20)
K 3.1 (3.1)	Hgb 135 (13.5)	Alb 38 (3.8)
Cl 95 (95)	ALT 0.42 (25)	Mg 1.1 (2.2)
HCO_3 20 (20)	WBC 8.9 × 10^9	MCV 105 (105)
Glu 6.1 (110)	(8.9 × 10^3)	T Bili 15 (0.9)
BUN 12 (35)	Plts 280 × 10^9	Ca 2.3 (9.4)
SCr 213 (2.8)	(280 × 10^3)	PO_4 1.03 (3.2)

Theophylline: 4 μg/mL

Digoxin: 0.7 ng/mL

ABG: pH 7.4, PO_2 52, PCO_2 50

ECG: Irregularly irregular

Pulmonary function tests: Prebronchodilator FEV_1: 1.5 L; post-bronchodilator FEV_1: 2 L

PROBLEM LIST

Identify principal problems from the scenario in priority order [completed Problem List and SOAP Note at end of casebook]

SOAP NOTE

To be completed by student

QUESTIONS

[Answers at end of casebook]

1. The therapeutic range for theophylline is: (EO-5)
   a. 4–8 μg/mL
   b. 5–15 μg/mL
   c. 15–25 μg/mL
   d. 25–40 μg/mL

2. Which of the following is *not* a factor that would predispose to digoxin toxicity? (EO-4, 6, 8)
   a. Renal dysfunction
   b. Hypokalemia
   c. Decreased liver function
   d. Hypomagnesemia

3. Effervescent aspirin tablets should be discontinued, because: (EO-8, 9, 10)
   a. Not indicated for MM
   b. Induces digoxin toxicity
   c. Decreases absorption of other drugs
   d. Contains high sodium content, which should be avoided in patients with hypertension and congestive heart failure

4. Describe the mechanisms of action of the pharmacologic and nonpharmacologic interventions in this case. (EO-7)

5. Which of the following is *not* a sign or symptom of digoxin toxicity? (EO-2)
   a. Anorexia
   b. Tachycardia
   c. Fatigue, weakness
   d. PVC

6. Which of the following factors is irrelevant when determining whether MM should receive antibiotic therapy? (EO-8, 12)
   a. Hospital stay less than 48 hours
   b. White blood cell count is not elevated
   c. Afebrile
   d. No infiltrates on chest x-ray films

7. Which of the following is *not* a reason that MM should be started on daily potassium supplementation? (EO-11, 12)
   a. MM will continue to take diuretics
   b. Hypokalemia can induce atrial fibrillation
   c. If patient remains hypokalemic, hypomagnesemia cannot be corrected
   d. Hypokalemia can predispose to digoxin toxicity

8. List the pharmacologic and nonpharmacologic treatment problem(s) present in MM's treatment plan. (EO-11)

9. MM should be educated for all of the following, *except:* (EO-14)
   a. Smoking cessation
   b. Proper use of MDI
   c. That he requires nursing home services
   d. Importance of compliance to her medications

10. What psychosocial factors may affect MM's adherence to both pharmacologic and nonpharmacologic therapy? (EO-15)

11. Evaluate the pharmacoeconomic considerations relative to MM's plan of care. (EO-17)

12. Summarize pathophysiologic, therapeutic, and disease management concepts for a given condition utilizing a key points format. (EO-18)

CASE 56
Kevin M. Sowinski
Topic: Cardiac Arrhythmias
Level 1
EDUCATIONAL MATERIALS
Chapter 41: Cardiac Arrhythmias; Chapter 44: Thromboembolic Disease

SCENARIO

Patient and Setting

GH, 67-year-old male; anticoagulation clinic

Chief Complaint

Frequent nosebleeds (three in the last week), easy bruising, palpitations, weakness, abdominal discomfort, and a lack of appetite; had a cold last week which has since resolved.

Past Medical History

Atrial fibrillation (Afib); has maintained normal sinus rhythm (NSR) with procainamide for 3 years; history of alcohol abuse—heavy use recently; nocturnal heartburn relieved with OTC cimetidine

Past Surgical History

Noncontributory

Family/Social History

Family History: Noncontributory

Social History: Smoking: 15 pack-years; quit 10 years ago; alcohol use: binge drinking for the past month

Medication History

Warfarin, 6 mg QD

Digoxin, 0.25 mg QD

Procainamide SR, 500 mg QID

Cimetidine, 200 mg BID PRN

Pseudoephedrine SR, 120 mg BID PRN for recent cold symptoms

Allergies

NKDA

Physical Examination

GEN: Well-developed, well-nourished male in distress

VS: HR 125, irregularly irregular; BP 175/96, RR 25; Wt 96 kg, Ht 174cm

HEENT: WNL

CHEST: WNL

ABD: (+) bowel sounds

GU: Deferred

RECT: Heme (−)

EXT: Bruising on arms and knees

NEURO: A & O × 3

Results of Pertinent Laboratory Tests, Serum Drug Concentrations, and Diagnostic Tests

Na 143 (143)   BUN 4.3 (12)   Hct 0.43 (43)
K 4.8 (4.8)   Cr 79 (0.9)   INR 3.9
Cl 98 (98)   Hgb 140 (14.0)

Procainamide 6 µg/mL

Digoxin 1.8 ng/mL

ECG: Atrial fibrillation

ECHO: slight atrial enlargement, ejection fraction 45%

PROBLEM LIST

Identify principal problems from the scenario in priority order [completed Problem List and SOAP Note at end of casebook]

SOAP NOTE

To be completed by student

QUESTIONS

[Answers at end of casebook]

1. Which of the following is least likely to have contributed to the increased INR in this patient? (EO-1, 9, 15)
   a. OTC cimetidine
   b. Binge alcohol consumption
   c. Taking his warfarin inappropriately (i.e., he took too much warfarin)
   d. Addition of pseudoephedrine therapy

2. Each of the following are signs and symptoms associated with atrial fibrillation *except:* (EO-2)
   a. Ventricular rate of 125
   b. Palpitations
   c. Bruising on arms and legs
   d. Irregularly irregular rhythm

3. Each of the following are potential causes of this patient's atrial fibrillation exacerbation *except:* (EO-1, 3)
   a. Binge drinking
   b. Pseudoephedrine use
   c. Atrial enlargement
   d. Elevated INR

4. If this patient's ventricular rate cannot be controlled with digoxin, which of the following may be used as an alternative for ventricular rate control? (EO-8, 11, 12)
   a. Amlodipine
   b. Atenolol
   c. Quinidine
   d. Ibutilide

5. Which of the following is an adverse effect of procainamide therapy? (EO-10)
   a. Hypertension
   b. Bradycardia
   c. Drug-induced lupus erythematosus syndrome
   d. Corneal microdeposits

6. What is the target INR values in each of the following three patients receiving anticoagulation therapy with warfarin? (EO-5, 12)
   a. Nonrheumatic atrial fibrillation
   b. Mechanical prosthetic heart valves
   c. Patient being discharged from the hospital following treatment of deep vein thrombosis

7. Each of the following are monitoring parameters for digoxin therapy in this patient, *except:* (EO-5)
   a. Ventricular rate
   b. Renal function
   c. Development of gastrointestinal tract symptoms (nausea, vomiting, etc.)
   d. ESR (erythrocyte sedimentation rate)

8. Which of the following drugs does not increase digoxin concentrations? (EO-9)
   a. Verapamil
   b. Amiodarone
   c. Cholestyramine
   d. Quinidine

9. Which of the following drugs used to treat atrial fibrillation and to maintain normal sinus rhythm would be an alternative to procainamide in this patient? (EO-8, 11, 12)
   a. Amiodarone
   b. Digoxin
   c. Verapamil
   d. Atenolol

10. List the pharmacologic and nonpharmacologic treatment problems present in this patient's treatment plan. (EO-11)

11. Describe what psychosocial factors may affect this patient's adherence to both pharmacologic and nonpharmacologic therapy. (EO-15)

12. Evaluate the pharmacoeconomic considerations relative to this patient's plan of care. (EO-17)

13. Utilizing a key points format, describe the treatment of atrial fibrillation. (EO-18)

CASE 57
Kevin M. Sowinski, James M. Holt, Greta K. Gourley
Topic: Congestive Heart Failure
Level 2
EDUCATIONAL MATERIALS
Chapter 40: Congestive Heart Failure (diagnosis and clinical findings, vasodilators, diuretics)

SCENARIO

Patient and Setting
ED, 72-year-old female; cardiology clinic

Chief Complaint
Increasing shortness of breath (SOB) requiring a sitting position to sleep, swollen legs, malaise, weakness, weight gain, and facial rash

History of Present Illness
Discontinued hydralazine and lisinopril (new medications) 2 days ago due to facial rash; increasing SOB; ankle edema, malaise, weakness, and weight gain

Past Medical History
EF (ejection fraction, 26%; New York Heart Association Class III); orthopnea; sustained ventricular tachycardia; coronary artery disease (CAD) with angina for 20 years; hypertension (HTN) for 30 years; four myocardial infarctions (MIs); chronic renal insufficiency

Past Surgical History
Three coronary artery bypass grafts (CABGs)

Family/Social History
Family History: Mother died at age 62 with HF

Social History: Former cigarette smoker 1 PPD × 25 years; no alcohol intake

Medication History
Amiodarone, 300 mg PO QD

Digoxin, 0.125 mg PO every day

Furosemide, 80 mg PO q AM and 40 mg PO q PM

Maxzide, 2 tab PO q AM

Lisinopril, 5 mg PO QD

Nitroglycerin (NTG), 0.4 mg sublingual PRN for chest pain

Hydralazine, 50 mg PO TID for 7 months

Allergies

NKDA

Physical Examination

GEN: Well-developed, well-nourished female with noticeable SOB

VS: BP 150/92, HR 84, RR 26, T 37.8°C, Wt 64 kg (Wt 2 months earlier 59 kg), Ht 157 cm

HEENT: WNL

COR: +S_3, displaced PMI

CHEST: Bibasilar rales

ABD: WNL

GU: Deferred

RECT: Deferred

EXT: 1+ edema bilateral LE

NEURO: Alert, O × 4

Results of Pertinent Laboratory Tests, Serum Drug Concentrations, and Diagnostic Tests

Na 136 (136)	Plts 200 × 10^9	Glu 6.1 (110)
K 4.0 (4.0)	(200 × 10^3)	Ca 2.2 (8.8)
Cl 98 (98)	MCV 80 (80)	PO$_4$ 0.92 (3.0)
HCO$_3$ 26 (26)	T Bili 3.4 (0.2)	Mg 1.2 (2.5)
BUN 7.5 (21)	AST 0.50 (30)	Uric Acid 190 (3.2)
Cr 143 (1.7)	ALT 0.50 (30)	Dig 1.3 (0.9)
Hct 0.35 (35)	LDH 1.7 (100)	ANA +
Hgb 130 (13)	Alk Phos 1.5 (90)	ESR 100 (100)
Lkcs 8.2 × 10^9	Alb 40 (4.0)	
(8.2 × 10^3)		

Lkc differential: WNL

Urinalysis: 2+ protein

Chest x-ray films: Enlarged cardiac silhouette

ECG: Paced rhythm 84, wide complex

PROBLEM LIST

Identify principal problems from the scenario in priority order

SOAP NOTE

To be completed by student

QUESTIONS

1. The probable cause for ED's HF exacerbation: (EO-1)
   a. Use of amiodarone for control of her atrial fibrillation
   b. Discontinuing hydralazine and lisinopril on her own
   c. Use of digoxin every 3 days
   d. Her obesity

2. ED presents with all the following signs and symptoms of right-sided and left-sided HF exacerbation *except:* (EO-2)
   a. 2+ edema bilateral lower extremities
   b. Orthopnea
   c. Bibasilar rales
   d. HR 84

3. All of the following disease processes listed in ED's medical history probably contributed to ED's HF *except:* (EO-1)
   a. Coronary artery disease
   b. Hypertension
   c. Myocardial infarction
   d. Chronic renal insufficiency

4. Physical assessment findings apparent in ED that point to left-sided heart failure include all the following *except:* (EO-5)
   a. S_3 heart sounds
   b. Orthopnea
   c. Bibasilar rales
   d. S_1 and S_2 heart sounds

5. Describe the mechanisms of action of the pharmacologic interventions for this patient's heart failure. (EO-7)

6. ED should be monitored for factors that would predispose her to digoxin toxicity. Which of the following may increase risk for this problem? (EO-4, 6, 8)
   a. Hypokalemia
   b. Decreased liver function
   c. CrCl >60 mL/min
   d. Hyponatremia

7. ED appears to have drug-induced lupus. This may be due to which one of her medications? (EO-10)
   a. Amiodarone
   b. Furosemide
   c. Maxzide
   d. Hydralazine

8. List the pharmacologic and nonpharmacologic treatment problem(s) present in ED's treatment plan. (EO-11)

9. Metolazone may be indicated in ED when the following occurs: (EO-4, 6, 8, 12)
   a. Creatinine clearance >80 mL/min
   b. Renal function is reduced
   c. HR 90
   d. JVD (+)

10. ED is placed on isosorbide dinitrate TID to assist in lowering her blood pressure as it remains elevated despite further increases in the doses of her antihypertensives. ED should be instructed to take the medication as ordered to allow for a nitrate-free interval to avoid: (EO-10, 14)
    a. Hypotension
    b. Nitrate tolerance
    c. Bradycardia
    d. Rebound hypertension

11. What psychosocial factors may affect ED's adherence to both pharmacologic and nonpharmacologic therapy? (EO-15)

12. Describe the health care provider's role relative to the proposed psychosocial factors identified. (EO-16)

13. Evaluate the pharmacoeconomic considerations relative to ED's plan of care. (EO-17)

14. Utilizing a key points format, summarize the pathophysiologic, therapeutic, and disease management concepts for a given condition. (EO-18)

CASE 58
Kevin M. Sowinski
Topic: Hypertension
Level 1
EDUCATIONAL MATERIALS
Chapter 41: Cardiac Arrhythmias; Chapter 39: Hypertension; Chapter 20: Hyperlipidemia

SCENARIO

Patient and Setting
CC, 62-year-old male; emergency department

Chief Complaint
Lightheadedness, palpitations, and shortness of breath, which has lasted for 2 days

History of Present Illness
Walks 2 miles daily and rides an exercise bicycle three times a week; has previously felt palpitations associated with exercise that usually went away with rest; 2 days ago, while washing the dishes, began feeling short of breath and felt that heart was "racing"; hoped that the palpitations would go away as usual, but came to the hospital as they continued.

Past Medical History
History of hypertension for 20 years, hyperlipidemia for 5 years and rheumatic heart disease (mitral valve) as a child; reports adhering to a step 2 diet for the last 2 years.

Past Surgical History
Noncontributory

Family/Social History
Family History: Noncontributory

Social History: Smoked 15 pack-years; quit 5 years ago; social drinker

Medication History
Lisinopril, 20 mg PO QD

Furosemide, 20 mg PO QD

Gemfibrozil, 600 mg PO BID

Allergies
NKDA

Physical Examination
GEN: Well-developed male in moderate distress

VS: BP 145/90 (clinic visit 1 month ago 145/85), HR 146, RR 22, T 37.2°C, Wt 80 kg, Ht 177.8 cm

HEENT: PERRLA, (−) JVD, mild AV nicking

COR: Rate irregularly irregular, no murmurs or gallops

CHEST: CTA

ABD: Soft, nontender, active bowel sounds

GU: Deferred

RECT: WNL

EXT: No edema, normal pulses throughout

NEURO: A & O × 3

Results of Pertinent Laboratory Tests, Serum Drug Concentrations, and Diagnostic Tests

Na 136 (136)	MCV 90 (90)	Mg 1.05 (2.1)
K 4.5 (4.5)	WBC 8 × 10⁹	Alb 51 (5.1)
Cl 97 (97)	(8 × 10³)	Glu 6.1 (120)
CO$_2$ 22 (22)	Plts 175 × 10⁹	Cholesterol 6.2 (240)
BUN 7.1 (20)	(175 × 10³)	Triglycerides 2.03 (180)
Cr 106 (1.2)	Alk Phos 1.08 (65)	HDL 0.88 (34)
Hct 0.38 (38)	AST 0.58 (35)	LDL 4.4 (170)
Hgb 135 (13.5)	ALT 0.5 (30)	

WBC differential: WNL

INR 1.1

Chest X-ray: clear

ECG: atrial fibrillation, no P waves, variable R-R interval, normal QRS

Echocardiogram: enlarged atria, mild left ventricular hypertrophy, no thrombi

PROBLEM LIST
Identify principal problems from the scenario in priority order [completed Problem List and SOAP Note at end of casebook]

SOAP NOTE
To be completed by student

QUESTIONS
[Answers at end of casebook]

1. Which of the following characteristics in this patient is NOT a risk factor for the development of coronary artery disease? (EO-1, 3)
   a. 20-year history of hypertension
   b. History of rheumatic heart disease
   c. He is a 62-year-old male
   d. HDL of 34 mg/dL

2. Given this patient's history of atrial fibrillation during exercise, which of the following drugs is likely to be least effective at controlling this patient's rapid ventricular response? (EO-8, 12)
   a. Digoxin
   b. Verapamil
   c. Diltiazem
   d. Atenolol

3. All of the following findings are associated with atrial fibrillation in this patient *except:* (EO-1, 2)
   a. Heart rate of 146 bpm
   b. AV nicking
   c. Atrial enlargement
   d. No P waves on the ECG

4. To ensure that this patient has been following and adhering to a Step II diet, in explaining it to him, which of the following are the characteristics of a Step II diet? (EO-11, 12)
   a. <25 % of total calories from fat, 8–10 % of total calories from saturated fat and < 200 mg cholesterol/day.
   b. <30 % of total calories from fat, ≤7 % of total calories from saturated fat and <200 mg cholesterol/day.
   c. <30 % of total calories from fat, ≤8–10 % of total calories from saturated fat and <300 mg cholesterol/day.
   d. <30 % of total calories from fat, ≤7 % of total calories from saturated fat and <300 mg cholesterol/day.

5. Which of the following therapeutic options is most appropriate for the treatment of this patient's hyperlipidemia? (EO-8, 12)
   a. Continue gemfibrozil
   b. D/C gemfibrozil and initiate fenofibrate therapy
   c. D/C gemfibrozil and initiate fluvastatin therapy
   d. Continue gemfibrozil and add fenofibrate therapy

6. Prior to either pharmacologic or electrical cardioversion for atrial fibrillation, which of the following is the appropriate time frame for warfarin therapy? (EO-8, 12)
   a. Three days
   b. One week
   c. Three weeks
   d. Three months

7. Intravenous verapamil is used initially to treat this patient's atrial fibrillation and thus oral verapamil is chosen for long-term control of ventricular rate. Due to the addition of verapamil for atrial fibrillation therapy, which of the following is the most appropriate treatment of this patient's hypertension? (EO-8, 10, 12)
   a. Continue lisinopril and furosemide
   b. Continue lisinopril and D/C furosemide
   c. Continue lisinopril
   d. Continue lisinopril, D/C furosemide, and add hydrochlorothiazide

8. List adverse effects associated with chronic verapamil therapy for rate control in atrial fibrillation. (E0-10)

9. Which of the following medications may decrease the effect of warfarin? (EO-7, 9)
   a. Phenytoin
   b. NSAIDs (e.g., ibuprofen, naproxen)
   c. Cimetidine
   d. Phytonadione

10. List the nonpharmacologic treatment problems present in this patient's treatment plan. (EO-11)

11. Describe what psychosocial factors may affect this patient's adherence to both pharmacologic and nonpharmacologic therapy. (EO-15)

12. Evaluate the pharmacoeconomic considerations relative to this patient's plan of care. (EO-17)

13. Utilizing a key points format, list the points related to the treatment of hypertension in this patient. (EO-18)

CASE 59
Kevin M. Sowinski
Topic: Cardiac Arrhythmias (Atrial Fibrillation)
 Level 2
EDUCATIONAL MATERIALS
Chapter 41: Cardiac Arrhythmias; Chapter 44: Thromboembolic Disease

---

SCENARIO

Patient and Setting
MB, a 68-year-old female, emergency department

Chief Complaint
Sudden onset of right-sided weakness and inability to speak

History of Present Illness
Unknown

Past Medical History
Atrial fibrillation (Afib) since 1990; osteoarthritis; hypothyroidism; mild osteoporosis

Past Surgical History
Hysterectomy 5 years ago

Family/Social History
Family History: Lives alone
Social History: Financially independent

Medication History
Digoxin, 0.125 mg PO QD
Naproxen, 375 mg PO BID
Levothyroxine, 0.2 mg PO QD
Calcium carbonate, 1250 mg PO QD
Conjugated estrogens, 0.625 mg PO QD

Allergies

NKDA

Physical Examination

GEN: Lethargic, weak-appearing elderly female unable to speak, respond to questions, or walk

VS: BP 100/80, P 110 irreg irreg, R 18, T 36.5°C, Wt 58 kg

HEENT: Thin hair, patches of baldness

COR: Irregularly irregular; Grade II/VI SEM

CHEST: Clear to P and A

ABD: Benign

GU: Deferred

RECT: Guaiac negative

EXT: R-sided weakness, mild deformities hands/fingers

NEURO: Consistent with acute ischemic stroke

Results of Pertinent Laboratory Tests, Serum Drug Concentrations, and Diagnostic Tests

Electrolyte levels:	INR 1.0	TSH 3 mU/L (3 μM/dL)
WNL	APTT 26 sec	RT3U 0.3 (30%)
CBC: WNL	ESR 65 mm/hr	FT4I 3.6
PO$_4$ 1.2 (3.75)	Thyroxine (TT4)	
Cr 50 (0.6)	150 nmol/L	
Ca 2.5 (9.4)	(12 μg/dL)	

ECG: Afib, ventricular rate 110

MRI scan: Evidence consistent with acute embolic stroke

Echocardiogram: Large left ventricular thrombus

PROBLEM LIST

Identify principal problems from the scenario in priority order [completed Problem List and SOAP Note at end of casebook]

SOAP NOTE

To be completed by student

QUESTIONS

[Answers at end of casebook]

1. Which of the following characteristics in this patient is a sign or symptom of acute ischemic stroke? (EO-2)
   a. Mild deformities in the hands and fingers
   b. Echocardiographic findings of a large left ventricular thrombus
   c. Pulse of 110 bpm
   d. Aphasia

2. Which of the following characteristics in this patient is NOT a sign and symptom of hyperthyroidism? (EO-2)
   a. Thin hair with patches of baldness
   b. Lethargic
   c. TT$_4$ 150
   d. Heart rate of 110 bpm

3. Which of the following is the mechanism of the interaction between NSAIDs and warfarin? (EO-7, 9)
   a. Protein binding displacement of warfarin from albumin, resulting in transient increases in warfarin effect (i.e., increased INR)
   b. NSAID-induced inhibition of CYP3A4, resulting in increases in warfarin effect (i.e., increased INR)
   c. NSAID-induced induction of CYP3A4, resulting in decreases in warfarin effect (i.e., decreased INR)
   d. Increased warfarin bioavailability, resulting in increased warfarin effect (i.e., increased INR)

4. Which of the following drug regimens is the most appropriate for the treatment of this patient's osteoarthritis? (EO-11, 12)
   a. D/C naproxen, start ECASA 650 mg q6h
   b. D/C naproxen, start ibuprofen 400 mg TID
   c. D/C naproxen, start APAP 650 mg q6h
   d. Continue naproxen

5. Which of the following factors may enhance the removal of vitamin K-dependent clotting factors and increase warfarin's effect? (EO-7, 9)
   a. Hyperthyroidism
   b. Decreased ingestion of vitamin K in the diet
   c. NSAID use
   d. Increased ingestion of vitamin K in the diet

6. Which of the following describes why this patient is not a candidate for thrombolytic therapy for acute ischemic stroke? (EO-8, 11, 12)
   a. She has suffered a hemorrhagic stroke and thus is at risk for bleeding
   b. She is receiving a NSAID and thus is at risk for gastrointestinal tract bleeding
   c. The time since the onset of her symptoms is uncertain
   d. Her condition is too unstable for the administration of a thrombolytic

7. Which of the following regimens and monitoring parameters is most appropriate during the initiation of warfarin therapy in this patient? (EO-12)
   a. Warfarin 5 mg PO × 3 days, adjust based on INR goal of 2–3
   b. Warfarin 10 mg PO × 3 days, adjust based on INR goal of 2–3
   c. Warfarin 5 mg PO × 3 days, adjust based on an INR goal of 2.5–3.5
   d. Warfarin 10 mg PO × 3 days, adjust based on an INR goal of 2.5–3.5

8. Which of the following are the most appropriate daily monitoring parameters for heparin therapy in this patient? (EO-5, 12)
   a. Platelets, Hgb/Hct, aPTT, and INR
   b. Platelets, Hgb/Hct, aPTT
   c. Platelets, Hgb/Hct, and serum creatinine
   d. aPTT and INR

9. List the nonpharmacologic treatment problems present in this patient's treatment plan. (EO-11)

10. Describe what psychosocial factors may affect this patient's adherence to both pharmacologic and nonpharmacologic therapy. (EO-15)

11. Utilizing a key points format, list the points related to the treatment of atrial fibrillation in this patient. (EO-18)

12. Following a year of therapy with estrogen replacement therapy for osteoporosis, this patient is initiated on alendronate 10 mg daily. How should the health care provider counsel the patient to take this therapy? (EO-10, 14)

13. Evaluate the pharmacoeconomic considerations relative to this patient's plan of care. (EO-17)

CASE 60
Kevin M. Sowinski
Topic: Hypertension

Level 2

EDUCATIONAL MATERIALS
Chapter 44: Thromboembolic Disease; Chapter 39: Hypertension; Chapter 20: Hyperlipidemia

---

SCENARIO

Patient and Setting
JF, 29-year-old white male; hypertension clinic

Chief Complaint
Patient states he takes his medication as prescribed but has been unable to comply with the low-salt, low-cholesterol diet recommended 6 months ago.

History of Present Illness
Two previous high blood pressure readings; increasing headaches, dark stools, polyuria, polydipsia, and general weakness; noticed spots of blood on the tissue after the last few bowel movements, but no other bleeding; recently ran out of chemstrips, has not checked his blood glucose for 1 week; noted regular insulin not its usual color.

Past Medical History
Type 1 diabetes mellitus (DM) since age 23
Iron deficiency anemia
Hypercholesterolemia

Past Surgical History
Mitral valve replacement (3 months ago, secondary to rheumatic heart disease, St. Jude valve)

Family/Social History
Family History: Unknown
Social History: Smokes 1 PPD; no alcohol intake

Medication History
$FeSO_4$, 325 mg PO QD for 1 month
Warfarin, 7.5 mg PO QD
Insulin Reg and NPH SC (unknown doses), recently switched from pork to human
Ibuprofen, PO PRN for headache

Allergies
Sulfonamides

Physical Examination
GEN: Well-developed, well-nourished male
VS: BP 190/98, HR 76, T 37°C, RR 18, Wt 80 kg, Ht 173 cm
HEENT: AV nicking; remainder of examination within normal limits
COR: NL S_1 & S_2
CHEST: WNL
ABD: Soft without masses
GU: WNL
RECT: Small external hemorrhoid
EXT: WNL
NEURO: Oriented × 3

Results of Pertinent Laboratory Tests, Serum Drug Concentrations, and Diagnostic Tests

Na 143 (143)	Hct 0.34 (34)	LDH 1.6 (95)
K 4.5 (4.5)	Hgb 142 (14.2)	Alk Phos 0.8 (45)
Cl 103 (103)	Lkcs 9.0×10^9	Alb 40 (4.0)
HCO_3 24 (24)	(9.0×10^3)	T Bili 17.1 (1.0)
BUN 7.9 (22)	Plts 200×10^9	INR 4.9
Cr 70.1 (0.8)	(200×10^3)	TG 3.6 (320)
Glu (Fasting)	MCV 84 (84)	Chol 7.24 (280)
22.2 (400)	AST 0.5 (30)	LDL 1.81 (186)
HbA_{1C} 13.5	ALT 0.37 (22)	HDL 0.78 (30)

Urinalysis: (−) protein; (−) ketones; 0 RBCs/hpf; 2+ glucose
Chest x-ray: Moderate cardiomegaly; bilateral fluffy infiltrates
ECG: WNL

PROBLEM LIST
Identify principal problems from the scenario in priority order [completed Problem List and SOAP Note at end of casebook]

SOAP NOTE

To be completed by student

QUESTIONS

[*Answers at end of casebook*]

1. Six weeks after JF is initiated on enalapril therapy he develops a dry nonproductive cough that keeps him awake at night. Which of the following changes to his antihypertensive regimen is most appropriate for treating his hypertension, alleviating his cough, and slowing the progression of diabetic nephropathy? (EO-10, 11, 12)
   a. Continue enalapril and add dextromethorphan at bedtime
   b. D/C enalapril and initiate lisinopril therapy
   c. D/C enalapril and initiate diltiazem therapy
   d. D/C enalapril and initiate terazosin therapy

2. Which of the following is a long-term complication of uncontrolled diabetes? (EO-8, 10)
   a. Hypertension
   b. Renal disease
   c. Atrial fibrillation
   d. Hypercholesterolemia

3. Which of the following antihypertensive medications should be used with caution in this patient, secondary to his diabetes? (EO-5, 8, 11, 12)
   a. Atenolol
   b. Prazosin
   c. Enalapril
   d. Diltiazem

4. Which of the following laboratory parameters is the most appropriate to assess his long-term diabetes control? (EO-5, 8, 12)
   a. Blood glucose concentrations
   b. Urinary protein
   c. HbA_{1C}
   d. Serum creatinine

5. If JF were not taking iron, which of the following would be the most likely cause of his melena? (EO-10)
   a. Hypertension
   b. Insulin Regular
   c. Warfarin-induced rectal bleeding
   d. NSAID-induced gastritis

6. This patient is very concerned about the development of "sexual problems" due to his antihypertensive medications. Which of the following antihypertensive drugs is associated with the lowest incidence of sexual dysfunction? (EO-10)
   a. Propranolol
   b. Clonidine
   c. HCTZ
   d. Diltiazem

7. Which of the following antihypertensive drugs may worsen left ventricular hypertrophy? (EO-10)
   a. Atenolol
   b. Hydralazine
   c. Enalapril
   d. Labetalol

8. Based on JNC VI guidelines, the goal blood pressure for this patient is: (EO-5, 12)
   a. <150/90 mmHg
   b. <140/90 mmHg
   c. <130/85 mmHg
   d. <135/90 mmHg

9. Based on ADA guidelines, the goal LDL-C for this patient is: (EO-5, 12)
   a. <100 mg/dL
   b. <200 mg/dL
   c. <130 mg/dL
   d. <160 mg/dL

10. Summarize the nonpharmacologic treatment for this patient's hypertension and dyslipidemia. (EO-11)

11. List the risk factors that this patient has for the development of cardiovascular disease. (EO-1, 3)

12. Utilizing the key points format, list the points related to the treatment of hypertension in this patient. (EO-18)

13. In the treatment of hypertension in patients with the following coexistent disease states, list one antihypertensive which would be preferred first-line therapy and one agent which would *not* be preferred as first-line therapy. Briefly explain your answers. (EO-14)
    a. Congestive heart failure
    b. Diabetes mellitus

14. Evaluate the pharmacoeconomic considerations relative to this patient's plan of care. (EO-17)

CASE 61
Kevin M. Sowinski
Topic: Angina Pectoris

EDUCATIONAL MATERIALS
Chapter 41: Cardiac Arrhythmias; Chapter 39: Hypertension; Chapter 40: Congestive Heart Failure; Chapter 42: Ischemic Heart Disease

---

SCENARIO

Patient and Setting
TA, 55-year-old male; hypertension clinic

Chief Complaint
Patient being seen for hypertension (HTN) follow-up

History of Present Illness
HTN follow-up visit

Past Medical History
30-year history of HTN; 10-year history of coronary artery disease (CAD), poorly controlled due to poor compliance;

2 years ago had an inferior wall myocardial infarction (MI) and developed sustained ventricular tachycardia (SVT) 2 months after hospitalization; treated with amiodarone; subsequent to the MI, had symptoms of heart failure (HF), controlled on furosemide; angina worsened over the past 6 months; currently 3 to 5 episodes of chest pain per week; history of degenerative joint disease

Past Surgical History

None

Family/Social History

Family History: Noncontributory

Social History: Smoked 1 PPD × 40 years; currently smokes 1–2 packs per week and on average drinks a six-pack of beer per week

Medication History

Amiodarone, 400 mg PO daily

Furosemide, 20 mg PO BID

Nitroglycerin, 0.4 mg PO PRN for chest pain

Ketoprofen, 75 mg PO TID

Allergies

NKDA

Physical Examination

GEN: TA is an anxious male, appearing older than his stated age

VS: BP 120/90, HR 105, T 38.2°C, RR 20, Wt 68 kg

HEENT: AV nicking and narrowing, corneal microdeposits

COR: Normal S_1, S_2, and + S_4

CHEST: CTA

ABD: WNL

GU: WNL

RECT: Guaiac negative

EXT: 1+ ankle edema, bluish-gray skin discoloration on sun-exposed areas

NEURO: Alert and Oriented × 3

Results of Pertinent Laboratory Tests, Serum Drug Concentrations, and Diagnostic Tests:

Na 134 (134)	Hgb 140 (14)	AST 0.70 (42)
K 3.9 (3.9)	Lkcs 8.3 × 10⁹	ALT 0.64 (38)
Cl 102 (102)	(8.3 × 10³)	LDH 3.18 (192)
HCO₃ 28 (28)	Plts 186 × 10⁹	Alk Phos 0.8 (45)
BUN 6.1 (17)	(186 × 10³)	Alb 38 (3.8)
Cr 106 (1.2)	MCV 88 (88)	ESR 43 mm/hr
Hct 0.38 (0.38)		

Lkc differential: WNL

Urinalysis: WNL

ECG: Shows evidence of old inferior wall MI; voltage changes consistent with LVH; currently is in sinus tachycardia with a rate of 100 bpm

PROBLEM LIST

Identify principal problems from the scenario in priority order

SOAP NOTE

To be completed by student

QUESTIONS

1. Which of the following is an amiodarone adverse effect observed in this patient? (EO-10)
   a. Blue-gray skin on sun-exposed areas
   b. 1+ ankle edema
   c. AV nicking and narrowing
   d. Guaiac-positive stools

2. Which of the following anti-ischemic drugs has been shown to affect long-term outcome in patients with heart failure? (EO-8, 12)
   a. Carvedilol
   b. Amlodipine
   c. Isosorbide mononitrate
   d. Diltiazem

3. Which of the following monitoring parameters is NOT important in the early assessment of ACE inhibitor therapy in this patient? (EO-5, 8, 12)
   a. Serum potassium
   b. Serum creatinine
   c. Serum sodium
   d. Liver function tests

4. Over the course of the following 6 months this patient develops two episodes of sustained ventricular tachycardia. Which of the following treatment options is most appropriate? (EO 8, 12)
   a. Continue amiodarone therapy; these episodes are expected
   b. Consider implantable cardioverter defibrillator therapy
   c. Add quinidine therapy to the patient's current regimen
   d. D/C amiodarone and add sotalol

5. Which of the following describes how NSAIDs decrease the efficacy of heart failure medications? (EO-7, 10)
   a. Decreased blood pressure
   b. Increased renal function
   c. Enhanced fluid retention
   d. Reduced angiotensin II formation

6. Upon your recommendation, enalapril is initiated. Four months later, TA returns to the clinic complaining of a new-onset persistent cough that is extremely bothersome, especially at night. The cough prevents TA from sleeping.

Which of the following is the most likely explanation? (EO-1, 3, 7, 10)
a. Amiodarone pulmonary toxicity
b. Enalapril-induced cough
c. Cough induced by the K-Dur being caught in the patient's throat
d. Interaction between aspirin and enalapril, resulting in increased bradykinin concentrations

7. Which of the following therapies is an appropriate vasodilator regimen for heart failure treatment in a patient with bilateral renal artery stenosis? (EO-7, 10, 12)
a. Isosorbide dinitrate and hydralazine
b. Metoprolol
c. Enalapril
d. Losartan

8. Your medical team decides that digoxin should be initiated in this patient. Which of the following doses is the most appropriate maintenance dose for this patient? (EO-4)
a. 0.375 mg PO QD
b. 0.25 mg PO QD
c. 0.125 mg PO BID
d. 0.125 mg PO every other day

9. ACE inhibitor therapy is to be initiated in this patient. Which of the following regimens is an appropriate ACE inhibitor initiation regimen? (EO-12)
a. Enalapril 10 mg PO BID
b. Captopril 6.25 mg PO TID
c. Enalaprilat 1.25 mg IV q6h
d. Lisinopril 10 mg PO BID

10. TA is having difficulty swallowing the KCl tablet (K-Dur) because of its large size. The intern is considering switching to the liquid preparation. What is your response to the physician? (EO-11, 12)

11. What patient education would you give TA about the proper use of his sublingual nitroglycerin tablets? (EO-12, 14, 15)

12. Summarize the risk factor reduction therapies for this patient's ischemic heart disease. (EO-12, 14, 15)

13. Describe what psychosocial factors are important to discuss with this patient and his family. (EO-15)

14. Utilizing the key points format, list the points related to the treatment of ischemic heart disease in this patient. (EO-18)

15. Evaluate the pharmacoeconomic considerations relative to this patient's plan of care. (EO-17)

CASE 62
Kevin M. Sowinski
Topic: Angina Pectoris

EDUCATIONAL MATERIALS
Chapter 41: Cardiac Arrhythmias; Chapter 39: Hypertension; Chapter 40: Congestive Heart Failure; Chapter 42: Ischemic Heart Disease

---

SCENARIO
Patient and Setting
RS, 58-year-old female; cardiology clinic

Chief Complaint
Follow-up evaluation of angina pectoris

History of Present Illness
At last visit, started on a nitroglycerin (NTG) transdermal patch, 0.4 mg/hr q24h, and sublingual NTG, 0.4 mg PRN; states that during the first week of this therapy the number of anginal episodes decreased from 4–5 episodes/week to 1–2 episodes/week; thereafter the episodes returned to 4 to 5 times/week; all anginal episodes occurred during physical exertion and were relieved by rest and administration of one sublingual NTG; able to walk 4 or 5 blocks before developing chest pains; denies fatigue, shortness of breath (SOB), orthopnea, and paroxysmal nocturnal dyspnea (PND)

Past Medical History
Lateral myocardial infarction (MI) 6 years ago; history of mild congestive heart failure (CHF); chronic atrial fibrillation (failed conversion to normal sinus rhythm with quinidine, procainamide, and propafenone); hypercholesterolemia; previous history of medication noncompliance; does not understand why nitroglycerin patch should be removed at night; attends an anticoagulation clinic regularly for adjustments to warfarin therapy

Past Surgical History
Noncontributory

Family/Social History
Family History: Mother died at age 65 from an acute myocardial infarction, father died at age 80
Social History: Social drinker

Medication History
Digoxin, 0.125 mg PO QD
Furosemide, 40 mg PO QD
Warfarin, 5 mg PO QD
Lovastatin, 20 mg PO q PM, initiated 1 month ago
Captopril, 12.5 mg PO TID
KCl, 20 mEq PO BID
Nitroglycerin, 0.4 mg SL PRN
Nitroglycerin patch, 0.4 mg/hr q24h

Allergies

No known drug allergies

Physical Examination

GEN: Adult female in NAD
VS: BP 136/82, P 62 (irregular), RR 18, Wt 53.2 kg, Ht 165 cm
HEENT: PERRLA, EOM
COR: S_1, S_2, and S_3 heart sound, no JVD or HJR, no murmur
CHEST: CTA and P
ABD: Soft, nontender with bowel sounds
GU: WNL
RECT: WNL
EXT: Normal pulses throughout, no peripheral edema
NEURO: Cranial nerves II–XII grossly intact, oriented × 3

Results of Pertinent Laboratory Tests, Serum Drug Concentrations, and Diagnostic Tests

Na^+ 142 (142)   Hgb 136 (13.6)   TC 5.20 (200)
K^+ 4.8 (4.8)   Lkcs 7.8 × 10^9 LDL 3.00 (115)
Cl 103 (103)   (7.8 × 10^3)   VLDL 0.98 (38)
HCO_3 25 (25)   Plts 333 × 10^9 HDL 1.2 (47)
BUN 60 (18)   (333 × 10^3)   Trig 2.14 (190)
SCr 100 (1.1)   RBC 4.64 × 10^{12} Digoxin 1.8 (1.4)
Hct 0.40 (40.9)   (4.64 × 10^6)   INR 2.1

Lkc differential: segs 0.64 (64), bands 0.04 (4), lymphs 0.29 (29), monos 0.03 (3), eos 0 (0), baso 0 (0)

ECG: Atrial fibrillation with ventricular rate of 65 bpm, with Q-wave

PROBLEM LIST

Identify principal problems from the scenario in priority order [completed Problem List and SOAP Note at end of casebook]

SOAP NOTE

To be completed by student

QUESTIONS

[Answers at end of casebook]

1. Which of the following is the most appropriate therapy for managing this patient's nitrate tolerance? (EO-7, 8, 12)
   a. *N*-Acetylcysteine
   b. Increase the captopril dose to 50 mg TID
   c. Hydrochlorothiazide
   d. Provide a 10–12-hour nitrate-free period

2. RS is currently receiving captopril 12.5 mg TID. Which of the following goal ACE inhibitor regimens will provide this patient with a dose shown to reduce mortality in controlled clinical trials? (EO-8, 10, 12)
   a. Captopril 25 mg TID
   b. Enalapril 5 mg BID
   c. Lisinopril 20 mg daily
   d. Benazepril 10 mg daily

3. Which of the following physical assessment findings is consistent with a prior myocardial infarction? (EO-2)
   a. ECG findings
   b. S_3 heart sound
   c. Irregular pulse
   d. Chest pain with exertion

4. Given the patient's risk factors and previous myocardial infarction, which of the following is the most appropriate LDL goal in this patient? (EO-5, 12)
   a. <70 mg/dL
   b. <100 mg/dL
   c. <130 mg/dL
   d. <160 mg/dL

5. Which of the following medications that this patient is receiving is LEAST likely to affect potassium homeostasis? (EO-7, 10)
   a. Furosemide
   b. Captopril
   c. KCl
   d. Nitroglycerin

6. The medical resident wants to obtain a digoxin serum concentration in this patient. The patient receives her daily dose at 7 AM and daily labs are obtained at 8 AM. While reviewing the chart prior to morning work rounds, it is noted that the resident ordered the "digoxin level" to be obtained with the daily labs. Which of the following is the most appropriate advice for the resident? (EO-6, 12)
   a. Serum concentrations obtained 1 hour after a digoxin dose are likely to be falsely low.
   b. Serum concentrations obtained 1 hour after a digoxin dose are likely to be falsely elevated.
   c. Although the serum concentration is likely to be falsely elevated the order does not need to be changed since you will be able to correct the concentration using a formula.
   d. This is the most appropriate time to obtain a digoxin serum concentration.

7. While receiving counseling about her prescription medications from her health care provider, RS asks which OTC analgesic is the best one to use for an occasional headache. The health care provider correctly replies: (EO-11, 12)
   a. Naproxen
   b. Enteric coated aspirin
   c. Goody's headache powders
   d. Acetaminophen

8. When communicating medication instructions to this patient, which of the following is NOT a reason to immediately contact her health care provider? (EO-14, 15, 16)
   a. Shortness of breath that does not go away with rest
   b. Weight gain of 2–3 pounds in 1 week

c. Swelling in ankles, feet, and/or legs

d. Persistent cough and/or wheezing

9. Summarize the nonpharmacologic therapies for this patient's heart failure. (EO-11)

10. List the pharmacologic treatment problems present in this patient's treatment plan. (EO-11)

11. Describe what psychosocial factors may affect this patient's adherence to both pharmacologic and nonpharmacologic therapy. (EO-15)

12. Utilizing a key points format, list the points related to the treatment of angina/heart failure in this patient. (EO-18)

13. Evaluate the pharmacoeconomic considerations relative to this patient's plan of care. (EO-17)

CASE 63
Kevin M. Sowinski
Topic: Thromboembolic Disorders
Level 3

EDUCATIONAL MATERIALS
Chapter 41: Cardiac Arrhythmias; Chapter 44: Thromboembolic Disease

---

SCENARIO

Patient and Setting

JO, 38-year-old female; emergency department

Chief Complaint

Intense sudden-onset pleuritic chest pain

History of Present Illness

Intense pleuritic chest pain came suddenly; difficulty breathing, coughed up some bright red blood; before this time felt fine

Past Medical History

History of "palpitations"; mitral valve prolapse (MVP); paroxysmal supraventricular tachycardia (PSVT) controlled with atenolol; irritable bowel syndrome (IBS); and iron deficiency anemia

Past Surgical History

Noncontributory

Family/Social History

Family History: Noncontributory

Social History: No ethanol use; smokes 1 PPD

Medication History

Atenolol, 50 mg PO QD

Psyllium, 2 tablespoons PO QD

Ferrous sulfate, 1 tablet PO QD

Oral contraceptives (35 mg ethinyl estradiol/1 mg norethindrone, PO 21 days per month)

Allergies

NKDA

Physical Examination

GEN: Anxious-appearing young woman, sitting upright, complaining of shortness of breath and chest pain

VS: BP 155/95, P 110 reg, RR 25, T 37.8°C, Wt 62 kg

HEENT: WNL

COR: S_1 midsystolic click heard best along the left lower sternal border; NL S_2, negative S_3, S_4

CHEST: Decreased breathing sounds

ABD: Slight guarding

GU: Deferred

RECT: Guaiac negative

EXT: No clubbing, cyanosis, or edema

NEURO: Intact, alert, and oriented × 3

Results of Pertinent Laboratory Tests, Serum Drug Concentrations, and Diagnostic Tests

Chem 7 WNL	Lkcs 6 × 10⁹	Plts 240 × 10⁹
LFTs WNL	(6 × 10³)	(240 × 10³)
Hct 0.33 (33)		MCV 85 (85)
Hgb 110 (11)		

Chest x-ray: Slight density in lower lobes

ECG: Sinus tachycardia with normal intervals

Ventilation perfusion scan (V/Q): Shows a ventilation perfusion mismatch; high probability for pulmonary embolism

Pulmonary angiography: Confirms diagnosis and localizes clot to a large pulmonary artery

PROBLEM LIST

Identify principal problems from the scenario in priority order [completed Problem List and SOAP Note at end of casebook]

SOAP NOTE

To be completed by student

QUESTIONS

[Answers at end of casebook]

1. Which of the following signs and symptoms is *not* associated with pulmonary embolism in this patient? (EO-1, 2)
   a. Midsystolic click heard best along the left lower sternal border
   b. Decreased breath sounds
   c. Shortness of breath
   d. Chest pain

2. Which of the following problems in this patient is most likely to complicate iron therapy for the treatment of this patient's anemia? (EO-8, 10, 12)
   a. Contraception
   b. Mitral valve prolapse
   c. Paroxysmal supraventricular tachycardia
   d. Constipation

3. Which of the following is *not* true regarding heparin therapy? (EO-7, 10, 11, 12,)
   a. Weight-based heparin dosing should be based on ideal body weight.
   b. Goal aPTT is 1.5–2.5 times the control value.
   c. Thrombocytopenia is a common adverse effect secondary to heparin therapy.
   d. Platelets and Hct/Hgb should be measured daily during the initiation of heparin therapy.

4. Which of the following is the likely etiology for the development of pulmonary embolism in this patient? (EO-1)
   a. Oral contraceptive use
   b. Irritable bowel syndrome
   c. Atenolol therapy
   d. Embolism secondary to paroxysmal supraventricular tachycardia

5. Due to the history of mitral valve prolapse this patient's cardiologist decides she is a candidate for dental prophylaxis. Which of the following is the most appropriate recommendation for this patient? (EO-8, 12)
   a. Penicillin VK 2 g PO × 1
   b. Azithromycin 500 mg PO × 1
   c. Clindamycin 900 mg PO × 1
   d. Amoxicillin 2 g PO × 1

6. This patient has been previously diagnosed with PSVT. All of the following are types of PSVT *except:* (EO-3)
   a. Ventricular fibrillation
   b. AV nodal reentrant tachycardia
   c. AV reentrant tachycardia
   d. Wolff-Parkinson-White syndrome

7. Given the patient's current history, which of the following contraceptives would be inappropriate for this patient? (EO-8, 12)
   a. Condoms
   b. Spermicidal gel
   c. Oral contraceptives
   d. Sponge

8. Which of he following is the appropriate duration of warfarin therapy in this patient? (EO-12)
   a. Until discharge from the hospital
   b. At least 3 weeks
   c. At least 3 months
   d. Lifelong therapy

9. List the nonpharmacologic treatment problems present in this patient's treatment plan. (EO-11)

10. Describe the risks associated with warfarin use in pregnancy and what alternatives are available for chronic treatment of venous thromboembolism. (EO-8, 10, 12)

11. Describe what psychosocial factors may effect this patient's adherence to both pharmacologic and nonpharmacologic therapy. (EO-15)

12. Evaluate the pharmacoeconomic considerations relative to this patient's plan of care. (EO-17)

CASE 64
Kevin M. Sowinski
Topic: Congestive Heart Failure

EDUCATIONAL MATERIALS
Chapter 39: Hypertension;
Chapter 40: Congestive Heart Failure

SCENARIO

Patient and Setting
AR, 69-year-old male; cardiology clinic

Chief Complaint
Feeling nauseated and extremely fatigued

History of Present Illness
2-week history of nausea and fatigue

Past Medical History
Congestive heart failure (CHF) × 6 months; hypertension (HTN) × 10 years

Past Surgical History
None

Family/Social History
Noncontributory

Medication History
Digoxin, 0.375 mg PO QD
Furosemide, 40 mg PO q AM

Enalapril, 5 mg PO q AM
KCl, 10 mEq PO BID

Allergies
NKDA

Physical Examination

GEN: Well-developed, well-nourished, appearing pale and fatigued
VS: BP 160/95, HR 48, RR 18, Wt 70 kg, Ht 183 cm
HEENT: WNL
COR: Displaced PMI, nl S_1, S_2, (+) S_3
CHEST: Clear
ABD: (+) Bowel sounds
GU: Slightly enlarged prostate
RECT: Deferred
EXT: Trace ankle edema,
NEURO: A & O $\times$ 3

Results of Pertinent Laboratory Tests, Serum Drug Concentrations, and Diagnostic Tests

Na 145 (145)   Hgb 140 (14)   Alk Phos 1.5 (90)
K 3.0 (3.0)   Lkcs 8.5 $\times$ 10^9 Alb 50 (5.0)
Cl 96 (96)   (8.5 $\times$ 10^3)   Ca 2.2 (8.8)
HCO$_3$ 22 (22)   Plts 350 $\times$ 10^9 PO$_4$ 0.97 (3.0)
BUN 3.5 (10)   (350 $\times$ 10^3)   Mg 1.0 (2.0)
Cr 106 (1.3)   AST 0.5 (30)   Uric Acid 172 (2.9)
Glu 6.1 (110)   ALT 0.5 (30)   Digoxin 3.2 (2.5)
Hct 0.39 (39)   LDH 1.7 (100)

Urinalysis: WNL

Chest x-ray: Enlarged cardiac silhouette

ECG: First-degree AV block, bradycardia

PROBLEM LIST

Identify principal problems from the scenario in priority order

SOAP NOTE

To be completed by student

QUESTIONS

1. Which of the following laboratory findings in this patient predisposes him to the development of digoxin toxicity? (EO-5, 10)
   a. Potassium: 3.0 mEq/L
   b. Hct: 39%
   c. BP: 160/95
   d. Uric acid: 2.9

2. Each of the following physical findings in this patient are signs/symptoms of digoxin toxicity *except:* (EO-2, 10)
   a. AV block
   b. Nausea
   c. Bradycardia
   d. Enlarged cardiac silhouette

3. Each of the following are signs and/or symptoms of heart failure in this patient, *except:* (EO-2)
   a. Enlarged cardiac silhouette
   b. Displaced PMI
   c. Trace ankle edema
   d. First-degree AV block

4. Which of AR's heart failure medications have been shown to reduce mortality in long-term controlled clinical trials? (EO-8, 12)
   a. Digoxin
   b. Furosemide
   c. Enalapril
   d. Potassium chloride

5. To appropriately manage this patient's heart failure an estimate of left-ventricular ejection fraction would be useful. Which of the following methods is NOT used to estimate ejection fraction? (EO-5)
   a. Echocardiography
   b. Radionuclide ventriculography
   c. Contrast ventriculography
   d. Chest x-ray

6. After maximizing this patient's ACE inhibitor, which of the following heart failure therapies should be considered as additional therapy for this patient's heart failure? (EO-8, 12)
   a. Metolazone to furosemide therapy
   b. Carvedilol therapy
   c. Amlodipine therapy
   d. Hydralazine therapy

7. Which of the following ACE inhibitor doses is equivalent to enalapril 5 mg BID? (EO-5, 8, 12)
   a. Captopril 6.25 mg TID
   b. Lisinopril 20 mg QD
   c. Benazepril 40 mg QD
   d. Lisinopril 10 mg QD

8. Which of the following is NOT a common adverse effect from acute administration of oral potassium therapy? (EO-10)
   a. Cardiac arrhythmias
   b. Nausea
   c. Bad taste
   d. Diarrhea

9. List the criteria for Digibind therapy for the treatment of digoxin toxicity. (EO-12)

10. Summarize the nonpharmacologic treatment options for this patient's heart failure. (EO-11)

11. Describe what psychosocial factors may affect this patient's adherence to both pharmacologic and nonpharmacologic therapy. (EO-15)

12. Utilizing a key points format, list the points related to the treatment of acute ischemic stroke in this patient. (EO-18)

13. Evaluate the pharmacoeconomic considerations relative to this patient's plan of care. (EO-17)

CASE 65
Kevin M. Sowinski
Topic: S/P Acute Myocardial Infarction/
Heart Failure

EDUCATIONAL MATERIALS
Chapter 40: Congestive Heart Failure; Chapter 42:
Ischemic Heart Disease; Chapter 43: Acute
Myocardial Infarction

SCENARIO

Patient and Setting
DA, 57-year-old female; medicine clinic

Chief Complaint
Follow-up clinic appointment

History of Present Illness
Complains of leg edema, nocturia, and SOB

Past Medical History
Came to the ED 30 days ago with an anterior wall myocardial infarction (MI); immediately after the MI, experienced intermittent bradycardia with occasional PVCs; has experienced multiple episodes of Crohn's disease since age 25; currently Crohn's disease in remission; last flare-up resolved 6 months ago; long history of uncontrolled hypertension

Past Surgical History
Appendectomy, age 22; intestinal resection for enterocutaneous fistula, age 45

Family/Social History
Family History: Mother died at age 55 of lung cancer, and father died at age 61 of heart failure; has three children, all alive and well

Social History: Smokes 1.5 PPD × 43 years; continues to smoke; drinks alcohol occasionally

Medication History
Aspirin, 325 mg PO QD

Metoprolol, 25 mg PO BID

Nitroglycerin, 0.4 mg SL PRN for chest pain

Hydrochlorothiazide (HCTZ), 50 mg PO BID

KCl, 10 mEq PO QD

Sulfasalazine, 500 mg PO QID

Prednisone, 7.5 mg PO QD

Beclomethasone nasal inhaler

Allergies
PCN and "novocaine"

Physical Examination
GEN: Slightly obese female with round face, in moderate distress, increased leg edema, nocturia, and SOB

VS: BP 150/100, HR 110, T 37.3°C, RR 24, Wt 70 kg, Ht 158 cm

HEENT: AV nicking and narrowing, retinal exudates

COR: Normal S_1, S_2, + S_3, and + S_4 with gallop, + JVD, –HJR

CHEST: Bilateral rales

ABD: Soft, nontender, hepatomegaly, abdominal striae

GU: Deferred

RECT: Heme (−)

EXT: 2+ ankle edema

NEURO: WNL

Results of Pertinent Laboratory Tests, Serum Drug Concentrations, and Diagnostic Tests

Na 137 (137)	Hct 0.37 (37)	AST 0.42 (25)
K 4.7 (4.7)	Hgb 123 (12.3)	ALT 0.32 (19)
Cl 103 (103)	Lkcs 4.8×10^9	LDH 1.30 (78)
HCO$_3$ 23 (23)	(4.8×10^3)	Ca 2.27 (9.1)
BUN 8.57 (24)	Plts 220×10^9	PO$_4$ 1.0 (3.2)
SCr 177 (2.0)	(220×10^3)	Mg 0.9 (1.8)
Glu 7.05 (127)		

ECG: Shows evidence of anterior wall MI, voltage changes consistent with LVH, currently in sinus tachycardia at a rate of 110 bpm with occasional multiform premature ventricular contractions

PROBLEM LIST
Identify principal problems from the scenario in priority order [completed Problem List and SOAP Note at end of casebook]

SOAP NOTE
To be completed by student

QUESTIONS
[Answers at end of casebook]

1. Each of the following is evidence of end-organ damage secondary to hypertension in this patient, *except:* (EO-1, 2)

a. AV nicking

b. Renal insufficiency

c. Left-ventricular hypertrophy

d. +JVD

2. Which of the following is a sign or symptom of left-sided heart failure? (EO-2)

a. Bilateral rales

b. +JVD

c. Hepatomegaly

d. Splenomegaly

3. Which of the following is the most likely etiology of this patient's heart failure? (EO-1, 3)

a. Coronary artery disease

b. Renal insufficiency

c. Crohn's disease

d. Hypertension

4. All of the following are evidence of adverse effects of long-term corticosteroid use in this patient *except:* (EO-10)

a. Abdominal striae

b. Round face

c. Allergic rhinitis

d. Congestive heart failure

5. All of the following are potential causes of the recent exacerbation of this patient's heart failure *except:* (EO-1, 2)

a. Uncontrolled hypertension

b. Steroid use

c. Sulfasalazine

d. Metoprolol

6. Which of the following is an equivalent glucocorticoid dose to the prednisone this patient is receiving? (EO-8, 12)

a. Hydrocortisone 20 mg QD

b. Methylprednisolone 6 mg QD

c. Prednisolone 10 mg QD

d. Cortisone 25 mg QD

7. Which of the following steroid regimens is appropriate for the management of severe stress in this patient? (EO-8, 12)

a. Hydrocortisone 100 mg IV q8h until the stress resolves

b. Continue the prednisone 7.5 mg QD

c. Change prednisone to hydrocortisone 30 mg PO

d. Change prednisone to hydrocortisone 60 mg PO

8. Your medical team wants to initiate digoxin therapy in DA. What is an appropriate maintenance dose for this patient? (EO-6, 8, 12)

a. 0.125 mg PO every other day

b. 0.125 mg PO QD

c. 0.25 mg PO QD

d. 0.375 mg PO QD

9. To help DA stop smoking, DA is started on nicotine gum. What should you tell DA about the proper use of nicotine gum? (EO-14, 16)

10. Summarize the nonpharmacologic treatment options for this patient's congestive heart failure. (EO-11)

11. What pharmacoeconomic considerations may be included in this patient's plan of care? (EO-17)

12. Utilizing a key points format, list the points related to the treatment of heart failure/S/P myocardial infarction in this patient. (EO-18)

CASE 66
Kevin M. Sowinski
Topic: Acute Myocardial Infarction
 Level 3
EDUCATIONAL MATERIALS
Chapter 42: Ischemic Heart Disease; Chapter 43: Acute Myocardial Infarction; Chapter 39: Hypertension; Chapter 20: Hyperlipidemia

SCENARIO

Patient and Setting

SK, 45-year-old male; emergency department

Chief Complaint

Chest pain nonresponsive to NTG

History of Present Illness

Brought to the emergency department Sunday at 8 PM by two friends; confused and severely short of breath but able to complain loudly of crushing chest pain radiating to neck, jaw, and left arm; had 2 sublingual nitroglycerin (SLNTG) prior to arrival which have not relieved pain.

Past Medical History

Coronary artery disease (CAD) with previous hospitalization 2 years ago and positive workup. Angiography revealed 70% occlusion of the left anterior descending (LAD) artery, and 50 to 60% occlusion of the circumflex coronary artery. Type 1 diabetes (DM); questionable control with history of ketoacidosis. Hypertension (HTN); hypercholesterolemia

Past Surgical History

None

Family/Social History

Family History: Unknown

Social History: Nonsmoker, does not consume alcohol

Medication History

Insulin human regular, 10 units SC q AM and q PM

Insulin human NPH, 10 units SC q AM and q PM

Verapamil SR, 120 mg PO QD for 1 year

Furosemide, 40 mg PO BID for 6 months

Nitroglycerin, 0.4 mg SL PRN for chest pain for 2 years

Isosorbide dinitrate, 10 mg PO TID for 6 months

Cholestyramine, 4 g PO TID for 8 years

Lovastatin, 20 mg PO QD for 2 years

Allergies

NKDA

Physical Examination

GEN: Confused, anxious, red-faced, well-developed, well-nourished male in moderate distress; tachypneic, diaphoretic, and complains of severe (9 out of 10) chest pain radiating to neck, jaw, and left arm.

VS: BP 140/90, HR 120, RR 45, T 38.3°C, Wt 78 kg

HEENT: AV nicking and narrowing

COR: Positive S_3 and S_4 gallop

CHEST: Clear to auscultation (CTA) and percussion

ABD: Central obesity

GU: WNL

RECT: Guaiac negative

EXT: Edema to mid-calf

NEURO: Mildly confused, alert, and oriented ×3

ECG: Sinus tachycardia; S-T segment elevation to 6 mm in leads I, II, V_1 to V_6; flattened T waves

Results of Pertinent Laboratory Tests, Serum Drug Concentrations, and Diagnostic Tests

Na 135 (135)

K 3.0 (3.0)

Cl 105 (105)

HCO_3 20 (20)

BUN 8.6 (24)

Cr 110 (1.3)

Hct 0.40 (40)

Hgb 130 (13)

Lkcs 12×10^9 (12×10^3)

Plts 170×10^9 (170×10^3)

AST 0.08 (48)

ALT 0.38 (23)

LDH 7.3 (440)

PT 11.5

PTT 34.8

Glu 23.3 (420)

Ca 4.15 (8.3)

PO_4 1.03 (3.2)

Mg 0.55 (1.0)

HbA_{1C} 11.0

Cholesterol 6.21 mmol/L (240)

Triglycerides 1.5 mmol/L (135)

HDL 0.80 mmol/L (30)

LDL 4.73 (183)

O_2 saturation 85%

Lkc differential: WNL, no bands

Urinalysis: 2+ glucose, (−) ketones, (−) protein

Chest x-ray: WNL

Time	CK	CK-MB	CK-MB Fract	LDH	LDH$_1$ Fract	LDH$_2$ Fract
2000	7.84 (472)	0.55 (33)	0.07 (7)	7.33 (440)	0.43 (43)	0.28 (28)
0400	15.5 (930)	1.86 (111)	0.12 (12)	14.0 (840)	0.48 (48)	0.34 (34)
1200	39.7 (2380)	7.93 (476)	0.20 (20)	22.0 (1320)	0.53 (53)	0.31 (31)

PROBLEM LIST

Identify principal problems from the scenario in priority order

SOAP NOTE

To be completed by student

QUESTIONS

1. Each of the following are signs or symptoms of acute myocardial infarction in this patient *except:* (EO-2)
   a. Chest pain unrelieved by nitroglycerin (NTG) tablets
   b. S-T segment elevation to 3 mm in leads I, V_1 to V_4
   c. AV nicking and narrowing
   d. Diaphoresis

2. Which of the following is the most appropriate regimen to administer nitroglycerin to this patient? (EO-8, 12)
   a. NTG at 5 to 10 mg/min and increase by 10 mg/min every 10 minutes, titrating to resolution of chest pain; continue infusion for 24 to 48 hours.
   b. Administer SL NTG until chest pain is resolved.
   c. NTG at 5 to 10 mg/kg/min and increase by 10 mg/kg/min every 10 minutes, titrating to resolution of chest pain; continue infusion for 24 to 48 hours.
   d. NTG at 5 to 10 mg/min and increase by 10 mg/min every 10 minutes, titrating to resolution of chest pain; continue infusion for 24 to 48 hours. Convert to ISDN therapy and continue indefinitely for prevention of a future myocardial infarction.

3. Which of the following is the appropriate LDL goal in this patient? (EO-5, 12)
   a. <70 mg/dL
   b. <100 mg/dL
   c. <130 mg/dL
   d. <160 mg/dL

4. Which of the following is true regarding the etiology as well as treatment of this patient's constipation? (EO-8, 10, 12)
   a. Constipation is likely caused by verapamil; however, the drug cannot be discontinued because it is needed chronically to prevent the development of future myocardial infarctions.
   b. Constipation is most likely caused by cholestyramine and verapamil. Both drugs can be discontinued and alternatives used.
   c. Constipation is most likely caused by cholestyramine and verapamil. Continue both and add docusate sodium to treat the constipation.
   d. None of the drugs received prior to admission cause constipation.

5. This patient is initiated on tPA therapy administered as 100 mg given over 90 minutes. Which of the following anticoagulant regimens is most appropriate in this patient? (EO-8, 12)
   a. Heparin 75 U/kg bolus, followed by 18 U/kg infusion, initiated after the tPA administration
   b. Heparin 7,500 U SC q12h initiated immediately upon tPA administration
   c. Warfarin 5 mg daily initiated immediately upon tPA administration
   d. Heparin 75 U/kg bolus, followed by 18 U/kg infusion, given concomitantly with tPA

6. Treatment of hypokalemia and hypomagnesemia is

necessary to prevent which of the following complications? (EO-10)
a. Arrhythmias
b. Severe hypotension
c. Renal dysfunction
d. Hypocalcemia

7. Therapy with captopril is initiated on the day following the myocardial infarction. All of the following are appropriate reasons for adding captopril to this patient's drug regimen *except:* (EO-7)
a. Lower blood pressure
b. Prevent diabetic nephropathy
c. Increase potassium concentrations
d. Prevent myocardial remodeling

8. Which of the following is the most appropriate information to provide to this patient related to his lovastatin therapy? Take: (EO-8, 9, 14)
a. In the morning
b. At bedtime
c. With evening meal
d. With lunch

9. Explain why relief of pain and anxiety is important. What other benefits are derived from using a narcotic analgesic in this patient? (EO-7)

10. Summarize the risk factor reduction therapies and their rationale in preventing another myocardial infarction. (EO-14, 15)

11. What pharmacoeconomic considerations may be included in this patient's plan of care? (EO-17)

12. Utilizing a key points format, summarize pathophysiologic, therapeutic, and disease management concepts for acute myocardial infarction. (EO-18)

CASE 67
Kevin M. Sowinski
Topic: Thromboembolic Disease

Level 3

EDUCATIONAL MATERIALS
Chapter 44: Thromboembolic Disease; Chapter 41: Cardiac Arrhythmias

---

SCENARIO

Patient and Setting
WM, 57-year-old male; medicine clinic

Chief Complaint
Swelling in right calf and thigh accompanied by tenderness and redness

History of Present Illness
Recently returned from a trip to the Middle East. After arriving home noted swelling in right calf and thigh accompanied by tenderness and redness; noted swelling in both legs recently, right leg is definitely more swollen than the left; denies chest pain or shortness of breath; exercises very little and is approximately 40 pounds overweight.

Past Medical History
Wolff-Parkinson-White (WPW) syndrome currently controlled with amiodarone. Obesity with decreased exercise tolerance; abnormal liver function tests (LFTs)

Past Surgical History
Noncontributory

Family/Social History
Family History: Noncontributory
Social History: A heavy drinker (several martinis with lunch and dinner plus two to three glasses of wine per day)

Medication History
Amiodarone, 200 mg PO QD × 5 years
Diphenhydramine, 25 to 50 mg PO q6h PRN for itching
Alka Seltzer, PO PRN for headache pain

Allergies
NKDA

Physical Examination
GEN: Obese male with smell of alcohol on breath
VS: BP 110/70, HR 60, RR 16, Wt 125 kg, Ht 183 cm
HEENT: Large neck, EOM intact, PERRLA, icteric sclera
COR: Sustained impulse, nl S_1, S_2
CHEST: Clear to P and A
ABD: Obese, enlarged and palpable liver
GU: WNL
RECT: Guaiac negative
EXT: Enlarged, red, painful R leg greater than L, 3+ pitting edema both lower extremities, decreased pulses bilaterally
NEURO: Alert and oriented × 3, cranial nerves intact

Results of Pertinent Laboratory Tests, Serum Drug Concentrations, and Diagnostic Tests

Na 138 (138)	Hct 0.38 (38)	AST 7.26 (220)
K 3.5 (3.5)	Hgb 130 (13)	ALT 7.0 (200)
Cl 96 (96)	Lkcs 3.8 × 10⁹	LDH 2.66 (150)
HCO₃ 24 (24)	(3.8 × 10³)	Alb 35 (3.5)
BUN 5.5 (18)	Plts 200 × 10⁹	
Cr 110 (1.2)	(200 × 10³)	
Glu 6.1 (105)	MCV 103 (103)	

INR 1.3; aPTT 30.2 sec

Venogram: Consistent with filling defect in right calf and thigh

ECG: NSR

Chest x-ray: Slightly enlarged heart, normal lung fields

PROBLEM LIST

Identify principal problems from the scenario in priority order [completed Problem List and SOAP Note at end of casebook]

SOAP NOTE

To be completed by student

QUESTIONS

[Answers at end of casebook]

1. Which of the following is a sign or symptom of alcoholic liver disease in this patient? (EO-2)
   a. Icteric sclera
   b. Red painful right leg larger than left
   c. Cranial nerves intact
   d. Obesity

2. Which of the following is a life-threatening adverse effect associated with chronic amiodarone therapy? (EO-10)
   a. Hyperthyroidism
   b. Hypothyroidism
   c. Pulmonary fibrosis
   d. Corneal microdeposits

3. Which of the following arrhythmias do patients with Wolff-Parkinson-White syndrome most commonly manifest? (EO-4)
   a. Paroxysmal supraventricular tachycardia
   b. Ventricular tachycardia
   c. Ventricular fibrillation
   d. Atrial fibrillation

4. Which of the following is *not* a risk factor for development of DVT? (EO-4, 10)
   a. Oral contraceptives
   b. Immobilization
   c. Malignancies
   d. Hypertension

5. What is the appropriate duration of antithrombotic therapy in this patient? (EO-12)
   a. 3 weeks
   b. 6 weeks
   c. 3 months
   d. Lifelong

6. Six hours after initiating heparin therapy in this patient the aPTT is 40 sec. Which of the following is most appropriate? (EO-8, 12)
   a. Increase the infusion rate by 200 U/hr
   b. Re-bolus at 40 U/kg and increase the infusion rate by 2 U/kg
   c. Discontinue heparin and initiate warfarin at 5 mg daily
   d. Maintain the current infusion rate

7. Which of the following best describes the mechanism of the increased INR in this patient? (EO-3, 8)
   a. Use of Alka-Seltzer
   b. Ethanol-induced decreased degradation of vitamin K-dependent clotting factors
   c. Vegetarian diet resulting in decreased availability of vitamin K
   d. Reduced synthesis of vitamin K-dependent clotting factors by the liver

8. Which of the following is NOT a routine monitoring parameter for spironolactone? (EO-5, 10, 12)
   a. Serum potassium concentrations
   b. Urinary output
   c. Plasma aldosterone concentrations
   d. Abdominal girth

9. Describe the effects of alcohol on warfarin therapy. (EO-10)

10. List the nonpharmacologic treatment problems present in this patient's treatment plan. (EO-11)

11. Describe what psychosocial factors may affect this patient's adherence to both pharmacologic and nonpharmacologic therapy. (EO-15)

12. Utilizing a key points format, list the points related to the treatment of venous thromboembolism in this patient. (EO-18)

CASE 68
Ted L. Rice
Topic: Allergic Diseases of the Skin
Level 2
EDUCATIONAL MATERIALS
Chapter 45: Allergic and Drug-Induced Skin Disease (skin structure and function, contact dermatitis, etiology, pathogenesis, diagnosis and clinical findings, treatment)

SCENARIO

Patient and Setting

AM, 54-year-old female; medicine clinic

Chief Complaint

Itchy rash over hands, arms, and forehead

History of Present Illness

Rash began yesterday on abdomen and front of legs; cleaned out brush and weeds along the fence 3 days ago; two days ago, worked in the garage wearing clothes from previous day because already dirty

Past Medical History

Type 2 diabetes identified over a year ago, adequately treated with glyburide; HTN since age 45, previously controlled with hydrochlorothiazide but switched to enalapril after diabetes diagnosed; PUD by endoscopy 2 years ago (biopsy negative for *H. pylori*); successfully treated with cimetidine, and currently on maintenance therapy

Past Surgical History

None

Family/Social History

Family History: Noncontributory

Social History: Nonsmoker; occasional alcohol consumption

Medication History

Glyburide, 2.5 mg PO q AM

Enalapril, 10 mg PO q AM

Cimetidine, 400 mg PO HS

Allergies

NKDA

Physical Examination

GEN: Obese female who appears restless and agitated and complains of itching

VS: BP 135/95, HR 85, RR 19, T 37.2°C, Wt 72 kg, Ht 155 cm

HEENT: Several small patches of erythematous vesicles are located on the forehead, with a few vesicles on each side of the neck

COR: WNL

CHEST: Clear

ABD: No masses or tenderness, areas of vesicles developing on skin

GU: WNL

RECT: Deferred

EXT: Arms and hands have numerous erythematous vesicular and bullous areas, with some in a linear configuration; several of these areas are weeping; the fronts of the thighs show erythematous areas with some swelling and beginning development of vesicles; no open, oozing areas noted

NEURO: WNL

Results of Pertinent Laboratory Tests, Serum Drug Concentrations, and Diagnostic Tests (from clinic visit 1 month ago)

Fasting plasma glucose (FPG): 6.4 mmol/L (115 mg/dL)

HbA$_{1C}$ 8%

PROBLEM LIST

Identify principal problems from the scenario in priority order

SOAP NOTE

To be completed by student

QUESTIONS

1. Usual causes of *allergic* contact dermatitis include all of the following *except:* (EO-1)
   a. Metallic salts
   b. Plants
   c. Latex
   d. Detergents

119

2. A typical delayed hypersensitivity reaction requires all of the following *except:* (EO-1)
   a. Penetration of the stratum corneum by the allergen
   b. Interaction with epidermal or dermal cells
   c. Interaction with the neurovascular system
   d. Activation of the inflammatory response

3. Sensitizing agents (haptens) are usually: (EO-1)
   a. Water-soluble
   b. High molecular weight
   c. Eicosanoids
   d. Highly reactive

4. In contrast to allergic contact dermatitis, the pathogenesis of *irritant* contact dermatitis includes: (EO-1, 5)
   a. A latent period
   b. Direct cellular damage
   c. An elicitation dose
   d. A sensitizing dose

5. Acute contact dermatitis involves all of the following *except:* (EO-1, 2, 5)
   a. Erythema
   b. Edema
   c. Papules and vesicles
   d. Hematomas

6. Severe, acute contact dermatitis may require: (EO-8)
   a. Systemic corticosteroids
   b. Topical corticosteroids
   c. Photochemotherapy
   d. Lubricating cream

7. Calamine, topical antihistamines, and topical anesthetics are avoided in contact dermatitis because of all the following *except:* (EO-7, 8)
   a. Modest benefit
   b. Potential sensitization
   c. Preservatives
   d. Inadequate skin penetration

8. Contact allergy to topical corticosteroids occurs more frequently with: (EO-10)
   a. Budesonide
   b. Betamethasone
   c. Dexamethasone
   d. Mometasone

9. Why does the rash from poison ivy involve areas of unexposed skin? (EO-1)

10. Will administration of prednisone affect AM's HTN? (EO-9)

11. Describe the pharmacotherapeutic rationale for treating AM's HTN with an angiotensin converting enzyme inhibitor (ACEI). (EO-1, 2, 8)

12. What psychosocial factors may influence AM's adherence to both pharmacologic and nonpharmacologic therapy? (EO-15)

13. Evaluate the pharmacoeconomic considerations relative to AM's plan of care. (EO-17)

14. Summarize the pathophysiologic, therapeutic, and disease management concepts of allergic contact dermatitis utilizing a key points format. (EO-18)

CASE 69
Ted L. Rice
Topic: Drug-Induced Skin Diseases
Level 3
EDUCATIONAL MATERIALS
Chapter 45: Allergic and Drug-Induced Skin Disease (skin structure and function, contact dermatitis, etiology, pathogenesis, diagnosis and clinical findings, and treatment)

SCENARIO

Patient and Setting
SA, 55-year-old female; hospital

Chief Complaint
My breathing is better now, but my skin really itches

History of Presenting Illness
Admitted to hospital 1 week ago with respiratory failure due to pneumonia/bronchitis requiring mechanical ventilation; after extubation on hospital day 3, became tachypneic and experienced seizure activity; computed tomographic (CT) scan of head showed a left frontal meningioma; treated with various medications during this admission, including methylprednisolone, ampicillin/sulbactam, gentamicin, furosemide, theophylline, and phenytoin; 3 days ago, began oral amoxicillin/clavulanate (IV antibiotics discontinued), and continues cimetidine, furosemide, and phenytoin; developed moderate diarrhea on hospital day 6, with 4–6 small volume (<300 mL), heme-negative liquid stools per day; a diffuse, erythematous, maculopapular, pruritic rash is now noted on back, buttocks, and thighs

Past Medical History
Chronic obstructive lung disease/chronic obstructive pulmonary disease (COPD): long-standing restrictive lung disease secondary to cigarette smoking; intubation during this admission (first time required mechanical ventilation)

Past Surgical History
None

Family/Social History
Family History: Married; three children, all in good health

Social History: Ex-smoker (quit 6 months ago); no ethanol intake; works as a secretary

Medication History

In hospital:

    Methylprednisolone, 75 mg IV q6h (days 1 to 3)

    Methylprednisolone, 8 mg PO q6h (days 4 to 7)

    Ampicillin/sulbactam, 3 g IV q6h (days 1 to 4)

    Furosemide, 20 mg IV QD (days 1 to 7)

    Cimetidine, 300 mg IV BID (days 1 to 3)

    Cimetidine, 300 mg PO BID (days 4 to 7)

    Theophylline, 25 mg/hr IV Infusion (days 1 to 3)

    Theophylline SR, 300 mg PO BID (days 4 to 7)

    Phenytoin loading dose (15mg/kg), 1000 mg IV over 60 min (day 3)

    Phenytoin capsules, 100 mg PO TID (days 4 to 7)

    Amoxicillin/clavulanate, 875/125 mg PO q12h (days 5 to 7)

    Albuterol sulfate nebulization q6h (days 1 to 3)

    Ipratropium bromide nebulization q6h (days 1 to 3)

    Albuterol sulfate/ipratropium bromide MDI, 2 inhalations QID (days 4 to 7)

Medications prior to admission:

    Azithromycin, 250 mg PO QD

    Theophylline SR, 300 mg PO BID

    Albuterol sulfate/ipratropium bromide MDI, 2 inhalations QID

Allergies

Sulfa drugs

Physical Examination

    GEN: Well-developed, well-nourished patient in moderate distress due to pruritic rash

    VS: BP 125/82, HR 80, RR 22, T 38.2°C, Wt 65 kg, Ht 168 cm

  HEENT: WNL

    COR: WNL

  CHEST: Occasional rales, wheezes

    ABD: Nontender, no masses

    GU: Deferred

  RECT: Deferred

  SKIN: Diffuse, erythematous, maculopapular rash over back, buttocks, thighs

NEURO: A, O × 4

Results of Pertinent Laboratory Tests, Serum Drug Concentrations and Diagnostic Tests

Na 143 (143)	BUN 4.28 (12)	Hgb 141 (14.1)
K 4.2 (4.2)	Cr 80 (0.9)	Lkcs 10.8 × 10^9
Cl 105 (105)	Glu 7.4 (134)	(10.8 × 10^3)
CO_2 35 (35)	Hct 0.41 (41)	AST 0.90 (54)
ALT 1.04 (63)	T Bili 24 (1.4)	PO_4 0.90 (2.7)
LDH 4.08 (245)	Mg 0.74 (1.8)	Plts 195 × 10^9
Alb 32 (3.2)	Ca 2.05 (8.2)	(195 × 10^3)

Lkc differential: Neutrophils 0.62, bands 0.01, lymphs 0.22, monos 0.04, eos 0.08.

Arterial Blood Gases: (Day 1) − pH 7.28, PO_2 5.8 kPa (44 mm Hg), PCO_2 10.0 kPa (75 mm Hg), HCO_3 34 (34), FIO_2 0.6; (Day 7) − pH 7.35, PO_2 10.7 kPa (80 mm Hg), PCO_2 7.3 kPa (55 mm Hg), HCO_3 30 (30), FIO_2 0.21 {room air}

Serum theophylline concentration (day 6): 38.85 (7)

Serum phenytoin concentration (day 6): 71.35 (18)

Sputum culture: *Moraxella catarrhalis*–susceptible to: amoxicillin/clavulanate, ampicillin/sulbactam, cephalothin, ceftriaxone, erythromycin, clarithromycin, azithromycin, piperacillin, gentamicin, cotrimoxazole, and ofloxacin

PROBLEM LIST

Identify principal problems from the scenario in priority order [completed Problem List and SOAP Note at end of casebook]

SOAP NOTE

To be completed by student

QUESTIONS

[Answers at end of casebook]

1. The greatest risk of cutaneous reactions from immunologic sensitization to drugs occurs with: (EO-1)
   a. Topical application
   b. Oral administration
   c. Intravenous administration
   d. Rectal administration

2. A nonimmunologic mechanism associated with cutaneous drug reactions is: (EO-1)
   a. Antibody production
   b. Complement inhibition
   c. Drug interaction
   d. Homeopathic dosing

3. Activation of effector pathways can involve all of the following *except:* (EO-1)
   a. Mediator release
   b. Complement activation
   c. Alteration of arachidonic acid metabolism
   d. IgE production

4. Exanthems comprise approximately ___ % of cutaneous drug reactions. (EO-3)
   a. 20
   b. 30

c. 40

d. 50

5. Drug exanthems are generally all of the following *except:* (EO-2)

   a. A morbilliform or maculopapular eruption

   b. Start on the trunk

   c. Erythematous pustules

   d. Pruritic

6. Drug exanthems are often associated with: (EO-1, 2)

   a. Eosinophilia

   b. A discrete, localized lesion

   c. Asymmetry

   d. Nonpressure points

7. A drug-induced exanthem would not usually occur: (EO-1, 2)

   a. With the first dose of therapy

   b. Within the first 3 days of therapy

   c. Within the first week of therapy

   d. Within 3 weeks of therapy

8. After discontinuation of therapy, most drug-induced exanthems will disappear: (EO-1)

   a. Within the first day

   b. Within 3 days

   c. Within 1–2 weeks

   d. Within 2–3 weeks

9. What clinically significant drug interactions are possible in SA? (EO-9)

10. Explain the method of serum phenytoin concentration assessment in the setting of hypoalbuminemia. (EO-5, 6)

11. What psychosocial factors may influence SA's adherence to both pharmacologic and nonpharmacologic therapy? (EO-15)

12. Evaluate the pharmacoeconomic considerations relative to SA's plan of care. (EO-17)

13. Summarize the pathophysiologic, therapeutic, and disease management concepts of drug-induced skin diseases utilizing a key points format. (EO-18)

CASE 70
Ted L. Rice and S.E. Taylor
Topic: Psoriasis
Level 2
EDUCATIONAL MATERIALS
Chapter 46: Common Skin Disorders (psoriasis)

SCENARIO

Patient and Setting

BF, 37-year-old female; dermatology clinic

Chief complaint

Red, scaling skin on her knees and elbows; anxious and frustrated about not being able to stop smoking

History of Present Illness

Noticed scaling plaques on elbows and knees for several weeks, which seem to have become increasingly red and itchy; also notes no previous similar symptoms and admits being afraid to put any lotions on the area for fear of making it worse; attempted to quit smoking for the third time this year, but each time has returned to smoking after experiencing anxiety, insomnia, hunger, irritability, depression, and the craving for cigarettes

Past Medical History

Severe dysmenorrhea before initiation of oral contraceptives 10 years ago

Past Surgical History

None

Family/Social History

Family History: Unmarried, lives alone

Social History: Smokes 2 PPD × 10 years; drinks wine socially

Medication History

Oral contraceptive (35 µg ethinyl estradiol, 1 mg norethindrone), 1 tab PO QD × 10 years

Allergies

Penicillin: rash

Physical Examination

    GEN: Well-developed, well-nourished female in no acute distress

      VS: BP 120/70, HR 72, RR 16, T 37.1°C, Wt 50 kg, Ht 165 cm

  HEENT: WNL

    COR: RRR, S_1, S_2, no murmurs

  CHEST: Clear to auscultation

    ABD: Soft, nontender, nondistended

     GU: WNL

  RECT: Deferred

     XT: Erythematous, dry, scaling psoriatic plaques on elbows and knees bilaterally

NEURO: Alert, O × 3, cranial nerves II–XII intact

Results of Pertinent Laboratory Tests

Na 142 (142)	Lkcs 6.0 × 10⁹	LDH 1.2 (70)
K 4.1 (4.1)	(6.0 × 10³)	Alk Phos 1.17 (70)
Cl 98 (98)	Plts 210 × 10⁹	Alb 40 (4.0)
HCO₃ 26 (26)	(210 × 10³)	Glu 5.6 (100)
BUN 4.3 (12)	MCV 85 (85)	Ca 2.3 (9.2)
Cr 76 (1.0)	T Bili 17.1 (1.0)	PO₄ 1.2 (3.6)
Hct 0.4 (40)	AST 0.38 (23)	Mg 1.1 (2.1)
Hgb 130 (13.0)	ALT 0.43 (25)	

PROBLEM LIST

Identify principal problems from the scenario in priority order [completed Problem List and SOAP Note at end of casebook]

SOAP NOTE

To be completed by student

QUESTIONS

[Answers at end of casebook]

1. The demographic epidemiology of psoriasis is: (EO-3)
   a. Equal frequency in women and men
   b. More frequent in men
   c. More frequent in women
   d. Unable to be identified

2. The age of most patients when they develop the initial lesions of psoriasis is: (EO-3)
   a. Adolescence
   b. 20s
   c. 30s
   d. 40s

3. Psoriasis can cause all of the following *except:* (EO-1, 2, 15)
   a. Functional impairment
   b. Skin disfigurement
   c. Emotional distress
   d. Melanoma

4. Psoriatic lesions are commonly observed on all of the following *except:* (EO-1, 2, 5)
   a. Knees
   b. Axillae
   c. Elbows
   d. Scalp

5. All of the following statements regarding the etiology of psoriasis are true *except:* (EO-1)
   a. Inflammation is usually not observed
   b. An increase in epidermal cell proliferation is usually not observed
   c. Cell proliferation in psoriatic lesions is 12 times the normal rate
   d. Epidermal turnover and transit times are significantly reduced

6. Emollient agents: (EO-7)
   a. Hydrate the stratum corneum and prevent the increased transepidermal water loss observed in patients with psoriasis
   b. Dehydrate the stratum corneum and prevent the increased transepidermal water loss observed in patients with psoriasis
   c. Promote fissuring and scaling in hyperkeratotic areas in patients with psoriasis
   d. Increase epidermal cell proliferation, which promotes desquamation of scales

7. Keratolytic agents include: (EO-7)
   a. Salicylic acid
   b. Pyrrolidone carboxylic acid
   c. Urea
   d. Coal tar

8. All of the following statements regarding the use of topical corticosteroids are true *except:* (EO-7)
   a. Topical corticosteroids can be used alone or in combination with other agents for psoriasis therapy
   b. Local side effects of topical steroids include striae and atrophy, skin fragility producing bruising, and poor wound healing
   c. Topical corticosteroids may mask clinically nonapparent dermatophyte infections
   d. HPA-axis suppression is generally irreversible after short-term use of potent topical corticosteroids

9. Coal tar is more effective for psoriasis when combined with: (EO-7, 12)
   a. Psoralen
   b. Trioxsalen
   c. UVA
   d. UVB

10. If BF returns to clinic in 5 days saying she is still experiencing withdrawal symptoms and has begun to smoke again, what can be done? (EO-12, 14)

11. If BF had decided to use nicotine gum, what dose and schedule should be recommended, and how would you counsel her on the use of nicotine gum? (EO-7, 9, 14)

12. What psychosocial factors may influence BF's adherence to both pharmacologic and nonpharmacologic therapy? (EO-15)

13. Describe the health care provider's role relative to the psychosocial factors identified. (EO-16)

14. Evaluate the pharmacoeconomic considerations relative to BF's plan of care. (EO-17)

15. Summarize the pathophysiologic, therapeutic, and disease management concepts of psoriasis utilizing a key points format. (EO-18)

CASE 71
Ted L. Rice, S.E. Taylor
Topic: Acne

EDUCATIONAL MATERIALS FOR CASE ADAPTATION
Chapter 46: Common Skin Disorders (acne, summary of treatment strategies)

SCENARIO

Patient and Setting

LP, 18-year-old female; dermatology clinic

Chief Complaint

Worsening acne

History of Present Illness

Acne on face has worsened over the last 3 months and wants something to take to make it better; also of note, started taking birth control pills about 4 months ago

Past Medical History

None

Past Surgical History

None

Family/Social History

Family History: Lives at home with parents; starts college in the fall

Social History: Nonsmoker; denies alcohol use or IVDA

Medication History

Oral contraceptive (35 μg ethinyl estradiol, 1 mg norethindrone), 1 tab PO QD

Allergies

NKDA

Physical Examination

GEN: Well-developed, well-nourished teenage female in NAD
VS: BP 115/70, HR 72, RR 18, Wt 47.3 kg, Ht 165 cm
HEENT: PERRLA
COR: Normal S_1, S_2; no murmurs
CHEST: CTA
ABD: WNL
GU: Deferred
RECT: Deferred
SKIN: Moderate acne over the forehead, chin, and cheeks
NEURO: Alert, O × 4

Results of Pertinent Laboratory Tests

Na 140 (140)	Cr 70.4 (0.8)	AST 0.167 (10)
K 3.7 (3.7)	Hct 0.4 (40)	ALT 0.12 (7)
Cl 104 (104)	Hgb 160 (16)	T Bili 1.7 (0.1)
HCO_3 25 (25)	Plts 250 × 10^9	Glu 6.6 (120)
BUN 7.14 (20)	(250 × 10^3)	Chol 2.8 (110)

PROBLEM LIST

Identify principal problem(s) from the scenario in priority order

SOAP NOTE

To be completed by student

QUESTIONS

1. LP presents with moderate acne and should *not* have: (EO-1, 2)
   a. Pustules
   b. Cysts
   c. Open comedones (blackheads)
   d. Closed comedones (whiteheads)

2. Which of the following antibiotics is *not* applied topically for inflammatory acne? (EO-7)
   a. Erythromycin
   b. Clindamycin
   c. Trimethoprim/sulfamethoxazole
   d. Tetracycline

3. Which of the following drugs is most likely to aggravate acne? (EO-7, 10, 11)
   a. Rifampin
   b. Danazol
   c. Dicloxacillin
   d. Minocycline

4. In general, patients with acne should avoid all of the following *except:* (EO-1, 3)
   a. Oil-based cosmetics
   b. Chocolate
   c. Oil-based sun screens
   d. Greasy hair gels

5. All of the following nonpharmacological measures should be instituted by LP, *except:* (EO-11)
   a. Use a gentle soap with a low oil content
   b. Wash skin as frequently as possible to minimize sebum accumulation
   c. Ensure that cosmetics are water-based
   d. Use a mildly abrasive cleanser for her noninflammatory acne

6. A female patient starting isotretinoin capsules should be counseled about each of the following adverse effects *except:* (EO-10)
   a. Dry skin and eyes
   b. Teratogenic effects and the importance of avoiding pregnancy during therapy and for 1 month following discontinuation of therapy
   c. Mutagenic effects and the importance of avoiding pregnancy after stopping isotretinoin
   d. Hyperlipidemia

7. All of the following are appropriate scenarios for the consideration of isotretinoin, *except:* (EO-8)
   a. Treatment of resistant nodulocystic acne on a patient's back
   b. Patient with moderate acne that has not responded to topical therapy or systemic antibiotics
   c. Patient with moderate acne who is responding poorly to initial therapy with topical benzoyl peroxide, and has evidence of facial scarring

d. Patient with mild to moderate acne who requests initial therapy with "the most effective" product

8. Topical antibiotics are used: (EO-8)
   a. In mild to moderate inflammatory acne
   b. In noninflammatory acne
   c. As comedolytics
   d. In a low alcohol content vehicle to improve absorption

9. Describe the mechanism of action of benzoyl peroxide. (EO-7)

10. Describe the mechanism of action of tretinoin. (EO-7).

11. What psychosocial factors may affect LP's adherence to both pharmacologic and nonpharmacologic therapies? (EO-15)

12. Evaluate the pharmacoeconomic considerations relative to AM's plan of care. (EO-17)

13. Summarize the pathophysiologic, therapeutic, and disease management concepts of acne utilizing a key points format. (EO-18)

CASE 72
Ted L. Rice
Topic: Allergic Diseases of the Skin
Level 1
EDUCATIONAL MATERIALS
Chapter 45: Allergic and Drug-Induced Skin Disease (skin structure and function, atopic dermatitis, etiology, pathogenesis, diagnosis and clinical findings, and treatment)

SCENARIO

Patient and Setting
EM, 6-year-old female; dermatology clinic

Chief Complaint
Unable to sleep because of itching

History of Present Illness
For the last 4 nights, only 2–3 hours of sleep; awakens scratching left antecubital space, crying that it itches

Past Medical History
Asthma diagnosed at age 4; eczema diagnosed 1½ years ago but has had few exacerbations; recent *S. aureus* eczematous skin infection treated with mupirocin cream

Past Surgical History
None

Family/Social History
Family History: Mother has seasonal allergic rhinitis (hay fever)

Social History: Parents struggling to keep EM from scratching, especially at bedtime; suspect manipulative behavior due to sibling rivalry (newborn brother arrived 2 months ago)

Medication History
Hydrocortisone 1% cream

Moisturizing cream

Theophylline sprinkle, 125 mg PO BID

Albuterol MDI, PRN

Recently completed treatment with mupirocin 2.15% cream

Allergies
Food allergy to peanuts

Physical Examination
GEN: Well appearing, well-nourished female not in acute distress
VS: BP 95/64, HR 102, RR 16, T 38°C, Wt 23 kg, Ht 122 cm
HEENT: Perioral pallor; patches of erythematous, scaly rash in scalp, on forehead and neck
COR: Normal S1 and S2, no murmurs or rubs
CHEST: CTA with no rales, rhonchi, or wheezes
ABD: WNL
GU: WNL
RECT: Deferred
EXT: LUE has erythematous, scaly rash; smaller area of similar rash on RUE
NEURO: WNL

Results of Pertinent Laboratory Tests, Serum Drug Concentrations, and Diagnostic Tests
IgE 528 µg/L (220 IU/mL) determined at last visit

PROBLEM LIST
Identify principal problems from the scenario in priority order [completed Problem List and SOAP Note at end of casebook]

SOAP NOTE
To be completed by student

QUESTIONS

[Answers at end of casebook]

1. The most common symptom of eczema is: (EO-2)
   a. Urticaria
   b. Pain
   c. Erythema
   d. Pruritus

2. The etiology of eczema is multifactorial and includes the following factors *except:* (EO-1)
   a. Genetic
   b. Immunological
   c. Environmental
   d. Viral

3. Potent topical corticosteroids are used in an acute flare of eczema to: (EO-7, 8)
   a. Add moisture to the skin
   b. Reduce the inflammation and itching
   c. Keep the skin soft and supple
   d. Prevent the skin from becoming infected

4. The duration of potent topical corticosteroid use is limited to avoid: (EO-10)
   a. Hypertension
   b. HPA suppression
   c. Glaucoma
   d. Hypoglycemia

5. Because of prolonged scratching, eczematous skin may develop: (EO-1)
   a. Lichenoid plaques
   b. Erythematous areas
   c. Dryness
   d. Blisters

6. Why should eczema patients bathe daily? (EO-7)
   a. Hot water improves local blood flow
   b. Rubbing dry with a rough towel removes scales and crusting
   c. Bathing in conjunction with lubricant application helps prevent dry skin
   d. They shouldn't bathe; a shower is better

7. The clinical appearance of eczema can be similar to all of the following *except:* (EO-1)
   a. Pemphigus
   b. Contact dermatitis
   c. Psoriasis
   d. Seborrheic dermatitis

8. Flare factors in eczema include all of the following *except:* (EO-1)
   a. Having a pet dog
   b. Keeping the bedroom cool and using cotton bedding
   c. Keeping the bedroom warm and using synthetic bedding
   d. Wearing woolen gloves

9. Analyze the pharmacoeconomics of topical antimicrobial selection for the treatment of mildly infected eczematous rash. (EO-8, 17)

10. Review the psychosocial aspects of childhood eczema. (EO-15)

11. List antihistamine options if diphenhydramine causes adverse side effects. (EO-8)

12. Summarize the pathophysiologic, therapeutic, and disease management concepts of eczema utilizing a key points format. (EO-18)

CASE 73
Ted L. Rice
Topic: Burns

EDUCATIONAL MATERIALS
Chapter 47: Burns; Chapter 9: Fluid and Electrolyte Therapy and Acid-Base Balance; Chapter 103: Critical Care Therapy

---

SCENARIO

Patient and Setting
JD, 31-year-old male; Burn Center ICU

Chief Complaint
Unable to communicate

History of Present Illness
Rescued from house fire; 60% TBSA burn (40% full thickness); lactated Ringer's infusion at 500 mL/hr (1.5 L while in the ED); intubated/ventilated; laryngoscopy demonstrated inflammation, edema, and carbonaceous residue below vocal cords; received Td, thiamine 100 mg, morphine sulfate, midazolam, and mafenide acetate cream applied to burns; Foley catheter and NG tube inserted

Past Medical History
None

Past Surgical History
None

Family/Social History
Family History: Married, one young child

Social History: Works as electrician; history of alcohol abuse

Medication History
Occasional aspirin and antacid use; last tetanus and diphtheria toxoids, adsorbed (Td) immunization date unknown

Allergies

NKDA

Physical Examination

GEN: Critically injured well-developed male

VS: BP 110/64; HR 142; RR 26; T 38°C; Wt 73 kg; Ht 178 cm

HEENT: Eyebrows, eyelashes, and nasal hair singed; corneas uninjured; orotracheal tube in place

COR: Tachycardic with normal S1 and S2, no murmurs or rubs

CHEST: Circumferential full-thickness injury; rales and rhonchi heard over all lung fields; inspiratory and expiratory wheezes

ABD: Absence of bowel sounds in all four quadrants

GU: WNL, Foley catheter in place (current urine output = 15 mL/hr); the urine is brownish-red (evidence of hemochromogens)

RECT: Deferred

EXT: LUE: blisters and burns that are pink and blanch to pressure; RUE: dry and leathery; coagulated blood vessels visible under eschar; radial and ulnar pulses absent; RLE and LLE have intact blisters; uninjured below the ankle

NEURO: Does not respond to verbal stimuli; responds to and localizes pain; Glasgow Coma Scale (GCS)–7

Results of Pertinent Laboratory Tests, Serum Drug Concentrations, and Diagnostic Tests

Na 143 (143)	Hgb 175 (17.5)	T Bili 24 (1.4)
K 5.2 (5.2)	Plts 195 × 10⁹	Mg 0.74 (1.8)
Cl 110 (110)	(195 × 10³)	Ca 2.05 (8.2)
CO₂ 15 (15)	AST 0.90 (54)	PO₄ 0.30 (0.9)
BUN 2.14 (6)	ALT 1.04 (63)	MCV 92 (92)
Cr 80 (0.9)	LDH 4.08 (245)	Lkcs 4.5 × 10⁹
Glu 7.4 (134)	Alb 29 (2.9)	(4.5 × 10³)
Hct 0.51 (51)		

Lkc differential: Neutrophils 0.62, bands 0.10, lymphs 0.22, monos 0.04

Urinalysis: Specific gravity 1.022, pH 6.2, protein-positive, leukocyte esterase-negative, blood-positive, glucose-negative, ketones-negative, urobilinogen-normal

Blood ethanol: 45 (206)

Arterial blood gas: pH 7.27, PO₂ 9.6 kPa (72 mm Hg), PCO₂ 4.4 kPa (33 mm Hg), HCO₃ 14 mmol/L (14 mEq/L), FIO₂ 0.4, carboxyhemoglobin 0.37

Chest x-ray: Minor peribronchial cuffing; ET tube in adequate position

PROBLEM LIST

Identify principal problems from the scenario in priority order [completed Problem List and SOAP Note at end of casebook]

SOAP NOTE

To be completed by student

QUESTIONS

[Answers at end of casebook]

1. The highest priority for grafting of burned areas is: (EO-8)
   a. To preserve function
   b. To maintain life
   c. An optimal cosmetic result
   d. To avoid excising partial-thickness injuries

2. In general, the single procedure limit for excision of burn wounds is: (EO-8)
   a. 5–10 % TBSA
   b. 10–20 % TBSA
   c. 20–35 % TBSA
   d. 30–45 % TBSA

3. A burn that appears dry or leathery with visible sub-eschar coagulated blood vessels is: (EO-1)
   a. First-degree injury
   b. Superficial partial-thickness injury
   c. Deep partial-thickness injury
   d. Full-thickness injury

4. Excised burn wounds are permanently closed with: (EO-1, 12)
   a. Autograft
   b. Allograft
   c. Homograft
   d. Xenograft

5. The topical antimicrobial cream associated with metabolic acidosis is: (EO-8, 10)
   a. Silver sulfadiazine
   b. Silver sulfadiazine combined with chlorhexidine
   c. Mafenide acetate
   d. Nitrofurazone

6. Nutrition requirements for hypermetabolic burn patients are substantial, but carbohydrate administration should not exceed: (EO-8)
   a. 2 mg/kg/min
   b. 3 mg/kg/min
   c. 4 mg/kg/min
   d. 5 mg/kg/min

7. One-half of the resuscitation fluid requirement estimated by the Parkland formula is to be administered during the first: (EO-1, 8)
   a. 4 hours
   b. 8 hours
   c. 16 hours
   d. 24 hours

8. Opioid analgesics are the mainstay of burn pain

management but nonpharmacologic adjuncts for pain management include all of the following *except:* (EO-8, 12)
a. Hypnosis
b. Distraction therapy
c. Cognitive-behavioral therapy
d. Radiotherapy

9. The metabolic acidosis produced by mafenide acetate is due to: (EO-10)
a. Propylene glycol
b. Carbonic anhydrase inhibition
c. Renal tubular acidosis
d. Ketoacidosis

10. Would you recommend that JD receive tetanus immune globulin? Support your rationale. (EO-1, 11)

11. What are the preferred agents for sedation and neuromuscular blockade in burn patients, and what are the reasons for their preferred status? (EO-4, 7, 8, 12)

12. JD apparently has postburn ileus, since he has a nasogastric tube attached to suction and absent bowel sounds. What method of nutritional support would you recommend? (EO-12)

13. The current topical antimicrobial is silver sulfadiazine. If JD develops leukopenia (Lkcs $< 2.0 \times 10^9$) on postburn day 2 or 3, what is the likely explanation? (EO-8, 10)

14. What psychosocial factors may influence JD's adherence to both pharmacologic and nonpharmacologic therapy? (EO-15)

15. Evaluate the pharmacoeconomic considerations relative to JD's plan of care. (EO-17)

16. Summarize the pathophysiologic, therapeutic, and disease management concepts of burn trauma utilizing a key points format. (EO-18)

CASE 74
J. Douglas Wurtzbacher
Topics: Conjunctivitis and Keratitis
Level 2
EDUCATIONAL MATERIALS
Chapter 48: Common Eye Disorders
(disorders of the conjunctiva and sclera)

SCENARIO

Patient and Setting

GT, 78-year-old male; clinic

Chief Complaint

Painful, red, left eye with both eyelids "sticking together" upon awakening

History of Present Illness

Brought to clinic today; nasal congestion for 3 days; taking triprolidine and pseudoephedrine; began self-treating with sulfacetamide eye drops (prescribed for a previous eye infection) 2 days ago

Past Medical History

Hypertension for 20 years (well controlled until this visit); eye infection 2 years ago, treated with sulfacetamide eye drops

Past Surgical History

Unremarkable

Family/Social History

Family History: Wife died 6 months ago, lives alone
Social History: Drinks alcohol occasionally; no tobacco use

Medication History

Triprolidine and pseudoephedrine, 2 tablets PO QID × 2 days
Hydrochlorothiazide, 25 mg PO QD
Sulfacetamide eye drops, 2 drops both eyes q6h × 2 days
Potassium chloride tablets, 10 mEq 2 tablets PO BID (stopped taking it several months ago)

Allergies

Penicillin (rash)

Physical Examination

GEN: Well-groomed gentleman, appears slightly malnourished and dehydrated; red left eye with purulent discharge accumulated on the lashes
VS: BP 155/96, HR 85 (supine); BP 130/80, HR 100 (standing); RR 23, T 37.2°C, Wt 57 kg, Ht 183 cm
HEENT: Left eye, brilliant red appearance, more intense at the limbus, with a mucopurulent discharge; right eye marginally red; both eyelids moderately swollen; no evidence of trauma, but a gray, well-circumscribed corneal lesion can be seen with fluorescein stain. Pupils react mildly to light, slightly dilated.
COR: Sinus tachycardia
CHEST: WNL
ABD: Soft, tender, nondistended
GU: Deferred
RECT: Deferred
EXT: WNL
NEURO: A&O × 3

Results of Pertinent Laboratory Tests, Serum Drug Concentrations, and Diagnostic Tests

Na 144 (144)	Cr 150 (1.7)	Plts 350 × 10⁹
K 3.0 (3.0)	Hct 0.44 (44)	(350 × 10³)
Cl 85 (85)	Hgb 2.3 (15)	Glu 5.6 (101)
HCO₃ 30 (30)	Lkcs 11.4 × 10⁹	LFT: WNL
BUN 14 (39.1)	(11.4 × 10³)	CXR: WNL

Conjunctival swab: Gram's stain: gram-positive lancet-shaped cocci in pairs; culture and sensitivities pending

PROBLEM LIST

Identify principal problems from the scenario in priority order

SOAP NOTE

To be completed by student

QUESTIONS

1. GT should be counseled about the proper administration of erythromycin ophthalmic ointment. All of the following points should be made *except:* (EO-14)

a. Gently massage the eyelids to spread the ointment

b. Be careful not to touch any part of the eye with tip of the tube

c. Continue using the medication until it is finished

d. Discard any unused portion of the ointment after 30 days

2. Prior to this visit, GT's blood pressure has been well-controlled. Which of the following is most likely to have caused an increase in GT's blood pressure? (EO-1, 10)

a. Discontinuation of potassium supplementation

b. Use of high doses of triprolidine and pseudoephedrine

c. Acute bacterial conjunctivitis

d. Excessive diuretic doses

3. All of the following are typical signs and symptoms of bacterial conjunctivitis *except:* (EO-2)

a. Excessive tearing and irritation

b. Mucopurulent discharge from the eye

c. Excessive eyelid crusting upon awakening

d. Eyelid edema

4. In a patient presenting with conjunctivitis that has an onset within 12 hours, extremely profuse mucopurulent discharge, and a Gram's stain positive for gram-negative diplococci, which type of conjunctivitis should be suspected? (EO-1, 5)

a. Gonococcal

b. Meningococcal

c. Fungal

d. Viral

5. List problems from this case that can be attributed to self-medication and noncompliance. (EO-15)

6. Develop an educational plan including pharmacologic and nonpharmacologic interventions for treatment of GT's hypertension. (EO-14)

7. Bacterial keratitis should be considered a medical emergency because it: (EO-1)

a. Can lead to severe upper respiratory infections

b. Is often caused by resistant microorganisms

c. Can lead to loss of sight if not properly treated

d. Does not need to be considered a medical emergency; most cases will spontaneously resolve

8. Systemic therapy with erythromycin should be used in GT's case to: (EO-8, 12)

a. Reduce the systemic side effects of the topical erythromycin

b. Prevent upper respiratory infection and ensure adequate therapy for bacterial keratitis

c. Prevent microorganism resistance

d. Ensure medication compliance

9. All of the following are physical or laboratory signs or symptoms of dehydration in GT *except:* (EO-5)

a. Tachycardia

b. Decreased serum sodium value

c. Increased blood urea nitrogen value

d. Poor skin turgor

10. List and describe laboratory values which may be altered by hydrochlorothiazide therapy. (EO-10, 11)

11. Why shouldn't the clinician use oral amoxicillin in GT's case? (EO-8)

a. It is significantly more expensive than oral erythromycin

b. It interacts with GT's antihypertensive therapy

c. It has ocular side effects that may worsen GT's condition

d. GT has a documented penicillin allergy

12. What measures can the health care provider provide to help ensure proper medication compliance in this case? (EO-15, 16)

13. Why is it important to consider psychosocial factors when referring a patient with bacterial keratitis to an ophthalmologist? (EO-16)

14. How would the etiology of a patient's conjunctivitis affect pharmacoeconomic considerations associated with treatment? (EO-17)

15. Summarize the key points of therapeutic, pathophysiologic, and disease management concepts for the treatment of bacterial conjunctivitis and keratitis. (EO-18)

CASE 75
J. Douglas Wurtzbacher
Topic: Acute Angle-Closure Glaucoma

EDUCATIONAL MATERIALS
Chapter 50: Glaucoma (angle-closure glaucoma, drug-induced glaucoma, recommended therapeutic strategies); Chapter 42: Angina Pectoris (therapeutic strategies)

SCENARIO

Patient and Setting
MC, 64-year-old male; emergency department

Chief Complaint
Severe chest pain

History of Present Illness
Complains of chest pain not relieved by two nitroglycerin (NTG) sublingual (SL); received one tablet NTG SL in the emergency department, with complete relief of pain; had been working outside in the garden when the pain occurred; usually experiences 2–3 anginal episodes per year; last episode was 10 months ago and resolved following one SL NTG. Nitroglycerin is "about 2 years old"; complains of increasing heartburn for 2 weeks, not relieved by antacids; experiencing blurred vision for several weeks; ran out of propranolol and has not been able to get it refilled; troponin levels and AcG were negative for MI; his endoscopy showed no ulcerations in the gastric mucosa; ophthalmic examination of his fundus completed one day after admission to evaluate blurred vision; atropine drops used to dilate eyes;

5 minutes after administration of atropine, developed extreme eye pain, red steamy-appearing corneas, and an intraocular pressure (IOP) of 50 mm Hg

Past Medical History

Exertional angina usually relieved by SL NTG; hypertension (HTN) controlled with propranolol

Past Surgical History

None

Family/Social History

Family History: Lives with wife of 42 years, mother died of myocardial infarction (MI) age 49; father died prostate cancer age 77

Social History: Alcohol: 2 drinks/day; smokes 1 PPD × 42 years

Medication History

NTG 0.4 mg SL PRN for chest pain

Magnesium/aluminum antacid PRN for heartburn

Propranolol 20 mg PO BID

Saw Palmetto for "prostate"

Allergies

Sulfa (Stevens-Johnson syndrome)

Physical Examination

GEN: Well-developed, well-nourished man in moderate distress
VS: BP 150/95, HR 100, RR 20, T 37°C, Wt 80 kg
HEENT: Papilledema
COR: Tachycardic
CHEST: Clear
ABD: Positive bowel sounds, slight tenderness without guarding
GU: Deferred
RECT: WNL
EXT: Small abrasion on left forearm
NEURO: WNL

Results of Pertinent Laboratory Tests, Serum Drug Concentrations, and Diagnostic Tests

Na 140 (140)	BUN 8.9 (25)	Lkcs 7.0 × 10^9
K 3.8 (3.8)	SCr 97.2 (1.1)	(7.0 × 10^3)
Cl 101 (101)	Hct 0.40 (40)	Troponin I 1.1 (1.1)
HCO$_3$ 24 (24)	Hgb 143 (14.3)	UA: WNL

Endoscopy: No visible gastric ulcerations

Helicobacter pylori culture: pending

Fundoscopic exam: Unable to complete due to severe eye pain following administration of atropine; tonometry measurements demonstrated IOP of 50 mm Hg

PROBLEM LIST

Identify principal problems from the scenario in priority order [completed Problem List and SOAP Note at end of casebook]

SOAP NOTE

To be completed by student

QUESTIONS

[Answers at end of casebook]

1. Which of the following describes pilocarpine's mechanism of action in controlling intraocular pressure? (EO-7)
   a. Blocks alpha-1 receptors, causing decrease in aqueous humor outflow
   b. Miotic activity causes increase in aqueous humor outflow
   c. Blocks carbonic anhydrase causing a decrease in aqueous humor production
   d. Beta-blocking activity decreases aqueous humor outflow

2. How can systemic absorption of glaucoma medications be minimized? (EO-6, 10)
   a. Use oral formulations of agents, such as acetazolamide
   b. Have the patient occlude the nasolacrimal duct for approximately 3–5 minutes following instillation of eye drops
   c. Have the patient tilt his head back during instillation of eye drops
   d. Instruct the patient to pull the lower lid down during administration of eye drops

3. List the problem(s) present in this case that can be attributed to noncompliance. (EO-11, 15)

4. Describe the anatomical differences between open-angle closure and angle-closure glaucoma in terms of the eye. (EO-1)

5. Which of the following medications is known to precipitate angle-closure glaucoma in susceptible individuals? (EO-1, 9)
   a. Pilocarpine
   b. Oral contraceptives
   c. Propranolol
   d. Scopolamine or atropine

6. If MC's *Helicobacter pylori* test returns positive, analyze the factors that should be considered when choosing eradicative therapy in this patient. (EO-8)

7. MC should be told all of the following regarding his sublingual nitroglycerin therapy *except:* (EO-14)
   a. He should keep the tablets in a cool, dry place
   b. He should allow for a nitrate-free interval of at least 4 hours a night
   c. If he takes a tablet and has no improvement, he may repeat two times
   d. He may experience a headache following use of the sublingual product

8. Why should acute angle-closure glaucoma be considered a medical emergency? (EO-1)
   a. It may lead to hypertensive crisis
   b. It may cause open-angle glaucoma
   c. Patients commonly do not experience symptoms; therefore, acute angle-closure glaucoma may go unnoticed for long periods of time
   d. It may lead to blindness if not corrected

9. Which of the following enzymes can be monitored to help diagnose myocardial infection in MC? (EO-5)
   a. Troponin I
   b. Creatinine
   c. ESR
   d. WBC

10. Which of the following is curative therapy for the treatment of acute angle-closure glaucoma? (EO-12)
    a. Laser iridotomy or peripheral trabeculoplasty
    b. IV infusion of mannitol
    c. Instillation of pilocarpine eye drops
    d. Use of oral acetazolamide

11. All of the following should be monitored regarding MC's propranolol therapy *except:* (EO-10)
    a. Blood pressure and heart rate
    b. Central nervous system effects such as depression
    c. Serum troponin I levels
    d. Control of anginal attacks

12. Describe how psychosocial factors that may occur in cases of acute angle-closure glaucoma differ from those occurring in open-angle glaucoma. (EO-15)

13. What pharmacoeconomic outcomes are likely if a patient with acute angle-closure glaucoma does not receive appropriate medical therapy? (EO-17)

14. Summarize therapeutic, pathophysiologic, and disease management concepts for acute angle-closure glaucoma utilizing a key points format. (EO-18)

CASE 76
J. Douglas Wurtzbacher
Topic: Open-Angle Glaucoma

EDUCATIONAL MATERIALS
Chapter 50: Glaucoma (open-angle glaucoma, drug-induced glaucoma, recommended therapeutic strategies); Chapter 19: Diabetes (type 2 diabetes); Chapter 37: Chronic Obstructive Pulmonary Disease (clinical presentation and diagnosis, goals of therapy, specific therapy)

SCENARIO

Patient and Setting
KW, 54-year-old female; emergency department

Chief Complaint
Increasing shortness of breath (SOB) for 3 weeks; also C/O increasing fatigue, depression, polyuria, polydipsia, and polyphagia for 2 weeks

History of Present Illness
Denies noncompliance, recent illness, fever, cough, or sputum production; admits to increasing her prednisone dose 2 weeks ago from 10 mg PO QD to 20 mg PO QD because of increasing SOB that was "not controlled by my inhalers."

Past Medical History
Type 2 diabetes mellitus (DM) which has been moderately controlled (SMBGs 8.8–11.1 [150–170]) with glipizide; open-angle glaucoma × 2 years treated with pilocarpine; approximately 3 weeks ago, timolol was added to her glaucoma therapy because of an IOP measurement of 30 mm Hg; chronic obstructive pulmonary disease (COPD) diagnosed 4 years ago

Past Surgical History
Partial hysterectomy 6 years ago

Family/Social History
Family History: Adopted; unknown family history
Social History: Negative alcohol; smoked 2 PPD × 10 years, quit 2 years ago

Medication History
Glipizide, 5 mg PO QD
Metaproterenol MDI, 2 puffs QID PRN for SOB
Ipratropium MDI, 2 puffs QID PRN for SOB
Prednisone, 10 mg PO QD for 2 years (increased to 20 mg QD 2 weeks ago by patient)
Chlorpheniramine, 4 mg PO QID PRN
Timolol, 0.5% one GTTS OU BID × 3 weeks
Pilocarpine, 1% two GTTS OU QID

Allergies
NKDA

Physical Examination
GEN: Obese, cushingoid-appearing woman in mild respiratory distress
VS: BP 140/90, HR 85, RR 26, T 37.5°C, Wt 100 kg, Ht 167 cm
HEENT: IOP 35 mm Hg, moon facies, microaneurysms visible; sputum is nonpurulent

COR: NL S1, S2; no murmurs
CHEST: Bilateral expiratory/inspiratory wheezes
ABD: Positive bowel sounds, abdominal striae, truncal obesity
SKIN: Facial acne lesions
GU: Deferred
RECT: Refused
EXT: Slight edema of both ankles
NEURO: Alert, O × 3

Results of Pertinent Laboratory Tests, Serum Drug Concentrations, and Diagnostic Tests

Na 144 (144)	Cr 167 (1.9)	Lkcs 5.8 × 10^9
K 3.6 (3.6)	Glu 10.5 (190)	(5.8 × 10^3)
Cl 98 (98)	Hct 0.4 (40)	Ca 2.39 (4.8)
HCO$_3$ 24 (24)	Hgb 142 (14.2)	PO$_4$ 1.45 (4.5)
BUN 14.3 (40)		Mg 1.05 (2.1)

Urinalysis: specific gravity 1.020, pH 5.5, negative est. & nit., gluc 16.65 (3%), negative ketones
ABG: pH 7.35, PCO$_2$ 6.7 (50), SaO$_2$ 10.7 (80)

PROBLEM LIST

Identify principal problems from the scenario in priority order

SOAP NOTE

To be completed by student

QUESTIONS

1. Because KW's IOP remains elevated, you decide to reevaluate her glaucoma therapy. Which of the following should be done first? (EO-12)
   a. Add latanoprost drops
   b. Increase pilocarpine to 2% two GTTS OU QID
   c. Evaluate KW's administration technique and medication compliance
   d. Discontinue pharmacologic therapy and consider surgical management

2. List medical problems present in KW that may be attributed to, or exacerbated by oral corticosteroid therapy. (EO-10)

3. How should KW's COPD exacerbation be managed medically? (EO-12)

4. Describe reasons why a monoamine oxidase inhibitor should *not* be considered for the treatment of KW's depression. (EO-8, 12)

5. KW presents with common signs and symptoms of COPD. Which of the following is *not* a common sign/symptom of COPD: (EO-2)
   a. Moon facies
   b. Expiratory wheezing
   c. PaO$_2$ of 70 or less
   d. Cyanosis

6. Which of the following is a common complication of chronic renal failure? (EO-1)
   a. Hypernatremia
   b. Hypokalemia
   c. Hyperphosphatemia
   d. Renal artery stenosis

7. Which of the following psychosocial factors may be reasons for decreased compliance with glaucoma therapy? (EO-15)
   a. Patients typically do not exhibit symptoms of glaucoma
   b. Surgical therapy may be necessary if medications are not effective
   c. Glaucoma may be associated with genetic abnormalities
   d. Medications such as corticosteroids may induce glaucoma in susceptible patients

8. Which of KW's current medications is appropriately dosed on an as-needed basis? (EO-11, 12)
   a. Ipratropium
   b. Glipizide
   c. Prednisone
   d. Metaproterenol

9. Once KW's therapy is controlled, she notices some rather bothersome side effects such as nausea, diarrhea, lacrimation, and excessive salivation. Which of her therapies is most likely to cause these effects? (EO-10)
   a. Pilocarpine
   b. Glipizide
   c. Theophylline
   d. Ipratropium

10. Describe the mechanism of the IOP-lowering effect caused by pilocarpine. (EO-7)

11. Which of the following should *not* be included as part of patient education provided to KW? (EO-14)
    a. Pilocarpine may cause decreased night vision
    b. KW should close her eyes and press lightly in the corner of the eye for 3–5 minutes following pilocarpine administration
    c. Since pilocarpine is given in the eyes, its side effect profile is limited to blurred vision and other ocular effects
    d. KW's glaucoma therapy is important to reduce risk of damage to her vision and loss of eyesight

12. KW is started on theophylline to try to improve her shortness of breath. Which of the following statements is *incorrect* regarding theophylline therapy? (EO-8, 9, 10)
    a. Patients receiving theophylline should be advised about the importance of checking nonprescription medications for possible drug–drug interactions
    b. Adverse effects such as nervousness, shaking, and irritability are signs of theophylline toxicity
    c. Theophylline can increase intraocular pressure
    d. Patients who consume char-grilled beef should be advised that this may decrease theophylline blood levels and lead to inadequate therapy

13. How can proper administration of eye drops reduce overall costs of treatment of glaucoma? (EO-17)

14. Summarize therapeutic, pathophysiologic, and disease management concepts for open-angle glaucoma utilizing a key points format. (EO-18)

CASE 77
J. Douglas Wurtzbacher
Topic: Otitis Media
Level 1
EDUCATIONAL MATERIALS
Chapter 49: Common Ear Diseases (otitis media, microbiology, signs and symptoms, therapeutic plan)

SCENARIO

Patient and Setting

NK, 8-month-old male infant; outpatient clinic

Chief Complaint

Fever, runny nose, and "continual crying" for 2 days per the infant's mother

History of Present Illness

NK's older sister was recently with PO amoxicillin followed by PO erythromycin/sulfisoxazole for otitis media; NK began having a runny nose and "became irritable" 5 days ago; two days before this visit, NK developed a fever (37.7°C [(99.9°F)]); via the telephone, the physician's office suggested a course of acetaminophen liquid and a clinic visit if this did not help; NK has been pulling on left ear during this time period

Past Medical History

Healthy (no previous episodes of otitis media)

Past Surgical History

None

Family/Social History

Family History: NK lives at home with his parents and 4-year-old sister who attends preschool

Social History: Nonapplicable

Medication History

Acetaminophen liquid, PRN for fever

Immunizations are current

Allergies

NKDA

Physical Examination

GEN: Well-developed, well-nourished male infant; crying and inconsolable

VS: BP 100/50, HR 96, RR 26, T 37.4°C, Wt 8 kg

HEENT: Left tympanic membrane (TM) is erythematous, opaque, and slightly bulging; reduced mobility noted on pneumatic otoscopy; no discharge is present; rhinorrhea present (clear in color); mucous membranes are slightly dry, no pharyngeal erythema or lesions noted

COR: Regular rate and rhythm; no murmurs or gallops noted

CHEST: Tachypneic, otherwise clear to auscultation

ABD: Soft, nontender, no guarding; normoactive bowel sounds

GU: Normal genitalia

RECT: Deferred

EXT: Moves all extremities, no cyanosis noted

NEURO: Alert, responds to pain

Results of Pertinent Laboratory Tests, Serum Drug Concentrations, and Diagnostic Tests

Na 141 (141)	HCO$_3$ 22 (22)	Hgb 131 (13.1)
K 3.6 (3.6)	BUN 4.3 (12)	Lkcs 12.4 × 10^9
Cl 96 (96)	Cr 17.7 (0.2)	(12.4 × 10^3)
	Hct 0.40 (40)	

Lkc differential: Segs 0.76 (76), bands 0.12 (12), monos 0.6 (6), lymphs 0.6 (6)

PROBLEM LIST

Identify principal problems from the scenario in priority order [completed Problem List and SOAP Note at end of casebook]

SOAP NOTE

To be completed by student

QUESTIONS

[Answers at end of casebook]

1. Which of the following organisms is the most likely cause of acute otitis media in NK? (EO-1)
   a. *Staphylococcus aureus*
   b. *Pseudomonas aeruginosa*
   c. *Streptococcus pneumoniae*
   d. Beta-hemolytic streptococci, group A

2. Which common symptoms of acute otitis media does NK exhibit in this case? (EO-2)

3. Which of the following statements is *false* regarding

supportive treatment for patients with acute otitis media? (EO-8, 10, 12)
   a. Aspirin should be used to reduce fever and pain
   b. Antihistamines and decongestants are ineffective at improving outcomes of disease
   c. The dose of ibuprofen should not exceed 40 mg/kg/day
   d. The use of oral corticosteroids as adjunct therapy is controversial

4. Which of the following is considered first-line therapy for acute otitis media? (EO-8, 12)
   a. Erythromycin/sulfisoxazole
   b. Cefpodoxime proxetil
   c. Clarithromycin
   d. Amoxicillin

5. Describe considerations in which an alternative to first-line therapy should be prescribed. (EO-8)

6. Which of the following is *not* a risk factor for the development of otitis media? (EO-1, 3)
   a. Male gender
   b. Child care outside the home
   c. Previous exposure to amoxicillin
   d. Exposure to secondhand smoke

7. What anatomic changes in infants and children increase the incidence of otitis media in this population? (EO-1)

8. Which of the following psychosocial factors is at least somewhat responsible for overprescribing of antibiotics for otitis media in children at low risk for complications? (EO-15)
   a. Financial ability of the parent to obtain medication
   b. Fussiness and inconsolability of the infant or child causes parents to ask physicians for "something" to alleviate the condition
   c. Insurance plans attempt to increase medication use to improve patient satisfaction
   d. Antibiotics have been shown to only have a modest effect on the overall course of disease

9. Which of the following is *not* a reason for reserving combination products such as amoxicillin/clavulanic acid or erythromycin/sulfisoxazole as second-line therapy? (EO-8, 10)
   a. These agents are considerably more expensive than first-line therapy
   b. These agents may unnecessarily expose a child to broad-spectrum antibiotics
   c. These agents may be given less frequently and therefore have better compliance
   d. Amoxicillin/clavulanate has an increased incidence of diarrhea when compared to amoxicillin alone

10. NK's physician is unaware that decongestants are of no value in patients with acute otitis media. He prescribes phenylephrine nasal spray. Which of the following are adverse effects that could be caused by inappropriate use of this agent? (EO-10)
   a. Rebound congestion if used for periods of greater than 3 days
   b. Hypotension
   c. Drowsiness
   d. Decreased heart rate

11. Which of the following should *not* be considered when attempting to improve patient compliance to therapy? (EO-15)
   a. Simplicity of medication therapy regimen
   b. Palatability of the medication chosen
   c. Antimicrobial resistance patterns of the medication(s) chosen
   d. Cost of the medication regimen

12. What pharmacoeconomic considerations should be evaluated prior to choosing oral or topical antimicrobial treatment for acute otitis media? (EO-17)

13. Summarize therapeutic, pathophysiologic, and disease management concepts for acute otitis media utilizing a key points format. (EO-18)

CASE 78
J. Douglas Wurtzbacher
Topic: Acute Otitis Externa

EDUCATIONAL MATERIALS
Chapter 49 Common Ear Diseases (otitis externa, pathophysiology, treatment, patient education)

SCENARIO

Patient and Setting
LR, 16-year-old male; primary care clinic

Chief Complaint
Painful "raw" left ear

History of Present Illness
SR states that he "spent the day at the lake about a week ago" and experienced a "feeling of water in my left ear," unable to remove; the left ear now increasingly erythematous and painful with clear fluid draining for 3 days

Past Medical History
Seasonal allergies

Past Surgical History
None

Family/Social History
Family History: Lives at home with his parents and younger sister

Social History: Denies alcohol or tobacco use; no illicit drug use; avid water skier who spends considerable time in the water during the summer months

Medication History

Astemizole, 10 mg PO QD PRN for seasonal allergies

Allergies

Ragweed, pollen

Physical Examination

GEN: Well-developed, well-nourished male in mild distress secondary to pain; complains of pain and discharge from left ear

VS: BP 120/70, HR 96, RR 18, T 37.0°C

HEENT: Left auricle erythematous and tender to palpation; external auditory canal is macerated with a small amount of serous fluid present; tympanic membranes (TMs) intact and normal in appearance

The remainder of the physical examination is unremarkable

Results of Pertinent Laboratory Tests, Serum Drug Concentrations, and Diagnostic Tests

Culture of fluid in left ear: pending

PROBLEM LIST

Identify principal problems from the scenario in priority order [completed Problem List and SOAP Note at end of casebook]

SOAP NOTE

To be completed by student

QUESTIONS

[Answers at end of casebook]

1. Which of the following conditions is most likely to increase a patient's risk of developing otitis externa? (EO-1)
   a. Acute otitis media
   b. Scuba diving
   c. Upper respiratory infection
   d. Use of corticosteroid ear drops

2. List the most common causative organisms in cases of otitis externa. (EO-1)

3. Which of the following adverse events is *not* associated with chloramphenicol ear drops? (EO-10)
   a. Overgrowth of resistant organisms
   b. Ototoxicity
   c. Bone marrow suppression
   d. Hypoalbuminemia

4. Describe key points which should be discussed with patients regarding the proper administration of ear drops. (EO-14)

5. Seasonal allergy sufferers may take _____ beginning approximately 2–4 weeks before allergy season to reduce nasal symptoms. (EO-12)
   a. Cromolyn sodium
   b. Albuterol
   c. Terbutaline
   d. Theophylline

6. What is the purpose of isopropyl alcohol 70% when used in patients with otitis externa? (EO-7)
   a. It exerts antibacterial activity
   b. It prevents fungal overgrowth
   c. It is used as a drying agent
   d. It exerts anti-inflammatory activity

7. What psychosocial factors in this case could contribute to treatment failure? (EO-15)

8. Which of the following situations would require oral antibiotic therapy? (EO-12)
   a. For chronic, persistent otitis externa limited to the auditory canal
   b. For prophylactic use in patients with recurrent otitis externa
   c. For all patients in which culture and sensitivity data are available
   d. For cases when the infection has spread to surrounding tissues of the ear

9. Patients with _____ should be instructed that antihistamine products can worsen their disease severity. (EO-8)
   a. Hypertension
   b. Benign prostatic hyperplasia symptoms
   c. Rheumatoid arthritis
   d. Otitis media

10. Which of the following structures of the ear is *not* involved in otitis externa? (EO-1)
    a. External auditory canal
    b. Tissue surrounding the auditory canal
    c. Bone surrounding the auditory canal
    d. Tympanic membrane

11. Physical assessment findings apparent in LR that suggest otitis externa include all of the following *except:* (EO-5)
    a. Painful, erythematous left ear
    b. Clear fluid draining from the ear
    c. Perforated tympanic membrane
    d. Inflamed external auditory canal

12. From a pharmacoeconomic focus, justify prophylactic use of OTC drying agents to prevent acute otitis externa. (EO-17)

13. Summarize therapeutic, pathophysiologic, and disease management concepts for otitis externa utilizing a key points format. (EO-18)

CASE 79
Melanie P. Swims
Topic: Headache—Migraine
Level 2
EDUCATIONAL MATERIALS
Chapter 51: Headache

SCENARIO

Patient and Setting

SA, 35-year-old female; emergency department

Chief Complaint

Sudden onset headache pain, nausea and vomiting, and chest pain for 1.5 days

History of Present Illness

Reports 3–4 headache episodes per month with one to two of these episodes usually before the onset of menses; this headache episode began 1.5 days ago; described as unilateral, intense, throbbing pain so severe that she is unable to work; no relief with 2–3 ibuprofen 200 mg tablets every 6 hours; a worsening in her regular GERD chest pain is also noted

Past Medical History

Distal vein thrombosis in left lower calf–9 months ago (no long-term anticoagulation required), GERD

Past Surgical History

None

Family/Social History

Family History: Mother died of breast cancer at age 73; father died of myocardial infarction (MI) at age 70

Social History: Smokes 2 PPD; drinks 4 cups of coffee per day; no alcohol

Medication History

Ibuprofen, 200 to 300 mg PO q6h PRN for headache pain

Aluminum hydroxide gel, 40 mL PO q4–6h PRN for heartburn

Allergies

Sulfa drugs cause hives

Chlorpromazine causes dystonia

Physical Examination

GEN: Obese female in moderate distress
VS: BP 128/82, HR 70, RR 26, T 36.0°C, Wt 90 kg, Ht 172 cm
HEENT: PERRLA, photophobia, normocephalic, atraumatic, erythematous oropharynx
COR: Normal S1 and S2, regular rate and rhythm
CHEST: Clear to auscultation and palpation, no rales or rhonchi
ABD: Soft, nontender, no hepatosplenomegaly, no lymphadenopathy
RECT: Guaiac negative
EXT: + clubbing, no evidence of cyanosis; no evidence of swelling or erythema in lower extremities
NEURO: Oriented to time, place, and person; cranial nerves intact; normal deep tendon reflexes

Results of Pertinent Laboratory Tests, Serum Drug Concentrations, and Diagnostic Tests

Na 140 (140)	Hgb 120 (12)	Cr 88 (1)
K 3.8 (3.8)	Lkcs 5×10^9	Glu 6.1 (110)
Cl 109 (109)	(5×10^3)	Ca 2.2 (8.9)
HCO_3 22 (22)	Plts 290×10^9	PO_4 0.64 (2)
BUN 10 (30)	(290×10^3)	Mg 1.75 (3.5)
Hct 0.34 (34)		

Chest x-ray: Normal
ECG: Normal

PROBLEM LIST

Identify principal problems from the scenario in priority order [completed Problem List and SOAP Note at end of casebook]

SOAP NOTE

To be completed by student

QUESTIONS

[Answers at end of casebook]

1. What role does stress play as a precipitating factor in exacerbation of SA's GERD? (EO-1)

2. List the criteria noted for the diagnosis of migraine. (EO-2)

3. Why is drug acquisition cost only a simplistic model to consider in the treatment of acute and chronic migraine? (EO-17)

4. Prophylactic migraine therapy is: (EO-8)
   a. Reserved for patients who have the most severe attacks
   b. Selected for patients dependent on factors such as attack frequency and impact on quality of life
   c. Reserved for hemiplegic migraine
   d. Often avoided due to the lack of effective choices

5. What factors limit the use of ergotamines in SA? (EO-8)
   a. Status post deep venous thrombosis
   b. Nausea
   c. Prior use of NSAIDs
   d. Risk of pregnancy in a female patient

6. If SA is started on propranolol, what monitoring parameters are appropriate? (EO-5)

7. What is the mechanism of action of the sumitriptan? (EO-7)
   a. 5HT1B/1D Agonist
   b. Selective serotonin reuptake inhibitor
   c. 5HT2C Antagonist
   d. Selective vasodilation of trigeminal nucleus

8. What nondrug measures may help to relieve SA's reflux chest pain? (EO-12)
   a. Lower the head of bed
   b. Avoid large meals especially before bed
   c. Psychological counseling
   d. Physical therapy

9. What is the unique pharmacokinetic property of naratriptan that may offer an advantage in some patients? (EO-4)
   a. No protein binding
   b. Renal elimination
   c. First order kinetics
   d. Longer half-life

10. Which prophylactic antimigraine medications, if any, should be avoided in SA? (EO-9)

11. Acute migraine treatment should be limited to: (EO-12, 18)
    a. Two to three times per week
    b. Nonnarcotic agents only
    c. One health care provider, so as to limit drug-seeking patients
    d. Monotherapy

12. Which acute treatment provides the fastest relief? (EO-6, 8)
    a. Intranasal sumitriptan
    b. Naratriptan
    c. Valproic acid
    d. SC sumatriptan

13. What factors should be considered in the diagnosis of migraine? (EO-2)
    a. Abusive family history
    b. Alcohol abuse
    c. Associated symptoms
    d. Personality type

14. Summarize therapeutic, pathophysiologic, and disease management concepts for migraine headache utilizing a key points format. (EO-18)

CASE 80
Melanie P. Swims
Topic: Seizure
Level 1
EDUCATIONAL MATERIALS
Chapter 52: Seizure Disorders

SCENARIO

Patient and Setting
MJ, 62-year-old male; emergency department

Chief Complaint
Tonic–clonic seizure with loss of consciousness

History of Present Illness
Tonic–clonic seizure, witnessed by the nurse at the skilled nursing facility (SNF); nurse reports that this is MJ's third seizure in the last 30 minutes; seizures characterized by jerking movements of his upper extremities, muscle rigidity, urinary incontinence, and loss of consciousness lasting approximately 2 minutes; first seizure was then immediately followed by another lasting 4 minutes; then a third seizure occurred on the way to the hospital which lasted approximately 2 minutes

Past Medical History
One-year history of secondarily generalized tonic–clonic seizures after a stroke 2 years ago, residual left-sided body weakness as well as mild mental deficiency; resides at a skilled care facility; approximately 3 months noted to have some new difficulty swallowing; physician changed phenytoin sodium extended release 300 mg QHS to 300 mg QHS of the chewable tablets

Past Surgical History
None

Family/Social History
Noncontributory

Medication History
Phenytoin chewable tablets, 300 mg PO QHS
Aspirin, 325 mg PO QD
Ibuprofen, 400 mg PO PRN for back pain

Allergies
NKDA

Physical Examination

VS: BP 170/100, HR 105, RR 26, T 38.0°C, Wt 60 kg, Ht 175 cm

HEENT: PERRLA, poor dentition

CHEST: Clear to auscultation

COR: Sinus tachycardia, S_1, S_2, no S_3 or S_4

EXT: Thin with minimal muscle development, especially lower extremities

NEURO: Unresponsive to deep pain, 1/5 upper and lower extremity weakness prior to admission

Results of Pertinent Laboratory Tests, Serum Drug Concentrations, and Diagnostic Tests

Na 140 (140)	Hgb 160 (16)	AST 0.5 (31)
K 5.2 (5.0)	Hct 0.4 (40)	ALT 0.4 (25)
Cl 100 (100)	Plts 150×10^9	Alb 44 (4.4)
HCO_3 20 (20)	(150×10^3)	T Bili 9 (0.5)
BUN 6.5 (18)	Lkcs 8.8×10^9	Ca 1.95 (7.8)
Cr 67 (0.8)	(8.8×10^3)	Phos 0.80 (2.5)
Glu 6.1 (110)	RBC 5.0×10^{12}/L	Mg 1.1 (2.5)
Phenytoin 16 (4)	(5.0×10^6)	Alk Phos 2.0 (120)

ECG: Sinus tachycardia

Blood gases showed acidosis

PROBLEM LIST

Identify principal problems from the scenario in priority order

SOAP NOTE

To be completed by student

QUESTIONS

1. If the seizures continue following benzodiazepine and phenytoin administration what is the next step in the status epilepticus protocol? (EO-12)
   a. IV valproate
   b. Rectal diazepam
   c. IM fosphenytoin
   d. IV phenobarbital

2. Why are MJ's seizures referred to as "secondarily generalized" seizures? (EO-1)

3. Which phenytoin preparation(s) is/are approved as once daily formulations? (EO-8)

4. Choose the phenytoin preparation below that is 100% phenytoin. (EO-8)
   a. Phenytoin oral suspension
   b. Fosphenytoin
   c. Parenteral phenytoin
   d. Phenytoin sodium, extended

5. What pharmacokinetic property does phenytoin exhibit? (EO-6)

   a. First order kinetics
   b. Autoinduction
   c. Michaelis-Menten kinetics
   d. Zero order kinetics

6. What is the normal half-life of phenytoin? (EO-6)

7. What food/drug interaction is important with phenytoin? (EO-9)
   a. Enteral feeds
   b. Grapefruit juice
   c. Apple juice
   d. Calcium containing products

8. If MJ is diagnosed with a new embolic stroke and put on warfarin, what may happen to the phenytoin levels? (EO-9)

9. MJ is described as having mild cognitive impairment from the previous stroke. Which antiepileptic drug below is the least likely to impair cognition? (EO-10, 15)
   a. Phenobarbital
   b. Clonazepam
   c. Primidone
   d. Phenytoin

10. If MJ is found to have a new thrombotic stroke, what antiplatelet agent might be best for him? (EO-8)
    a. Ticlopidine
    b. Clopidogrel
    c. Dipyridamole
    d. Aspirin

11. What are the disadvantages of the chewable phenytoin tablet? (EO-15)

12. What is the proper approach for the family to take to a patient/individual discovered having a seizure? (EO-14)
    a. Put a spoon in the patient's mouth to prevent swallowing of the tongue
    b. Restrain the patient's movements
    c. Put cold water on the patient's face at once to bring him or her out of the seizure
    d. Observe the patient and intervene only if his or her movements may cause injury

13. MJ's seizure disorder is likely: (EO-1)
    a. Autosomal recessive
    b. Triggered by a focal brain lesion
    c. Triggered by poor nursing home care
    d. Autosomal dominant

14. Summarize therapeutic, pathophysiologic, and disease management concepts for seizure disorder utilizing a key points format. (EO-18)

CASE 81

Melanie P. Swims

Topic: Seizure

Level 3

EDUCATIONAL MATERIALS

Chapter 52: Seizure Disorders

SCENARIO

Patient and Setting

HK, 59-year-old male; neurology clinic

Chief Complaint

Recurrent seizures

History of Present Illness

HK reports an increase in number of seizures up to four monthly as well as nausea, anorexia, occasional epigastric distress unrelated to food intake; recently experiencing greater sleepiness and unsteady gait

Past Medical History

22-year history of idiopathic generalized tonic–clonic seizures that have occurred sporadically in the past; however, presently reports about 4 seizures monthly; hypertension (HTN); peptic ulcer disease (PUD) and gastritis diagnosed by endoscopy 1 week ago

Past Surgical History

None

Family/Social History

Family History: Noncontributory

Social History: Smokes 33 pack/year; drinks $1\frac{1}{2}$ pints of liquor daily; divorced and lives alone

Medication History

Phenytoin, 500 mg PO QD × 22 years

Cimetidine, 800 mg PO QHS

Hydrochlorothiazide, 12.5 mg PO QD

Allergies

NKDA

Physical Examination

GEN: Poorly groomed male appearing somnolent and with slurred speech

VS: BP 160/90, HR 70, RR 20, T 37.0°C, Wt 74 kg, Ht 175 cm

HEENT: Gingival hyperplasia

COR: RRR, nl S1, S2

RECT: Guaiac positive

NEURO: (+) bilateral nystagmus on lateral gaze (at 45 degrees); ataxia; (+) Romberg sign

Results of Pertinent Laboratory Tests, Serum Drug Concentrations, and Diagnostic Tests

Na 144 (144)	Cr 97 (1.1)	ALT 0.83 (50)
K 3.1 (3.1)	Hct 0.33 (33)	Alb 32 (3.2)
Cl 102 (102)	Hgb 110 (11)	T Bili 18.8 (1)
HCO_3 26 (26)	MCV 108 (108)	Glu 6.0 (108)
BUN 5.0 (14)	AST 1.3 (78)	Phenytoin 130 (32.5)

PROBLEM LIST

Identify principal problems from the scenario in priority order [completed Problem List and SOAP Note at end of casebook]

SOAP NOTE

To be completed by student

QUESTIONS

[*Answers at end of casebook*]

1. HK's measured phenytoin concentration is 32.5 mg/L. Calculate an adjusted phenytoin level for low albumin. (EO-6)

2. Explain the mechanism by which HK's serum phenytoin level became elevated. (EO-9)

3. What signs/symptoms presented by HK are indicative of phenytoin toxicity? (EO-2, 10)
   a. Ataxia
   b. Low hematocrit
   c. Anorexia
   d. Guaiac positive

4. In what ways specifically does alcoholism influence the physical health of HK? (EO-12, 14, 15)

5. Would polytherapy for HK's seizures be the most advantageous plan? (EO-12, 14, 15, 18)

6. How would you advise HK on nonpharmacologic and pharmacologic approaches to decrease the number of seizures? (EO-14)

7. What aggravating factor likely contributed to HK's gastritis? (EO-1)
   a. Low weight
   b. Phenytoin prescription
   c. Alcoholism
   d. Seizure disorder

8. Which of the following options is appropriate to treat HK's gastritis? (EO-12)
   a. 30 mL of extra strength antacid daily and PRN for heartburn pain
   b. Maximum dose proton pump inhibitor therapy
   c. Bismuth subsalicylate PRN for pain
   d. Full dose H_2 antagonist

9. What lab/physical exam parameters provide evidence that HK's gastritis is not under control? (EO-5)
   a. Albumin and weight are low
   b. Guaiac positive, low hematocrit

c. Ataxia and nystagmus

d. Lack of seizure control and high phenytoin level

10. Which of the following nonpharmacologic treatment plans listed below may help HK's gastritis symptoms? (EO-12)
    a. Discontinue smoking
    b. Eating well to get weight back up
    c. Avoidance of seizure triggers
    d. Proper rest

11. Select the non–dose-related side effect of phenytoin. (EO-10)
    a. Nystagmus
    b. Positive Romberg
    c. Cerebellar ataxia
    d. Gingival hyperplasia

12. Which side effect listed below is attributable to cimetidine? (EO-10)
    a. Gynecomastia
    b. Ataxia
    c. Neuropathic pain
    d. Hepatic hypertrophy

13. Which of the following steps may help the clinician in objectifying seizure control? (EO-12)
    a. Nurse to check on patient weekly
    b. Use of pill box
    c. Seizure diary
    d. Compliance counseling by pharmacy

14. Summarize therapeutic, pathophysiologic, and disease management concepts for seizure disorder utilizing a key points format. (EO-18)

CASE 82

Melanie P. Swims

Topic: Seizure

Level 2

EDUCATIONAL MATERIALS

Chapter 52: Seizure Disorders

SCENARIO

Patient and Setting

JZ, 38-year-old female; emergency department

Chief Complaint

Tonic–clonic seizure with loss of consciousness

History of Present Illness

Upon arrival at JZ's home, paramedics noted a generalized tonic–clonic seizure in JZ characterized by loss of consciousness, tongue biting, urinary incontinence, muscle rigidity, and subsequent jerking movements of all extremities; duration 3 minutes and quickly followed by another seizure lasting 5 minutes; paramedics administered diazepam, 10 mg IV causing seizure termination but full alertness did not ensue; while waiting to be seen in the ER, another generalized tonic–clonic seizure occurred

Past Medical History

Numerous episodes of recurrent epigastric pain with anorexia, vomiting, and weight loss over the past several years; last seen in the GI clinic 3 days ago, denied abdominal pain and other GI distress but reported a 3-week history of arthralgias, fatigue, and mild fever; 7-year history of posttraumatic epilepsy with seizures preceded by an aura described as a rising epigastric sensation followed by a tingling sensation progressing from neck to head followed by loss of consciousness and a stereotypical generalized tonic–clonic seizure; poor compliance; 12-year history of systemic lupus erythematosus (SLE); and chronic pancreatitis of unknown cause

Past Surgical History

None

Family/ Social History

Family History: Aunt with SLE diagnosed at age 27

Social History: Denies alcohol and tobacco use

Medication History

Carbamazepine, 200 mg PO TID

Naproxen, 550 mg PO BID

Allergies

NKDA

Physical Examination

VS: BP 168/98, HR 110, RR 20, T 37.5°C, Wt 63 kg, Ht 160 cm

HEENT: Bite wound on tongue; erythematous malar rash

CHEST: Clear

COR: Normal S1, S2; no S3 or S4

EXT: Moderate joint swelling of hands and feet

NEURO: Unresponsive to deep pain

Results of Pertinent Laboratory Tests, Serum Drug Concentrations, and Diagnostic Tests

Na 135 (135)	Hgb 120 (12)	T Bili 17.1 (1.0)
K 4.8 (4.8)	Plts 45 × 10⁹	Glu 6.8 (122)
Cl 95 (95)	(45 × 10³)	Amylase 3.67 (220)
HCO₃ 26 (26)	AST 0.5 (30)	Carbamazepine 13 (3)
BUN 13.6 (38)	ALT 0.6 (36)	ESR 50 (50)
Cr 212 (2.4)	Alb 42 (4.2)	ANA titer 1:480
Hct 0.34 (34)		

PROBLEM LIST

Identify principal problems from the scenario in priority order [*completed Problem List and SOAP Note at end of casebook*]

SOAP NOTE

To be completed by student

QUESTIONS

[*Answers at end of casebook*]

1. An additional dose of diazepam (10 mg IV) and a full loading dose of phenytoin (1200 mg IV) were given in the ER and seizures were terminated. JZ was then admitted to the neurology service. The physician would like to continue maintenance anticonvulsant therapy by the intravenous route until oral medications can be given. Which option is appropriate for JZ? (EO-4)
   a. IV phenytoin 100 mg q8h
   b. IV carbamazepine 100 mg q8h
   c. IV ethosuximide 100 mg q8h
   d. IV phenobarbital 100 mg q8h

2. How should JZ's hematological status be monitored for the potential adverse effects of carbamazepine therapy? (EO-10)
   a. Baseline CBC and if pretreatments are normal then periodically
   b. Weekly CBC indefinitely
   c. Hematological monitoring is unnecessary
   d. Monthly CBC for duration of treatment

3. How do NSAIDs adversely affect the kidney? (EO-10)

4. What are the most commonly associated dose-related side effects of carbamazepine? (EO-2, 10)
   a. Diplopia, nausea, ataxia
   b. Renal failure, rash, decreased WBC
   c. Pulmonary toxicity, liver failure, autoimmune syndromes
   d. Angina, urticaria, vomiting

5. If JZ's lupus worsens and she is begun on hydroxychloroquine, what monitoring will be required? (EO-8,10)

6. What aids may the pharmacist provide for JZ to assist in strengthening her compliance? (EO-14)

7. Once JZ is able to take oral medications, if she has been off of her carbamazepine during the time that she was on IV therapy, how would you reinitiate the carbamazepine? (EO-11, 12)
   a. Carbamazepine, 800 mg PO load
   b. Carbamazepine suspension, 200 mg PO BID
   c. Carbamazepine extended release, 400 mg, take two tablets every day
   d. Carbamazepine 100 mg twice daily for 3 days, then 200 mg twice daily for 1 week, then 200 mg of extended release product twice daily with titration to therapeutic levels

8. What unique pharmacokinetic property does carbamazepine exhibit? (EO-4, 6)
   a. Michaelis-Menten kinetics
   b. Dose-dependent absorption
   c. Autoinduction
   d. No protein binding

9. Which of the following antiepileptic agents is a hepatic enzyme inhibitor? (EO-9)
   a. Valproate
   b. Carbamazepine
   c. Gabapentin
   d. Phenytoin

10. The physician treating JZ is worried that the hematological toxicity of carbamazepine is adversely affecting her SLE. What agent listed below is least likely to be associated with hematological or hepatic toxicity? (EO-11)
    a. Gabapentin
    b. Phenytoin
    c. Carbamazepine
    d. Valproate

11. After the addition of hydroxychloroquine, if JZ's lupus continues to worsen, what would be the best new agent to add to her drug therapy regimen? (EO-12)
    a. Prednisone
    b. Narcotic analgesics
    c. Intra-articular injections
    d. Azathioprine

12. Describe the mechanism of action of naproxen in the treatment of SLE. (EO-7)

13. Summarize therapeutic, pathophysiologic, and disease management concepts for seizure disorder utilizing a key points format. (EO-18)

CASE 83
Melanie P. Swims
Topic: Parkinson's Disease

Level 3

EDUCATIONAL MATERIALS
Chapter 53: Parkinsonism

SCENARIO

Patient and Setting

FM, 72-year-old male; geriatric clinic

Chief Complaint

Decreased functional status

History of Present Illness

Exhibiting signs of declining function over the past 6 weeks; since last clinic visit increased tremor, more rigidity, and more slowness of movements with two falls noted

Past Medical History

Hypertension (HTN); chronic mild renal insufficiency; chronic obstructive pulmonary disease (COPD); S/P MI 1996; Parkinson's disease; constipation; and degenerative joint disease (DJD)

Past Surgical History

None

Social/Family History

Family History: Mother died of a stroke at 82; father died of an MI at age 70

Social History: No alcohol; former smoker 20 pack/year

Medication History

Carbidopa/levodopa, 25/100 mg, 1 tablet PO TID

Amantadine, 100 mg PO TID

Naproxen, 250 mg PO TID

Triamcinolone inhaler, 3 puffs QID

Ipratropium bromide inhaler, 2 puffs q6h

Albuterol inhaler, 2 puffs q6h

Reserpine, 0.25 mg PO QD

Verapamil, sustained release, 240 mg PO QD

Nitroglycerin, sustained release, 9.0 mg, 1 capsule PO q8h

Nitroglycerin SL, 0.4 mg every 5 minutes for 3 doses PRN for angina

Multivitamin tablet, 1 PO QD

Allergies

Penicillin

Physical Examination

GEN: Well-nourished male with decreasing mobility in no apparent distress

VS: BP 175/95, HR 100, RR 32, T 37.5°C, Wt 70 kg, Ht 180 cm

HEENT: No evidence of trauma, PERRLA, neck supple, no bruits, no JVD

COR: Irregular rhythm with occasional PVC, normal rate, normal S_1, S_2, no S_3 or S_4

CHEST: Diffuse expiratory wheezes bilaterally

ABD: Soft, distended, nontender; liver small, 6 cm; no spleen palpable

GU: Normal male genitalia, prostate enlarged, nonnodular

RECT: Brown, heme-negative stool

EXT: Pulses decreased in lower extremities, decreased ROM and pain of left knee

NEURO: Cranial nerves II–XII within normal limits, strength 4/5 bilaterally upper extremities, 5/5 lower extremities, unsteady gait with small steps and reduced armswing, (+) cog-wheeled rigidity upper and lower extremities, (+) pill-rolling tremor upper extremities, (+) bradykinesia, sensory intact, A and O × 4

Results of Pertinent Laboratory Tests, Serum Drug Concentrations, and Diagnostic Tests

Na 135 (135)	Hct 0.40 (40)	ALT 0.2 (12)
K 3.9 (3.9)	Lkcs 9.8 × 10^9	Alb 41 (4.1)
Cl 96 (96)	(9.8 × 10^3)	Glu 6.0 (108)
HCO$_3$ 27 (27)	Plts 305 × 10^9	Ca 2.3 (9.2)
BUN 13.6 (38)	(305 × 10^3)	PO$_4$ 1.07 (3.3)
Cr 185.6 (2.1)	AST 0.28 (17)	Mg 0.75 (1.5)

PROBLEM LIST

Identify principal problems from the scenario in priority order

SOAP NOTE

To be completed by student

QUESTIONS

1. What drug is worsening FM's Parkinson's disease? (EO-9)
   a. Naproxen
   b. Nitroglycerin
   c. Triamcinolone inhaler
   d. Reserpine

2. What pair below includes 2 of the cardinal features of Parkinson's disease? (EO-2)
   a. Bradykinesia, rigidity
   b. Tremor, shortness of breath
   c. Tachycardia, dementia
   d. Seborrhea, gastritis

3. What answer below correctly describes the neurotransmitter imbalance found in Parkinson's disease? (EO-1)
   a. Increased acetylcholinesterase, decreased serotonin
   b. Increased glutamic acid, decreased norepinephrine
   c. Increased acetylcholine, decreased dopamine
   d. Increased dopa decarboxylase, decreased GABA

4. What factors place FM at high risk for falls and subsequently fractures? (EO-1)

5. Which drug listed below is the most likely cause of drug-induced Parkinsonism? (EO-9)
   a. Metoclopramide
   b. Hydroxyzine
   c. Gold
   d. Ketorolac

6. What is the mechanism of the naproxen-induced renal insufficiency in FM? (EO-10)

7. What is the most common serious complication of NSAID therapy? (EO-10)
   a. Renal failure
   b. Serum sickness
   c. Rash
   d. Gastrointestinal bleeding

8. Why does the nitroglycerin sustained-release formulation need to be dosed during the day rather than every 8 hours? (EO-11)

9. What dietary component can interfere with the proper effect of carbidopa/levodopa? (EO-14)
   a. Zinc
   b. Protein
   c. Saturated fats
   d. Sodium

10. How should FM be counseled as to the prognosis of Parkinson's disease? (EO-14, 16)

11. Which enzyme does carbidopa inhibit? (EO-7)
    a. Dopacholinesterase
    b. Catechol-O-methyl transferase
    c. MAO-B
    d. Dopa decarboxylase

12. What pharmacological treatment listed below is NOT proven to improve Parkinson's disease when added to carbidopa/levodopa? (EO-8)
    a. Trihexyphenidyl
    b. Bromocriptine
    c. Pemoline
    d. Selegiline

13. Summarize therapeutic, pathophysiologic, and disease management concepts for Parkinson's disease utilizing a key points format. (EO-18)

CASE 84
Melanie P. Swims
Topic: Parkinson's Disease
Level 2
EDUCATIONAL MATERIALS
Chapter 53: Parkinsonism

SCENARIO

Patient and Setting
AJ, 70-year-old female; neurology clinic

Chief Complaint
"My medicine is wearing off on me. I am getting some odd movements about 30 minutes after a dose of my medication for Parkinson's disease, and I am seeing things that I know are not there."

History of Present Illness
AJ has noted wearing off manifested as increased tremor, more rigidity, and more slowness of movements with some freezing spells; dyskinetic writhing movements are noted one half hour after carbidopa/levodopa administration; late in the day AJ sometimes has visual hallucinations

Past Medical History
Parkinson's disease (for 5 years); osteoporosis; hypertension (HTN); and obesity

Past Surgical History
Total abdominal hysterectomy

Family/Social History
Family History: Noncontributory
Social History: No alcohol intake; nonsmoker

Medication History
Carbidopa/levodopa, 25/250 mg, 1 tablet PO BID
Conjugated estrogens, 0.625 mg PO QD
Atenolol, 25 mg PO QD
Multivitamin, 1 tablet PO QD
Calcium carbonate, 500 mg PO TID

Allergies
Sulfa

Physical Examination
GEN: Well-nourished female with decreasing mobility in no apparent distress
VS: BP 166/90 (last clinic visit 180/92), HR 60, RR 22, T 37.5°C, Wt 80 kg, Ht 165 cm
HEENT: No evidence of trauma, PERRL, neck supple, no bruits, no JVD
COR: WNL
CHEST: WNL
ABD: Soft, distended, nontender
GU: WNL
RECT: Brown, heme-negative stool
EXT: Pulses decreased in lower extremities
NEURO: Cranial nerves II–XII within normal limits, strength 5/5 bilaterally upper extremities, 5/5 lower extremities, gait with small steps and reduced arm swing, (+) cog-wheeled rigidity upper and lower extremities, (+) pill-rolling tremor upper extremities, (+) bradykinesia, sensory intact, alert and oriented × 4, mini mental state exam = 29/30

Results of Pertinent Laboratory Tests, Serum Drug Concentrations, and Diagnostic Tests

Na 135 (135)   Hct 0.36 (36)   AST 0.28 (17)
K 3.9 (3.9)   Lkcs 9.8×10^9 ALT 0.2 (12)
Cl 96 (96) (9.8×10^3) Glu 6.0 (108)
HCO_3 27 (27)   Plts 305×10^9 Ca 2.3 (9.2)
BUN 4 (11) (305×10^3) PO_4 1.07 (3.3)
Cr 88.4 (1)

PROBLEM LIST

Identify principal problems from the scenario in priority order [completed Problem List and SOAP Note at end of casebook]

SOAP NOTE

To be completed by student

QUESTIONS

[Answers at end of casebook]

1. AJ's tremor, as seen in most patients with Parkinson's disease, is characterized as a: (EO-2)
   a. Involuntary resting tremor
   b. Voluntary kinetic tremor
   c. Postural tremor
   d. Familial tremor

2. Which pair describes some of the more common side effects seen in patients that are taking carbidopa/levodopa? (EO-10)
   a. Urinary retention, dry mouth
   b. Diarrhea, excessive tearing
   c. Nausea, abnormal movements
   d. Itching, paresthesias

3. The etiology of AJ's Parkinson's disease is best described as: (EO-1)
   a. Genetic
   b. Environmental
   c. Drug induced
   d. Idiopathic

4. Which pharmacological option listed has *not* been helpful in treating on/off syndrome? (EO-12)
   a. Selegiline
   b. Diphenhydramine
   c. Cisapride
   d. Pergolide

5. The physician states he may utilize amantadine in AJ if the current therapy does not provide optimal control. What labs would you order and why? (EO-6)

6. One of the physicians at the clinic asks you for the mechanism of action of selegiline. You correctly reply that this agent is a: (EO-7)
   a. COMT inhibitor
   b. MAO-B inhibitor
   c. Dopamine decarboxylase inhibitor
   d. MAO-A inhibitor

7. Selegiline must be dosed twice daily every AM and at noon. Why? (EO-6, 10)

8. How could giving AJ hydrochlorothiazide for her hypertension potentially improve her osteoporosis? (EO-8)

9. Which antipsychotic listed below would be the best choice to treat AJ's hallucinations? (EO-8)
   a. Haloperidol
   b. Chlorpromazine
   c. Prochlorperazine
   d. Olanzapine

10. What is the mechanism of action of bromocriptine? (EO-7)
    a. Dopamine agonist
    b. COMT inhibitor
    c. Increases release of dopamine
    d. Increases synthesis of dopamine

11. What advantages might a dopamine agonist have in end-stage Parkinson's disease? (EO-8)

12. How does carbidopa/levodopa sustained-release formulation differ from immediate-release carbidopa/levodopa? (EO-6)
    a. Bioavailability
    b. Protein binding
    c. Excretion
    d. Route of administration

13. How would you counsel AJ regarding her hallucinations and their relationship to the potential occurrence of dementia at a later stage? (EO-14, 15, 16)

14. Summarize therapeutic, pathophysiologic, and disease management concepts for Parkinson's disease utilizing a key points format. (EO-18)

CASE 85
Jeff Hulstein
Topic: Pain Management

EDUCATIONAL MATERIALS
Chapter 54: Pain Management (treatment goals, epidemiology, modulation and interruption of central pain processing, clinical presentation and diagnosis, psychosocial, therapeutic plan, pharmacotherapy, nonopioid analgesics, analgesic adjuncts, special considerations in analgesic pharmacotherapy)

SCENARIO

Patient and Setting

FF, 14-year-old African American male; pediatric clinic

Chief Complaint

Recent onset of pain in the back and chest; low grade fever

History of Present Illness

Pain and fever began last night after a school field trip; in moderate pain today; complaints are similar to previous sickle-cell exacerbation; teacher informed mother of FF's "day-dreaming" episodes in class that occur 6–7 times a week (3–5 seconds each) with some eye blinking; continues use of inhaler 3–4 times daily; compliant with other medications

Past Medical History

Sickle-cell anemia; vaso-occlusive pains resulting from compromised blood circulation (4 admissions within last year for parenteral narcotic treatment of vaso-occlusive crises); generalized absence seizures (petit mal) for past 4 years; childhood asthma (controlled with β-agonist and theophylline); fractured collar bone from sports injury; moderate acne diagnosed 1 week ago by dermatologist

Past Surgical History

Four stitches to forehead after a car accident

Family/Social History

Family History: Neither parent has sickle cell anemia; 8-year-old sister is asthmatic

Social History: Noncontributory

Medication History

Ethosuximide, 250 mg PO TID

Sustained-release theophylline, 200 mg PO BID

Albuterol MDI, 1 to 2 puffs PRN for shortness of breath

Folic acid, 1 mg PO QD

Benzoyl peroxide gel 5%, applied once daily in the evening (first prescribed 1 week ago)

Allergies

Aspirin (induces bronchospasm)

PROBLEM LIST

Identify principal problems from the scenario in priority order

SOAP NOTE

To be completed by student

QUESTIONS

1. The reason hemoglobin takes on the "sickle-cell" shape: (EO-1)
   a. Low blood volume
   b. State of deoxygenation in Hgb
   c. Faulty bone marrow
   d. Prenatal complications

2. Identify other signs and symptoms often seen at presentation of sickle-cell anemia. (EO-2)

3. The gene for sickle-cell anemia is most prominent in which ethnic group? (EO-3)
   a. Greeks
   b. Italians
   c. Arabians
   d. African Americans

4. Which one of FF's current medications has the greatest potential to precipitate seizure activity? (EO-10)
   a. Albuterol inhaler
   b. Folic acid
   c. Theophylline
   d. Benzoyl peroxide

5. List common causes of analgesic failure in pain management. (EO-11)

6. After increasing FF's ethosuximide dose, what therapeutic range is desired? (EO-5)
   a. 45–100 ng/mL
   b. 40–100 μg/mL
   c. 10–20 ng/mL
   d. 100–150 μg/mL

7. Describe the pharmacologic and nonpharmacologic treatments that would help treat FF's moderate acne. (EO-12)

8. Analyze psychosocial factors that may affect FF's adherence to nonpharmacologic and pharmacologic therapies of his problem list. (EO-15)

9. FF's pain from the vaso-occlusion can be managed with all of the following oral agents *except:* (EO-8)
   a. Morphine
   b. Hydrocodone
   c. Tramadol
   d. Piroxicam

10. List signs and symptoms of pain that FF may present with and create a technique to grade his pain. (EO-2)

11. Appropriate monitoring for a patient on a high-dose narcotic includes all of the following *except:* (EO-11)
    a. Respiratory rate
    b. Bowel sounds
    c. Blood concentration levels
    d. Blood pressure

12. Maximum therapy duration is limited to 5 days because of GI complications in which of the following analgesics: (EO-8)
    a. Etodolac
    b. Indomethacin
    c. Ketorolac
    d. Ketoprofen

13. For the treatment of absence seizures, what is another alternative to ethosuximide? (EO-8)
    a. Valproic acid
    b. Phenytoin
    c. Clonazepam
    d. Carbamazepine

14. How can pharmacists reduce the economic burdens of chronic pain to patients and hospitals? (EO-17)

15. Summarize pathophysiologic, therapeutic, and disease management concepts for pain management utilizing a key points format. (EO-18)

CASE 86
Jeff Hulstein
Topic: Pain Management
Level 1
EDUCATIONAL MATERIALS
Chapter 54: Pain Management (treatment goals, epidemiology, modulation and interruption of central pain, clinical presentation at diagnosis, psychosocial, therapeutic plan, treatment-pharmacotherapy, non-opioid analgesics, analgesic adjuncts, special considerations in analgesic pharmacotherapy)

SCENARIO

Patient and Setting
KM, 60-year-old female; hospital

Chief Complaint
Tonic–clonic seizure following attempted pain control with meperidine PCA S/P hip replacement surgery

History of Present Illness
Total hip replacement was performed 3 days ago and KM was immediately placed on meperidine PCA for pain control; experienced tonic-clonic seizure this morning and was treated with 500 mg IV phenytoin and 5 mg IV lorazepam; currently on meperidine IM and phenytoin PO and experiencing more pain

Past Medical History
Hospitalized 4 years ago for fall down flight of stairs; dislocated hip in fall; developed seizures from head injury in fall; last seizure was 1 year ago

Past Surgical History
None

Family/Social History
Family History: Father with hypertension
Social History: No alcohol use; no tobacco use

Medication History
Phenytoin, 300 mg PO HS
Acetaminophen/codeine, 30 mg PO QID PRN for hip pain

Current Medications
Meperidine, 75 mg IM q4h PRN for pain
Enoxaparin, 30 mg SC BID
Phenytoin, 400 mg PO HS
Ibuprofen, 600 mg PO QID PRN for pain

Allergies
Penicillin (rash)

PROBLEM LIST
Identify principal problems from the scenario in priority order [completed Problem List and SOAP Note at end of casebook]

SOAP NOTE
To be completed by student

QUESTIONS
[Answers at end of casebook]

1. KM appears to be toxic from which metabolite of meperidine? (EO-1, 10)
   a. *N*-Demethyl
   b. Normeperidine
   c. L-Meperidine
   d. Meperidinic acid

2. KM is later switched to IV morphine 10 mg/hr. Calculate an equivalent oral dose that would be given in sustained-release tablets. (EO-6, 12)

3. When should prophylactic therapy with enoxaparin be initiated? (EO-8)

4. Which lab test and therapeutic range for anticoagulation are recommended for KM's hip replacement? (EO-5)
   a. PTT at 1.5–2.5 times control
   b. Monitoring anticoagulation tests not required
   c. INR at 2.5–3.5
   d. Both a and c

5. Which of the following analgesics, like meperidine, has a renally cleared metabolite that can cause CNS irritability? (EO-4, 8)
   a. Hydrocodone
   b. Oxycodone
   c. Morphine
   d. Fentanyl

6. Identify the narcotic that could be substituted for morphine to reduce nausea, vomiting, sedation, constipation, or euphoria. (EO-8, 11, 12)

a. Hydromorphone
b. Fentanyl
c. Butorphanol
d. Methadone

7. Calculate KM's estimated creatinine clearance using the Cockroft & Gault equation. (EO-5, 6)

8. Would it be appropriate to dose adjust KM's meperidine therapy? (EO-8, 11)

9. Which NSAID would be safest to use for pain because of its limited effect on platelet activity? (EO-7, 8)
   a. Naproxen
   b. Aspirin
   c. Ibuprofen
   d. Salate

10. Which of the following is *not* a factor to predisposing KM to seizures when using meperidine? (EO-8)
    a. Doses >400–600 mg/day
    b. Previous seizures
    c. Phenytoin metabolism
    d. Poor renal function

11. All of the following agents have anti-inflammatory properties *except:* (EO-7, 8)
    a. Acetaminophen
    b. Diclofenac
    c. Indomethacin
    d. Tolmentin

12. Identify psychosocial factors that health care providers may encounter when treating a patient in pain. (EO-15)

13. What would be the immediate treatment of choice if KM was excessively somnolent and suddenly developed respiratory depression from her morphine therapy? (EO-10)
    a. Naltrexone
    b. Pentazocine
    c. Naloxone
    d. Flumazenil

14. What would be the economic and medical benefits of rechecking another phenytoin level 12–24 hours after KM's seizure? (EO-17)

15. Summarize therapeutic concepts for KM's pain management utilizing a key points format. (EO-18)

CASE 87
Bob L. Lobo
Topic: Generalized Anxiety Disorder
Level 2
EDUCATIONAL MATERIALS
Chapter 55: Anxiety Disorders (diagnosis and clinical findings, nonpharmacologic approaches, antianxiety medications)

SCENARIO

Patient and Setting

TB, a 27-year-old female; clinic

Chief Complaint

"I feel that I am anxious and always on edge, and my stomach is giving me more trouble."

History of Present Illness

Worried about career as an accountant, "love life," and father who has been ill for several years; worries increased over the past few months since taking on more responsibility at work, has broken up with her boyfriend, and father has been more ill; stomach trouble has worsened over the past few months

Past Medical History

Atopic eczema for the past 4 years; improved since her last vacation over 1 year ago; heavy menstrual periods and dysmenorrhea

Past Surgical History

None

Family/Social History

Family History: Father with coronary artery disease

Social History: Drinks "2 pots" of coffee every day; avoids alcohol and denies illicit drug use

Medication History

OTC Hydrocortisone 0.5% cream PRN rash (according to TB, "Doesn't help")

OTC Ibuprofen or naproxen PRN dysmenorrhea symptoms

Hydroxyzine PRN nerves (according to TB, "It doesn't do anything")

Allergies

NKDA

Physical Examination

GEN: Slender female, mildly anxious, hypervigilant, diaphoretic
VS: BP 110/65, HR 85, RR 20, T 37.0°C, Wt 47 kg
HEENT: WNL except for pale conjunctiva
COR: RRR without murmurs
CHEST: CTA
ABD: WNL
GU: WNL
RECT: Stool guaiac positive
EXT: Several mild eczematous lesions on R and L anticubital fossae and face; pale nail beds
NEUR: A and O $\times$ 4

Results of Pertinent Laboratory Tests, Serum Drug Concentrations, and Diagnostic Tests

BUN 2.5 (7)	Plts 270×10^9 (270×10^3)	Ferritin 110 (110)
Cr 61 (0.8)	MCV 70 (70)	TSH 3 (3)
Hct 0.32 (32)	RBC 3.1×10^{12} (3.1×10^6)	T-3 2.3 (150)
Hgb 90 (9)	Glu 4.7 (85)	T-4 23 (1.8)
Lkcs 5.5×10^9 (5.5×10^3)	TIBC 82 (460)	

PROBLEM LIST

Identify principal problems from the scenario in priority order [completed Problem List and SOAP Note at end of casebook]

SOAP NOTE

To be completed by student

QUESTIONS

[Answers at end of casebook]

1. What is the most probable cause of TB's anxiety? (EO-1)
   a. Endorphin deficiency
   b. Excessive noradrenergic activity
   c. Use of NSAIDs
   d. Iron deficiency

2. Which of the following signs and symptoms of anxiety is TB experiencing? (EO-5)

    a. Hypervigilance
    b. Bradycardia
    c. Constipation
    d. Decreased MCV

3. Which of the following is true concerning the pharmacokinetics of diazepam? Diazepam has: (EO-6)
    a. A slow onset of action
    b. A rapid onset of action
    c. A short half-life
    d. Nonlinear kinetics

4. Physical assessment findings in TB that are consistent with generalized anxiety disorder include: (EO-5)
    A. Diaphoresis
    b. Pale conjunctiva
    c. Guaiac-positive stool
    d. Eczematous lesions

5. Describe the mechanisms of action of diazepam. (EO-7)

6. Which of the following potential adverse effects of diazepam should be monitored for in TB? (EO-10)
    a. Vomiting
    b. Anxiety
    c. Insomnia
    d. Memory impairment

7. Which of the following may predispose TB to excessive central nervous system depression in combination with diazepam? (EO-9)
    a. Alcohol use
    b. Caffeine use
    c. Betamethasone cream
    d. Ferrous sulfate

8. List the pharmacologic and nonpharmacologic treatment problem(s) present in TB's treatment plan. (EO-11)

9. If TB developed hepatic impairment, she should be changed to which of the following benzodiazepines: (EO-4, 5, 8, 9)
    a. Chlordiazepoxide
    b. Clorazepate
    c. Lorazepam
    d. Prazepam

10. Which of the following nonpharmacologic treatments would be most appropriate to reduce TB's anxiety? (EO-12)
    a. Counseling
    b. Long vacation
    c. Career change
    d. Find new boyfriend

11. What psychosocial factors may improve or worsen TB's anxiety disorder? (EO-15)

12. Evaluate the pharmacoeconomic considerations relative to TB's plan of care. (EO-17)

13. Using a key points format, summarize pathophysiologic, therapeutic, and disease management concepts for TB's anxiety disorder. (EO-18)

CASE 88
Bob L. Lobo
Topic: Eating Disorders

EDUCATIONAL MATERIALS
Chapter 60: Obesity and Eating Disorders (etiology and incidence, diagnosis, complications, recognizing eating disorders, psychotherapy, pharmacotherapy)

SCENARIO

Patient and Setting
RF, a 36-year-old female; clinic

Chief Complaint
Frequent, painful urination, lower abdominal pain, foul-smelling urine, intense vulvar burning, and flu

History of Present Illness
Wants to obtain refills on imipramine, ampicillin, and tetracycline; history of recurrent UTI (four UTIs this year); recently treated with ampicillin 250 mg PO QID × 10 days; missed follow-up appointment because asymptomatic; 4 weeks later, returns to clinic complaining of frequent, painful urination; reports despite fact treated with acyclovir for recurrent genital herpes last month, now experiencing the same symptoms (vulvar burning and white vaginal discharge) again

Past Medical History
Recurrent UTI

Genital herpes

Chronic acne

Bulimia—on imipramine

Noncompliance with medications

Past Surgical History
None

Family/Social History
Family History: Noncontributory

Social History: Heavy alcohol use on weekends, several sexual partners over the past year

Medication History
Ampicillin, 250 mg PO QID × 10 days (last dose was taken 4 weeks ago)

Acyclovir, 200 mg PO QID × 5 days (admits to not finishing the 5-day course)

Imipramine, 200 mg PO QHS

Tetracycline, 250 mg PO BID

Ortho-Novum 7/7/7, PO QD

Allergies

NKDA

Physical Examination

GEN: Thin and anxious female in no acute distress

VS: T 38.0°C, BP 120/76, HR 89, Wt 51 kg, Ht 150 cm

HEENT: WNL

COR: RRR without murmurs/gallops/rubs

CHEST: CTA

ABD: Soft, nontender

GU: Multiple papules and vesicles, cottage cheese-like vaginal discharge

RECT: Stool guaiac negative

EXT: Normal

NEURO: A and O × 3

Results of Pertinent Laboratory Tests, Serum Drug Concentrations, and Diagnostic Tests

BUN 5.3 (15)   HCO$_3$ 25 (25)   Hct 36 (36)
Na 135 (135)   Cr 0.9 (79.5)   Hgb 190 (19)
K 3.9 (3.9)   Plts 190×10^9 (190×10^3)   Alb 49 (4.9)
Cl 99 (99)

Urinalysis: Gram-negative rods (consistent with previous Gram stain), cloudy, pH 8.0, SG 1.015, WBC 10/mm; 3 RBC; WBC esterase +

Urine culture: Pending

Culture of vesicles: Pending

Microscopic exam of lesion exudate: + herpes infection

PROBLEM LIST

Identify principal problems from the scenario in priority order

SOAP NOTE

To be completed by student

QUESTIONS

1. What is the most probable cause of RF's eating disorder? (EO-1)
   a. Depression
   b. Desire to be thin
   c. Nausea from tetracycline
   d. Euphoria associated with vomiting

2. Which of the following is a method of purging used by bulimics such as RF? (EO-2)
   a. Laxative use
   b. Prayer
   c. Avoidance of food
   d. Excessive sexual activity

3. Which of the following is true concerning the pharmacokinetics of imipramine in the treatment of RF? The dose should be reduced if RF began taking: (EO-6, 9)
   a. Phenobarbital
   b. Co-trimoxazole
   c. Fluoxetine
   d. Ciprofloxacin

4. Physical assessment finding in RF that would be consistent with bulimia would include: (EO-5)
   a. Weight gain
   b. Excessive hair growth
   c. ACE-face
   d. "Chipmunk face"

5. Describe the epidemiologic characteristics of bulimia. (EO-3)

6. Which of the following are potential adverse effects of imipramine in RF? (EO-10)
   a. Orthostatic hypotension
   b. Excessive salivation
   c. Anorexia
   d. Hirsutism

7. Which of the following antidepressants should be avoided in RF? (EO-8)
   a. Fluoxetine
   b. Desipramine
   c. Bupropion
   d. Sertraline

8. List the pharmacologic and nonpharmacologic treatment problems present in RF's treatment plan. (EO-11)

9. Which of the following nonpharmacologic treatments would be most appropriate for RF's bulimia? (EO-12)
   a. Psychotherapy
   b. Relaxation therapy
   c. Assertiveness training
   d. Alcohol rehabilitation

10. What psychosocial factors may improve or worsen RF's bulimia? (EO-15)

11. Evaluate the pharmacoeconomic considerations relative to RF's treatment plan. (EO-17)

12. Summarize pathophysiologic, therapeutic, and disease management concepts for RF's eating disorder utilizing a key points format. (EO-18)

CASE 89
Bob L. Lobo
Topic: Mood Disorders
Level 1

EDUCATIONAL MATERIALS
Chapter 56: Mood Disorders (major depressive disorder, therapeutic plan, treatment of depressive disorders)

SCENARIO

Patient and Setting

MK, a 34-year-old man; admitted to psychiatric care unit of hospital

Chief Complaint

None

History of Present Illness

Admitted following attempted suicide; was successful aerospace engineer; laid off from job; unemployed 8 months; drinking heavily recently; lapsed into deep depression contemplating suicide; wife left him recently; has ingested an unknown number of (propoxyphene/acetaminophen); treated successfully for the propoxyphene overdose in the emergency department (ED); now admitted to the hospital for observation and further treatment.

Past Medical History

Asthma

Past Surgical History

None

Family/Social History

Family History: Nonapplicable

Social History: Drank a bottle of gin each day for the past 3 days; smoked 1 PPD × 10 years (quit 2 years ago)

Medication History

Alupent inhaler (metaproterenol), 2 to 4 puffs q4h PRN

Allergies

Sulfa drugs (rash)

Physical Examination

GEN: Thin, lethargic male complaining of mild nausea
VS: BP 110/80, HR 80, RR 18, T 37.4°C, Wt 68 kg
HEENT: Unremarkable
COR: Percusses at midclavicular line without murmur or gallop
CHEST: Clear to percussion and auscultation
ABD: Thin and soft without masses, tenderness, or organomegaly
GU: WNL
RECT: WNL
EXT: WNL
NEURO: A and O × 3

Results of Pertinent Laboratory Tests, Serum Drug Concentrations, and Diagnostic Tests

Glu 6.11 (110)	HCO$_3$ 25 (25)	ALT 1.17 (70)
BUN 6.43 (18)	Cr 70.7 (0.8)	LDH 3.33 (200)
Na 140 (140)	Hct 0.40 (40)	Alk Phos 1.67 (100)
K 4.0 (4.0)	Hgb 160 (16)	T Bili 17.1 (1.0)
Cl 106 (106)	AST 1.0 (60)	PT 14.0

Acetaminophen 2 hours; postingestion 330 (5)

Lkc differential, urinalysis, chest x-ray, ECG: all WNL

PROBLEM LIST

Identify principal problems from the scenario in priority order [completed Problem List and SOAP Note at end of casebook]

SOAP NOTE

To be completed by student

QUESTIONS

[Answers at end of casebook]

1. What is the most likely cause of MK's suicidal gesture? (EO-1)
   a. Personality disorder
   b. Serotonin deficiency
   c. Loss of wife
   d. Combination of personal losses with genetic predisposition

2. What is the most significant risk factor for suicidal ideation in MK? (EO-3)
   a. Smoking history
   b. Heavy drinking
   c. Asthma
   d. Propoxyphene use

3. Which of the following is true concerning the pharmacokinetics of fluoxetine in MK? (EO-6, 9)
   a. Use of alcohol will decrease fluoxetine absorption
   b. Fluoxetine will decrease the absorption of propoxyphene
   c. Fluoxetine will increase the metabolism of metaproterenol
   d. Fluoxetine will inhibit the metabolism of tricyclic antidepressants

4. Physical assessment findings in MK that would be consistent with depression include: (EO-5)
   a. Weight loss
   b. Animated affect
   c. Tachycardia
   d. Muscle weakness

5. Describe the epidemiology of depression as it pertains to suicide. (EO-3)

6. Which of the following is a potential adverse effect of fluoxetine in MK? (EO-10)
   a. Reflex tachycardia
   b. Exacerbation of asthma

c. Insomnia

d. Craving for cigarettes

7. Which of the following antidepressants should be avoided in MK due to risk of toxicity in overdose? (EO-8)

a. Sertraline

b. Paroxetine

c. Fluvoxamine

d. Doxepin

8. List the pharmacologic and nonpharmacologic treatment problems present in MK's treatment plan. (EO-11)

9. Which of the following nonpharmacologic treatments would be most appropriate for MK at this time? (EO-12)

a. Supportive psychotherapy

b. Drug rehab

c. Stress management group

d. Hypnotherapy

10. What psychosocial factors may increase or decrease MK's risk for suicide? (EO-15)

11. Evaluate the pharmacoeconomic considerations relative to MK's treatment plan. (EO-17)

12. Using a key points format, summarize pathophysiologic, therapeutic, and disease management concepts for MK's depression. (EO-18)

CASE 90
Bob L. Lobo
Topic: Alcoholism
Level 3
EDUCATIONAL MATERIALS
Chapter 62: Substance Abuse (epidemiology, treatment goals, sedative, hypnotics and anxiolytics)

SCENARIO

Patient and Setting

TR, a 64-year-old male; ED

Chief Complaint

"My belly is swollen and it hurts."

History of Present Illness

Admitted through the ED of community hospital for a workup of a 1-month history of anorexia, nausea, abdominal distress, fatigue, and abdominal swelling. Has been drinking a fifth of bourbon daily since wife died 5 years ago; has been in alcohol rehab treatment centers on 3 occasions, and was discharged from a program 9 months ago.

Past Medical History

Has had numerous admissions for GI bleeds, all of which were associated with coagulopathy and alcohol; has long-standing COPD, hypertension, and degenerative joint disease (DJD) of his hips; has experienced delirium tremens (DTs) several times during previous admissions.

Past Surgical History

None

Family/Social History

Family History: Alcoholism in his father and uncle

Social History: Smokes 1 PPD; drinks a fifth of bourbon daily

Medication History

Albuterol MDI, 2 puffs q4–6h PRN wheezing

Aspirin, 325 mg (OTC) 2 tablets PO PRN hip pain (almost daily)

Cimetidine, 200 mg (OTC) 2 tablets PO for stomach pain daily

Methyldopa, 500 mg PO TID (takes occasionally)

Allergies

NKDA

Physical Examination

GEN: Obese, lethargic male in moderate respiratory distress

VS: BP 170/110, HR 95, RR 20, T 37.0°C, Wt 98 kg

HEENT: PERRLA

COR: RRR

CHEST: Faint rales, rhonchi. Several spider angiomas on chest

ABD: Moderately distended, taut, liver palpable 2 cm below costal margin, positive fluid wave

GU: Testicles atrophied

RECT: Pale, guaiac-positive stool

EXT: 2+ pitting edema around ankles

NEURO: A and O × 2, cranial nerves intact, moderately decreased DTR's, asterixis

Results of Pertinent Laboratory Tests, Serum Drug Concentrations, and Diagnostic Tests

Cr 80 (0.9)	Hct 0.296 (29.6)	ALT 0.28 (17)
K 3.4 (3.4)	Lkcs 2.7 × 10⁹	Alk Phos 10.6 (638)
Cl 98 (98)	(2.7 × 10³)	Alb 30 (3.0)
HCO₃ 27 (27)	Plts 76 × 10⁹	T Bili 10 (0.6)
BUN 3.2 (9)	(76 × 10³)	GGT 29.17 (1750)
Na 132 (132)	MCV 102 (102)	Ca 2.15 (8.6)
Glu 7 (125)	AST 0.67 (40)	Mg 0.7 (1.7)
Hgb 102 (10.2)		

PROBLEM LIST

Identify principal problems from the scenario in priority order

SOAP NOTE

To be completed by student

QUESTIONS

1. What is the most likely etiology for delirium tremens? (EO-1)
   a. Thiamine deficiency
   b. Hepatic encephalopathy
   c. Downregulated GABA receptors
   d. Dopaminergic hypersensitivity

2. Which of the following are signs and symptoms of Wernicke's encephalopathy? (EO-2)
   a. Anxiety, diaphoresis, tremor
   b. Visual disturbance, ataxia, confusion
   c. Agitation, paranoia, fever
   d. Dizziness, hallucinations, delusions

3. Which of the following benzodiazepines would be most appropriate to treat TR's alcohol withdrawal? (EO-4,5)
   a. Oxazepam
   b. Clorazepate
   c. Clonazepam
   d. Chlordiazepoxide

4. Which of the following is the most sensitive indicator of alcohol abuse and dependence in TR? (EO-5)
   a. MCV
   b. GGT
   c. Abdominal girth
   d. Magnesium

5. Describe the relative advantages and disadvantages of scheduled versus PRN benzodiazepines for the treatment of alcohol withdrawal. (EO-8)

6. Which of the following is an adverse effect of spironolactone? (EO-10)
   a. Hypoglycemia
   b. Gout
   c. Gynecomastia
   d. Priapism

7. Which of the following antihypertensives should be avoided in TR? (EO-8)
   a. Losartan
   b. Verapamil
   c. Nicardipine
   d. Metoprolol

8. List the pharmacologic and nonpharmacologic treatment problems present in TR's treatment plan. (EO-11)

9. Which of the following nonpharmacologic treatments would be most appropriate for TR's hepatic encephalopathy? (EO-12)
   a. Low sodium diet
   b. Low protein diet
   c. Low potassium diet
   d. Low phosphorus diet

10. What psychosocial factors may improve or worsen TR's alcohol dependence? (EO-15)

11. Evaluate pharmacoeconomic considerations relative to TR's treatment plan. (EO-17)

12. Which of the following drugs would not be effective in reducing the risk of alcohol withdrawal seizures in TR?
    a. Lorazepam
    b. Diazepam
    c. Chlordiazepoxide
    d. Phenytoin

13. Utilizing a key points format, summarize pathophysiologic, therapeutic, and disease management concepts for TR's alcoholism. (EO-18)

CASE 91
Bob L. Lobo
Topic: Anxiety Disorders-Panic Disorder
 Level 1
EDUCATIONAL MATERIALS
Chapter 55: Anxiety Disorders (etiology and pathophysiology, epidemiology, panic disorder)

SCENARIO

Patient and Setting
JM, a 35-year-old female; ED

Chief Complaint
"I think I might have a serious heart condition."

History of Present Illness
6-month history of episodic events which have increased recently; characterized by smothering sensations, trembling, lightheadedness, shortness of breath, and heart pounding

Past Medical History
Migraine headaches that occur 2–3 times per month

Past Surgical History
None

Family/Social History
Family History: Migraine headaches on mother's side of the family

Social History: Noncontributory

Medication History

Naproxen, 500 mg PO for mild-to-moderate migraine
headaches

Sumatriptan, 25 mg PO at the onset of each severe
migraine headache

Allergies

NKDA

Physical Examination

GEN: Well-developed, slightly anxious appearing,
well-nourished female in no apparent distress
VS: BP 140/80, HR 85, RR 18, T 37.2°C
HEENT: WNL
COR: WNL
CHEST: Clear to auscultation
ABD: WNL
GU: Deferred
RECT: Deferred
EXT: Warm and moist skin, pale complexion
NEURO: A and O × 3, cranial nerves intact

Results of Pertinent Laboratory Tests, Serum Drug Concentrations, and Diagnostic Tests

Na 138 (138)
K 3.7 (3.7)
Cl 98 (98)
HCO$_3$ 25 (25)
BUN 3.6 (10)
Cr 70 (0.8)
Hct 0.37 (37.2)
Hgb 112 (11.2)

Lkcs 8 × 10^9
  (8 × 10^3)
Plts 158 × 10^9
  (158 × 10^3)
MCV 86 (86)
MCHC 310 (31)
AST 0.17 (10)
ALT 0.40 (24)

Alk Phos 0.7 (40)
Alb 30 (3.0)
T Bili 5 (0.3)
Glu 4.1 (73)
PO$_4$ 0.97 (3.0)
Mg 0.6 (1.2)
Uric Acid 360 (6)
PT 14.2
PTT 39.2

Lkcs differential: WNL

Urinalysis: WNL

Urine Drug Screen: Negative

ECG: Normal

Chest x-ray: Normal

PROBLEM LIST

Identify principal problems from the scenario in priority order

SOAP NOTE

To be completed by student

QUESTIONS

1. Which of the following is true of the noradrenergic hypothesis of anxiety disorders? There is an abnormal: (EO-1)

   a. Increase in locus ceruleus activity
   b. Decrease in norepinephrine secretion
   c. Noradrenergic innervation in periaqueductal gray area
   d. Increase in adrenal norepinephrine

2. Which of the following is most likely to be a symptom of panic disorder? (EO-2)

   a. Excessive worry about multiple different life situations
   b. Abrupt onset of fear that one is going to die
   c. Recurrent obsessions about having been contaminated
   d. Recurrent flashbacks of an especially traumatic event

3. If JM developed an upper respiratory infection and was prescribed clarithromycin 500 mg BID, which of the following interventions would be most appropriate? (EO-9)

   a. Decrease dose of alprazolam
   b. Decrease dose of imipramine
   c. Increase dose of alprazolam
   d. Increase dose of imipramine

4. JM experienced signs and symptoms of imipramine toxicity (serum imipramine concentration of 300 ng/mL) at a dosage of 250 mg. What dosage should she be changed to if a serum imipramine level around 150 ng/mL is desired? (EO-6)

   a. 175 mg
   b. 150 mg
   c. 125 mg
   d. 75 mg

5. Describe the mechanism of action of benzodiazepines in the treatment of anxiety disorders. (EO-7)

6. Which of the following may be an unwanted adverse effect of imipramine in JM? (EO-10)

   a. Physical dependence
   b. Weight gain
   c. Hypertensive crisis when combined with cheese
   d. Bradycardia

7. Which of the following agents would reduce the frequency of JM's panic attacks? (EO-8)

   a. Propranolol
   b. Phenytoin
   c. Paroxetine
   d. Buspirone

8. List the pharmacologic and nonpharmacologic treatment problems present in JM's treatment plan. (EO-11)

9. Which of the following nonpharmacologic treatments should JM receive adjunctively with her medications? (EO-12)

   a. 12-step program
   b. Cognitive-behavioral therapy
   c. Relaxation therapy
   d. Assertiveness training

10. What psychosocial factors may increase or decrease JM's adherence to therapy? (EO-15)

11. Evaluate the pharmacoeconomic considerations relative to JM's treatment plan. (EO-17)

12. Summarize the pathophysiologic, therapeutic, and disease management concepts for JM's panic disorder utilizing a key points format. (EO-18)

CASE 92
Bob L. Lobo
Topic: Sleep Disorders
Level 3

EDUCATIONAL MATERIALS
Chapter 58: Sleep Disorders

SCENARIO

Patient and Setting

SF, a 47 year-old man; hospital

Chief Complaint

"I really need something to help me sleep. I just can't get to sleep unless I am in my own bed."

History of Present Illness

SF was admitted for cardiac catheterization and coronary arteriography due to angina pectoris. While in the hospital the second night, SF complains of difficulty sleeping. SF reports frequent symptoms of insomnia when he is in a new environment. SF was sleeping fairly well prior to admission, approximately 6–7 hours per night, and he usually wakes up refreshed. His chest pain was exacerbated this week when he decided to begin a new exercise program.

Past Medical History

Significant for chronic stable angina, hypertension, COPD, hypercholesterolemia, and gout

Past Surgical History

Appendix removed at age 8

Family/Social History

Family History: Father died of a heart attack at age 56
Social History: Smokes 2 PPD × 28 years

Medication History

Allopurinol, 300 mg PO QD

Nitroglycerin, 0.4 mg SL PRN

Isosorbide dinitrate, 10 mg PO q6–8h

Verapamil SR, 240 mg PO QD

Hydrochlorothiazide, 50 mg PO QD × 20 years

Ipratropium inhaler, 2 puffs q4–6h

Albuterol inhaler, 2 puffs q4–6h

Theophylline, 200 mg PO BID

Potassium chloride, 40 mEq PO QD

Allergies

Cholestyramine and colestipol–severe nausea and vomiting

Physical Examination

GEN: Moderately obese, somewhat anxious male
VS: BP 160/90, HR 70, RR 12, Wt 90 kg
HEENT: WNL
COR: Normal S1, S2; no S3, S4, or murmurs
CHEST: Bilateral rales and rhonchi
ABD: Benign
GU: Deferred
RECT: Deferred
EXT: No peripheral edema, yellow nicotine stains on fingers
NEURO: WNL

Results of Pertinent Laboratory Tests, Serum Drug Concentrations, and Diagnostic Tests

Na 138 (138)	Lkcs 6 × 10^9	Alb 40 (4)
K 5.0 (5.0)	(6 × 10^3)	Glu 8.3 (150)
Cl 102 (102)	Plts 300 × 10^9	Ca 2.25 (9)
HCO$_3$ 24 (24)	(300 × 10^3)	PO$_4$ 1.3 (4)
BUN 6.4 (18)	ALT 0.5 (30)	Mg 1 (2)
Cr 115 (1.3)	LDH 3.34 (200)	Uric Acid 416 (7)
Hct 0.48 (48)	Alk Phos 1.3 (80)	Chol 8.3 (320)
Hgb 160 (16)		TG 1.35 (120)

Lkcs differential: WNL

Urinalysis: WNL

Chest x-ray: WNL

ECG: NSR

Theophylline: Pending

Pulmonary function tests: WNL, with reversible component

PROBLEM LIST

Identify principal problems from the scenario in priority order [completed Problem List and SOAP Note at end of casebook]

SOAP NOTE

To be completed by student

QUESTIONS

[Answers at end of casebook]

1. What is the most probable cause of SF's insomnia? (EO-1)
   a. Angina
   b. Change in environment
   c. Nitroglycerin
   d. COPD

2. Which of the following types of insomnia is SF experiencing? (EO-2)
   a. Transient
   b. Chronic

c. Short-term

d. Drug-related

3. Which of the following is true concerning the pharmacokinetics of triazolam in SF? (EO-4)

a. Effects should not persist into the next day

b. Effects should persist into the next day and cause hangover

c. Effects should be detectable for 1 week

d. Effects of 0.25 mg in SF will be negligible

4. Which of the following would suggest a drug-related cause of insomnia in SF? (EO-2, 5, 10)

a. Theophylline level of 20 μg/dL

b. Verapamil-induced bradycardia

c. Hydrochlorothiazide-induced hypokalemia

d. Albuterol-induced tremor

5. Describe the mechanism of action of benzodiazepines for sleep induction. (EO-7)

6. Which of the following conditions may complicate use of triazolam use in SF? (EO-9)

a. Angina

b. COPD

c. Hypertension

d. Hypercholesterolemia

7. Which of the following drugs is most likely to decrease the metabolism of triazolam in SF? (EO-8)

a. Verapamil

b. Atenolol

c. Isosorbide dinitrate

d. Erythromycin

8. List pharmacologic and nonpharmacologic treatment problems present in SF's treatment plan. (EO-11)

9. Which of the following nonpharmacologic treatments would be most appropriate for SF's insomnia? (EO-12)

a. Psychotherapy

b. Exercise before bed

c. Eliminate daytime nap

d. Skip evening meal

10. What psychosocial factors may improve or worsen SF's insomnia? (EO-15)

11. Evaluate the pharmacoeconomic considerations relative to SF's treatment plan. (EO-17)

12. Summarize the pathophysiologic, therapeutic, and disease management concepts for SF utilizing a key points format. (EO-18)

CASE 93
Bob L. Lobo
Topic: Substance Abuse
Level 2

EDUCATIONAL MATERIALS
Chapter 62: Substance Abuse
(opioids, pharmacologic effects, recognition, management, treatment)

SCENARIO

Patient and Setting

LB, a 34-year-old male, ED

Chief Complaint

Patient unresponsive

History of Present Illness

Brought in to the ED by ambulance after wife found unresponsive on the bathroom floor; enrolled in a methadone detoxification clinic for several weeks, but recently purchased some "Mexican tar" and has been shooting up for the last few days

Past Medical History

Asthma since childhood, opiate dependence 8 years

Past Surgical History

Tonsils removed at age 6

Family/Social History

Family History: Noncontributory

Social History: Smoked 1–2 PPD × 15 years, drinks occasionally

Medication History

Methadone, 60 mg PO QD

Theophylline, 300 mg PO BID

Albuterol tablets, 2 mg PO PRN

Allergies

Penicillin causes hives

Codeine causes nausea

Physical Examination

GEN: Groggy, in some respiratory distress, pinpoint pupils noted

VS: BP 80/50, HR 49, RR 8, T 37.8°C, Wt 75 kg

HEENT: Pupils pinpoint and symmetrical

COR: Sinus bradycardia

CHEST: Decreased respirations, decreased breath sounds on the right, moderate wheezing

ABD: Decreased bowel sounds

GU: Normal

RECT: Normal, guaiac negative

EXT: Skin cool to touch, needle-track marks noted on both arms

NEURO: Responsive to pain, A and O × 0

Results of Pertinent Laboratory Tests, Serum Drug Concentrations, and Diagnostic Tests

Glu 4.4 (80)   Cr 71 (0.8)   Hct 0.45 (45)
HCO$_3$ 23 (23)   Lkcs 18.4 × 10^9 Alk Phos 2.2 (133)
Na 140 (140)   (18.4 × 10^3)   AST 0.58 (35)
K 3.7 (3.7)   Plts 140 × 10^9 ALT 0.58 (35)
Cl 96 (96)   (140 × 10^3)   T Bili 20.5 (1.2)
BUN 7.1 (20)   Hgb 160 (16)   Alb 24 (2.4)

Urinalysis: WNL

Theophylline: 5.5 μmol/L (1 mg/L)

Tox screen: (+) morphine

Chest x-ray: RLL infiltrate

Sputum gram stain: Gram-positive cocci in pairs and chains

PROBLEM LIST

Identify principal problems from the scenario in priority order [completed Problem List and SOAP Note at end of casebook]

SOAP NOTE

To be completed by student

QUESTIONS

[Answers at end of casebook]

1. Which of the following signs are consistent with opiate overdose in LB? (EO-2)
   a. Heart rate 49
   b. WBC 18.4
   c. Decreased breath sounds in RLL
   d. Wheezing

2. Which of the following is a reason why heroin injection is becoming less common in the United States? (EO-3)
   a. Increased use by lower socioeconomic classes
   b. Decreasing purity of heroin
   c. Increased use of other routes of administration
   d. Greater "rush" with intranasal route

3. Which of the following is true concerning naloxone treatment of LB? (EO-4, 6)
   a. Naloxone is likely to accumulate, leading to opiate withdrawal
   b. Naloxone is likely to wear off before methadone, leading to re-sedation
   c. Naloxone may inhibit theophylline metabolism
   d. Levofloxacin may inhibit naloxone metabolism

4. Which of the following findings in LB is most consistent with a pattern of long-term IV heroin abuse? (EO-5)
   a. Positive UDS for methadone
   b. Pinpoint pupils
   c. Needle-track marks
   d. Altered mental status

5. Describe the mechanism of action of naloxone in the treatment of opiate overdose. (EO-7)

6. Which of the following is the most likely adverse effect of naloxone in LB? (EO-10)
   a. Hepatotoxicity
   b. Opiate withdrawal
   c. Aspiration
   d. Wheezing

7. After successful treatment of LB's overdose, he complains of pain associated with his pneumonia. Which of the following drugs would be *inappropriate* to treat his pain? (EO-8)
   a. Morphine
   b. Oxycodone
   c. Propoxyphene
   d. Nalbuphine

8. List the pharmacologic and nonpharmacologic treatment problems in LB's treatment plan. (EO-11)

9. Which of the following pharmacologic or nonpharmacologic treatments would be most beneficial if LB did not want to discontinue use of opiates? (EO-12)
   a. Methadone maintenance
   b. Cognitive psychotherapy
   c. Methadone detoxification
   d. Group psychotherapy

10. What psychosocial factors may increase or decrease LB's risk of relapse? (EO-15)

11. Evaluate the pharmacoeconomic considerations relative to LB's treatment plan. (EO-17)

12. Summarize the pathophysiologic, therapeutic, and disease management concepts for LB's opiate dependence. (EO-18)

CASE 94
Bob L. Lobo
Topic: Smoking Cessation

Level 2

EDUCATIONAL MATERIALS
Chapter 63: Smoking Cessation
(pharmacologic and physiologic effects of nicotine, effects of smoking on drug therapy, pharmacist's role, nicotine replacement therapy)

SCENARIO

Patient and Setting

TT, a 66-year-old male; clinic

Chief Complaint

"I'm short of breath all the time, and I have been coughing up green junk all week." "I think I'm ready to quit smoking now, can you help?" "I just can't get around the way I used to."

History of Present Illness

Experienced increasing shortness of breath over the past several weeks and has a chronic productive cough

Past Medical History

Chronic bronchitis, S/P AMI 6 months ago, hypertension

Past Surgical History

None

Family/Social History

Family History: Father died of heart attack at age 55, mother still living

Social History: Smokes 2 PPD × 50 years

Medication History

Epinephrine MDI, 2 puffs q4h PRN SOB

Triamterene, 37.5 mg PO QD

Hydrochlorothiazide, 25 mg PO QD

Allergies

Penicillin

Physical Examination

      GEN: A chronically ill-appearing elderly gentleman in moderate respiratory distress
        VS: BP 170/80, HR 85, RR 18, T 39.5°C
   HEENT: mild AV nicking
      COR: RRR
   CHEST: Barrel chest, increased use of accessory muscles
      ABD: Soft, nontender
        GU: WNL
     RECT: Guaiac negative
      EXT: Normal
   NEURO: A and O × 3, cranial nerves intact

Results of Pertinent Laboratory Tests, Serum Drug Concentrations, and Diagnostic Tests

HCO_3 22 (22)   Hct 0.49 (49)   Ca 2.3 (9.4)

Glu 8.1 (145)   Hgb 160 (16) PO_4 1.1 (3.5)

Na 137 (137)   Lkcs 18.5 × 10^9   Chol 3.95 (152)

K 3.7 (3.7)   (18.5 × 10^3)

Cl 103 (103)

ECG: Normal

CXR: Clear, moderate cardiomegaly

PROBLEM LIST

Identify principal problems from the scenario in priority order
[completed Problem List and SOAP Note at end of casebook]

SOAP NOTE

To be completed by student

QUESTIONS

[Answers at end of casebook]

1. Which is the correct incidence of smoking in the United States? (EO-3)
   a. 15% of adults
   b. 25% of adults
   c. 40% of adults
   d. 50% of adults

2. Which of the following is a potential sequela from cigarette smoking? (EO-1)
   a. Cerebrovascular disease
   b. Cancer of the liver
   c. Chronic renal failure
   d. Gout

3. Which of the following is true concerning the pharmacokinetics of nicotine replacement therapies (NRT)? (EO-4)
   a. The patch has the most rapid absorption
   b. Nasal spray has the most rapid absorption
   c. Gum has the most rapid absorption
   d. Gum provides the most consistent blood levels of nicotine

4. Which of the following should be assessed in the patient who is withdrawing from nicotine? (EO-5)
   a. Appetite
   b. Bladder function
   c. Neurologic exam
   d. Pulmonary function

5. Describe the mechanism of nicotine's dependence-producing potential. (EO-7)

6. Which of the following is the most common adverse effect seen with a nicotine replacement patch? (EO-10)
   a. Dizziness
   b. Skin irritation
   c. Vivid dreams
   d. Headache

7. Which of the following drugs would require more intensive therapeutic drug monitoring in TT due to his change in smoking habit? (EO-9)
   a. Lithium
   b. Vancomycin
   c. Theophylline
   d. Cyclosporine

8. List pharmacologic and nonpharmacologic treatment problems present in TT's treatment plan. (EO-11)

9. Which of the following nonpharmacologic treatments would be most appropriate for TT's goal of smoking cessation at this time?

a. Behavioral modification
b. Stress management
c. Group therapy
d. Hypnotherapy

10. Which of the following is a recommended alternative to nicotine replacement therapy in TT?
a. Bupropion
b. Clonidine
c. Diazepam
d. Naltrexone

11. What psychosocial factors may increase or decrease TT's risk for relapse back into his smoking habit? (EO-15)

12. Evaluate the pharmacoeconomic considerations relative to TT's treatment plan. (EO-17)

13. Using a key points format, summarize pathophysiologic, therapeutic, and disease management concepts for TT's smoking cessation. (EO-18)

CASE 95
Bob L. Lobo
Topic: Mood Disorders—Bipolar
Level 2
EDUCATIONAL MATERIALS
Chapter 56: Mood Disorders (bipolar disorders, pharmacotherapy)

SCENARIO

Patient and Setting
RS, a 30-year-old obese male; ED (brought to the ED by the police after he was found walking on the freeway, shouting obscenities at the oncoming traffic)

Chief Complaint
"Leave me alone, I am the perfect physical specimen."

History of Present Illness
RS is a graduate student and was under treatment for bipolar disorder for the past 6 years with good results until several weeks ago. His roommate reports that he has been "up all night" for the past few days, and has a "harebrained scheme to win the Nobel prize."

Past Medical History
Bipolar disorder; hypercholesterolemia

Past Surgical History
None

Family/Social History
Family History: Mother with chronic depression
Social History: Drinks 5–6 beers daily

Medication History
Lithium carbonate, 600 mg TID
Imipramine, 50 mg TID

Allergies
Sulfa drugs

Physical Examination
GEN: Obese, well-developed, well-nourished male, appears agitated and hostile
VS: BP 140/90, HR 95, RR 20, T 38.0°C, Wt: 100 kg
HEENT: PERRLA, EOMI
COR: RRR
CHEST: CTA
ABD: Soft, nontender, nondistended
GU: WNL
RECT: Guaiac negative
EXT: WNL
NEURO: CNS intact, no focal findings

Results of Pertinent Laboratory Tests, Serum Drug Concentrations, and Diagnostic Tests

HCO₃ 26 (26)	Cr 88.4 (1.0)	LDH 2.5 (150)
Na 137 (137)	Hct 0.42 (42)	Alk Phos 1.67 (100)
K 3.4 (3.4)	Hgb 150 (15)	Glu 6.7 (120)
Cl 100 (100)	AST 1.0 (60)	Cholesterol 7.7 (300)
BUN 7.14 (20)	ALT 1.33 (80)	Lithium 0.5 (0.5)

Imipramine pending
Lkcs differential, urinalysis, chest x-ray, ECG: all WNL
Cholesterol 4 months ago 7.5 (290)

PROBLEM LIST
Identify principal problems from the scenario in priority order

SOAP NOTE
To be completed by student

QUESTIONS

1. Which of the following is true concerning the natural history of bipolar disorder? (EO-1)

a. Improves over time

b. Antidepressants may increase frequency of mania

c. Onset of mania is usually slow and gradual

d. Some bipolar patients never experience mania

2. Which of the following signs or symptoms of mania does RS display? (EO-2)

a. Grandiosity

b. Increased need for sleep

c. Hallucinations

d. Poor appetite

3. Which of the following is true concerning the pharmacokinetics of lithium? (EO-4)

a. Elimination is increased with enzyme inducers

b. Elimination is decreased by enzyme inhibitors

c. Increased concentrations are seen with dehydration

d. Decreased concentrations are seen with diarrhea

4. On the second day of hospitalization, RS woke up and began yelling at other patients. Which of the following actions would be most appropriate at this time? (EO-8)

a. Increase lithium dosage

b. Resume imipramine

c. Administer haloperidol

d. Obtain serum lithium concentration

5. One week after admission, RS has a serum lithium concentration of 1.6 that was drawn 4 hours after his morning dose. There are no significant signs of toxicity noted. Which of the following is the most appropriate action to take? (EO-5, 6)

a. Maintain present dosage

b. Hold lithium for 1 day, then resume at one-half previous dose

c. Change lithium to valproic acid

d. Repeat lithium level in am, 12 hours after the previous dose

6. Which of the following is a potential adverse effect of lithium in RS? (EO-10)

a. Polydipsia

b. Hyperthyroidism

c. Weight loss

d. Tachycardia

7. Explain why lorazepam and haloperidol are used in combination to treat RS's mania. (EO-7)

8. List the pharmacologic and nonpharmacologic treatment problems present in RS's treatment plan. (EO-11)

9. Which of the following pharmacologic or nonpharmacologic treatments would be most appropriate for RS to follow up with upon discharge? (EO-12)

a. Naltrexone

b. Disulfiram

c. Alcoholics Anonymous

d. Cardiac rehab program

10. What psychosocial factors may increase the likelihood of RS's adherence to treatment recommendations? (EO-15)

11. Evaluate pharmacoeconomic considerations relative to RS's treatment program. (EO-17)

12. Utilizing a key points format, summarize therapeutic, pathophysiologic, and disease management concepts for RS's bipolar disorder. (EO-12)

CASE 96

Stephen Cooke

Topic(s): ADHD, Asthma

Level 1

EDUCATIONAL MATERIALS

Chapter 59: Attention-Deficit/Hyperactivity Disorder (ADHD)

SCENARIO

Patient and Setting

KR, an 8-year-old asthmatic patient; ED

Chief Complaint

"Falling further and further behind in class."

Past Medical History

Taken to the ED during winter recess for SOB and blue skin color; appeared to have a fainting spell on the way to the hospital, but no other episodes were observed; ED personnel told parents to contact their family physician to r/o asthma; parents decided, on their own, to initiate a treatment regimen using over-the-counter (OTC) asthma inhalers; prior to episode, had a history of atopic dermatitis in the antecubital and popliteal fossae; latter episodes of atopic dermatitis have responded to OTC topical hydrocortisone and moisturizing lotion.

Past Surgical History

None

Family/Social History

Problem was brought to his family's attention by second-grade teacher. Teacher concerned that KR was falling further and further behind academically. Parents agreed to a school-based educational evaluation that identified significant speech and language problems, thought to be secondary to KR's recurring bouts with chronic bilateral serous otitis media; cognitive potential measured well within the average range; however, a discrepancy of more than 20 standard score points noted between reading comprehension achievement scores and cognitive potential, indicating learning disabilities; distractibility and impulsivity are also contributing to his academic limitations and worsening social status with peers.

Medication History

OTC epinephrine MDI PRN

Hydrocortisone cream 0.5% PRN

Moisturizing lotion applied after bath/shower

Allergies

NKDA

Physical Examination

GEN: Male child (8 years old), normal physical development, adequate diet/nourishment

VS: BP 104/64, HR 72, RR 20, T 37°C, Wt 23.1 kg, Ht 132 cm

HEENT: Normocephalic, bilateral myringotomy with P.E. tubes, language therapy initiated for frontal lisp and concept formation

COR: Normal S1 and S2; no murmurs, rubs, or gallop

CHEST: Clear to auscultation and percussion, but slight indication of hyperinflation

ABD: Soft, nontender, with no masses

EXT: Eczema

NEURO: Oriented $\times$ 3; DTRs and cranial nerves normal

Results of Pertinent Laboratory Tests, Serum Drug Concentrations, and Diagnostic Tests

HCO_3 22 (22)	Hct 0.49 (49)	PO_4 1.1 (3.5)
Na 137 (137)	Hgb 160 (16)	Lkcs 8.5 $\times$ 10^9
K 3.7 (3.7)	Glu 8.1 (145)	(8.5 $\times$ 10^3)
Cl 103 (103)	Ca 2.3 (9.4)	Chol 3.95 (152)

Lkcs differential: Eos 700/mm^3

Pulmonary function tests: RV 3.1 L, $FEV_{1.0}$ 1.9 L, FVC 3.4 L, $FEV_{1.0}$/FVC(%) 65%

Urinalysis: WNL

PROBLEM LIST

Identify principal problems from the scenario in priority order [completed Problem List and SOAP Note at end of casebook]

SOAP NOTE

To be completed by student

QUESTIONS

[Answers at end of casebook]

1. If KR was prescribed phenytoin, the addition of this medication to his current methylphenidate regimen would most likely: (EO-9)
   a. Increase phenytoin metabolism
   b. Decrease phenytoin metabolism
   c. Result in additive CNS excitation
   d. Increase the anorectant effects of methylphenidate

2. Which of the following strategies has been shown to minimize the extent of growth suppression associated with psychostimulants? (EO-10, 12, 5)
   a. Increasing the stimulant dose
   b. Co-administration of amantadine
   c. Dividing daily stimulant dose QID
   d. Utilization of drug holidays

3. One potential advantage that tricyclic antidepressants have over stimulants in the treatment of ADHD is: (EO-10, 12)
   a. Low abuse potential
   b. Greater efficacy
   c. Less cardiotoxicity
   d. Norepinephrine stimulation

4. Diagnostic criteria for ADHD include all of the following, *except:* (EO-2)
   a. Recognition of symptoms before age 7
   b. Impairment in at least two environmental settings
   c. Presence of symptoms for greater than two months
   d. Abnormal thyroid function

5. Counsel a patient diagnosed with ADHD who has just received his/her first prescription for methylphenidate. (EO-16)

6. The most logical step to take upon the therapeutic failure with one of the stimulants is: (EO-12)
   a. Initiate another stimulant
   b. Initiate a tricyclic antidepressant
   c. Monitor blood level of stimulant
   d. Clonidine augmentation

7. The stimulant with the highest degree of abuse potential is: (EO-10)
   a. Methylphenidate
   b. Pemoline
   c. Dextroamphetamine
   d. Diethylpropion

8. Associated features of ADHD include: (EO-1, 2)
   a. Mood disorders
   b. Sexual dysfunction
   c. Potts's syndrome
   d. Gingival hyperplasia

9. Family counseling in ADHD is intended to: (EO-15)
   a. Positively reinforce good behaviors
   b. Teach avoidance of distractors
   c. Reduce resentment toward child with ADHD
   d. Decrease hyperactivity

10. Summarize the psychosocial factors associated with positive outcomes in the treatment of ADHD. (EO-15, 16)

11. Describe the necessary monitoring parameters associated with pemoline usage. (EO-10)

12. Summarize pathophysiologic, therapeutic, and disease

management concepts for KR's ADHD using key point format. (EO-18)

13. Pharmacoeconomic considerations in the treatment of ADHD include all of the following, *except:* (EO-17)
    a. Monthly cost of methylphenidate
    b. Indirect societal costs such as absenteeism
    c. Frequent clinic visits
    d. CNS hyperstimulation

CASE 97
Stephan Cooke
Topic: Polysubstance Abuse
Level 3
EDUCATIONAL MATERIALS
Chapter 62: Substance Abuse

SCENARIO

Patient and Setting

RS, a 25-year-old female; ED

Chief Complaint

Brought into ED by friend, remains unresponsive after multidrug abuse on previous night

History of Present Illness

Per girlfriend, with whom partying, during the previous night RS "shot an eight ball of snow," drank vodka, and ingested large amounts of oral diazepam; had two incidents of blacking out after partying within the past week; well-known to the county ED for her drug-seeking behavior and frequent run-ins with the police.

Past Medical History

Single grand mal seizure 15 years ago; history of noncompliance with her seizure medication.

Past Surgical History

None

Family/Social History

Family History: Single parent; lives with her 4-year-old son in a motel located downtown

Social History: Smokes 1 PPD × 12 years; drinks alcohol almost daily (mostly vodka and gin); uses intravenous cocaine ("whenever I can afford it"); also takes oral diazepam 5 times a week, usually consuming between 5–30 mg at any given time; diazepam originally prescribed when she was a teenager in psychotherapy

Medication History

Diazepam, 5–30 mg PO QD PRN anxiety

Phenytoin, 300 mg PO QHS

Allergies

NKDA

Physical Examination

GEN: Skinny, emaciated adult female in acute distress.
VS: BP 80/50, HR 55 Reg, RR 6, T 37.6°C, Current Wt 54 kg, Dry Wt 52 kg, Ht 152 cm
HEENT: Pupils fixed and dilated to 7 mm
COR: Normal S_1 and S_2, no S_3 or S_4 or murmurs
CHEST: BS decreased, no rales, rhonchi, or wheezes
ABD: Distended, nontender, bowel sounds decreased but audible
GU: WNL
RECT: Guaiac positive
EXT: Decreased DTRs, + asterixis
NEURO: Oriented × 0, responsive only to painful stimuli

Results of Pertinent Laboratory Tests, Serum Drug Concentrations, and Diagnostic Tests

HCO_3 27 (27)	Hct .35 (35)	T Bili 27.4 (1.6)
Na 132 (132)	Hgb 115 (11.5)	AST 1.75 (105)
K 3.7 (3.7)	Glu 3.8 (70)	ALT 7.8 (470)
Cl 100 (100)	Alk Phos 2.5 (150)	Lkcs 10 × 10^9
BUN 6.8 (19)	Alb 25 (2.5)	(10 × 10^3)
Cr 88.4 (1.0)		

INR 1.3

Ethanol 20.6 (95)

Phenytoin 0 (0)

Urinalysis: + EtOH, + cocaine, + ecgonine, + benzodiazepine

Chest x-ray: Clear, no signs of pneumonia, mild cardiomegaly

PROBLEM LIST

Identify principal problems from the scenario in priority order [completed Problem List and SOAP Note at end of casebook]

SOAP NOTE

To be completed by student

QUESTIONS

[Answers at end of casebook]

1. A simple 4-point questionnaire used to easily and effectively identify patients with alcohol abuse and dependence would be the: (EO-5)
   a. CAGE
   b. BPRS
   c. AUDIT
   d. Brief MAST

2. Wernicke's encephalopathy secondary to alcohol withdrawal is associated with depletion of which of the following: (EO-10)
   a. Thiamine
   b. Glucose
   c. GABA
   d. Pyridoxine

3. Withdrawal seizures are most likely to occur in patients who have chronically used which of the following drugs: (EO-8)
   a. Diazepam
   b. Heroin
   c. Desipramine
   d. Theophylline

4. Acute cocaine abuse is likely to produce symptoms similar to which of the following: (EO-2)
   a. Paranoid schizophrenia
   b. Major depression
   c. Obsessive compulsive disorder
   d. Huntington's chorea

5. Contraindications to nicotine gum include: (EO-8)
   a. Lactation
   b. Peptic ulcer
   c. COPD
   d. Epilepsy

6. Which of the following drugs is responsible for three times as many deaths every year as alcohol, heroin, and cocaine combined? (EO-3)
   a. Nicotine
   b. Marijuana
   c. PCP
   d. LSD

7. Substance dependence is characterized by all of the following, *except:* (EO-1)
   a. Tolerance
   b. Withdrawal symptoms upon stopping substance
   c. Compulsive substance use
   d. Positive quality of life

8. Substance abuse is least likely to occur in which of the following groups: (EO-3)
   a. Males
   b. Females
   c. Health care professionals
   d. Psychiatric patients

9. The primary goal of substance abuse treatment is: (EO-7, 11, 12)
   a. To allow patient to socially use desired substance
   b. Total abstinence
   c. Psychiatric stabilization
   d. Minimize familial discord

10. The most common current route of administration of heroin in the U.S. is: (EO-1, 2)
    a. Oral
    b. Nasal
    c. Intravenous
    d. Intramuscular

11. Describe the psychosocial parameters associated with substance abuse. (EO-15)

12. List the desired positive treatment outcomes associated with substance abuse treatment. (EO-12, 18)

13. A smokable form of cocaine, created by heating a mixture of baking soda and water, is: (EO-3)
    a. Monkey morphine
    b. Ganja
    c. Crack
    d. Vitamin P

14. Acute marijuana intoxication is characterized by all of the following, *except:* (EO-1, 2)
    a. Conjunctival injection
    b. Diminished reaction time
    c. Dry mouth
    d. Gingival hyperplasia

15. Which of the following hallucinogens is synthetically derived? (EO-1, 2)
    a. Peyote
    b. Mescaline
    c. Psilocybin
    d. LSD

16. Which of the following is a pharmacoeconomic consideration in the treatment of substance abuse?
    a. Crack lung
    b. Decreased morbidity
    c. Disproportionate health care utilization
    d. Esophageal varicies

17. Summarize pathophysiological, therapeutic, and disease state management utilizing a key point format.

CASE 98
Stephen Cooke
Topic: Eating Disorders
 Level 3

EDUCATIONAL MATERIALS
Chapter 60: Obesity and Eating Disorders

SCENARIO

Patient and Setting
TD, a 16-year-old female; hospital

Chief Complaint
"Fatigue and weakness"

History of Present Illness
Over the past several months has been involved with a rigorous exercise program (daily 3–5 mile runs and aerobics) to get in shape for cheerleading try outs and to "fit in more with her friends"; she has lost a total of 10 kg over the last

month and is concerned about not making the cheerleading squad because she thinks she is "too fat"; parents have noticed a progressive decrease in the amount of food intake and an increased amount of time spent by herself. TD states she routinely vomits after eating and her last menses was over 4 months ago.

Past Medical History

Unremarkable

Past Surgical History

None

Family/Social History

Unremarkable

Medication History

Admits to taking her mother's water-pill (hydrochlorothiazide) and various nonprescription laxatives to help maintain her weight; denies the use of alcohol, tobacco, or any other medications.

Allergies

NKDA

Physical Examination

GEN: Quiet, emaciated, young female with noticeable hip, knee, and elbow joints; despite pronounced weight loss, perceives herself as being overweight.

VS: BP 85/60, HR 54, RR 24, T 37.0°C, Wt 36.5 kg (less than 35% ideal body weight), Ht 165 cm

HEENT: Dry mucous membranes, mild acne on face and back, fetid breath, tooth enamel degradation with dental caries evident in three teeth

COR: Bradycardia; hypotension

CHEST: Clear to auscultation and percussion

ABD: Soft, nontender with no masses found

GU: Not performed

RECT: Not performed

SKIN/EXT: Dry, flaky skin; cold extremities; comedones on face and back

NEURO: A and O × 3

Results of Pertinent Laboratory Tests, Serum Drug Concentrations, and Diagnostic Tests

Na 121	Cr 53 (0.6)	HCO_3 36
BUN 18.5 (52)	Cl 70	WBC 4 × 10^9 (4 × 10^3)
K 2.7		

Thyroid screen (TSH, T_4, T_3 Uptake, FTI): WNL

Amylase: WNL

Catecholamine levels: WNL

Arterial blood gases: pH 7.58; PCO_2 40; PO_2 90; HCO_3 36; BE +11

PROBLEM LIST

Identify principal problems from the scenario in priority order [completed Problem List and SOAP Note at end of casebook]

SOAP NOTE

To be completed by student

QUESTIONS

[Answers at end of casebook]

1. Anorexia nervosa is a syndrome characterized by all of the following *except:* (EO-1, 2)
   a. Self starvation
   b. Extreme weight loss
   c. Purging
   d. Fear of obesity despite being severely underweight

2. Bulimia nervosa is characterized by the following: (EO-1, 2)
   a. Binge eating
   b. Avoidance of exercise
   c. Self-induced vomiting
   d. Laxative and diet pill abuse

3. One-third of bulimic patients have a history of anorexia *or:* (EO-3)
   a. Major depressive disorder
   b. Bipolar disorder
   c. Generalized anxiety disorder
   d. Schizophrenia

4. Anorexia is most commonly first seen in: (EO-3, 5)
   a. Females age 30–40 years old
   b. Males age 18–35 years old
   c. Postmenopausal females
   d. Females age 13–18 years old

5. The following classifications concerning anorexia nervosa patients are true, *except:* (EO-3)
   a. Patients are often Caucasian
   b. 95% of patients are female
   c. Incidence of anorexia decreases with increased economic status
   d. 5–10% of young women are affected to some degree

6. Medical conditions consistent with anorexia nervosa include: (EO-3, 5)
   a. Increased LFTs
   b. Amenorrhea
   c. Cyanosis
   d. Seizure disorders

7. The most common cause of death in anorexia nervosa patients is: (EO-1)
   a. Status epilepticus
   b. Renal failure
   c. Cardiac complications
   d. Starvation

8. Bulimic patients characteristically present with all of the following *except*: (EO-3, 1, 5)
   a. Complaints of sore throats
   b. Increased infections
   c. Papulomacular rash
   d. Dental caries

9. Russell's sign, an indication of chronic vomiters, is characterized by: (EO-1, 3, 8)
   a. Irritation of oral mucosal tissue
   b. Swollen extremities
   c. Red eyes
   d. Abrasions or calluses on the dorsum of the dominant hand

10. The medication carrying FDA approval for bulimia nervosa is: (EO-8)
    a. Fluoxetine
    b. Amitriptyline
    c. Sertraline
    d. Phenelzine

11. Dosing of an SSRI for treatment of an eating disorder is generally: (EO-7, 8)
    a. Lower than those recommended for depression
    b. Higher than those recommended for depression
    c. The same as those recommended for depression
    d. Not comparable to those recommended for depression

12. Phenelzine, an MAOI that has an unlabeled indication for treatment of bulimia, is not considered first-line therapy due to: (EO-7, 8)
    a. High dosage requirements
    b. Expense of treatment
    c. Side effect profile and drug interactions
    d. Incidence of rebound binging

13. Discuss the major objectives of psychotherapy in the treatment of eating disorders. (EO-14)

14. Discuss common side effects experienced with the use of SSRI antidepressants. (EO-7, 8, 10)

15. Discuss aspects of normal-weight bulimia that make it a difficult disorder to detect. (EO-15, 16)

16. Outline important facts to include during patient counseling on an SSRI antidepressant. (EO-10, 18)

17. Pharmacoeconomic considerations of eating disorder management include all of the following, *except*: (EO-17)
    a. Loss of self-esteem
    b. Increased health care utilization
    c. Cost of fluoxetine
    d. Insurance coverage of psychotherapy

18. Summarize pathophysiological, therapeutic, and disease state management in key point format.

CASE 99
Stephen Cooke
Topic: Schizophrenia

EDUCATIONAL MATERIALS
Chapter 57: Schizophrenia (diagnosis, therapeutic goals, pharmacotherapy)

SCENARIO

Patient and Setting

MJ, a 62-year-old female; ambulatory care clinic

Chief Complaint

Thirst, lethargy, constipation; began 1 month ago

History of Present Illness

Presents to clinic for prescription refills; speech slurred, tongue sticking out of mouth; eyes appeared to blink frequently, and arms and legs moved in a writhing, involuntary manner; states that she has been hearing some voices again for the past 2 weeks and needs some ear plugs to shut them out

Past Medical History

30-year history of schizophrenia; seizure activity secondary to head injury 5 years ago

Past Surgical History

None

Family/Social History

Family History: Mother has history of depression
Social History: Unremarkable

Medication History

Haloperidol, 4 mg PO TID × 20 years (dose recently decreased)
Benztropine, 1 mg PO BID
Docusate sodium, 100 mg PO QD
Phenytoin, 100 mg PO TID
Ibuprofen, 200 mg PO q4–6h
Conjugated estrogens, 0.625 mg PO QD
Multivitamins, 1 PO QD

Allergies

Thioridazine (rash)

Physical Examination

GEN: Lethargic, thin, anxious, and depressed-looking woman
VS: BP 100/60, HR 70, RR 18, T 38.0°C
HEENT: PERRLA; EOMs intact
COR: Regular, without murmurs or extra sounds
CHEST: Lungs clear bilaterally to auscultation and percussion
ABD: Soft, tender, no palpable masses
GU: Deferred
RECT: Deferred
EXT: No clubbing, cyanosis, or edema
NEURO: Normal

Results of Pertinent Laboratory Tests, Serum Drug Concentrations, and Diagnostic Tests

Cr 62 (0.7)   Alb 20 (2)   Phenytoin 27.7 (7)

PROBLEM LIST

Identify principal problems from the scenario in priority order [completed Problem List and SOAP Note at end of casebook]

SOAP NOTE

To be completed by student

QUESTIONS

[Answers at end of casebook]

1. Considering MJ's thioridazine allergy, which of the following would *not* be an appropriate antipsychotic for her to take? (EO-7)
   a. Mesoridazine
   b. Thiothixene
   c. Fluphenazine
   d. Olanzapine

2. Gender differences in schizophrenia can be described as: (EO-3)
   a. Males develop schizophrenia twice as often as females
   b. Females develop schizophrenia twice as often as males
   c. Males have a better prognosis
   d. Males tend to develop schizophrenia earlier than females

3. Risk factors for suicide in schizophrenics include all of the following *except:* (EO-1)
   a. Female gender
   b. Male gender
   c. Unemployment
   d. Comorbid depressive symptoms

4. DSM-IV diagnostic criteria for schizophrenia require all of the following criteria *except:* (EO-2)
   a. Hallucinations
   b. Delusions
   c. Significant social dysfunction
   d. Paranoia

5. The most common type of hallucination seen in schizophrenia is: (EO-2)
   a. Visual
   b. Auditory
   c. Tactile
   d. Olfactory

6. Which of the following symptoms is MJ experiencing? (EO-1)
   a. Delusions
   b. Auditory hallucinations
   c. Ideas of reference
   d. Avolition

7. Which of the following statements concerning antipsychotics is true? (EO-6, 8, 11)
   a. Atypical antipsychotics should always be used prior to any other drug therapy.
   b. Antipsychotic drug selection should be based on MHPG plasma levels.
   c. QID dosing diminishes adverse effects, thereby increasing compliance.
   d. Depot preparations are indicated in the chronically non-compliant.

8. MJ's eventual haloperidol dose is 10 mg PO BID. Convert this to an approximate equivalent of haloperidol decanoate. (EO-12)

9. If MJ reports to the nursing station with her head pulled sharply to the side and rear, complaining of severe pain in the neck and back area, the most appropriate diagnosis and subsequent treatment would be: (EO-2, 11)
   a. Akathisia–propranolol 20 mg IM until resolution
   b. Dystonic reaction–diphenhydramine 50 mg IM every 30 minutes until resolution
   c. Tardive dyskinesia–physical therapy
   d. Dystonic reaction–lorazepam 2 mg IM every 30 minutes until resolution

10. Your patient is receiving fluphenazine 10 mg PO TID. What is the appropriate dose to convert to fluphenazine decanoate? (EO-12)
    a. 300 mg IM every 2 weeks
    b. 37.5 mg IM every 2 weeks
    c. 300 mg IM every 4 weeks
    d. 37.5 mg IM every 4 weeks

11. Agranulocytosis associated with clozapine is defined as: (EO-10)
    a. WBC <4,000 and neutrophil count <2,000
    b. WBC >4,000 and eosinophil count <2,000
    c. WBC <3,500 and neutrophil count <1,500
    d. WBC <3,500 and PMNC of 45%

12. Explain why or why not MJ would be a good candidate for clozapine. (EO-12)

13. What psychosocial factors limit medication compliance in the schizophrenic population? (EO-15)

14. Which of the following antipsychotics is classified as a Pregnancy Category B agent? (EO-9)
    a. Perphenazine
    b. Chlorpromazine
    c. Clozapine
    d. Haloperidol

15. Which of the following is an important pharmacoeconomic consideration for patients receiving clozapine? (EO-17)
    a. Cost of concomitant risperidol use that is commonly required
    b. Cost of frequent monitoring of serum liver enzymes
    c. Cost of frequent monitoring of complete blood count
    d. Cost of additional therapy commonly required to control negative schizophrenic

16. Summarize pathophysiologic, therapeutic, and disease management concepts for MJ's schizophrenia using a key points format. (EO-18)

CASE 100
Stephen Cooke
Topic: Depression
Level 2
EDUCATIONAL MATERIALS
Case 56: Mood Disorders

SCENARIO

Patient and Setting

DR, a 65-year-old female; family physician's office

Chief Complaint

"I've been depressed lately . . . I've had some numbness and tingling in left foot."

History of Present Illness

Depression and numbness/tingling in left foot began 4 months ago; denies any current signs and symptoms of hyper- or hypoglycemia; admits to occasional hypoglycemic episodes when not eating on time; noncompliant with checking her blood glucose levels

Past Medical History

Type 1 diabetes for 40 years

Past Surgical History

Cataract surgery 10 years ago

Family/Social History

Family History: Father, mother, and brother all have a history of Type 1 diabetes
Social History: Unremarkable

Medication History

Regular human insulin, 20 units SC q AM and 10 units SC QHS

NPH human insulin, 20 units SC q AM and 10 units SC QHS
Nitroglycerin, 0.4 mg SL PRN chest pain
Levothyroxine, 0.1 mg PO QD
Conjugated estrogen, 0.625 mg PO QD
Docusate sodium, 100 mg PO BID
Clonidine, 0.1 mg PO BID
Hydrochorothiazide (HCTZ), 50 mg PO BID
Cholestyramine, 4 g PO BID

Allergies

Aspirin (stomach pain)

Physical Examination

GEN: Nervous, thin, depressed female
VS: BP 100/60, HR 70, RR 18, T 37.0°C, Wt 60 kg
HEENT: WNL, except for complaints of blurred vision
COR: Normal S1, S2; no S3, S4, or murmurs
CHEST: WNL
ABD: Soft, no palpable masses
GU: WNL
RECT: Guaiac negative
EXT: Tingling/numbness, left foot
NEURO: Cranial nerves intact; A and O × 3

Results of Pertinent Laboratory Tests, Serum Drug Concentrations, and Diagnostic Tests

Na 142 (142)	Hct 0.38 (38)	LDH 2.0 (120)
K 5.2 (5.2)	Lkcs 4 × 10⁹	Alk Phos 1.67 (100)
Cl 108 (108)	(4 × 10³)	HbA₁C 10
HCO₃ 28 (28)	Plts 300 × 10⁹	TSH 5.2 (5.2)
BUN 7.14 (20)	(300 × 10³)	Free T₄ Index 1.2
Cr 310 (3.5)	AST 38 (38)	Chol 3.9 (150)
Glu 5.6 (100)	ALT 36 (36)	TG 40 (350)
Hgb 130 (13)		

HDL chol 0.52 (20)
Lkc differential, chest x-ray, ECG: all WNL
Urinalysis: pH 1.020, glucose (−), protein (3+), casts (+)

PROBLEM LIST

Identify principal problems from the scenario in priority order [completed Problem List and SOAP Note at end of casebook]

SOAP NOTE

To be completed by student

QUESTIONS

[Answers at end of casebook]

1. Most depressed individuals who present to a general practitioner for the first time have a chief complaint of: (EO-1)
   a. Depression
   b. Midlife crisis
   c. Sexual inadequacies
   d. Physical ailments

2. Which of the following factors should be considered when recommending antidepressant therapy? (EO-7)
   a. Gender
   b. Marital status
   c. Number of previous episodes of depression
   d. Previous response to antidepressants

3. Discuss the psychosocial factors that are prevalent in depression. (EO-15)

4. DSM-IV criteria for major depression require that a person have: (EO-1)
   a. Crying spells
   b. Suicide attempt
   c. Anhedonia
   d. Past history of depression

5. A new customer presents to your pharmacy with a prescription for phenelzine. In the past, she has been treated unsuccessfully with trials of nortriptyline, bupropion, and fluoxetine. She desperately hopes this agent will relieve her symptoms. Which of the following questions is most important to ask? (EO-9)
   a. Do you have hypertension?
   b. How long were you treated with each of the previous antidepressants?
   c. What doses of each of the previous antidepressants did you receive?
   d. When did you last take fluoxetine?

6. Which of the following combination of agents is contraindicated? (EO-9)
   a. Fluoxetine and trazodone
   b. Nefazodone and astemizole
   c. Nortriptyline and propranolol
   d. Sertraline and alprazolam

7. The most common adverse effect of the SSRIs is: (EO-10)
   a. Nausea
   b. Torsades-de-pointes
   c. Narcolepsy
   d. Edema

8. The long half-life of the SSRIs may facilitate which of the following therapeutic and pharmacoeconomic advantages in certain patients: (EO-4, 17)
   a. Every other day dosing
   b. Less anticholinergic side effects
   c. Sublingual medication delivery
   d. More rapid antidepressant response

9. All of the following are common adverse effects of tricyclic antidepressants except: (EO-10)
   a. Dry mouth
   b. Constipation
   c. Peripheral edema
   d. Tachycardia

10. Risk factors for suicide include all of the following except: (EO-3)
    a. Psychiatric illness
    b. Feelings of hopelessness
    c. Older age
    d. Female gender

11. Educating the depressed patient who is prescribed amitriptyline should include the following point: (EO-10)
    a. Possible insomnia
    b. May be habit forming
    c. May cause weight gain, so weigh self regularly
    d. May cause diarrhea

12. Which of the following antidepressants cannot be administered once daily? (EO-4, 10)
    a. Bupropion
    b. Fluoxetine
    c. Nortriptyline
    d. Paroxetine

13. Which of the following statements about suicide is true? (EO-2)
    a. Talking about suicide will often put the idea into someone's head
    b. Most persons who attempt suicide communicate their intention
    c. Suicide is rare in patients who have AIDS
    d. Persons who attempt suicide are at decreased risk for future suicide attempts

14. Which of the following is most likely to cause constipation? (EO-8, 10)
    a. Clomipramine
    b. Fluoxetine
    c. Fluvoxamine
    d. Sertraline

15. Which of the following antidepressants is least likely to cause withdrawal symptoms upon abrupt discontinuation? (EO-4, 6)
    a. Fluoxetine
    b. Imipramine
    c. Paroxetine
    d. Venlafaxine

16. Depression should be diagnosed according to: (EO-2)
    a. Family opinion
    b. DSM-IV criteria
    c. Laboratory workup
    d. Hamilton Rating Scales

17. Summarize medication counseling information for sertraline. Include possible adverse effects, length of time until full benefits can be expected, and duration of treatment. (EO-14)

18. Summarize therapeutic, pathophysiologic, and disease management concepts for depression using a key points format. (EO-18)

CASE 101
Lorianne Wright
Topic: Immunization Therapy
Level 1
EDUCATIONAL MATERIALS
Chapter 65: Immunization Therapy

SCENARIO

Patient and Setting
BG, 4½-year-old male; clinic visit

Chief Complaint
Well-care visit

History of Present Illness
Has been in good health; scheduled for a routine physical exam and immunizations; mother is anxious regarding the administration of immunizations; mother states he had a "bad reaction" to his last shot

Past Medical History
Born at 38 weeks gestation; birth weight 4.9 kg; multiple episodes of acute otitis media in the past, last episode 2 years ago; chickenpox at 15 months

Past Surgical History
None

Family/Social History
Family History: Lives with both parents and a 20-month-old sister; both parents and sister healthy

Social History: Attends daycare 3 days a week; starting kindergarten in 2 months; mother reports calling poison control last month after her daughter was found with an open bottle of BG's vitamins

Medication History
Multivitamins, 1 tab PO QD

HBV and HiB series completed; three doses of OPV given at 2, 4, and 12 months; one dose of MMR at 15 months; four doses of DTwP with the last dose administered at 15 months of age; mother reports that "he was crying and fussy for hours" and had a fever of 40°C after his last DTwP

Allergies
NKDA

Physical Examination
GEN: Well-developed, well-nourished male
VS: BP 105/65, HR 95, RR 22, T 37°C, Wt 19.5 kg (90th %), Ht 105 cm (75th %)
HEENT: Normocephalic, conjunctiva clear, PERRL, tympanic membranes clear
COR: RRR, no murmurs
CHEST: Clear to auscultation
ABD: Soft, nontender, bowel sounds present
GU: Normal male
RECT: Deferred
EXT: Normal
NEURO: Alert and oriented, DTRs normal

Results of Pertinent Laboratory Tests, Serum Drug Concentrations, and Diagnostic Tests
UA: Normal
CBC: Normal

PROBLEM LIST
Identify principal problems from the scenario in priority order [completed Problem List and SOAP Note at end of casebook]

SOAP NOTE
To be completed by student

QUESTIONS
[Answers at end of casebook]

1. Describe the difference between a toxoid and a vaccine. (EO-7)

2. Routine pediatric immunizations provide prevention against diseases associated with the following pathogen: (EO-1)
   a. Respiratory syncytial virus
   b. *Neisseria meningitidis*
   c. *Haemophilus influenzae* type B
   d. Hepatitis C

3. BG should receive the DTP vaccination by which of the following routes? (EO-12)
   a. IM
   b. IV

c. SC

d. ID

4. The DPT is used to prevent diseases associated with the following pathogens: (EO-7)

   a. *Salmonella typhi, Bordetella pertussis, Mycobacterium tuberculosis*

   b. *Corynebacterium diphtheriae, Bordetella pertussis, Clostridium tetani*

   c. *Corynebacterium diphtheriae, Vibrio cholerae, Clostridium perfringens*

   d. *Salmonella typhi, Borrelia burgdorferi, Clostridium tetani*

5. Which of the following routine vaccinations will BG need to receive during his 11–12 year visit? (EO-12)

   a. MMR

   b. Td

   c. DTaP

   d. HBV

6. If BG suffers a severe reaction to either the IPV or the DTP immunization, who should be notified of the reaction? (EO-10)

   a. AAP

   b. ACIP

   c. VAERS

   d. WHO

7. Children less than 2 years of age do not mount an adequate immune response to which of the following immunization types? (EO-8)

   a. Live, attenuated vaccines

   b. Polysaccharide vaccines

   c. Killed vaccines

   d. Toxoids

8. If BG was diagnosed with sickle cell disease, which vaccines should he receive in addition to the routine immunizations? (EO-12)

9. If BG's mother was undergoing chemotherapy for Hodgkin's disease, which of the following should BG not receive at this visit? (EO-12)

   a. IPV

   b. DTaP

   c. DT

   d. OPV

10. Which of the following vaccines is a live, attenuated vaccine? (EO-7)

    a. Td

    b. Varicella vaccine

    c. HiB vaccine

    d. HBV vaccine

11. IPV has the following advantage over OPV: (EO-8)

    a. IPV is less expensive

    b. IPV has not been associated with VAPP

    c. IPV provides better GI mucosal immunity

    d. IPV is a live, attenuated vaccine

12. Describe the psychosocial factors that may affect parents' willingness to have their child immunized. (EO-15)

13. Summarize pathophysiologic, therapeutic, and disease prevention concepts for immunization therapy in this patient utilizing a key points format. (EO-18)

CASE 102
Lorianne Wright
Topic: Immunization Therapy

EDUCATIONAL MATERIALS
Chapter 65: Immunization Therapy; Chapter 66: Upper Respiratory Infections (otitis media)

SCENARIO

Patient and Setting

AH, a 12-month-old female; clinic

Chief Complaint

Follow-up visit for recent episode of acute otitis media

History of Present Illness

Seen in clinic 7 days ago for acute otitis media (AOM) with right tympanic membrane (TM) that was bulging, red, and opacified; given amoxicillin; scheduled for a follow-up visit for reevaluation and scheduled immunizations; mother reports AH is having some loose stools but is otherwise "doing much better"

Past Medical History

One episode of AOM at 10 months; treated with amoxicillin; gastroesophageal reflux disease (GERD); started cisapride and ranitidine 1 month ago

Past Surgical History

None

Family/Social History

Family History: Lives with her mother and father who are healthy; cared for in the home by the mother and a grandmother; grandmother recently received a kidney transplantatio–receiving prednisone and cyclosporine

Social History: Noncontributory

Medication History

Amoxicillin, 200 mg PO TID (~60 mg/kg/day)– completed 7 of 10-day course

Cisapride, 2 mg PO TID (0.6 mg/kg/day)

Ranitidine, 20 mg PO BID (4 mg/kg/day)

Immunizations: HBV, DTwP/HiB at 2, 4, and 6 months; IPV at 2 and 4 months

Allergies

NKDA

Physical Examination

GEN: Well-developed, well-nourished female

VS: BP 100/64, HR 121, RR 28, T 37.0°C, Wt 10.5 kg (75th %), Ht 75 cm (50th %)

HEENT: Neck supple; conjunctiva clear; R-TM effusion present, color normal; L-TM WNL

COR: WNL, no murmur

CHEST: Good breath sounds, no rales or rhonchi

ABD: Soft, nontender, no distention, positive bowel sounds

GU: Normal female, mild erythema and inflammation of diaper area; no lesions

RECT: Deferred

EXT: WNL

NEURO: Awake and alert with no focal findings

Results of Pertinent Laboratory Tests, Serum Drug Concentrations, and Diagnostic Tests

Na 140 (140)
K 4.5 (4.5)
Cl 99 (99)
HCO_3 26 (26)
BUN 4.3 (12)

Cr 35 (0.4)
RBC 4.2×10^{12}
  (4.2×10^6)
Hct 0.42 (42)
Hgb 130 (13)

Lkc 7.3×10^9
  (7.3×10^3)
Plts 230×10^9 (230×10^3)
Glu 4.4 (80)

PROBLEM LIST

Identify principal problems from the scenario in priority order

SOAP NOTE

To be completed by student

QUESTIONS

1. All of the following are live, attenuated vaccines, *except*: (EO-7)
   a. MMR
   b. Varicella
   c. HiB
   d. OPV

2. If AH had a documented case of meningitis due to *H. influenzae* type B at 11 months of age, which of the following would be true? AH should: (EO-8)
   a. Receive his final HiB shot at this visit
   b. Not receive any further doses of HiB since he has developed immunity as a result of the infection
   c. Receive his final HiB shot 6 months after the episode of meningitis
   d. Receive the entire HiB series over again

3. What percentage of patients will develop a mild maculopapular rash or varicelliform rash after receiving the varicella vaccine? (EO-10)

   a. 2%
   b. 8%
   c. 20%
   d. 35%

4. Describe the adverse effects that AH may experience from the MMR vaccine. (EO-10)

5. Which of the following immunizations are administered subcutaneously? (EO-7)
   a. DTaP, rotavirus, IPV
   b. MMR, varicella, yellow fever
   c. HBV, HiB, varicella
   d. Hepatitis A, MMR, IPV

6. Precautions associated with the use of the DTaP immunization include all of the following *except:* (EO-10)
   a. Seizure within 72 hours of the immunization
   b. Persistent uncontrollable crying for 3 hours within 48 hours of immunization
   c. Hypotonic-hyporesponsive state after immunization
   d. Fussiness and crying for 3 hours after the immunization

7. If AH had a history of hypersensitivity to egg products, which of the following would be the most appropriate choice regarding administration of the MMR? (EO-10)
   a. MMR should be deferred until AH can be desensitized
   b. AH should receive the measles and mumps vaccines individually without receiving the rubella vaccine
   c. MMR should be administered and AH should be observed for 90 minutes for adverse reactions
   d. AH should not receive the MMR but should receive IGIV if she is exposed to individuals with measles or rubella

8. Routine pediatric vaccinations prevent against infections associated with all of the following pathogens *except:* (EO-1)
   a. Paramyxovirus
   b. *Clostridium tetani*
   c. Nontypeable *Haemophilus influenzae*
   d. Hepatitis B virus

9. List factors that should be taken into consideration when choosing the product to be used to vaccinate an individual. (EO-8)

10. Describe the pharmacoeconomic factors that should be taken into consideration when incorporating new vaccines into the universal immunization schedule. (EO-17)

11. Summarize therapeutic, pathophysiologic, and disease prevention concepts for immunization therapy in this patient utilizing a key points format. (EO-18)

CASE 103

Robert C. Stevens

Topic: Upper Respiratory Infections— Viral and Bacterial

EDUCATIONAL MATERIALS

Chapter 66: Upper Respiratory Infections

SCENARIO

Patient and Setting

LW, a 12-month-old female; clinic

Chief Complaint

"Cold," lethargy, and irritability

History of Present Illness

Mother brought LW to the clinic because she has a "cold"; LW has a mild, nonproductive cough, nasal congestion, runny nose, and sore throat with increasing lethargy and irritability over the past 3 days; she began pulling on her right earlobe this morning; LW's appetite is very poor, and she is slightly warm to the touch; LW had her first bout of otitis media 8 days ago, which responded to antibiotic therapy

Past Medical History

Nonsignificant

Past Surgical History

None

Family/Social History

Family History: LW lives with her mother and father, who are both recovering from the "flu"

Social History: LW has no siblings and does not attend daycare but lives in a community with a high prevalence of penicillin-nonsusceptible *Streptococcus pneumoniae*

Medication History

Vitamin supplement, 1 mL PO QD

Amoxicillin, 250 mg PO TID (50 mg/kg/day); completed a 5-day course 3 days ago

Immunizations are up-to-date

Allergies

NKDA

Physical Examination

GEN: Well-developed, well-nourished girl, crying, in moderate distress, tugging on right earlobe

VS: BP 100/68, HR 124, RR 30, T 39°C, Wt 15 kg (90th %)

HEENT: Pale skin; right tympanic membrane red and bulging, no exudate seen; throat is erythematous; neck supple; clear, watery nasal discharge

COR: WNL, no murmur

CHEST: Good breath sounds, no rales or rhonchi

ABD: Soft, nontender; no distention; positive bowel sounds

GU: Erythema, tenderness, and inflammation over entire diaper area; vesicular satellite lesions on periphery of redness

RECT: Deferred

EXT: WNL

NEURO: Awake and alert with no focal findings

Results of Pertinent Laboratory Tests, Serum Drug Concentrations, and Diagnostic Tests

No laboratory tests ordered for this outpatient clinic visit

PROBLEM LIST

Identify principal problems from the scenario in priority order [completed Problem List and SOAP Note at end of casebook]

SOAP NOTE

To be completed by student

QUESTIONS

[Answers at end of casebook]

1. Describe the pathophysiologic events that make a child susceptible to middle ear infections. (EO-1)

2. Identify the age at which the peak incidence for acute otitis media occurs. (EO-1, 3)
   a. Newborn to 3 months
   b. 6 months to 1 year
   c. Years 1 to 2
   d. Years 2 to 4

3. Select the most important risk factor for developing otitis media. (EO-1, 3)
   a. Day-care settings
   b. High socioeconomic status
   c. Breast-fed infants
   d. Children who live in rural environments

4. Identify the peak season for acute otitis media. (EO-3)
   a. Summer
   b. Fall
   c. Winter
   d. Spring

5. List the possible etiologic pathogens of otitis media in LW. (EO-1, 3)

6. Indicate the recommended duration of therapy of amoxicillin/clavulanate for acute otitis media in LW. (EO-8, 11)
   a. Single dose
   b. 3–5 days
   c. 10 days
   d. 14 days

7. Explain the rationale for treatment with an antibiotic (amoxicillin/clavulanate) if the cause of otitis media in LW is viral. (EO-3, 5, 8, 11)

8. Choose the adverse event that is associated more with amoxicillin/clavulanate than amoxicillin. (EO-10)
   a. Macular rash
   b. Diarrhea
   c. Headaches
   d. Difficulty in swallowing

9. Describe the differences of amoxicillin/clavulanate compared with amoxicillin. (EO-7, 12)

10. After 10 days of therapy with amoxicillin/clavulanate, LW is afebrile and her appetite and energy returned to baseline. Select the appropriate follow-up. (EO-5, 8, 12)
    a. Return to clinic; obtain culture if tympanic membranes are inflamed
    b. Complete a total of 14 days of decongestants to relieve eustachian tube congestion
    c. Return to clinic for evaluation of prophylactic antibiotics for chronic otitis media
    d. No follow-up is required as long as LW remains asymptomatic

11. Select the best reason for not using aspirin for fever and pain in LW. (EO-3, 5, 8, 9)
    a. Association of aspirin use and Reye's syndrome in children with influenza
    b. Antipyretic effect of aspirin is inferior to that of acetaminophen in infants and toddlers
    c. Anticytokine activity of aspirin interferes with host-defense mechanisms activated during viral infections
    d. GI intolerance from aspirin is augmented with amoxicillin/clavulanate

12. Cardec-DM pediatric drops yield all of the following pharmacologic responses *except:* (EO-7)
    a. Decongestant
    b. Antihistamine
    c. Antipyretic
    d. Cough suppressant

13. Provide educational instruction to LW's mom about proper care for diaper rash. (EO-14)

14. Summarize pathophysiologic, therapeutic, and disease management concepts for upper respiratory infections utilizing a key points format. (EO-18)

CASE 104
Robert C. Stevens
Topic: Upper Respiratory Infections— Bacterial (Acute Sinusitis)
 Level 1

EDUCATIONAL MATERIALS
Chapter 66: Upper Respiratory Infections

SCENARIO
Patient and Setting
LM, a 36-year-old woman; family medicine clinic

Chief Complaint
Congestion, "pain around my nose and eyes," "runny nose," and headache

History of Present Illness
LM was in her normal state of health until 10 days ago when she developed an upper respiratory infection characterized by greenish/yellowish-colored nasal discharge, sinus tenderness, headache, mild fever, sneezing, nasal congestion, and cough; the latter two symptoms were only mildly relieved by over-the-counter drugs; LM denies any recent viral illness and has no history of respiratory allergies; no other household family members are ill

Past Medical History
Gestational diabetes with last pregnancy (13 months ago) that resolved post-partum; OB: grav 2, para 2; both deliveries were by normal vaginal delivery

Past Surgical History
Noncontributory

Family/Social History
Family History: Mother has Type 2 diabetes mellitus; father died of acute MI at age 63

Social History: Full-time mom at home with 2 children ages 2.5 and 1 year; denies cigarette smoking; drinks alcohol socially

Medication History
Multivitamin with iron, 1 tablet PO QD

Oral contraceptive (Nordette) (30 μg ethinyl estradiol and 3 mg norethindrone), 1 tablet PO QD

Ibuprofen, 600 mg PO TID PRN fever and pain

Robitussin, 1 tablespoon PO QID PRN cough

Tavist-D, 1 tablet PO QID PRN nasal congestion and runny nose

Allergies
NKDA

Physical Examination
GEN: Well-developed, well-nourished woman experiencing discomfort from headache and sinus pain/congestion

VS: BP 108/66, HR 79, RR 20, T 37.7°C, Wt 65 kg
HEENT: PERRLA; extraocular movement intact; sinus tenderness (maxillary > frontal); sinus pressure; postnasal discharge; periorbital swelling; pharyngeal erythema; no nasal polyps; no impacted or abscessed teeth or evidence of periodontal disease
COR: RRR, normal S_1 and S_2, no murmur
CHEST: Clear to auscultation and percussion
ABD: Soft, nontender, nondistended, positive bowel sounds
GU: Examination deferred
RECT: No masses, guaiac negative
EXT: Full ROM, deep tendon reflexes intact
NEURO: Alert, O × 3; cranial nerves intact

Results of Pertinent Laboratory Tests, Serum Drug Concentrations, and Diagnostic Tests

Na 141 (141)	Cr 70.7 (0.8)	Plts 257×10^9
K 4.2 (4.2)	Hct 0.39 (39)	(257×10^3)
Cl 98 (98)	Hgb 160 (16)	AST 0.67 (40)
HCO$_3$ 26 (26)	Lkcs 10.6×10^9	ALT 0.53 (32)
BUN 3.2 (9)	(10.6×10^3)	Alb 49 (4.9)

Glu 9.2 (165) (fasting glucose since LM only consumed water this morning)

Lkc differential: PMN 0.70 (70%), bands 0.7 (7%), lymphs 0.19 (19%)

Otoscope with nasal speculum: thick, greenish-yellowish, mucopurulent nasal secretions observed primarily in the middle meatus

Gram stain of sinus lavage: >75 Lkcs/HPF; many gram-positive cocci in pairs; few gram-negative cocci-bacillus

PROBLEM LIST

Identify principal problems from the scenario in priority order

SOAP NOTE

To be completed by student

QUESTIONS

1. All of the following are true statements regarding acute sinusitis, *except:* (EO-1)
   a. It is a common upper respiratory infection accounting for millions of physician visits annually
   b. Viruses are the most common etiology
   c. The most practical and cost-effective method to assess a patient consists of the history and physical examination
   d. Antibiotics are appropriate for treatment

2. Select the most common cause of community-acquired acute sinusitis. (EO-1)
   a. *Streptococcus pneumoniae*
   b. *Haemophilus influenzae*
   c. Rotavirus
   d. *Viridans streptococci*

3. Identify the condition that is *least* likely to differentiate acute sinusitis from viral upper respiratory infection in LM. (EO-1, 2, 3, 5)
   a. Worsening of symptoms over 10 days
   b. Colored, purulent nasal discharge
   c. No other family members have upper respiratory tract symptoms
   d. Fever

4. Choose the most likely pathogen causing acute sinusitis in LM. (EO-1)
   a. *Streptococcus pneumoniae* and *Haemophilus influenzae*
   b. *Moraxella catarrhalis* and *Staphylococcus aureus*
   c. *Streptococcus pneumoniae* and *Staphylococcus aureus*
   d. *Peptostreptococcus* and *Bacteroides melaninogenicus*

5. Explain the rationale for selecting trimethoprim/sulfamethoxazole (TMP-SMX) as initial therapy for acute sinusitis in LM. (EO-6, 8, 11, 17)

6. Choose the best reason for avoiding use of oral pseudoephedrine for relief of nasal congestion in LW. (EO-9, 10, 11)
   a. Efficacy is inferior to nasal spray
   b. May enhance TMP-SMX central nervous system toxicity
   c. Can increase blood glucose
   d. Potential drug interaction with ibuprofen

7. Provide educational instruction to LM regarding how she should evaluate her clinical response to TMP-SMX. (EO-2, 14)

8. Provide educational information to LM about potential adverse events associated with TMP-SMX. (EO-10, 14)

9. After 2 doses of TMP-SMX, LM calls the pharmacy and complains that her "tummy gets upset" within 1 hr of taking TMP-SMX. What advice would you provide to LM? (EO-10)
   a. Take with food to minimize nausea
   b. Administer with antacids
   c. Split the tablets in half and space administration over 4 hours
   d. Take with a cola soft drink to increase absorption and therefore decrease the amount of drug in the gut

10. LM is feeling "much better" since starting TMP-SMX 3 days ago. This morning, however, she observed a rash on her arms and around her neck and shoulders. Upon consultation with you at the pharmacy, the rash is macular and nonpruritic. Choose the best course of management. (EO-8, 10, 11)
    a. Continue TMP-SMX since the rash is not symptomatic
    b. Continue TMP-SMX since this is only a "Red Man's syndrome" reaction such as observed with vancomycin
    c. Discontinue TMP-SMX and switch to a different antibiotic to complete 10 days of therapy
    d. Discontinue therapy since LM received an appropriate duration of therapy

11. Identify a well-tolerated, cost-effective, and convenient-to-take alternative to TMP-SMX for acute sinusitis in LM. (EO-6, 8, 12, 17)
    a. Erythromycin
    b. Azithromycin
    c. Amoxicillin
    d. Cephalexin

12. List the common adverse events and laboratory monitoring parameters for the antibiotic you selected in question 11 above. (EO-5, 10)

13. Identify a psychosocial issue that is likely to evolve in this case. (EO-15)

14. Summarize pathophysiologic, therapeutic, and disease management concepts for acute sinusitis utilizing a key points format. (EO-18)

CASE 105
Robert C. Stevens
Topic: Pneumococcal Pneumonia
`Level 3`
EDUCATIONAL MATERIALS
Chapter 67: Pneumonia

SCENARIO

Patient and Setting
JS, a 60-year-old man; ED

Chief Complaint
Fevers, severe right-sided chest pain, increasing shortness of breath (SOB), and increased heart rate

History of Present Illness
JS was in his usual state of health until he presented to the ER today after 2 days of increasing malaise, SOB, spiking fevers, chest pain, rigors, tachycardia, and gastric pain; admitted for pneumonia and acute exacerbation of COPD

Past Medical History
JS has a long history of chronic obstructive pulmonary disease (COPD) that strongly correlates with his smoking history of 25 years; JS carries two inhalers, metaproterenol and ipratropium for SOB; prednisone was started during hospitalization for COPD 2 months ago; JS admits that prednisone upsets his stomach so he "misses a few doses here and there"; JS's alcohol problem has been complicated by several alcohol withdrawal seizures, the most recent occurring 2 years ago; JS currently takes phenytoin for seizure prophylaxis; JS diagnosed with degenerative joint disease (DJD) approximately 3 years ago for which he takes acetaminophen with no complaints

Past Surgical History
Noncontributory

Family/Social History
Family History: Noncontributory

Social History: Smoked for past 25 years; S/P alcohol abuse; enrolled in Alcoholics Anonymous and has not had a drink for more than 1 year

Medication History
Phenytoin, 400 mg PO QHS

Ipratropium inhaler, 2–4 puffs PRN

Metaproterenol inhaler, 2–4 puffs PRN

Prednisone, 30 mg PO QD

Acetaminophen, 650 mg PO TID

Allergies
Ampicillin (rash) "years ago"

Physical Examination
- GEN: Diaphoretic, agitated, weak-looking man with obvious SOB
- VS: BP 140/90, RR 28, HR 125, T 39.5°C, Wt 65 kg
- HEENT: Purulent, rust-colored sputum × 2 days
- COR: Normal S_1 and S_2; no murmurs
- CHEST: Prolonged expiratory phase, bilateral rales and rhonchi, RLL dullness
- ABD: Gastric pain
- GU: WNL
- RECT: Guaiac positive
- EXT: WNL
- NEURO: A and O × 3; appropriate affect, lethargic

Results of Pertinent Laboratory Tests, Serum Drug Concentrations, and Diagnostic Tests

Na 145 (145)	Hct 0.49 (49)	AST 0.67 (40)
K 3.7 (3.7)	Hgb 180 (18)	ALT 0.53 (32)
Cl 101 (101)	Lkcs 18.6×10^9	Alb 42 (4.2)
HCO_3 33 (33)	(18.6×10^3)	Phenytoin 80 (20)
BUN 59 (21)	Plts 300×10^9	
Cr 106.1 (1.2)	(300×10^3)	

Lkc differential: PMN 0.88 (88%), bands 0.10 (10%), lymphs 0.02 (2%)

ABG (on room air): PO_2 70, PCO_2 47, pH 7.35

PFTs: FEV_1–60% (pre-β_2-agonist), FEV_1/FVC–70% (post-β_2-agonist)

Sputum Gram's stain >50 Lkcs/HPF; 0–5 epithelium cells/HPF; gram-positive cocci in pairs (many)

Blood cultures: Pending

Chest x-ray: RLL consolidation consistent with right lower lobe pneumonia

PROBLEM LIST

Identify principal problems from the scenario in priority order [completed Problem List and SOAP Note at end of casebook]

SOAP NOTE

To be completed by student

QUESTIONS

[Answers at end of casebook]

1. Identify the least important drug factor when considering the most appropriate empiric antibiotic therapy for pneumonia. (EO-8, 12, 17)
   a. Clinical efficacy
   b. Cost
   c. Adverse effects
   d. Pharmacokinetic properties

2. All of the following can impair the activity of the mucociliary transport system, *except:* (EO-1)
   a. Chronic lung disease
   b. Aging
   c. Smoking
   d. Vitamin C deficiency

3. Identify the factor associated with diminished alveolar macrophage activity. (EO-1)
   a. Coronary artery disease
   b. Rheumatoid arthritis stabilized with NSAIDs
   c. Hypertension
   d. Diabetes mellitus

4. All of the following are risk factors in JS for developing pneumococcal pneumonia, *except:* (EO-3)
   a. COPD
   b. Alcoholic
   c. Seizures
   d. Prednisone use

5. JS has all of the classic clinical manifestations of pneumococcal pneumonia, *except:* (EO-3, 5)
   a. Purulent, rust-colored sputum
   b. Guaiac-positive stools
   c. Leukocytosis with a left shift
   d. Fever with chills

6. List the drug(s) of choice for pneumococcal pneumonia in the United States based on susceptibility data. (EO-5, 8)

7. Why was ceftriaxone and not aqueous penicillin-G used as empiric therapy in JS? (EO-5, 8, 11)

8. Select the first sign of improvement that you would predict in JS. (EO-2, 5, 11)
   a. Normal leukocyte count
   b. Resolution of chest x-ray
   c. De-effervescence
   d. Absence of polymorphonuclear cells on sputum smear

9. JS has improved clinically after 3 doses of ceftriaxone. Final sputum culture was positive for *S. pneumoniae* sensitive to penicillin (MIC < 0.1 mg/L). Blood cultures were negative. Construct a disease management plan for the remainder of pneumonia therapy in JS. (EO-2, 5, 8, 10, 18)

10. The nurse practitioner wants to switch ceftriaxone to oral ofloxacin in JS. Your advice is: (EO-9, 12)
    a. Switching to ofloxacin is appropriate
    b. Ofloxacin should be reserved for penicillin-resistant pneumococci
    c. Phenytoin may inhibit the metabolism of ofloxacin and ofloxacin should not be used
    d. Ofloxacin has unreliable pneumococcal sensitivities and should not be used

11. Three days after switching from ceftriaxone to oral antibiotic therapy, JS complains of chills, myalgias, diaphoresis, increased SOB, and dyspnea. What is the most likely explanation of these symptoms? (EO-2, 5, 10, 11)

12. Identify the patient in which pneumococcal vaccine is *not* necessary. (EO-3, 11)
    a. Type 1 diabetic patient
    b. CHF patient
    c. Patients with sickle cell anemia
    d. Elderly patients >65 years old

13. Instruct JS on the proper use of inhalers. (EO-14)

14. Identify a psychosocial issue that is least likely to be observed in this case presentation. (EO-15)
    a. Erectile dysfunction
    b. Communications with patient and family for follow-up care upon discharge from hospital
    c. Alleviate patient concerns on proper use of inhalers
    d. Patient's expressed need to have a cigarette

15. Summarize the pathophysiologic, therapeutic, and disease management concepts for pneumococcal pneumonia utilizing a key points format. (EO-18)

CASE 106
Robert C. Stevens
Topic: Atypical Pneumonia
Level 2
EDUCATIONAL MATERIALS
Chapter 67: Pneumonia

SCENARIO

Patient and Setting

RH, a 64-year-old male; general medicine clinic

Chief Complaint

Two-day history of "flu-like illness" including fever, anorexia, myalgia, headache, diarrhea, cough, and chest pain; presented at clinic because of flu-like symptoms and is admitted for evaluation and treatment of moderate respiratory distress

History of Present Illness

RH started a nonproductive cough 5 days ago without relief from OTC cough medicine; 3 days later he developed fever, diarrhea, myalgia, pleuritic chest pain, headaches, and confusion; these symptoms have worsened over the past 48 hours

Past Medical History

RH has a history of congestive heart failure (CHF) diagnosed 8 years ago; he also developed chronic renal insufficiency due to the progression of CHF; 1 month ago, RH experienced severe pain in his left great toe after walking for 30 minutes; RH's serum uric acid was found to be elevated and allopurinol was started

Past Surgical History

Total hip replacement 15 years ago

Family/Social History:

Family History: Noncontributory

Social History: Smokes 1.5 PPD × 25 years; no alcohol consumption

Medication History

Captopril, 12.5 mg PO TID

Hydrochlorothiazide, 25 mg PO QD

Allopurinol, 300 mg PO QD

Aspirin, 1 baby tablet PO QD

Robitussin, 1 tbsp q6h PRN cough

Allergies

NKDA

Physical Examination

GEN: Well-developed, well-nourished man in moderate respiratory distress

VS: BP 135/88, HR 78, RR 28, T 40.1°C, Wt 73 kg

HEENT: PERRLA; neck supple; (+) JVD 12 cm

COR: Normal S_1 and S_2, positive S_3, no murmurs

CHEST: Bilateral crackles and rales (R>L); pleural rub

ABD: Soft, nontender

GU: Deferred

RECT: Guaiac negative

EXT: 1+ pitting edema bilaterally, no clubbing or cyanosis

NEURO: A and O × 3; cannot recall what he ate for breakfast this AM; deep tendon reflexes intact

Results of Pertinent Laboratory Tests, Serum Drug Concentrations, and Diagnostic Tests

Na 125 (155)	Hct 0.37 (37)	AST 2.78 (167)
K 4.5 (4.5)	Hgb 110 (11)	ALT 3.47 (208)
Cl 101 (101)	Lkcs 18 × 10⁹	Alb 42 (4.2)
HCO₃ 26 (26)	(18 × 10³)	LDH 16.3 (975)
BUN 12.1 (34)	Plts 180 × 10⁹	Uric Acid 446 (7.5)
Cr 185.6 (2.1)	(180 × 10³)	
Glu 7.7 (140)		

Lkc differential: PMN 0.90 (90%), bands 0.08 (8%), lymphs 0.01 (1%)

Sputum: No organisms seen on Gram stain; many polymorphonuclear (PMN) cells with only a few squamous epithelial cells

ABG (on room air): PO_2 64, PCO_2 52, pH 7.38

Blood culture: Pending

Chest x-ray: Diffuse, patchy infiltrates bilaterally (R>L) with right-sided pleural effusion

ECG: Normal sinus rhythm

PROBLEM LIST

Identify principal problems from the scenario in priority order

SOAP NOTE

To be completed by student

QUESTIONS

1. All of the following statements describe *Mycoplasma pneumoniae*, except: (EO-1)
    a. *M. pneumoniae* is the smallest free living organism
    b. *M. pneumoniae* has a cell wall
    c. *M. pneumoniae* is a common cause of community-acquired pneumonia in young adults
    d. *M. pneumoniae* is a common cause of pharyngitis

2. Select the correct statement about *Legionella pneumoniae*. (EO-1)
    a. *L. pneumoniae* is a gram-positive cocci
    b. *L. pneumoniae* is ubiquitous to aquatic environments
    c. Peak incidence for *Legionella* pneumonia occurs in the winter
    d. *L. pneumoniae* can be spread from person to person

3. All of the following signs or symptoms are often associated with *Legionella* pneumonia, *except:* (EO-2)
    a. Increased serum creatinine
    b. Hyponatremia
    c. Diarrhea
    d. CNS changes

4. Based on results from the Gram stain, select the organism that is *not* the likely etiology of the pneumonia in RH. (EO-1, 5)
   a. *Legionella pneumoniae*
   b. *Mycoplasma pneumoniae*
   c. *Chlamydia* spp.
   d. *Haemophilus influenzae*

5. Identify the rationale of including cefotaxime with erythromycin for treatment of community-acquired pneumonia in RH. (EO-11)
   a. Empiric therapy for gram-positive or gram-negative organisms
   b. Synergistic with erythromycin for atypical pathogens
   c. Lack of organisms on Gram stain is predictive of a resistant bacterial pathogen
   d. Admitting medical resident thought RH was ill-appearing and looked like he was going to "crash"

6. Describe the etiology and risk factors associated with Legionnaires' disease. (EO-1, 3)

7. Select the most cost-effective therapy for Legionnaires' disease. (EO-17)
   a. Azithromycin
   b. Clarithromycin
   c. Erythromycin
   d. Gentamicin

8. During rounds on day 4 of erythromycin therapy, RH does not respond to verbal questions and complains that he has buzzing in his ears. Select the most likely explanation for this new event. (EO-4, 5, 8, 10)
   a. Worsening CNS symptoms indicates disease progression
   b. Persistent hyponatremia
   c. Erythromycin-induced ototoxicity
   d. Captopril "tinnitus"

9. Outline measures to minimize the adverse events associated with parenteral erythromycin. (EO-10, 12)

10. RH complains of his "vein hurting" on day 5 of erythromycin IV therapy. On physical examination the antecubital vein is tender, inflamed, and erythematous. RH is afebrile and O_2 saturation levels are in the 90% range. RH remains nauseous and has some diarrhea. The final report on all cultures is no growth. Choose the most appropriate antibiotic for continuation of therapy for Legionnaires' disease. (EO-5, 8, 10, 12)
    a. Rifampin
    b. Gentamicin plus ceftazidime
    c. Switch to erythromycin PO
    d. Azithromycin IV

11. Construct the plan for continued management of pneumonia in RH. (EO-12, 18)

12. Identify the condition in RH that increases his risk of developing hypotension caused by captopril. (EO-5, 8, 9, 10)
    a. Hypoxia
    b. Hyponatremia
    c. Pleural effusion
    d. Jugular venous distention

13. Provide RH with an education plan for management of acute gouty attack with colchicine. (EO-14)

14. Outline the psychosocial factors associated with this case. (EO-15)

15. Summarize pathophysiologic, therapeutic, and disease management concepts for atypical pneumonia utilizing a key points format. (EO-18)

CASE 107
Caroline S. Zeind
Topic: Tuberculosis
Level 3
EDUCATIONAL MATERIALS
Chapter 68: Tuberculosis (transmission and pathogenesis, diagnosis and clinical features, therapeutic strategies, antituberculous agents in current use, initial treatment regimens, drug monitoring parameters, evaluation of response to therapy, psychosocial aspects of the disease)

SCENARIO

Patient and Setting
RC, a 27-year-old female; ED

Chief Complaint
Several weeks of fatigue, weight loss, fevers, chills, night sweats, and a productive cough

History of Present Illness
Decrease in energy over the past few weeks, along with weight loss, fevers, chills, night sweats, and a productive cough

Past Medical History
Diagnosed with HIV infection (September 1998) with *Pneumocystis carinii* pneumonia (PCP) as AIDS-defining illness; last HIV clinic visit was 2 months ago (5/10/99); depression (September 1998)

Past Surgical History
None

Family/Social History
Family History: Heterosexual female with one sexual partner (also diagnosed with HIV infection); currently lives with him

Social History: Nonsmoker; occasional alcohol; works as accountant

Medication History

Nelfinavir, 1250 mg PO BID

Zidovudine 300 mg/lamivudine 150 mg (combination), 1 tablet PO BID

Trimethoprim/sulfamethoxazole, 1 DS tablet PO 3×/week

Sertraline, 50 mg PO QD

Oral contraceptive (30 μg ethinyl estradiol and 0.3 mg norgestrel), 1 tablet PO QD

Multivitamin with iron, 1 tablet PO QD

Allergies

NKDA

Physical Examination

GEN: Thin female with productive cough
VS: BP 110/72, HR 90, RR 22, T 37.5°C, Wt 50 kg (Wt 2 months ago was 55 kg), Ht 160 cm
HEENT: PERRLA, lymphadenopathy
COR: RRR
CHEST: Radiograph: apical fibrocavitary infiltrates
ABD: Nontender, no masses
GU: WNL
RECT: WNL, guaiac negative
EXT: WNL
NEURO: A and O × 4, no headache

Results of Pertinent Laboratory Tests, Serum Drug Concentrations, and Diagnostic Tests

Na 137 (137)	Hgb 100 (10)	LDH 1.7 (100)
K 3.6 (3.6)	Lkc 3.2 × 10⁹	Alk Phos 1.5 (90)
Cl 98 (98)	(3.2 × 10³)	Alb 36 (3.6)
HCO₃ 26 (26)	Plts 160 × 10⁹	T Bili 3.4 (0.2)
BUN 3.6 (10)	(160 × 10³)	Glu 6.1 (110)
Cr 70.7 (0.8)	MCV 115 (115)	Ca 2.2 (8.8)
Total Chol 4.65 (180)	RBC 3.6 × 10¹² (3.6 × 10⁶)	PO₄ 0.92 (3.0)
HDL 1.22 (47)	AST 0.37 (22)	Mg 1.2 (2.5)
Hct 0.30 (30)	ALT 0.38 (23)	Uric Acid 190 (3.2)

Pregnancy test: Negative

Glucose-6-phosphate dehydrogenase (G6PD) deficiency screening test: Negative (test results 9/98)

PPD tuberculin skin test: 8 mm

Three serial sputa for AFB stains and cultures were obtained:

AFB smear: Positive for mycobacteria

Culture and sensitivity: Pending

Blood, urine, and stool cultures and sensitivity: Pending

Induced sputum: Negative for *Pneumocystis carinii* pneumonia

Arterial oxygen: 90 mm Hg (on room air)

Date	Viral load (RT-PCR by Roche Amplicor)	CD4 count (cells/mm³)
Baseline 10/15/98	200,000 copies/mL	140
11/18/98	20,000 copies/mL	155
2/10/99	2,000 copies/mL	180
5/10/99	Undetectable	205

PROBLEM LIST

Identify principal problems from the scenario in priority order [completed Problem List and SOAP Note at end of casebook]

SOAP NOTE

To be completed by student

QUESTIONS

[Answers at end of casebook]

1. RC acquired tuberculosis: (EO-1)
   a. Inhaling airborne particles of *Mycobacterium tuberculosis* from an individual with active tuberculosis
   b. By touching the skin of an individual with active tuberculosis
   c. Following exposure to an individual with tuberculosis infection
   d. By touching an animal with active tuberculosis

2. List signs and symptoms of tuberculosis noted upon RC's presentation to the ED, as well as other signs and symptoms that are probable in patients co-infected with HIV infection. (EO-2)

3. Identify factor(s) present in RC that increases the risk that tuberculosis infection will progress to disease. (EO-3)

4. List RC's physical assessment findings, laboratory tests, and diagnostic tests that support the diagnosis of tuberculosis. (EO-5)

5. Which of the following statements regarding the use of rifabutin is true? (EO-6, 9)
   a. RC should be counseled to use alternative forms of birth control while receiving this agent
   b. The dose of rifabutin for treatment of tuberculosis should be increased while receiving nelfinavir
   c. The most toxic effect of this agent is nephrotoxicity
   d. Rifabutin is a more potent inducer of cytochrome P450 than rifampin

6. Which of the following statements regarding isoniazid is true? (EO-4, 6, 9, 10)
   a. Isoniazid is an inducer of several cytochrome P450 pathways
   b. Hyperuricemia occurs frequently with this drug and uric acid concentration should be checked frequently.
   c. RC should receive supplementation with pyridoxine while receiving isoniazid to reduce the occurrence of isoniazid-induced side effects in the central and peripheral nervous system
   d. The most toxic effect of isoniazid is optic neuritis and

baseline examination of visual acuity should be performed, followed by monthly eye examinations while receiving this agent

7. While receiving pyrazinamide, RC should be carefully monitored for the following dose-limiting toxicity: (EO-10)
   a. Nephrotoxicity
   b. Hepatotoxicity
   c. Optic neuritis
   d. Pulmonary fibrosis

8. Which of the following statements regarding ethambutol is true? (EO-4, 6, 9)
   a. Since the drug is metabolized primarily by the liver, baseline and monthly measurements of liver enzyme levels should be performed
   b. The most toxic effect of this agent is optic neuritis; thus, RC should receive baseline examination of visual acuity prior to initiation of therapy, followed by monthly eye examinations
   c. Ethambutol is a potent inducer of cytochrome P450 and should be avoided in RC since she is taking nelfinavir
   d. Ethambutol is a potent inhibitor of several cytochrome P450-dependent microsomal pathways

9. If streptomycin had been chosen as an antituberculous agent in RC's regimen, what monitoring parameters would be required? (EO-6)
   a. Baseline examination of visual acuity should be performed followed by monthly eye examinations
   b. A transaminase measurement such as aspartate aminotransferase (AST) should be obtained prior to initiation of therapy and monthly
   c. Monitor BUN and serum creatinine; baseline and periodic audiometric testing is also recommended
   d. Serum uric acid should be routinely monitored since acute gout is a common occurrence

10. The following statements regarding the mechanism of action of both pharmacologic and nonpharmacologic interventions in this case are true, *except:* (EO-7)
    a. Combination antituberculous therapy is necessary to cure tuberculosis since the organism harbors within various sites of the body
    b. By implementing directly observed therapy (DOT), patient adherence can be ensured
    c. Antituberculous therapy should not be initiated in a patient suspected of having tuberculosis until the diagnosis is confirmed by positive culture results
    d. RC's response to therapy should be evaluated by sputum cultures

11. RC is continuing her current antiretroviral regimen while treatment for tuberculosis is initiated. All of the following are appropriate treatment options for RC, *except:* (EO-12)
    a. Isoniazid, pyrazinamide, ethambutol, and streptomycin; pyridoxine should also be added
    b. Isoniazid, rifabutin, pyrazinamide, and ethambutol; pyridoxine should also be added
    c. Isoniazid, rifampin, pyrazinamide, and ethambutol; pyridoxine should also be added
    d. Isoniazid, rifabutin, pyrazinamide, and streptomycin; pyridoxine should also be added

12. List the pharmacologic and nonpharmacologic treatment problem(s) present in RC's treatment plan. (EO-11)

13. What psychosocial factors may affect RC's adherence to both pharmacologic and nonpharmacologic therapy? (EO-15)

14. What common emotional disorders may present in a patient diagnosed with tuberculosis?

15. Describe the health care provider's role relative to the proposed psychosocial factors identified. (EO-16)

16. Evaluate the pharmacoeconomic considerations relative to RC's plan of care. (EO-17)

17. Summarize therapeutic, pathophysiologic, and disease management concepts for tuberculosis utilizing a key points format. (EO-18)

CASE 108
Dawn Chandler-Toufieli
Topic: Urinary Tract Infections
Level 3

EDUCATIONAL MATERIALS
Chapter 69: Urinary Tract Infections (epidemiology, pathogenesis, clinical presentation and diagnosis, treatment, pharmacoeconomics)

SCENARIO

Patient and Setting
DL, a 72-year-old female; transferred to the hospital from assisted living facility

Chief Complaint
Two-day history of fever, anorexia, nausea, vomiting, and flank pain

History of Present Illness
During the past 2 weeks, increased difficulty voiding resulting in Foley catheter placement; increasing frequency of anginal attacks to several episodes a week

Past Medical History
RA for 30 years; angina for 15 years; HTN for 3 years; stroke 4 months ago; depression (diagnosed 3 weeks ago)

Past Surgical History
Unknown

Family/Social History
Family History: Adopted–unknown family history
Social History: No alcohol or tobacco intake; assisted living for 2 years

Medication History

Prednisone, 20 mg PO QD × 4 years

Propranolol, 20 mg PO BID × 2 years

Nitroglycerin, 0.4 mg SL PRN CP; MR q 5 min × 3

Aspirin, 325 mg PO QD × 4 months

Amitriptyline, 100 mg PO BID started 3 weeks ago

Allergies

NKDA

Physical Examination

GEN: Thin, ill-appearing elderly woman in moderate distress

VS: BP 163/94, HR 89, RR 28, T 39°C, Wt 55 kg, Ht 166 cm

HEENT: Moon facies

COR: Sinus tachycardia

CHEST: Clear

ABD: CVA tenderness, striae

GU: Foley catheter in place

RECT: Deferred

EXT: Thin, tissue-paper skin, mild swelling of MCP and MTP joints

NEURO: A and O × 3, left-sided partial paralysis, speech impairment

Results of Pertinent Laboratory Tests, Serum Drug Concentrations, and Diagnostic Tests

Na 140 (140)	Lkcs 18 × 10⁹	Alk Phos 1.85 (111)
K 4.2 (4.2)	(18 × 10³)	Alb 40 (4.0)
Cl 102 (102)	Plts 200 × 10⁹	T Bili 18 (1)
HCO₃ 26 (26)	(200 × 10³)	Glu 15.5 (280)
BUN 11.4 (32)	MCV 82 (82)	Ca 2.2 (8.9)
Cr 124 (1.4)	AST 0.58 (35)	PO₄ 0.97 (3)
Hct 0.33 (33)	ALT 0.58 (35)	Mg 0.8 (1.8)
Hgb 140 (14)	LDH 2.1 (126)	Uric Acid 178 (3)

Lkc differential: Neutrophils 76%, bands 10%, lymphs 13%, eos 1%

Urinalysis: >20 bacteria/HPF; >15 Lkcs/HPF

Chest x-ray: WNL; no infiltrates

PROBLEM LIST

Identify principal problems from the scenario in priority order

SOAP NOTE

To be completed by student

QUESTIONS

1. Which of the following disease processes listed in DL's medical history probably contributed to her development of a UTI? (EO-1)
   a. Rheumatoid arthritis
   b. Hypertension
   c. Angina
   d. Neurogenic bladder

2. DL presents with all of the following signs and symptoms of an upper UTI, *except:* (EO-2)
   a. Fever
   b. Nausea and vomiting
   c. Increased anginal attacks
   d. Flank tenderness

3. Which of the following microorganisms is most likely to be the cause of DL's UTI? (EO-3)
   a. *E. coli*
   b. *Proteus*
   c. *Enterobacter*
   d. *Klebsiella*

4. An objective finding in DL that points to a complicated UTI is: (EO-5)
   a. Moon facies
   b. Temperature 39°C
   c. Mild swelling of MCP and MTP joints
   d. A and O × 3

5. DL may have drug-induced urinary retention. Which of DL's following drugs has been reported to cause urinary retention? (EO-10)
   a. Prednisone
   b. Propranolol
   c. Nitroglycerin
   d. Amitriptyline

6. Describe the mechanisms of action of the pharmacologic and nonpharmacologic interventions in the treatment of DL's pyelonephritis. (EO-7)

7. Which of DL's medications is renally eliminated? (EO-6)
   a. Aspirin
   b. Nitroglycerin
   c. Ampicillin
   d. Prednisone

8. What is DL's calculated creatinine clearance? (EO-6)
   a. 16 mL/min or 0.96 L/hr
   b. 32 mL/min or 1.9 L/hr
   c. 64 mL/min or 3.8 L/hr
   d. 100 mL/min or 6 L/hr

9. What dose of gentamicin will achieve a peak of 7 mg/L and a trough < 2 mg/L in DL? (EO-6)
   a. 80 mg IV 8h
   b. 90 mg IV q12h
   c. 100 mg IV q8h
   d. 120 mg IV q12h

10. One day after admission, DL's urine culture returns with *Pseudomonas aeruginosa* as the causative organism. What antibiotics would provide adequate coverage? Should DL's therapy be changed? (EO-12)

11. After 3 days of intravenous antibiotic therapy, DL has been afebrile for 48 hr. Would you recommend a change to oral therapy? If so, what options are available? (EO-12)

12. List the pharmacologic and nonpharmacologic treatment problem(s) present in DL's treatment plan. (EO-11)

13. What psychosocial factors may affect DL's adherence to both pharmacologic and nonpharmacologic therapy? (EO-15)

14. Describe the health care provider's role relative to the proposed psychosocial factors identified. (EO-16)

15. Evaluate the pharmacoeconomic considerations relative to DL's plan of care. (EO-17)

16. Summarize pathophysiologic, therapeutic, and disease management concepts for a complicated UTI utilizing a key points format. (EO-18)

CASE 109
Dawn Chandler-Toufieli
Topic: Urinary Tract Infections
Level 1

EDUCATIONAL MATERIALS

Chapter 69: Urinary Tract Infections (epidemiology, pathogenesis, clinical presentation and diagnosis, treatment, pharmacoeconomics)

SCENARIO

Patient and Setting

AM, a 28-year-old female; outpatient clinic

Chief Complaint

Two-day history of frequency, burning, and pain upon urination; increased lower abdominal pain and vaginal discharge over the past week

History of Present Illness

Complains of urinary symptoms similar to those of previous urinary tract infections (UTIs) which started approximately 2 days ago; also experiencing increasingly severe lower abdominal pain and noted a brown, foul-smelling vaginal discharge after having unprotected sex with a former boyfriend

Past Medical History

Recurrent urinary tract infections (3 UTIs this year); gonorrhea × 2, Chlamydia × 1; Gravida IV, para III

Past Surgical History

Tubal ligation

Family/Social History

Family History: Single; history of multiple male sexual partners; currently lives with her new boyfriend and 3 children

Social History: denies smoking, alcohol use, and IVDA

Medication History

None

Allergies

Trimethoprim (TMP)/sulfamethoxazole (SMX), rash

Physical Examination

GEN: Female in moderate distress
VS: BP 100/80, HR 80, RR 16, T 99.7°F, Wt 60 kg, Ht 5'5"
HEENT: WNL
COR: WNL
CHEST: WNL
ABD: Soft, tender bilaterally, increased suprapubic tenderness
GU: Cervical motion tenderness, adnexal tenderness, foul-smelling vaginal drainage
RECT: WNL
EXT: WNL
NEURO: WNL

Results of Pertinent Laboratory Tests, Serum Drug Concentrations, and Diagnostic Tests

Na 136 (136)	Lkcs 6 × 10⁹	Alb 40 (4.0)
K 4.2 (4.2)	(6 × 10³)	T Bili 18 (1.0)
Cl 102 (102)	Plts 350 × 10⁹	Glu 5.6 (101)
HCO₃ 27 (27)	(350 × 10³)	Ca 2.2 (8.8)
BUN 3.9 (11)	MCV 86 (86)	PO₄ 1.28 (4.0)
Cr 80 (0.9)	ALT 0.58 (35)	Mg 1.0 (2.0)
Hct 0.38 (38)	LDH 2.66 (150)	Uric Acid 357 (6.0)
Hgb 126 (12.6)	Alk Phos 2.0 (120)	

Lkc differential: Neutrophils 0.68 (68%), bands 0.07 (7%), lymphs 0.13 (13%), monos 0.08 (8%), eos 0.02 (2%)

Urinalysis: Straw-colored, 1.015, 8.0 pH, prot-, gluc-, ket-, many bacteria, Lkcs 10–15, RBC 0–1

Urine Gram stain: Gram-negative rods

Vaginal discharge culture: Gram-negative diplococci, *Neisseria gonorrhoeae;* sensitivities pending

Positive monoclonal AB for *Chlamydia,* KOH preparation, wet preparation, and VDRL negative

PROBLEM LIST

Identify principal problems from the scenario in priority order [completed Problem List and SOAP Note at end of casebook]

SOAP NOTE

To be completed by student

QUESTIONS

[Answers at end of casebook]

1. AM presents with all of the following signs and symptoms of a cystitis *except:* (EO-2)
   a. Urinary frequency
   b. Urinary urgency
   c. Dysuria
   d. Vaginal discharge

2. All of the following factors identified in AM's medical history probably contributed to her UTI, *except:* (EO-1, 3)
   a. Sexual history
   b. Past history of UTIs
   c. Past history of tubal ligation
   d. Female sex

3. What microorganism is the most likely cause of AM's UTI? (EO-1)
   a. *Klebsiella*
   b. *Pseudomonas aeruginosa*
   c. *Proteus*
   d. *E. coli*

4. What made AM a candidate for prophylactic antibiotics for recurrent UTIs? (EO-3)
   a. The severity of her current UTI
   b. The number of UTIs she has had this year
   c. The number of STDs she has had this year
   d. The number of pregnancies she has had in her lifetime

5. What is another antibiotic that could have been used as a prophylactic antibiotic for AM? (EO-8, 12)
   a. Norfloxacin
   b. Amoxicillin
   c. Gentamicin
   d. Ampicillin

6. Describe the mechanisms of action of the pharmacologic and nonpharmacologic interventions in this case. (EO-7)

7. All of the following oral regimens are possible treatments for AM's gonorrhea, *except:* (EO-8, 12)
   a. Azithromycin 1 g PO × 1
   b. Cefixime 400 mg PO × 1
   c. Ciprofloxacin 500 mg PO × 1
   d. Ofloxacin 400 mg PO × 1

8. If doxycycline were used to treat AM's *Chlamydia*, what is the recommended length of therapy? (EO-12)
   a. Single dose
   b. 3 days
   c. 7 days
   d. 10 days

9. What would you include in your counseling session with AM if she had been prescribed doxycycline? (EO-9, 10)
   a. Take doxycycline with a full glass of milk to prevent esophagitis
   b. Avoid unnecessary and prolonged sun exposure
   c. Avoid sunscreen with UVA and UVB protection
   d. Take an antacid with doxycycline to prevent GI distress

10. Describe the health care provider's role relative to the proposed psychosocial factors identified. (EO-16)

11. What psychosocial factors may affect AM's adherence to both pharmacologic and nonpharmacologic therapy? (EO-15)

12. Summarize pathophysiologic, therapeutic, and disease management concepts for AM's recurrent UTIs utilizing a key points format. (EO-18)

CASE 110
Michelle Ceresia
Topic: Intra-abdominal Infections
 Level 2

EDUCATIONAL MATERIALS
Chapter 70: Intra-abdominal Infections (primary peritonitis) (definitions, treatment goals, epidemiology, pathophysiology, clinical presentation and diagnosis, psychosocial, treatment, improving outcomes, pharmacoeconomics)

SCENARIO

Patient and Setting
MS, a 42-year-old male; ED

Chief Complaint
Fever, chills, abdominal pain, nausea; weeks of fatigue and loss of appetite

History of Present Illness
Over the past 2 days: fever, chills, abdominal pain, and nausea; last few weeks: chronic fatigue and loss of appetite; for the last 2 years: intermittent fatigue, right upper quadrant pain, weakness, anorexia, ascites, bleeding gums, and occasional epistaxis

Past Medical History
Posttraumatic seizure disorder (9 years ago; last seizure 26 months ago); positive for hepatitis C virus (HCV) (4 years, infected from a blood transfusion for head trauma); liver biopsy positive for chronic active hepatitis (3 years ago); cirrhosis (3 years); ascites; primary peritonitis (8 months ago)

Past Surgical History
None

Family/Social History

Family History: Father alive and well; mother died in automobile accident 9 years ago

Social History: Denies alcohol or tobacco use; single, lives alone

Medication History

Spironolactone, 100 mg PO QD

Furosemide, 40 mg PO QD

Phenytoin, 300 mg PO QHS

Allergies

NKDA

Physical Examination

GEN: Tired-looking man in moderate distress

VS: BP 144/84, HR 84, RR 22, T 39°C, Wt 73 kg, Ht 183 cm

HEENT: PERRLA, EOMI, anicteric

COR: RRR with no S_3 or S_4, no m/g/r

CHEST: Lungs clear to auscultation and percussion

ABD: Increased girth, + hepatosplenomegaly, + fluid wave, + abdominal pain, + diffuse tenderness, hypoactive bowel sounds

GU: WNL

RECT: WNL

EXT: 2+ edema

NEURO: WNL, no asterixis

Results of Pertinent Laboratory Tests, Serum Drug Concentrations, and Diagnostic Tests

Na 129 (129)	Lkc 12.1 × 10⁹	Alb 35 (3.5)
K 3.7 (3.7)	(12.1 × 10³)	T Bili 36 (2.1)
Cl 105 (105)	Plts 84 × 10⁹	Glu 6.4 (115)
HCO₃ 24 (24)	(84 × 10³)	Ca 2.3 (9.3)
BUN 5.7 (16)	MCV 96 (96)	PO₄ 1.29 (4.0)
Cr 88.4 (1.0)	AST 3.72 (223)	Mg 0.9 (1.8)
Hct 0.42 (42)	ALT 2.87 (172)	PTT 34 (34)
Hgb 120 (12)	Alk Phos 0.58 (35)	PT 13.7 (13.7)
		INR 1.4

Lkc differential: Neutrophils 0.80 (80%), bands 0.09 (9%), lymphs 0.08 (8%)

Phenytoin serum concentration: 49.5 μmol/L (12.5 mg/L)

Anti-HCV positive

HCV-PCR quantitative: 1.2 million copies/mL

Urinalysis: WNL

Paracentesis: Cloudy ascitic fluid, pH 7.18, polymorphonuclear count (PMN) 540 cells/m³

Gram stain (ascitic fluid): Gram-negative rods

Ascites culture: Pending

Blood cultures: Pending

Chest x-ray: WNL

ECG: WNL

EEG: WNL

Liver biopsy: 20% bridging necrosis

PROBLEM LIST

Identify principal problems from the scenario in priority order [completed Problem List and SOAP Note at end of casebook]

SOAP NOTE

To be completed by student

QUESTIONS

[Answers at end of casebook]

1. Which of the following is a risk factor for MS's primary peritonitis? (EO-1)
   a. Epistaxis
   b. Ascites
   c. Seizures
   d. Phenytoin

2. List the signs and symptoms of primary peritonitis noted in MS. (EO-2)

3. List physical assessment findings, laboratory tests, and diagnostic tests that support the diagnosis of primary peritonitis in MS. (EO-5)

4. Which of the following statements regarding peritonitis is true? (EO-1, 3)
   a. A majority of secondary peritonitis cases are monomicrobial
   b. Pathogens most likely to cause primary peritonitis include *Escherichia coli*, *Klebsiella* spp., and other gram-negative bacilli
   c. Primary peritonitis may result from bacterial spread from the bloodstream, lymphatic system, or torn bowel
   d. Peritoneal dialysis is a risk factor for secondary peritonitis

5. List the pharmacologic and nonpharmacologic treatment problems present in MS's treatment plan. (EO-11)

6. All of the following are true regarding the treatment of primary peritonitis, *except:* (EO-8, 17)
   a. Primary peritonitis prophylaxis is recommended for high-risk cirrhotic patients
   b. Surgical debridement combined with appropriate antibiotic coverage is the standard of care
   c. Ability to penetrate the infected site, potential adverse reactions, and cost are factors that should be considered when selecting an antibiotic
   d. Duration of treatment for MS's primary peritonitis is not clearly defined

7. All of the following are appropriate initial treatment regimens for primary peritonitis, *except:* (EO-8)
   a. Gentamicin plus ampicillin
   b. Ceftizoxime
   c. Cefoxitin
   d. Clindamycin

8. All of the following statements regarding a detailed education plan for MS are true, *except:* (EO-14)
   a. MS should be counseled not take norfloxacin with food, multivitamins or antacids
   b. MS should be encouraged to purchase a pill box or mark a calendar to help address potential adherence problems
   c. MS should be instructed to ask his pharmacist before taking over the counter medications or herbal remedies to avoid hepatotoxic drugs
   d. MS should be assured that HCV is not communicable

9. A computed tomography (CT) scan reveals MS has an abscess. All of the following statements regarding intra-abdominal abscesses are true, *except:* (EO-1, 7, 8)
   a. Aminoglycosides are effective in the treatment of abscesses because of the low oxygen tension environment
   b. Intra-abdominal abscess may be associated with primary, secondary, or tertiary peritonitis
   c. Antibiotic therapy should include coverage for anaerobes
   d. Surgical drainage of the abscess is often necessary

10. Which of the following statements regarding the treatment of hepatitis and complications of hepatic failure is true? (EO-6, 7, 8, 10)
    a. Interferon therapy hasn't shown efficacy in the treatment of chronic HCV
    b. Furosemide is minimally protein bound therefore hepatic disease has little to no effect on its free fraction
    c. Spironolactone inhibits aldosterone-mediated retention of salt and water making it an effective agent in ascites
    d. Conversion of oral to IV furosemide is 1:1 since oral absorption is predictable and extensive

11. Which of the following statements regarding phenytoin is true? (EO-6, 9, 10)
    a. Phenytoin is 90% protein bound and should be adjusted in patients who are hypoalbuminemic and/or with severe renal failure
    b. Phenytoin-induced hepatotoxicity commonly occurs several years after the start of therapy
    c. Absorption of phenytoin is enhanced when co-administered with enteral nutrition
    d. Phenytoin steady state is usually attained within 3 days

12. What psychosocial factors may affect MS's adherence to both pharmacologic and nonpharmacologic therapy? (EO-15)

13. Evaluate the pharmacoeconomic considerations relative to MS's plan of care. (EO-17)

14. Summarize pathophysiologic, therapeutic, and disease management concepts for primary peritonitis utilizing a key points format. (EO-18)

CASE 111
Robert C. Stevens
Topic: Infectious Diarrhea

EDUCATIONAL MATERIALS
Chapter 71: Gastrointestinal Infections

SCENARIO

Patient and Setting
FT, a 59-year-old male; cruise ship infirmary

Chief Complaint
Diarrhea, abdominal cramps, headache, and malaise

History of Present Illness
FT presents with a 3-day history of diarrhea, abdominal cramps, headache, and malaise; he has been feeling feverish for about 24 hours; diarrhea, which looked clear on day 1, has become bloody and more voluminous

Past Medical History
FT has a 9-year history of angina and coronary artery disease; since becoming ill on the cruise, he has been experiencing frequent episodes of chest tightness and shortness of breath with exercise; history of congestive heart failure (CHF), first diagnosed 4 years ago after he experienced shortness of breath, dyspnea on exertion, and needing two pillows at night to breathe while sleeping

Past Surgical History
Two coronary artery bypass surgeries, the last being performed 6 months ago

Family/Social History
Family History: Noncontributory

Social History: Smoked 1 PPD since age 17, none in the past year; alcohol socially; drinks 8 cups of coffee per day

Medication History
Digoxin, 0.25 mg PO QD

Aspirin, 325 mg PO QD

Furosemide, 40 mg PO BID

Verapamil, 80 mg TID (started 1 week ago)

Isosorbide, 10 mg PO TID

Nitroglycerin, 0.4 mg SL PRN

Ibuprofen, 200 mg PO PRN headaches or pain

Allergies

NKDA

Physical Examination

GEN: Well-developed, well-nourished man in mild distress

VS: BP 150/85, HR 100, RR 24, T 38.9°C, Wt 95 kg (97 kg before the cruise)

HEENT: Dry mucous membranes, mild jugular venous distention

COR: Normal S_1 and S_2, presence of an S_3 gallop

CHEST: Clear

ABD: Soft and tender; positive hepatojugular reflux

GU: WNL

RECT: Perirectal tenderness, erythematous

EXT: 1+ ankle edema; normal skin turgor

NEURO: A and O × 3, cranial nerves intact

Results of Pertinent Laboratory Tests, Serum Drug Concentrations, and Diagnostic Tests

Na 129 (129) HCO_3 18 (18)   Cr 124 (1.4)

K 2.9 (2.9)   BUN 10.7 (30)   Ca 2.5 (10)

Cl 95 (95)

Stool: Mucoid, bloody; (+) fecal Lkcs

Stool culture: Comma-shaped gram-negative rods identified as *Campylobacter jejuni*

PROBLEM LIST

Identify principal problems from the scenario in priority order

SOAP NOTE

To be completed by student

QUESTIONS

1. All of the following are appropriate treatment goals of gastroenteritis, *except:* (EO-6, 8, 11)
   a. Recommend antidiarrhea agents in all cases of viral gastroenteritis
   b. Deliver adequate oral fluid and electrolyte rehydration based on degree of dehydration
   c. Determine need for antibiotics based, in part, on duration of disease
   d. Hospitalize patient with severe dehydration for intravenous fluid therapy

2. What is the usual incubation time of pathogens associated with bacterial gastroenteritis? (EO-1)
   a. Less than 4 hours
   b. 0.5–72 hours
   c. 5–7 days
   d. 7–14 days

3. Identify the bacterial gastroenteritic pathogen associated with shellfish ingestion. (EO-1)
   a. *Campylobacter jejuni*
   b. *Salmonella enteritidis*
   c. *Yersinia enterocolitica*
   d. *Vibrio cholerae*

4. Describe the most likely route of transmission of *Campylobacter jejuni* gastroenteritis in FT. (EO-1)

5. *Campylobacter jejuni* is most often implicated as a cause of: (EO-3)
   a. Sinusitis
   b. Traveler's diarrhea
   c. Pyelonephritis
   d. Otitis media

6. FT wants to know how many days it will take for the diarrhea to resolve. (EO-2)
   a. Within 24 hr
   b. 2–3 days
   c. 5–7 days
   d. 2 weeks

7. The primary reason a systemic antibiotic (erythromycin) was used to treat the infectious diarrhea in FT was: (EO-8)
   a. FT was at risk of developing spontaneous bacterial peritonitis
   b. Rapid resolution of diarrhea was necessary since FT has underlying cardiovascular conditions
   c. FT's stools were mucoid, bloody, and more voluminous; high temperature
   d. FT did not want his vacation compromised by having diarrhea

8. Highlight the psychosocial factors associated with FT's infections. (EO-15)

9. Choose the advantage of including bismuth subsalicylate (BSS) to treat *Campylobacter* diarrhea. (EO-8, 11, 12)
   a. BSS has antimicrobial activity against *Campylobacter*
   b. BSS helps to restore normal GI flora
   c. BSS reduces abdominal bloating and pain
   d. BSS restores the alimentary integument

10. Counsel FT about the side effects of erythromycin. (EO-9)

11. FT wants to take loperamide to alleviate his diarrhea because he does not want "this GI bug to ruin my vacation." Provide appropriate advice. (EO-8)

12. After 3 doses of erythromycin, FT returns to the clinic complaining of increased nausea with some vomiting within 30 minutes of erythromycin. He is adamant about continuing antibiotic therapy but wants a different drug. Select the most appropriate and cost-effective antibiotic. (EO-10, 11)
   a. Doxycycline
   b. Cephalexin
   c. Ofloxacin
   d. Chloramphenicol

13. Outline the issues you would discuss with FT regarding instructions on how to take the antibiotic you selected in question 8 and the potential side effects. (EO-10, 14)

14. Instruct FT and his wife on how to reduce one's exposure to enteropathogens. (EO-14)

15. Summarize pathophysiologic, therapeutic, and disease management concepts for gastroenteritis utilizing a key points format. (EO-18)

CASE 112
Robert C. Stevens
Topic: Viral Gastroenteritis
Level 1

EDUCATIONAL MATERIALS
Chapter 71: Gastrointestinal Infections

SCENARIO

Patient and Setting

JP, 3-year-old boy; clinic

Chief Complaint

Diarrhea, vomiting, fever, no appetite, lethargic, restless and irritable

History of Present Illness

JP developed diarrhea 3 days ago, which has increased in frequency to where he has had 8–10 loose, watery stools in the past 24 hours alone; mom states that JP has become more lethargic and does not care to interact with his siblings; he has consumed little food during this period but is thirsty and requests apple juice; other family members are in good health and have no gastrointestinal (GI) symptoms

Past Medical History

Usual childhood diseases including two episodes of otitis media (last occurrence 8 months ago)

Past Surgical History

None

Family/Social History

Family History: Lives at home with his mom and dad and 2 sisters age 7 and 6 years old

Social History: JP attends a day care where mom reports that several children have been "sick at home with diarrhea"

Medication History

Immunizations: up to date

Allergies

NKDA

Physical Examination

GEN: Pale, weak-appearing child in no acute distress who did not want to be examined but was otherwise cooperative

VS: BP 90/70 (supine), HR 125, RR 22, T 38.1°C, Wt 13.3 kg (1 month ago: Wt 14.5 kg, 75th%)

HEENT: Sunken eyes; dry mucous membranes; tympanic membranes normal; crying without tears

COR: Normal S_1 and S_2; tachycardia; no murmur

CHEST: Clear

ABD: Soft and tender; no guarding

GU: WNL

RECT: Perirectal erythema

EXT: Decreased skin turgor

NEURO: Oriented but not attentive or alert; normal deep tendon reflexes

Results of Pertinent Laboratory Tests, Serum Drug Concentrations, and Diagnostic Tests

Na 131 (131)	BUN 8.9 (25)	Lkcs 8.5 × 10⁹
K 3.0 (3.0)	Cr 106 (1.2)	(8.5 × 10³)
Cl 93 (93)	Glu 3.4 (61)	Plts 170 × 10⁹
HCO₃ 20 (20)	Hct 0.34 (34)	(170 × 10³)
	Hgb 110 (11)	

Urinalysis: pH 7.4, specific gravity (SG) 1.005; clear but dark yellow color; no organisms seen

PROBLEM LIST

Identify principal problems from the scenario in priority order [completed Problem List and SOAP Note at end of casebook]

SOAP NOTE

To be completed by student

QUESTIONS

[Answers at end of casebook]

1. Identify the virus referred to as the "winter vomiting disease." (EO-1)
   a. Rotavirus
   b. Norwalk virus
   c. Calicivirus
   d. Astrovirus

2. All of the following statements describe rotavirus, *except:* (EO-1)
   a. Seasonal appearance starting in the fall in western states then moving eastward by winter and spring
   b. Primarily affects infants and children less than 24 months of age
   c. Adults are immune to rotavirus gastroenteritis
   d. Transmitted by the fecal-oral route

3. Choose the virus that causes gastroenteritis but is not associated with respiratory tract symptoms. (EO-1)
   a. Rotavirus
   b. Norwalk virus
   c. Adenovirus
   d. Astrovirus

4. Identify the most common mode of transmission of viral gastroenteritis. (EO-1, 3)
   a. Fecal-oral contamination
   b. Shellfish
   c. Ingestion or handling of undercooked meats
   d. Ingestion of nonrefrigerated dairy products

5. Choose the time period of incubation and duration of symptoms for rotavirus. (EO-1, 8)
   a. 2 days; 3–8 days
   b. 8–10 days; 5–12 days
   c. 12–48 hr; 1–2 days
   d. 1–4 days; 4–5 days

6. Select the most common gastrointestinal virus that is likely causing diarrhea in JP. (EO-1, 3)
   a. Rotavirus
   b. Norwalk virus
   c. Calicivirus
   d. Astrovirus

7. Calculate the degree of dehydration in JP based upon weight loss and clinical presentation. (EO-5)
   a. Mild (<5%)
   b. Moderate (5–10%)
   c. Severe (>10%)

8. Oral rehydration solutions (ORS) provide all of the following advantages compared with IV fluid replacement, *except:* (EO-8)
   a. Less invasive
   b. Less costly
   c. Less likely to result in overhydration
   d. Comparable rate of rehydration in patients with severe dehydration (>10% fluid deficit)

9. Construct a therapeutic plan to replenish fluid and electrolytes with Pedialyte. (EO-5, 8, 12, 18)

10. Provide instructions to JP's mom about how to care for her child during his bout of viral gastroenteritis. (EO-14)

11. Outline the psychosocial factors that may affect JP's outcome. (EO-15)

12. Summarize pathophysiologic, therapeutic, and disease management concepts for viral gastroenteritis utilizing a key points format. (EO-18)

CASE 113
Robert C. Stevens
Topic: Infective Endocarditis

EDUCATIONAL MATERIALS
Chapter 72: Infective Endocarditis

SCENARIO

Patient and Setting
SF, a 65-year-old woman; hospital

Chief Complaint
Fever, chills, night sweats, weakness, headaches, and a decreased appetite

History of Present Illness
SF had mitral valve replacement 2 years prior to admission, secondary to severe mitral valve regurgitation; 4 weeks prior to admission, she underwent a dental procedure—SF received amoxicillin 2 g PO 1 hour before this procedure; SF started daily flossing 24 hours after the dental procedure; 2 weeks later (i.e., 2 weeks prior to admission) she developed fevers to 38°C, chills, night sweats, malaise, headache, and decreased appetite that resulted in a 3.5-kg weight loss

Past Medical History
SF had a long history of mitral valve regurgitation, discovered in childhood; underwent MVR 2 years ago; since this time, she has always taken prophylactic antibiotics prior to any high-risk procedure and has had no history of endocarditis or other infections; SF has been taking warfarin daily since her valve replacement and has been on benzodiazepines since her MVR for anxiety disorders and is now dependent on these agents

Past Surgical History
Mitral valve replacement 2 years PTA

Family/Social History
Family History: Noncontributory
Social History: No tobacco or alcohol use

Medication History
Warfarin, 2.5 mg QD
Diazepam, 5 mg PO TID
Alprazolam, 1 mg PO QHS PRN sleep

Allergies

NKDA

Physical Examination

GEN: Pale, elderly-appearing woman in no acute distress

VS: BP 120/70, HR 75, RR 13, T 39°C, Wt 60 kg, Ht 160 cm

HEENT: PERRLA, oral cavity without lesions or erythema, Roth spots seen upon ophthalmologic examination

COR: Systolic ejection murmur III/VI at the left sternal border, normal S_1 and S_2

CHEST: Clear to auscultation and percussion

ABD: Soft, nontender; no hepatosplenomegaly

GU: WNL

RECT: Guaiac positive

EXT: Embolic lesions seen on fingertips of both hands; bruising noticed on both legs from thigh to ankle and upper arms

NEURO: Oriented to time, place, and person; cranial nerves intact; normal deep tendon reflexes

Results of Pertinent Laboratory Tests, Serum Drug Concentrations, and Diagnostic Tests

Na 138 (138)	Lkcs 12 × 10⁹	Alb 51 (5.1)
K 4.2 (4.2)	(12 × 10³)	T Bili 13.7 (0.8)
Cl 98 (98)	Plts 170 × 10⁹	Glu 5.55 (100)
HCO₃ 22 (22)	(170 × 10³)	Ca 2.4 (9.7)
BUN 3.6 (10)	MCV 65 (65)	PO₄ 1.07 (3.3)
Cr 106 (1.2)	AST 0.58 (35)	Mg 1 (2)
Hct 0.30 (30)	ALT 0.33 (20)	PT 29
Hgb 120 (12)	LDH 1.7 (101)	INR 6.3
	Alk Phos 1.08 (65)	

Urinalysis: No organisms seen, clear, no RBC/lkcs/casts, pH 7.5, SG 1.020

Chest x-ray: Normal

Transesophageal echocardiogram: Vegetation 1 × 2 cm located on prosthetic mitral valve

Blood cultures: Pending

PROBLEM LIST

Identify principal problems from the scenario in priority order [completed Problem List and SOAP Note at end of casebook]

SOAP NOTE

To be completed by student

QUESTIONS

[Answers at end of casebook]

1. All of the following are treatment goals of bacterial endocarditis, *except:* (EO-6, 8, 11)
   a. Use bactericidal antibiotics
   b. Duration of therapy is 10–14 days
   c. Antibiotic doses need to be high in order to penetrate the infected valvular vegetation
   d. Combination therapy is required for enterococcal endocarditis

2. Identify the valve most commonly infected in an intravenous drug user. (EO-3)
   a. Aortic valve
   b. Mitral valve
   c. Pulmonary valve
   d. Tricuspid valve

3. Select the item that is *not* a risk factor for infective endocarditis in SF. (EO-1, 3)
   a. Dental procedure
   b. Prosthetic heart valve
   c. Mitral valve prolapse
   d. Angina

4. Describe the pathophysiologic mechanism as to how infective endocarditis developed in SF. (EO-1)

5. Select the most likely pathogen causing infective endocarditis in SF: (EO-1, 3, 5)
   a. Viridans streptococci
   b. *Staphylococcus aureus*
   c. Enterococci
   d. *Escherichia coli*

6. Explain the rationale of low-dose gentamicin for only the first 5 days of treatment. (EO-4, 7, 8, 11)

7. Choose the recommended duration of antimicrobial therapy in SF. (EO-11)
   a. 7–10 days
   b. 2 weeks
   c. 4 weeks
   d. At least 6 weeks

8. On hospital day 2, blood cultures were (+) methicillin-sensitive *Staphylococcus aureus*. Which of the following is appropriate at this time? (EO-8, 11, 12)
   a. Switch vancomycin to oxacillin
   b. Continue vancomycin
   c. Continue vancomycin but discontinue gentamicin
   d. Switch vancomycin to nafcillin and discontinue rifampin

9. List the therapeutic endpoints of antibiotic therapy in SF. (EO-8, 11, 18)

10. Select the most likely drug interaction in SF. (EO-9)
    a. Chlordiazepoxide can inhibit the metabolism of rifampin
    b. Rifampin will induce the metabolism of warfarin
    c. Vancomycin will increase the renal clearance of gentamicin
    d. Rifampin reduces the absorption of chlordiazepoxide

11. After 3 days of antistaphylococcal therapy the peripheral blood culture remains positive for *S. aureus*. Choose the most appropriate intervention at this point. (EO-11, 12)
    a. Continue current antibiotics and ask the microbiology lab to test the strain for tolerance

b. Change antibiotics to ciprofloxacin and rifampin

c. Change antibiotics to cefazolin, amikacin, and rifampin

d. Requires surgical replacement of infected prosthetic valve

12. How would you counsel SF about dental care? (EO-14)

13. Identify a psychosocial issue that must be considered in SF. (EO-15)

    a. SF is likely to be concerned about the need for surgical replacement of the prosthetic mitral valve

    b. SF thinks she is sick because her urine is orange

    c. SF feels fine and wants to go home

    d. There are no major psychosocial events to consider in this patient because she is addicted to benzodiazepines

14. Select the most cost-effective therapy for treatment of methicillin-sensitive *Staphylococcus aureus* in SF. (EO-17)

    a. Oxacillin

    b. Vancomycin

    c. Oxacillin plus rifampin

    d. Oxacillin plus amikacin

15. Summarize pathophysiologic, therapeutic, and disease management concepts for infective endocarditis utilizing a key points format. (EO-18)

CASE 114
Robert C. Stevens
Topic: CNS Infections—*Haemophilus influenzae* Type B Meningitis

 Level 3

EDUCATIONAL MATERIALS
Chapter 73: Central Nervous System Infections

SCENARIO

Patient and Setting
AC, a 66-year-old male; ED

Chief Complaint
Fever, confusion, and lethargy

History of Present Illness
AC has a 2-day history of fever and a painful headache unrelieved by Ascriptin; this morning AC complained of increasing lethargy and slept much of the day; several hours prior to admission AC was difficult to arouse and had three documented episodes of vomiting (no hematemesis) at home

Past Medical History
Rheumatoid arthritis (RA) × 16 years; S/P splenectomy and compound fracture of right humerus 8 years ago secondary to injuries sustained in a MVA; AC sustained no head trauma at that time

Past Surgical History
S/P splenectomy

Family/Social History
Family History: Retired small-business owner; lives at home with his wife and provides care during the weekdays for their 3 grandchildren ages 5, 3, and 2 years

Social History: Denies cigarette smoking for the past 20 years; alcohol 3–4 beers daily

Medication History
Diclofenac, 200 mg PO TID

Methotrexate, 15 mg PO weekly (last dose was 4 days PTA)

Folate, 1 mg PO QD

Allergies
NKDA

Physical Examination
GEN: Well-developed male in a state of stupor

VS: BP 135/72, HR 86, RR 30, T 40.5°C, Wt 62.5 kg (down 2.5 kg)

HEENT: Dilated poorly reactive pupils; normal vessels without papilledema; decreased neck mobility; positive Brudzinski's sign

COR: Normal S_1 and S_2, (−) S_3 or S_4

CHEST: Clear to auscultation and percussion

ABD: Soft, nontender; positive bowel sounds

GU: WNL

RECT: Guaiac positive

EXT: WNL

NEURO: Not oriented to person, place, or time; lethargic; reflexes were 3+ throughout and symmetrical; palsy of cranial nerve VI

Results of Pertinent Laboratory Tests, Serum Drug Concentrations, and Diagnostic Tests

Na 141 (141)	Cr 80 (0.9)	Plts 285 × 10⁹
K 4.2 (4.2)	Hct 0.34 (34)	(285 × 10³)
Cl 105 (105)	Hgb 148 (14.8)	Mg 1.05 (2.1)
HCO₃ 24 (24)	Lkcs 16.5 × 10⁹	Glu 5.0 (90)
BUN 6.4 (18)	(16.5 × 10³)	Alb 45 (4.5)

Cerebrospinal fluid: Opening pressure 15 mm Hg, Lkcs 1.8 × 10⁹ (18.5 × 10³), 90% PMN, Glu 1.7 (30), protein 1.25 (125)

CSF Gram's stain: Gram-negative coccobacillus

Blood and CSF cultures: Pending

CT scan of the head: No mass, abscess; evidence of increased cerebral edema

PROBLEM LIST

Identify principal problems from the scenario in priority order

SOAP NOTE

To be completed by student

QUESTIONS

1. All of the following are treatment goals for CNS infections, *except:* (EO-1, 6, 7, 8)
   a. Bacteriostatic antibiotics should be avoided
   b. Antibiotic dosing should be high enough to ensure adequate CSF concentrations
   c. Direct instillation of antibiotics into the CSF is recommended for all cases of bacterial meningitis
   d. Therapy should be initiated promptly

2. All of the following are pathways in which pathogens are thought to infect the meninges, *except:* (EO-1)
   a. Hematogenous seeding
   b. Direct inoculation through trauma
   c. Contiguous spread from a parameningeal focus
   d. Inflammation of the blood-brain barrier

3. List the predisposing factors in AC that place him at risk for HiB meningitis. (EO-1, 3)

4. What is a positive Brudzinski's sign? (EO-1, 2)

5. All of the following clinical signs and symptoms in AC are consistent with bacterial meningitis, *except:* (EO-2)
   a. CSF pleocytosis
   b. Hypoglycorrhachia
   c. Serum glucose 5.0 (90)
   d. Altered mental status

6. List the reasons that support use of adjunctive dexamethasone in AC. (EO-2, 5, 8, 12)

7. Identify the most significant parameter to determine efficacy of ceftriaxone. (EO-11)
   a. Sterilization of CSF
   b. Temperature
   c. White blood cells
   d. Serum glucose

8. Identify the adverse effect associated with high-dose ceftriaxone. (EO-10)
   a. Neutropenia
   b. Mental status changes
   c. Nephrotoxicity
   d. Cholelithiasis

9. The medical student asks your opinion about intrathecal (IT) administration of ceftriaxone to obtain higher concentrations in the CSF. Your response is: (EO-4, 6)
   a. Give ceftriaxone IT since the drug is highly protein bound
   b. Do not give ceftriaxone IT since the flow of CSF is unidirectional
   c. Do not give ceftriaxone IT because the drug can irritate the meningeal membrane and cause seizures
   d. No need to give ceftriaxone IT because the blood-brain barrier allows for passive diffusion of cephalosporins

10. Select the reason why chemoprophylaxis with rifampin is *not* indicated in AC. (EO-8)
    a. AC developed antibodies to HiB and cannot infect others
    b. Ceftriaxone eradicated nasopharyngeal carriage of HiB
    c. AC will not respond to rifampin because of his splenectomy
    d. Rifampin is not indicated because of AC's alcohol consumption

11. Choose the *correct* statement pertaining to rifampin chemoprophylaxis of AC's household contacts. (EO-3, 12)
    a. Only the grandchildren need chemoprophylaxis
    b. Only AC's wife needs chemoprophylaxis
    c. Only AC's wife and the grandchildren's mom and dad need chemoprophylaxis
    d. AC's wife and all three grandchildren need chemoprophylaxis

12. Describe the mechanism and time course for drug interactions with rifampin. (EO-6, 7, 9)

13. Select an issue that needs to be considered in assessing psychosocial aspects that may be associated with bacterial meningitis in AC. (EO-15)
    a. Reinforce to the family that altered mental status is not unusual in patients with bacterial meningitis
    b. Inform the patient that this disease has a high mortality and he and his family may need to consider end-of-life plans
    c. Counsel patient and family about whether patient desires life-saving interventions such as full code
    d. Indicate to the family that AC will not recover his mental wherewithal and they should plan accordingly

14. Select the most cost-effective chemoprophylaxis for *Haemophilus influenzae* meningitis. (EO-17)
    a. Ceftriaxone
    b. Dexamethasone
    c. Rifampin
    d. Rifabutin

15. Summarize pathophysiologic, therapeutic, and disease management concepts for CNS infections utilizing a key points format. (EO-18)

CASE 115
Dorthea Rudorf
Topic: Bone and Joint Infections
Level 2

EDUCATIONAL MATERIALS

Chapter 74: Bone and Joint Infections (osteomyelitis, definition, epidemiology, etiology, pathophysiology, clinical presentation and diagnosis, treatment)

SCENARIO

Patient and Setting

AM, a 43-year-old homeless, wheelchair-bound, paraplegic female; ED

Chief Complaint

Fever, chills, myalgias, starting this morning; worsening ulcer over right buttock; diarrhea; feeling drowsy and "not herself"

History of Present Illness

Found asleep in public bathroom of the hospital; when sighted left quickly; returned 2 hours later; picked up by security and brought to ER due to stated complaints

Past Medical History

Paraplegia S/P car accident (9 years ago); recurrent UTIs; indwelling catheter; decubiti for 2 years; depression

Past Surgical History

Unknown

Family/Social History

Family History: Husband deceased 7 years ago; 10-year-old son in foster care

Social History: Homeless for several years; alcohol abuse; smokes 1 PPD

Medication History

Loperamide, 16–20 mg PO QD for several days

Clindamycin, unknown oral dose for several weeks

Trazodone, 100 mg PO TID

Allergies

Bactrim causes "red spots"

Physical Examination

GEN: Disheveled and cachectic paraplegic female in moderate distress; lying on left side to avoid pressure to right-sided wounds

VS: BP 100/57, HR 107, RR 18, T 39.4°C

HEENT: PERRLA; dry mucous membranes; bad oral hygiene; missing teeth; nits in hair

COR: RRR, tachycardia

CHEST: CTA, no congestion, no wheezing

ABD: Nondistended; slightly tender upon touch; red diffuse rash noted

GU: Tender, red, erythematous areas around rectum

EXT/SKIN: 4 × 4 cm, about 10-cm-deep decubitus ulcer (Stage IV) exposing bone on right buttock with yellowish-green drainage; indicates little pain; redness; no edema

NEURO: A and O × 3; but "a little off" in conversation

Results of Pertinent Laboratory Tests, Serum Drug Concentrations, and Diagnostic Tests

Na 134 (134)	Hct 0.34 (34)	Lkcs 14.7 × 10^9
K 3.4 (3.4)	Hgb 114 (11.4)	(14.7 × 10^3)
Plts 543 × 10^9	Glu 5 (90)	BUN 2.14 (6)
(543 × 10^3)	HCO$_3$ 23 (23)	Cr 44.2 (0.5)

Erythrocyte sedimentation rate (ESR) 75 (75)

Diff: 82 neutrophils, 8 bands, 8 lymph, 2 mono, 0 eos, 0 basos

Deep wound specimen/Gram stain results: Gram-positive cocci in pairs/chains/clusters; gram-negative rods, many neutrophils; cultures pending

Urinanalysis: Gram stain; few bacteria, negative nitrite test, negative leukocyte esterase test

Stool culture sent for ova and parasites and for *Clostridium difficile;* results pending

Blood cultures sent; results pending

X-ray of hip and buttock area indicates osteomyelitis

PROBLEM LIST

Identify principal problems from the scenario in priority order [completed Problem List and SOAP Note at end of casebook]

SOAP NOTE

To be completed by student

QUESTIONS

[Answers at end of casebook]

1. Osteomyelitis can be categorized depending on the pathogenesis. Which of the following best describes AM's osteomyelitis based on clinical presentation? (EO-1)
   a. Hematogenous osteomyelitis
   b. Vascular osteomyelitis
   c. Contiguous osteomyelitis
   d. Lymphatic osteomyelitis

2. Which of the following statements regarding epidemiologic factors for the development of osteomyelitis is true? (EO-3)
   a. A contiguous soft tissue infection is the most common risk factor for children
   b. Adults frequently develop osteomyelitis from short-term use of indwelling vascular access catheters

c. In elderly patients, osteomyelitis may involve the vertebral bodies infected from foci in the gastrointestinal and urinary tract

d. The most common organism causing osteomyelitis in neonates (<1 month) is *Haemophilus influenzae* associated with acute pharyngitis

3. In the treatment of osteomyelitis, all of the following parameters are considered essential for a successful outcome, *except*: (EO-8, 12)
   a. Initiating appropriate antibiotic before the culture and sensitivity results are known
   b. Starting empiric therapy with high-dose parenteral antibiotics
   c. Achieving antibiotic steady-state bone concentrations higher than or comparable to those in the serum
   d. Achieving antibiotic bone concentrations considerably above the MIC of the infecting organism(s)

4. Identify the signs and symptoms associated with osteomyelitis in AM's clinical presentation, and other possible signs and symptoms. (EO-2)

5. The most common organism(s) associated with osteomyelitis in adults is (are): (EO-1, 5)
   a. *Staphylococcus aureus*
   b. *Pseudomonas aeruginosa*
   c. *Haemophilus influenzae*
   d. Streptococci (including enterococci)

6. Discuss the factors that should be considered in choosing pharmacologic and nonpharmacologic therapy for AM's osteomyelitis. (EO-8)

7. The serum bactericidal titer (SBT) is considered a useful parameter for the assessment of adequate antibiotic therapy in osteomyelitis. Which of the following statements is false? (EO-5)
   a. It is useful in the oral therapy of children with osteomyelitis due to *Staphylococcus aureus*
   b. It uses serial dilutions of the patient's serum to determine the ability of the antibiotic to kill the infecting organism
   c. Peak serum sample should target a SBT $\leq$ 1:8
   d. A trough titer $\geq$ 1:2 is recommended

8. List the pharmacologic and nonpharmacologic treatment problems present in AM's treatment plan. (EO-11)

9. All of the listed antibiotic regimens are good empiric choices for polymicrobial (aerobic + anaerobic) osteomyelitis, *except*: (EO-8, 12)
   a. Ciprofloxacin
   b. Imipenem/cilastatin
   c. Piperacillin/tazobactam
   d. Gentamicin + clindamycin + nafcillin

10. It is recommended that AM should receive metronidazole instead of clindamycin. The reasons for this change include all of the following *except*: (EO- 8,9,10,12)
    a. Metronidazole has an excellent anaerobic spectrum
    b. Clindamycin may be the cause for AM's suspected antibiotic-associated pseudomembranous colitis (AAPC) and should be avoided
    c. In contrast to clindamycin, metronidazole does not interact with alcohol
    d. Metronidazole is used for the treatment of AAPC

11. Patients with chronic osteomyelitis often need long-term suppressive therapy. Quinolones are promising agents; however, they may have limitations. The combination with rifampin may alleviate some of the problems. Indicate the rationale for using this regimen. (EO-7, 8)
    a. Synergic effect against gram-negative organisms
    b. Ability to use lower doses of quinolones
    c. Broader antimicrobial spectrum
    d. Minimizing development of resistance, especially against *Staphylococcus aureus*

12. What psychosocial factors may affect AM's adherence to both pharmacologic and nonpharmacologic therapy? (EO-15)

13. Describe the healthcare provider's role relative to the proposed psychological factors identified. (EO-16)

14. Evaluate the pharmacoeconomic considerations relative to AM's care plan. (EO-17)

15. Summarize therapeutic, pathophysiologic, and disease management concepts for osteomyelitis utilizing a key points format. (EO-18)

CASE 116
Caroline S. Zeind
Topic: Sexually Transmitted Diseases
Level 2

EDUCATIONAL MATERIALS
Chapter 75: Sexually Transmitted Diseases (definition, prevention guidelines, ulcerogenic genital infections, syphilis, improving outcomes, selected other sexually transmitted diseases, and trichomoniasis)

SCENARIO

Patient and Setting
CS, a 30-year-old female; HIV clinic

Chief Complaint
Development of a widespread rash that involves palms of hands and soles of feet; also complains of oral sores, vaginal irritation, and vaginal discharge

History of Present Illness
Widespread rash and oral sores have occurred over the past week; thought it might go away, but it has not; also noted vaginal discharge and itching over the past few days

Past Medical History
HIV positive, diagnosed 1 year ago (last clinic visit was 3 months ago); one episode of gonorrhea 2 years ago; one episode of an uncomplicated urinary tract infection 3 years ago

Past Surgical History

None

Family/Social History

Family History: Heterosexual female; lives with boyfriend, who is also HIV positive; states she has no other sexual partners; works as a sales representative for an interior design firm

Social History: Negative intravenous use; when diagnosed with HIV infection quit cocaine with the assistance of a medical specialist and psychosocial support

Medication History

Zidovudine 300 mg/lamivudine 150 mg (combination), 1 tablet PO BID

Indinavir, 800 mg PO q8h

Trimethoprim/sulfamethoxazole, 1 DS tablet PO QD

Oral contraceptive (20 μg ethinyl estradiol and 1 mg norethindrone acetate), 1 tablet PO QD

Multivitamin with iron, 1 tablet PO QD

Allergies

NKDA

Physical Examination

GEN: Patient in moderate distress due to widespread maculopapular rash, oral sores, and vaginal discharge and irritation

VS: BP 120/76, HR 90, RR 22, T 37.5°C, Wt 60 kg (Wt last clinic visit 61 kg), Ht 175 cm

HEENT: PERRLA, lesions in oral cavity, lymphadenopathy

COR: RRR

CHEST: WNL

ABD: Nontender, no masses

GU: Vaginal discharge (loose, yellow-green, and malodorous)

RECT: WNL, guaiac negative

SKIN: Widespread macular-papular rash that involves the palms of hands and soles of feet

NEURO: A and O × 4, no headache

Results of Pertinent Laboratory Tests, Serum Drug Concentrations, and Diagnostic Tests

Na 136 (136)	Total Chol 4.65	Lkc 4.1 × 10⁹
K 3.6 (3.6)	(180)	(4.1 × 10³)
Cl 98 (98)	HDL 1.16 (45)	Plts 170 × 10⁹
HCO₃ 26 (26)	ESR 55 (55)	(170 × 10³)
BUN 3.6 (10)	Hct 0.30 (30)	MCV 112 (112)
Cr 70.7 (0.8)	Hgb 100 (10)	

RBC 3.6 × 10¹²	LDH 1.7 (100)	Glu 6.1 (110)
(3.6 × 10⁶)	Alk Phos 1.5 (90)	Ca 2.2 (8.8)
AST 0.33 (20)	Alb 36 (3.6)	PO₄ 0.92 (3.0)
ALT 0.37 (22)	T Bili 3.4 (0.2)	Mg 1.0 (2.1)

Date	Viral load (RT-PCR by Roche Amplicor)	CD4 count (cells/mm³)
Baseline 12/15/98	200,000 copies/mL	185
1/25/99	23,000 copies/mL	225
4/30/99	Undetectable	240

VDRL: Positive (titer 1:32)

FTA-abs: Positive

Gram stain of vaginal discharge: Negative for gram-negative diplococci

Wet mount examination of vaginal discharge reveals numerous trichomonads, along with large number of white blood cells

Direct fluorescent antibody (DFA) test for chlamydia: Negative

Culture and sensitivity of cervical discharge: Pending

Blood and urine cultures and sensitivities: Pending

PROBLEM LIST

Identify principal problems from the scenario in priority order [completed Problem List and SOAP Note at end of casebook]

SOAP NOTE

To be completed by student

QUESTIONS

[*Answers at end of casebook*]

1. Syphilis can be acquired by all of the following mechanisms *except:* (EO-1)
   a. Sexual intercourse
   b. Inhaling airborne particles of the organism
   c. Placental transfer
   d. Kissing or touching active lesions

2. CS presents with which of the following features of syphilis that are characteristic of this particular stage of the disease: (EO-2)
   a. Vaginal itching and discharge
   b. Rash on the palms of the hands and soles of the feet
   c. Multiple chancres
   d. Hyperimmune granulomas

3. Identify risk factor(s) present in CS that increases the risk for syphilis. (EO-3)

4. List physical assessment findings, laboratory tests, and diagnostic tests that support the diagnosis of syphilis in CS. (EO-5)

5. Which laboratory test supports the diagnosis of trichomoniasis? (EO-5)
   a. Gram-negative diplococci on Gram stain
   b. Wet mount examination of vaginal discharge that reveals numerous trichomonads
   c. Positive VDRL
   d. Positive FTA-abs

6. The health care team asks for a recommendation for the proper treatment of syphilis in CS. You correctly recommend: (EO-12)
   a. Ceftriaxone, 125 mg IM single once
   b. Metronidazole, 2 g PO once
   c. Azithromycin, 1 g PO once
   d. Benzathine penicillin, 2.4 million units IM once

7. If CS had been allergic to the drug of choice for syphilis, what would you recommend? (EO-8, 12)
   a. Desensitize CS and treat with ceftriaxone
   b. Desensitize CS and treat with metronidazole
   c. Desensitize CS and treat with azithromycin
   d. Desensitize CS and treat with benzathine penicillin

8. CS's pregnancy test was negative and she has NKDA. If CS had been pregnant, which treatment regimen would you recommend for syphilis? (EO-8, 12)
   a. Spectinomycin, 2 g IM once
   b. Ceftriaxone, 125 mg IM once
   c. Benzathine penicillin, 2.4 million units IM once
   d. Ciprofloxacin, 500 mg PO once

9. Within the first 24 hours of initiation of therapy for syphilis, CS develops an acute febrile reaction, accompanied by headache and myalgias, known as the Jarisch-Herxheimer reaction. All of the following statements are true, *except:* (EO-10)
   a. This reaction is benign and normally spontaneously resolves in 18–24 hours
   b. This reaction is thought to be caused by release of treponemal antigens due to rapid lysis of the organism by antibiotics
   c. Antipyretics may be administered for symptomatic relief
   d. This is an allergic reaction to the therapeutic agent used

10. The health care team asks for a recommendation for proper treatment of trichomoniasis in CS. You correctly reply: (EO-12)
    a. Ceftriaxone, 125 mg IM once
    b. Azithromycin, 2 g PO once
    c. Metronidazole, 2 g PO once
    d. Benzathine penicillin, 2.4 million units IM once

11. How should CS's response to syphilis and trichomoniasis therapy be monitored? (EO-12)

12. What psychosocial factors may affect CS's adherence to both pharmacologic and nonpharmacologic therapy? (EO-15)

13. Describe the health care provider's role relative to psychosocial factors. (EO-16)

14. Evaluate the pharmacoeconomic considerations relative to CS's pharmaceutical plan of care. (EO-17)

15. Summarize therapeutic, pathophysiologic, and disease management concepts for syphilis and trichomoniasis utilizing a key points format. (EO-18)

CASE 117
Nicole Turcotte
Topic: Sexually Transmitted Diseases

EDUCATIONAL MATERIALS
Chapter 75: Sexually Transmitted Diseases
(prevention guidelines, urethritis syndromes)

SCENARIO

Patient and Setting
JC, a 25-year-old white female; family practice health center

Chief Complaint
Vaginal discharge; pain with urination

History of Present Illness
Developed vaginal discharge and dysuria 2–3 days prior to office visit; had vaginal intercourse with a new partner for the first time approximately 10 days prior

Past Medical History
Gonococcal urethritis (treated successfully 2 months ago); urinary tract infection (3 years ago)

Past Surgical History
None

Family/Social History
Family History: Single; lives alone in low income housing; multiple sex partners; medical insurance without prescription coverage

Social History: No tobacco use; drinks 4–5 alcoholic beverages per month; no illicit drug use

Medication History
Norethindrone, 0.5 mg; ethinyl estradiol, 35 μg PO QD
Ibuprofen, 200 mg PO q6h PRN for headache

Allergies
Ciprofloxacin (anaphylaxis)

Physical Examination

GEN: Well-developed woman complaining of vaginal discharge and pain with urination

VS: BP 100/80, HR 76, T 37°C, Wt 55 kg

HEENT: WNL

COR: Heart rate regular with no murmers

CHEST: WNL

ABD: Soft, nontender, nondistended, + bowel sounds

GU: Slight vaginal discharge

RECT: WNL

EXT: WNL

NEURO: A and O × 3

Results of Pertinent Laboratory Tests, Serum Drug Concentrations, and Diagnostic Tests

Na 142 (142) Hgb 105 (10.5) LDH 1.8 (110)

K 4.8 (4.8) Lkcs 7 × 10⁹ Alk Phos 1.6 (95)

Cl 101 (101) (7 × 10³) Alb 35 (3.5)

HCO₃ 24 (24) Plts 260 × 10⁹ T Bili 13.7 (0.8)

BUN 4.3 (12) (260 × 10³) Glu 6.5 (118)

Cr 79.6 (0.9) AST 0.5 (30) Ca 2.7 (10.8)

Hct 0.38 (38) ALT 0.5 (30) PO₄ 1.03 (3.2)

Lkc differential: WNL

Urinalysis: WNL

Cervical culture: Gram stain shows gram-negative diplococci, cultures pending

PROBLEM LIST

Identify principal problems from the scenario in priority order

SOAP NOTE

To be completed by student

QUESTIONS

1. *Neisseria gonorrhoeae* is a: (EO-5)
   a. Gram-negative aerobic coccus
   b. Yeast
   c. Spirochete
   d. Virus

2. Which of the following is *not* a risk factor for gonorrhea in JC? (EO-3)
   a. Single marital status
   b. Low socioeconomic status
   c. Race
   d. History of gonococcal infections

3. The probable cause for JC's episode of gonococcal urethritis is: (EO-1)
   a. History of a urinary tract infection
   b. Treatment failure from previous episode of gonococcal urethritis
   c. Reinfection
   d. Poor hygiene

4. Symptoms of gonococcal urethritis, such as vaginal discharge and dysuria, will typically develop within how many days of infection? (EO-2)
   a. 2 days
   b. 10 days
   c. 21 days
   d. 28 days

5. Ofloxacin is *not* a good therapeutic choice in JC because: (EO-8)
   a. Ofloxacin is expensive, compared with ceftriaxone
   b. Ofloxacin is not efficacious against gonorrhea
   c. JC would develop anaphylaxis to ofloxacin therapy
   d. Ofloxacin must be dosed several times a day

6. The cure rate of ceftriaxone 125 mg IM × 1 against noncomplicated gonorrhea is: (EO-8)
   a. 25%
   b. 50%
   c. 75%
   d. 100%

7. Which of the following is one of the most common adverse effects associated with IM ceftriaxone? (EO-10)
   a. Pain at the injection site
   b. Constipation
   c. Headache
   d. Sedation

8. Which of the following does the Centers for Disease Control and Prevention (CDC) recommend as empiric therapy against *Chlamydia trachomatis* in patients diagnosed with gonorrhea? (EO-8, 12)
   a. Cefixime
   b. Doxycycline
   c. Gentamicin
   d. Penicillin

9. The best form of contraception against sexually transmitted diseases is: (EO-8, 11)
   a. Oral contraceptive tablets
   b. Spermicides
   c. Lamb skin condoms
   d. Latex condoms

10. Describe the mechanisms of action of the pharmacologic and nonpharmacologic interventions in this case. (EO-7)

11. What psychosocial factors may affect JC's adherence to both pharmacologic and nonpharmacologic therapy? (EO-15)

12. Describe the health care provider's role relative to the proposed psychosocial factors identified. (EO-16)

13. Evaluate the pharmacoeconomic considerations relative to ED's plan of care. (EO-17)

14. Summarize pathophysiologic, therapeutic, and disease management concepts for gonorrhea utilizing a key points format. (EO-18)

CASE 118
Caroline S. Zeind
Topic: HIV Infection—Antiretroviral Therapy

EDUCATIONAL MATERIALS
Chapter 76: Human Immunodeficiency Virus (HIV) Infection—Antiretroviral Therapy (pathophysiology, diagnosis, monitoring viral assays, therapeutic plan, pharmacotherapy, future therapies, pharmacoeconomics)

SCENARIO

Patient and Setting
JR; a 35-year-old male; HIV clinic

Chief Complaint
Noticeable loss of fat in arms, legs, buttocks, and face; increase of fat in the abdominal area

History of Present Illness
Gradual thinning of face, limbs, and buttocks occurring over the past several months; noticeable accumulation of abdominal fat over the past months with abdominal fullness and bloating

Past Medical History
Diagnosed with HIV infection (November 1997) with *Pneumocystis carinii* pneumonia (PCP) as AIDS-defining illness; cryptococcal meningitis (March 1998); recurrent sinusitis

Past Surgical History
None

Family/Social History
Family History: Father died 3 years ago of leukemia; mother alive with no significant medical history

Social History: Homosexual male; university professor; frequently travels outside the U.S.; lives with significant other (HIV positive); nonsmoker; occasionally drinks alcohol socially; owns a cat

Medication History
Indinavir, 800 mg PO q8h
Lamivudine, 150 mg PO BID
Stavudine, 40 mg PO BID
Trimethoprim/sulfamethoxazole, 1 DS tablet PO QD
Fluconazole, 200 mg PO QD

Allergies
Augmentin (rash)

Physical Examination
GEN: Pleasant male, no apparent distress; noticeable protuberant abdomen with thin limbs, buttocks, and face
VS: BP 115/75, HR 80, RR 22, T 37.8°C, Wt 74 kg (last clinic visit Wt 74.5 kg), Ht 178 cm
HEENT: PERRLA, no lymphadenopathy
COR: RRR, normal S1 and S2, no murmurs or rubs
CHEST: Clear to auscultation
ABD: Increase in abdominal girth
GU: WNL
RECTAL: WNL
EXT: Peripheral wasting in arms and legs
NEURO: A and O × 4, no headache

Results of Pertinent Laboratory Tests, Serum Drug Concentrations, and Diagnostic Tests

Na 138 (138)	Hgb 115 (11.5)	Alk Phos 1.72 (103)
K 3.5 (3.5)	Lkcs 3.2 × 10⁹	Alb 40 (4.0)
Cl 98 (98)	(3.2 × 10³)	T Bili 8.5 (0.5)
HCO₃ 26 (26)	Plts 170 × 10⁹	Glu 6.1 (110)
BUN 3.6 (10)	(170 × 10³)	Ca 2.4 (9.7)
Cr 70.7 (0.8)	MCV 104 (104)	PO₄ 1.07 (3.3)
Total Chol 5.5 (220)	AST 0.46 (28)	Mg 1.0 (2.1)
HDL 1.16 (45)	ALT 0.38 (23)	Uric Acid 240 (4.0)
Hct 0.39 (39)	LDH 1.7 (100)	

Date	Viral load (RT-PCR by Roche Amplicor)	CD4 count (cells/mm³)
Baseline (12/1/97)	150,000 copies/mL	130
01/5/98	15,000 copies/mL	150
4/2/98	1,000 copies/mL	160
7/7/98	Undetectable	175
10/1/98	Undetectable	190
1/5/99	Undetectable	220
4/6/99	Undetectable	235
Current clinic visit (3 months after 4/6/99 visit)	Undetectable	250

PROBLEM LIST
Identify principal problems from the scenario in priority order [completed Problem List and SOAP Note at end of casebook]

SOAP NOTE
To be completed by student

QUESTIONS
[Answers at end of casebook]

Na 138 (138)

1. The most probable cause for JR's lipodystrophy syndrome is use of: (EO-1)
   a. Indinavir
   b. Lamivudine
   c. Stavudine
   d. Trimethoprim/sulfamethoxazole

2. List signs and symptoms of lipodystrophy syndrome noted upon JR's presentation to the clinic, as well as other signs and symptoms that are probable. (EO-2)

3. Describe the mechanism of action of each antiretroviral agent utilized in JR's antiretroviral regimen. (EO-7)

4. It is important for clinicians to avoid selection of an antiretroviral regimen that contains agents with similar toxicity profiles. Which regimen below contains at least two agents with similar toxicity profiles? (EO-10)
   a. Zidovudine, lamivudine, and indinavir
   b. Didanosine, zalcitabine, and nelfinavir
   c. Zidovudine, didanosine, and saquinavir
   d. Stavudine, lamivudine, and indinavir

5. Describe factors that should be considered when selecting an appropriate antiretroviral regimen. (EO-8)

6. Currently the results of JR's viral load studies support: (EO-5, 11)
   a. Continuation of the current antiretroviral regimen
   b. Changing the current antiretroviral regimen
   c. Discontinuation of all antiretroviral agents
   d. Discontinuation of the protease inhibitor

7. Following this clinic visit, viral load studies should be obtained for routine monitoring in: (EO-5)
   a. 2 weeks
   b. 4 weeks
   c. 12 weeks
   d. 36 weeks

8. While receiving stavudine, JR's condition should be carefully monitored for the following dose-limiting toxicity: (EO-10)
   a. Nephrolithiasis
   b. Aplastic anemia
   c. Peripheral neuropathy
   d. Optic neuritis

9. All of the following agents require dosage adjustment in renal insufficiency, *except:* (EO-6)
   a. Indinavir
   b. Stavudine
   c. Lamivudine
   d. Trimethoprim/sulfamethoxazole

10. Which of the following agents is an inhibitor of the cytochrome P450 system and may interact with other agents metabolized by the cytochrome P450 system? (EO-9)
    a. Indinavir
    b. Stavudine
    c. Lamivudine
    d. Trimethoprim/sulfamethoxazole

11. Indinavir is administered every 8 hours on an empty stomach. JR should be instructed that oral hydration with 1.5–2 L of noncaffeinated beverages daily is recommended to prevent: (EO-10)
    a. Esophagitis
    b. Nephrolithiasis
    c. Peripheral neuropathy
    d. Gout

12. List the pharmacologic and nonpharmacologic treatment problems present in JR's treatment plan. (EO-11)

13. What psychosocial factors may affect JR's adherence to both pharmacologic and nonpharmacologic antiretroviral therapy? (EO-15)

14. Describe the health care provider's role relative to the proposed psychosocial factors identified. (EO-16)

15. Evaluate the pharmacoeconomic considerations relative to JR's plan of care. (EO-17)

16. Summarize therapeutic, pathophysiologic, and disease management concepts for HIV infection utilizing a key points format. (EO-18)

CASE 119
Robert C. Stevens
Topics: Cytomegalovirus Retinitis; Disseminated *Mycobacterium avium* Complex

EDUCATIONAL MATERIALS
Chapter 77: Human Immunodeficiency Virus Infection–Associated Opportunistic Infections (definition, *Mycobacterium avium* complex, cytomegalovirus)

SCENARIO

Patient and Setting
OM, a 43-year-old HIV-infected male; hospital

Chief Complaint
Fevers, night sweats, malaise, abdominal pains, and a persistent sore throat; acute vision loss with headaches and occasional "floaters" in the left eye

History of Present Illness
Approximately 1 month prior to admission, OM experienced fevers and night sweats coupled with weakness, fatigue, and abdominal pain; OM experienced a 4.4-kg weight loss during this period; OM denies any cough and has had a 2-week history of decreased visual acuity and floaters in the left eye

Past Medical History
OM has a medical history of seizures since childhood, stabilized on phenytoin (last seizure 1 year ago); OM was diagnosed with HIV infection 2 years ago when he was

treated for oral candidiasis; OM has been in stable health prior to his recent presentation and is consistent with keeping his HIV clinic appointments and also claims to be compliant with antiretroviral regimen

Past Surgical History

Noncontributory

Family/Social History

Family History: Homosexual in a monogamous relationship for the past 4 years; partner is also HIV infected

Social History: Marine biologist; denies intravenous drug use and does not drink or smoke

Medication History

Zidovudine 300 mg/lamivudine 150 mg (combination), 1 tablet PO BID

Indinavir, 800 mg PO TID

Trimethoprim/sulfamethoxazole, 1 DS tablet PO QD

Rifabutin, 150 mg PO QD

Phenytoin, 300 mg PO HS

Allergies

NKDA

Physical Examination

GEN: Thin, ill-appearing man
  VS: BP 110/60, HR 70, T 39.3°C, RR 14, Wt 63 kg
HEENT: No oral thrush, positive cervical lymphadenopathy
COR: Normal S_1 and S_2; no murmurs, rubs, or gallops
CHEST: WNL
ABD: Positive bowel sounds, diffuse tenderness
GU: WNL
RECT: WNL; guaiac negative
EXT: WNL
NEURO: A and O × 3

Results of Pertinent Laboratory Tests, Serum Drug Concentrations, and Diagnostic Tests

Na 141 (141)	Hct 0.28 (28)	MCV 118 (118)
K 4.1 (4.1)	Hgb 82 (8.2)	AST 1.96 (118)
Cl 97 (97)	Lkcs 0.6 × 10⁹	ALT 1.52 (92)
HCO₃ 23 (23)	(0.6 × 10³)	Alk Phos 4.02 (240)
BUN 5.7 (16)	Plts 138 × 10⁹	Alb 36 (3.6)
SCr 106.1 (1.2)	(138 × 10³)	Phenytoin 24 (6)
Glu 4.96 (90)	ANC 550	

CD4 count: Current 44 cells/mm^3; 3 months ago 52 cells/mm^3

HIV-RNA (as measured by the RT-PCR Amplicor): Current 110,450 copies/mL; 3 months ago 154,389 copies/mL (note: OM has never had an undetectable HIV viral load)

Blood cultures: (+) CMV (+) MAC

Ophthalmic examination: (+) white exudates with hemorrhage in left eye

PROBLEM LIST

Identify principal problems from the scenario in priority order

SOAP NOTE

To be completed by student

QUESTIONS

1. Choose the most likely explanation as to how OM developed CMV retinitis. (EO-1)
   a. Poor hygiene
   b. Reactivation of latent infection due to profound immunosuppression
   c. Consumption of contaminated food
   d. Direct inoculation into the eye

2. Describe the psychosocial aspects associated with CMV retinitis. (EO-15)

3. Identify a limitation of intraocular ganciclovir for CMV retinitis. (EO-12)
   a. Sclerosis of the optic nerve
   b. No antiviral effect to the contralateral eye
   c. Requires biweekly intravitreal injections
   d. More than 50% of HIV-infected patients cannot tolerate ophthalmic ganciclovir

4. Identify a potential drug interaction in the medications OM was taking prior to admission. (EO-9)
   a. Trimethoprim/sulfamethoxazole impaired the absorption of rifabutin
   b. Zidovudine/lamivudine (Combivir) inhibited the metabolism of phenytoin
   c. Rifabutin induced the metabolic clearance of indinavir
   d. Phenytoin impaired the metabolism of zidovudine

5. Select the adverse event that was necessary to monitor in OM while he received indinavir and rifabutin prior to admission. (EO-10)
   a. Cholestatic hepatitis
   b. Hemolytic anemia
   c. Avascular necrosis
   d. Uveitis

6. Provide an objective criterion that supports OM's statement that he "complies with my HIV medicines." (EO-5, 8, 10)

a. Zidovudine-induced macrocytic anemia
b. HIV RNA viral load of 10^5 copies/mL
c. Keeps regular clinic appointments
d. Hypoalbuminemia

7. Select the most pertinent laboratory value to monitor for ganciclovir toxicity. (EO-10, 11)
   a. ANC
   b. Serum creatinine
   c. Hematocrit
   d. Platelets

8. Describe the advantage of azithromycin compared with clarithromycin in OM. (EO-8, 9, 10, 12)

9. Which drug interaction can occur should OM receive didanosine and ciprofloxacin as part of his antiretroviral and DMAC therapies, respectively? (EO-9)
   a. Ciprofloxacin decreases the AUC of didanosine
   b. Didanosine reduces the bioavailability of ciprofloxacin
   c. Ciprofloxacin inhibits the metabolism of didanosine
   d. There is no drug interaction between didanosine and ciprofloxacin

10. Choose the most appropriate laboratory value to monitor for ethambutol toxicity. (EO-8, 10, 11)
    a. Amylase
    b. ALT, AST
    c. ANC
    d. Uric acid

11. Describe the reason why OM needs chronic maintenance therapy indefinitely for CMV and MAC infections. (EO-8, 11, 12)

12. Summarize pathophysiologic, therapeutic, and disease management concepts for CMV and MAC infections utilizing a key points format. (EO-18)

CASE 120
Robert C. Stevens
Topic: *Pneumocystis carinii* Pneumonia

EDUCATIONAL MATERIALS
Chapter 77: Human Immunodeficiency Virus Infection–Associated Opportunistic Infections

---

SCENARIO

Patient and Setting

RT, a 25-year-old HIV-infected woman; hospitalized for *Pneumocystis carinii* pneumonia (PCP)

Chief Complaint

On admission RT complained, "I am tired, can't catch my breath, and I become winded when climbing stairs."

History of Present Illness

RT presented to the emergency department 5 days ago with a month-long history of shortness of breath, nonproductive cough, fatigue, loss of energy, and difficulty performing normal tasks such as climbing stairs; these events have progressively worsened during the past several weeks

Past Medical History

RT has been in good health until this current event and did not know of her HIV-seropositivity until this admission

Past Surgical History

Noncontributory

Family/Social History

Family History: Bisexual with multiple sexual partners

Social History: Admits to intravenous drug use (heroin) and crack cocaine; alcohol ingestion is "social"

Medication History

Trimethoprim/sulfamethoxazole, 20 mg/kg/day (based on TMP) IV evenly divided q6h

Prednisone, 40 mg PO BID × 5 days then taper

O_2 40% via nasal cannula

Allergies

Penicillin ("My mom said I got a rash when I took penicillin when I was a kid.")

Physical Examination

(Hospital Day 4)
  GEN: Ill-appearing woman in moderate respiratory distress complaining of feeling agitated and a throbbing headache
   VS: BP 113/62, HR 87, T 38.9°C, RR 22, Wt 66 kg
HEENT: (+) cervical lymphadenopathy
  COR: Tachycardia
CHEST: Diffuse rales bilaterally
  ABD: Soft, nontender
   GU: WNL, no evidence of any sexually transmitted disease(s)
 RECT: (−) fissures, anus is normal appearance
  EXT: IV track marks on antecubital veins; nonpruritic, erythematous macular rash on extremities and upper torso
NEURO: Alert and oriented to person, place, but not time; fine peripheral motor tremor in both hands

Results of Pertinent Laboratory Tests, Serum Drug Concentrations, and Diagnostic Tests

Na 138 (138)   SCr 79.6 (0.9)   Plts 121 × 10⁹
K 5.9 (5.9)   Glu 4.55 (82)   (121 × 10³)
Cl 102 (102)   Hct 0.34 (34)   AST 3.58 (215)
HCO₃ 25 (25)   Hgb 155 (15.5)   ALT 2.42 (145)
BUN 3.9 (11)   Lkcs 5.2 × 10⁹   Alk Phos 8.59 (515)
                  (5.2 × 10³)   Alb 42 (4.2)

CD4: 123 cells/mm³

HIV antibody: Pending

HIV-RNA: 238,910 copies/mL (as measured by RT-PCR Amplicor)

Chest x-ray: Diffuse patchy infiltrates bilaterally

Arterial blood gases on room air at admission: pH 7.39 (7.39); PaO₂ 8.67 (65); PCO₂ 4.93 (37)

Bronchoalveolar lavage: (+) *Pneumocystis carinii* cysts

Blood cultures: No growth after 72 hours

Urine toxicology screen: (+) opiates

PROBLEM LIST

Identify principal problems from the scenario in priority order [completed Problem List and SOAP Note at end of casebook]

SOAP NOTE

To be completed by student

QUESTIONS

[Answers at end of casebook]

1. All of the following are clinical manifestations of PCP in RT, *except:* (EO-2)
   a. Shortness of breath
   b. Lung infiltrates
   c. Headache
   d. Fatigue

2. Which one of the following identifies two laboratory parameters that are useful to determine the severity of PCP and response to therapy? (EO-5)
   a. Leukocyte count and alanine aminotransferase
   b. PaO₂ and LDH
   c. Serum creatinine and serum potassium
   d. Hematocrit and partial pressure of carbon dioxide (PCO₂)

3. What is the indication for prednisone (an immunosuppressant) in RT? (EO-8, 11, 12)

4. The most likely explanation for the adverse events RT experienced with TMP-SMX is: (EO-10)
   a. Concentration-dependent toxicity due to excessive TMP-SMX dose
   b. Profound immunosuppression made RT more susceptible to drug toxicity
   c. Underlying HIV infection caused these events
   d. Cytokine release following TMP-SMX lysis of *P. carinii* led to the events RT experienced

5. Which adverse event is *not* associated with TMP-SMX in an AIDS patient with PCP? (EO-10)
   a. Gastrointestinal distress
   b. Neutropenia
   c. Renal dysfunction
   d. Arrhythmias

6. Describe the mechanism of action of TMP-SMX-associated hyperkalemia. (EO-7)

7. Identify the most significant laboratory parameter to monitor for pentamidine toxicity in RT. (EO-5, 10)
   a. Bilirubin
   b. Serum creatinine
   c. Hematocrit
   d. Sodium

8. On day 9 of pentamidine therapy, RT complains of weakness, headache, shakiness, and palpitations 2 hours after completing the infusion of IV pentamidine. Select the best initial intervention to identify the etiology of these symptoms. (EO-5, 10, 11)
   a. Stat serum K⁺ to rule out pentamidine-induced hyperkalemia
   b. Stat electrocardiogram to rule out pentamidine-induced torsades de pointes
   c. Stat toxicology drug screen
   d. Stat Accu-check to determine blood glucose

9. Describe the mechanism of action of pentamidine-induced hypoglycemia. (EO-7, 10)

10. RT successfully completed acute PCP therapy with pentamidine. Select the most appropriate and cost-effective agent for secondary PCP prophylaxis in RT. (EO-5, 8, 10, 12, 17)
    a. TMP-SMX, 1 double-strength tablet PO q 3/week
    b. Atovaquone 750 mg PO with food TID
    c. Aerosolized pentamidine 300 mg monthly
    d. Dapsone 25 mg/week (with leucovorin)

11. RT has received 6 months of antiretroviral therapy. Her HIV RNA viral load has been undetectable for 3.5 months, and the CD4 cell count is 325/μL. The attending physician seeks your input regarding discontinuation of the drug you selected in question 10 for PCP prophylaxis. (EO-11)
    a. Continue PCP prophylaxis until the long-term outcome of withdrawing prophylaxis is established from clinical trials
    b. Continue PCP prophylaxis but decrease the frequency of TMP-SMX to once weekly
    c. Continue PCP prophylaxis but decrease the frequency of atovaquone to once daily
    d. Continue PCP prophylaxis but decrease the frequency of dapsone to once monthly

12. Describe the psychosocial aspects that RT may experience upon learning that she is infected with HIV. (EO-15)

13. Summarize pathophysiologic, therapeutic, and disease management concepts for *Pneumocystis carinii* pneumonia utilizing a key points format. (EO-18)

CASE 121
Michelle Ceresia
Topics: Mycotic Infections and Renal Transplant
Level 3
EDUCATIONAL MATERIALS
Chapter 78: Mycotic Infections (aspergillosis, epidemiology, clinical manifestations, pulmonary, disseminated, diagnosis, amphotericin B, treatment); Chapter 81: Infections in the Immunosuppressed Patient (pathophysiology, pharmacotherapy-antifungal); Chapter 104: Transplantation (kidney transplantation)

SCENARIO

Patient and Setting
RT, a 32-year-old female; general medicine floor

Chief Complaint
Fevers, dry cough, chest pain, and shortness of breath (SOB)

History of Present Illness
Over the past week worsening dyspnea, dry cough, pleuritic chest pain, and high fevers

Past Medical History
Transplant rejection 1 month prior to admission (PTA) treated with pulse high-dose steroids; Type 1 diabetes mellitus (DM) for 19 years; diabetic gastroparesis; end-stage renal disease (ESRD) for 1 year secondary to Type 1 DM (received hemodialysis 3×/week prior to transplant); baseline Cr post-transplant 212 (2.4); hypertension (HTN) for 1 year secondary to ESRD; hyperlipidemia and hypertriglyceridemia managed with diet modification

Past Surgical History
Status post (S/P) cadaveric renal transplant (CRT) 2 months PTA

Family/Social History
Family History: Father and mother alive and well

Social History: Nonsmoker; no alcohol intake; single, lives alone

Medication History
Cyclosporine, 300 mg PO BID
Prednisone, 20 mg PO q AM
Azathioprine, 100 mg PO QHS
Acyclovir, 800 mg PO QID
Insulin, 20 units NPH SC q AM/
   10 units regular SC q AM/q PM
Isradipine, 5 mg PO BID
Cisapride, 10 mg PO QID

Allergies
NKDA

Physical Examination
    GEN: Ill-appearing woman in apparent respiratory distress
      VS: BP 150/92, HR 80, RR 26, T 39.2°C, Wt 65 kg (63.8 kg 2 weeks PTA), Ht 171 cm
  HEENT: WNL
   COR: RRR, normal S1 and S2
 CHEST: Decreased breath sounds, rales
   ABD: Soft, nontender, positive bowel sounds
    GU: WNL
  RECT: Guaiac-negative stool
   EXT: WNL
NEURO: A and O × 4

Results of Pertinent Laboratory Tests, Serum Drug Concentrations, and Diagnostic Tests

Na 136 (136)	Hct 0.33 (33)	Alk Phos 1.45 (87)
K 4.8 (4.8)	Hgb 120 (12)	Alb 31 (3.1)
Cl 103 (103)	Lkcs 9.1 × 10⁹	T Bili 6.8 (0.4)
HCO₃ 21 (21)	(9.1 × 10³)	Glu 18.9 (342)
BUN 24.6 (69)	Plts 363 × 10⁹	Ca 2.2 (8.8)
Cr 221 (2.5)	(363 × 10³)	PO₄ 1.26 (3.9)
Total Chol 5.69 (220)	AST 0.5 (30)	Mg 1.0 (2.0)
Trig 3.16 (280)	ALT 0.32 (19)	

Lkc differential: Neutrophils 0.70 (70.0%), bands 0.07 (7.0%), monos 0.10 (10.0%)

Cyclosporine whole blood concentration (monoclonal RIA): 300 μg/L

Oxygen saturation (SaO$_2$): 0.9 (90%) on room air

SaO$_2$ 0.95 (95%) on 40% fraction of inspired oxygen (FiO$_2$)

Bronchoscopy culture: *Aspergillus fumigatus*

Urinalysis: Mild proteinuria, few WBC

Chest x-ray: RLL infiltrate

Ventilation perfusion (VQ) scan: Low probability for pulmonary embolism (PE)

Renal Biopsy: No cellular infiltrate, scarring consistent with other chronic form of renal failure

PROBLEM LIST

Identify principal problems from the scenario in priority order [completed Problem List and SOAP Note at end of casebook]

SOAP NOTE

To be completed by student

QUESTIONS

[Answers at end of casebook]

1. Which of the following is a risk factor for RT's aspergillus pneumonia? (EO-1)
   a. Isradipine
   b. Acyclovir
   c. Prednisone
   d. Renal failure

2. List signs and symptoms of acute invasive pulmonary aspergillosis noted in RT. (EO-2)

3. List physical assessment findings in RT, laboratory tests, and diagnostic tests, which support the diagnosis of aspergillus pneumonia. (EO-5)

4. All of the following statements regarding the use of lipid-formulated amphotericin B are true, *except:* (EO-8, 10, 17)
   a. Lipid-formulated amphotericin B does not cause nephrotoxicity
   b. Lipid-formulated amphotericin B is appropriate therapy for RT since her CR is 2.5 mg/dL
   c. Lipid-formulated amphotericin B is costly compared with conventional amphotericin B
   d. Lipid-formulated amphotericin B is indicated in patients who have infections that are refractory to conventional amphotericin B therapy

5. All of the following statements regarding itraconazole are true, *except:* (EO-8, 9, 12)
   a. Itraconazole is highly protein bound
   b. In contrast to fluconazole, itraconazole is highly lipid soluble
   c. Monitor LFTs while RT is receiving itraconazole
   d. RT should be advised to take itraconazole with an H2-antagonist, because the drug requires an alkalotic environment for adequate absorption

6. The following statements regarding the mechanism of action of both pharmacologic and nonpharmacologic interventions in this case are true, *except:* (EO-7)

   a. Amphotericin B binds to ergosterol in the cell wall of susceptible fungi, causing leakage of the cellular contents and subsequently cell death
   b. Lipid-formulated amphotericin B is taken up by monocytes, which migrate to alveoli in the lungs to become alveolar macrophages
   c. Itraconazole inhibits the synthesis of ergosterol in the cell membrane
   d. A standardized method for in vitro testing of molds is commonly performed to evaluate response to therapy

7. The following statements regarding the treatment of RT's HTN are true, *except:* (EO-8, 10)
   a. Calcium channel blockers may improve renal hemodynamics and are considered first-line agents for post-transplant HTN
   b. Angiotensin-converting enzyme (ACE) inhibitors in combination with cyclosporine increase glomerular filtration and are considered an effective treatment for RT's HTN
   c. ACE inhibitors aggravate hyperkalemia caused by cyclosporine
   d. Gingival hyperplasia may be more common in patients who are on both cyclosporine and a calcium channel blocker

8. List the pharmacologic and nonpharmacologic treatment problem(s) present in RT's treatment plan. (EO-11)

9. Which of the following risk factors does RT have for CAD? (EO-1)
   a. CRT
   b. Diabetes mellitus
   c. Immunosuppressant therapy
   d. Renal failure

10. If RT were started on lovastatin for the treatment of hyperlipidemia, which of the following adverse effects would be a major concern (while she is on cyclosporine)? (EO-10)
    a. Lactic acidosis
    b. Glucose intolerance
    c. Rhabdomyolysis
    d. CRT rejection

11. Upon hospital discharge, if RT were placed on itraconazole for the treatment of her aspergillus pneumonia, which of the following would be a major concern? (EO-8, 9)
    a. Itraconazole and cisapride are contraindicated because of the potential of causing life-threatening arrhythmias
    b. Itraconazole may decrease RT's blood/serum cyclosporine level, putting her at risk for CRT rejection
    c. Itraconazole has inadequate activity against *Aspergillus* spp. and is not an effective therapy for RT's aspergillus pneumonia
    d. Itraconazole is available intravenously for treatment of severe, life-threatening fungal infections

12. What psychosocial factors may affect RT's adherence to both pharmacologic and nonpharmacologic therapy? (EO-15)

13. Summarize pathophysiologic, therapeutic, and disease management concepts for acute invasive pulmonary aspergillosis utilizing a key points format. (EO-18)

CASE 122
Dawn Chandler-Toufieli
Topic: Parasitic Diseases
Level 2
EDUCATIONAL MATERIALS
Chapter 79: Parasitic Infections (definition, treatment goals, cryptosporidiosis, isosporiasis, microsporidiosis, cyclosporiasis, improving outcomes)

SCENARIO

Patient and Setting
ME, a 56-year-old male; clinic visit; cousin as an interpreter

Chief Complaint
"Diarrhea all the time"

History of Present Illness
ME recently immigrated to the United States from Brazil; has been on chronic suppressive paromomycin therapy in the past but forgot to mention this at his last appointment; diarrhea and abdominal cramping have markedly improved; denies any history of fevers or night sweats; 10–15 pound weight loss over the past year, but has gained 3 pounds since last clinic visit 1 month ago

Past Medical History
Chronic cryptosporidial infection, iron deficiency anemia, hyperuricemia, HTN

Past Surgical History
None

Family/Social History
Family History: Married and lives with wife and three children; farmed in the past
Social History: Smokes 1 PPD × 40 years; drinks alcohol, 1 mixed drink/week

Medication History
Triamterene (75 mg)/HCTZ (50 mg), 1 tab PO QD

Iron sulfate, 325 mg PO BID

Acetaminophen, 500 mg QID PRN headache

Paromomycin, 500 mg PO BID (has not been taking since leaving Brazil)

Allergies
Penicillin, difficulty breathing

Physical Examination
GEN: Thin male in NAD
VS: BP 150/92, HR 84, RR 16, T 37.2°C, Wt 133 lb
HEENT: Fundi normal; no lymphadenopathy
COR: Regular rate and rhythm without murmur
CHEST: Diffuse wheezing, decreased breath sounds throughout lung fields
ABD: Spleen not palpable
GU: WNL
RECT: Prostate WNL, stool heme-positive, no masses
EXT: No clubbing, cyanosis, or edema
NEURO: WNL

Results of Pertinent Laboratory Tests, Serum Drug Concentrations, and Diagnostic Tests

HCO$_3$ 24 (24)	Lkcs 8.6 × 10^9	T Bili 8.6 (0.5)
Na 139 (139)	(8.6 × 10^3)	Glu 6.1 (110)
K 3.5 (3.5)	Plts 296 × 10^9	Ca 2.5 (10.1)
Cl 100 (100)	(296 × 10^3)	PO$_4$ 1.1 (3.4)
BUN 6.5 (18)	MCV 77 (77)	Mg 1.05 (2.1)
Cr 110 (1.2)	AST 0.58 (35)	Uric Acid 725.6 (12.2)
Hct 0.364 (36.4)	ALT 0.58 (35)	Chol 5.2 (200)
Hgb 112 (11.2)	LDH 2.66 (150)	PT 12
	Alb 42 (4.2)	PTT 30

Chest x-ray: Hyperinflation consistent with COPD

KUB: No air fluid levels

Skin tests: PPD (−), Candida skin test (+), mumps skin test (+)

HIV test: Negative

PROBLEM LIST
Identify principal problems from the scenario in priority order

SOAP NOTE
To be completed by student

QUESTIONS
1. The probable cause for ME's parasitic infection: (EO-1)

a. Exposure to infected mosquitoes
b. Exposure through vaginal intercourse
c. Fecal-oral spread
d. Exposure to infected aerosolized droplets

2. ME presents with a history of all the following signs and symptoms of a chronic cryptosporidial infection *except:* (EO-2)
   a. Diarrhea
   b. Weight loss
   c. Heme-positive stools
   d. Abdominal cramping

3. All of the following social factors listed in ME's medical history probably contributed to his cryptosporidial infection, *except:* (EO-1)
   a. History of farming
   b. History of smoking
   c. Social alcohol use
   d. Exposure to American culture

4. *Cryptosporidium parvum* may cause disease in: (EO-1)
   a. Humans only
   b. Animals only
   c. Insects only
   d. Humans and animals

5. Describe the mechanisms of action of the pharmacologic and nonpharmacologic interventions in ME's case. (EO-7)

6. Although no uniformly effective therapy has been identified for the treatment of chronic cryptosporidial infection, all of the following macrolide antibiotics have been reported to be useful with varying degrees of success, *except:* (EO-8, 12)
   a. Erythromycin
   b. Spiramycin
   c. Azithromycin
   d. Roxithromycin

7. Which of the following adverse effects has been reported to occur with paromomycin's use and should be included in ME's patient counseling session? (EO-9, 10)
   a. Disulfiram reaction
   b. Metallic taste
   c. Diarrhea
   d. Lactose intolerance

8. ME appears to have drug-induced hyperuricemia. This may be due to which one of his medications? (EO-10)
   a. Iron sulfate
   b. Hydrochlorothiazide
   c. Triamterene
   d. Acetaminophen

9. List the pharmacologic and nonpharmacologic treatment problem(s) present in ME's treatment plan. (EO-11)

10. What psychosocial factors may affect ME's adherence to both pharmacologic and nonpharmacologic therapy? (EO-15)

11. Describe the health care provider's role relative to the proposed psychosocial factors identified. (EO-16)

12. Summarize pathophysiologic, therapeutic, and disease management concepts for ME's chronic cryptosporidial infection utilizing a key points format. (EO-18)

CASE 123
Dawn Chandler-Toufieli
Topic: Surgical Antibiotic Prophylaxis

EDUCATIONAL MATERIALS
Chapter 80: Surgical Antibiotic Prophylaxis (treatment goals, epidemiology, pathophysiology, treatment, surgical procedures and suggested antibiotic regimens, improving outcomes)

SCENARIO
Patient and Setting
CT, a 53-year-old male; clinic the day before surgery for pre-op evaluation

Chief Complaint
"Wet cough"

History of Present Illness
Has a left tonsillar carcinoma; MRI revealed no lymph node involvement; scheduled tomorrow for an excision of the left tonsillar carcinoma, left radical neck resection, and tracheostomy

Past Medical History
HTN; COPD, moderate-to-severe by recent PFTs; psoriasis

Past Surgical History
None

Family/Social History
Family History: Father died at age 70 with lung cancer; mother died at 78 of unknown causes

Social History: Smokes 50 pack/year; drinks alcohol, questionable alcohol abuse reported by CT's wife; he and his wife run a small family business

Medication History
HCTZ, 50 mg PO QD
Ipratropium bromide, 2 puffs QID
Albuterol, 2 puffs q4h PRN

Allergies
Codeine (hives)

Physical Examination

GEN: Thin male appearing 10 years older than his stated age

VS: BP 135/85; HR 78

HEENT: Ears normal; nose normal; pharynx—on left tonsillar fossa there is a white ulcerated lesion extending to the base of the tongue; no enlarged lymph nodes

COR: No murmurs

CHEST: Chronic wet cough; however, lungs are clear

ABD: Soft, nontender, nondistended

GU: Deferred

RECT: Deferred

EXT: No cyanosis or edema

NEURO: A and O × 3

Results of Pertinent Laboratory Tests, Serum Drug Concentrations, and Diagnostic Tests

HCO$_3$ 22 (22)   Cr 50 (0.6)   RBC 4.3 × 10^{12}
Na 136 (136)   Mg 0.9 (1.8)   (4.3 × 10^6)
K 4.2 (4.2)   Lkcs 6.0 × 10^9 Hgb 116 (11.6)
Cl 105 (105)   (6.0 × 10^3)   Hct 0.39 (39)
Glu 5.72 (103)   Plts 130 × 10^9 PT 12
BUN 3.0 (8)   (130 × 10^3)   PTT 28

PROBLEM LIST

Identify principal problems from the scenario in priority order [completed Problem List and SOAP Note at end of casebook]

SOAP NOTE

To be completed by student

QUESTIONS

[Answers at end of casebook]

1. All of the following are treatment goals with respect to CT's surgical antibiotic prophylaxis, *except:* (EO-11)
   a. Decrease the incidence of postoperative infections
   b. Decrease the incidence of postoperative bleeding
   c. Minimize the adverse effects of the antibiotics used for surgical prophylaxis
   d. Minimize overall bacterial resistance in the institution

2. All of the following are possible additional outcomes of CT's surgical antibiotic prophylaxis, *except:* (EO-11)
   a. Decreased length of hospital stay
   b. Reduce the overall cost of care
   c. Increase the overall percentage of nosocomial infections
   d. Decrease the percentage of postoperative surgical wound infections

3. CT's risk of developing a surgical wound infection depends on which of the following patient factors: (EO-1, 3)
   a. Age
   b. Gender

c. Race
d. Past surgical history

4. Based on the National Research Council Wound classification, what classification is CT's surgical wound? (EO-1, 3)
   a. Dirty
   b. Contaminated
   c. Clean-contaminated
   d. Clean

5. What bacteria are most likely to be encountered during CT's surgical procedure? (EO-1)
   a. *Staphylococcus epidermidis*
   b. *Staphylococcus aureus*
   c. Diphtheroids
   d. Gram-negative enterics

6. Which of the following drug regimens should be instituted preoperatively to decrease CT's risk of developing a postsurgical infection? (EO-8, 11)
   a. Cefazolin 1 g IV
   b. Cefazolin 1 g IV and clindamycin 600 mg IV
   c. Vancomycin 1 g IV and clindamycin 600 mg IV
   d. Clindamycin 600 mg IV

7. If CT were allergic to beta-lactam antibiotics, which of the following regimens would be preferred to be administered preoperatively? (EO-8, 11)
   a. Vancomycin 1 g IV
   b. Cefazolin 1 g IV and clindamycin 600 mg IV
   c. Vancomycin 1 g IV and clindamycin 600 mg IV
   d. Clindamycin 600 mg IV

8. When should CT's surgical prophylaxis regimen be administered? (EO-6, 14)
   a. Preinduction
   b. At the time of making the surgical incision
   c. At the time of closing the surgical incision
   d. Postinduction

9. What psychosocial factors may affect CT's adherence to both pharmacologic and nonpharmacologic therapy? (EO-15)

10. Describe the health care provider's role relative to the proposed psychosocial factors identified. (EO-16)

11. Evaluate the pharmacoeconomic considerations relative to CT's plan of care. (EO-17)

12. Summarize pathophysiologic, therapeutic, and disease management concepts for surgical antibiotic prophylaxis utilizing a key points format. (EO-18)

CASE 124
Robert C. Stevens
Topic: Infections in Febrile Neutropenic Cancer Patient

 Level 3

EDUCATIONAL MATERIALS
Chapter 81: Infections in the Immunosuppressed Patient

SCENARIO

Patient and Setting

BF, a 55-year-old man; hospital

Chief Complaint

Fever, nosebleeds, and painful oral lesions

History of Present Illness

BF was diagnosed with acute lymphocytic leukemia (ALL) 2 weeks prior to admission; he is currently receiving day 10 of his induction chemotherapy regimen; on day 7 of therapy, he became febrile, was pancultured, and empirically started on ceftazidime; on the evening of day 8 BF spiked a temperature to 39.8°C and complains of nosebleeds, fever, painful oral lesions, and nausea/vomiting

Past Medical History

BF was diagnosed with rheumatoid arthritis (RA) 2 years ago and has been managed with NSAIDs; BF had been otherwise healthy prior to the diagnosis of ALL

Past Surgical History

Hernia repair 3.5 years ago; double-lumen Hickman central catheter placed on hospital day 2 of this admission

Family/Social History

Family History: Father died from colon cancer

Social History: Smokes 25 pack/year; alcohol socially

Medication History

Methotrexate, 1.5 g/m^2 IV day 1, then adjust dose per rate of clearance

Daunorubicin, 100 mg IV days 1–3

Vincristine, 2 mg IV days 1, 8, 15, 22

Prednisone, 50 mg PO BID days 1–28

Asparaginase, 10,000 U SC days 17–28

TMP-SMX, 1 double-strength tablet PO Mon, Tues, Wed

Prochlorperazine, 10 mg IV q6h PRN N/V

Naproxen, 500 mg PO BID

Allopurinol, 300 mg PO QD

Allergies

NKDA

Physical Examination

GEN: Thin, ill-appearing man

VS: BP 130/82, HR 82, RR 21, T 39.8°C, Wt 57 kg, Ht 147 cm, BSA 1.68 m^2

HEENT: Neck supple, no conjunctival hemorrhage, positive white plaques on oral mucosa

COR: Normal S_1 and S_2; tachycardia

CHEST: Clear

ABD: Soft, nontender; positive bowel sounds; Hickman catheter site erythematous and tender

GU: WNL

RECT: Deferred secondary to thrombocytopenia

EXT: Multiple ecchymoses and petechiae

NEURO: Intact, nonfocal examination

Results of Pertinent Laboratory Tests, Serum Drug Concentrations, and Diagnostic Tests

Na 139 (139)	Hgb 94 (9.4)	Alk Phos 8.9 (532)
K 4.1 (4.1)	Lkcs 0.1 × 10⁹	Alb 41 (4.1)
Cl 100 (100)	(0.1 × 10³)	Glu 6.44 (116)
HCO₃ 26 (26)	Plts 13 × 10⁹	Ca 2.5 (10.1)
BUN 5.7 (16)	(13 × 10³)	PO₄ 0.97 (3.0)
Cr 141.4 (1.6)	AST 1.13 (68)	Mg 1.0 (2.1)
Hct 0.28 (28)	ALT 0.3 (19)	Uric acid 535 (9.0)

Lkc differential: N 0 (0%), promyeloblasts present

Urinalysis: WNL

Chest x-ray: Clear, no infiltrates or cavitary lesions

Cultures: Blood—no growth after 48 hours; red lumen—(+) 400 colonies of *Staphylococcus aureus*; white lumen—no growth after 48 hours; oral scraping culture—*Candida albicans*

PROBLEM LIST

Identify principal problems from the scenario in priority order [completed Problem List and SOAP Note at end of casebook]

SOAP NOTE

To be completed by student

QUESTIONS

[Answers at end of casebook]

1. Define fever and neutropenia in patients with cancer (all temperatures are oral). (EO-3)
   a. T >37.0°C ANC <100
   b. T >37.5°C ANC <500
   c. T >38.0°C ANC <1000
   d. T >38.3°C ANC <500

2. Empiric anti-infective therapy in a febrile, neutropenic cancer patient is directed at which category of pathogens? (EO-1)
   a. Bacteria
   b. Viruses

c. Fungi

d. Parasites

3. List the indications for vancomycin in febrile neutropenic cancer patients. (EO-2, 3)

4. Explain why vancomycin was used as empiric therapy in BF. (EO-5, 8)

5. Identify the role of TMP-SMX in BF. (EO-8, 11)
   a. Reduce bacterial flora of GI tract
   b. *Pneumocystis carinii* pneumonia prophylaxis
   c. Prevent infection with MRSA
   d. Prophylaxis against central line infections

6. Select the most common adverse effect in cancer patients receiving TMP-SMX for PCP prophylaxis. (EO-10)
   a. Elevated serum hepatic transaminases
   b. Gastrointestinal intolerance
   c. Elevated CR
   d. Neutropenia

7. Select the best rationale for why BF received monotherapy with ceftazidime on day 7. (EO-8)
   a. BF did not appear septic and had no focus initially for gram-positive infection
   b. Ceftazidime has potent activity against both gram-positive and -negative pathogens
   c. TMP-SMX acts synergistically with ceftazidime
   d. Low threshold for anaerobic infection

8. Select the recommended time for starting empiric anti-fungal therapy in patients with fever and neutropenia. (EO-12)
   a. Febrile after 3 days of broad-spectrum antibiotics
   b. Febrile after 5–7 days of broad-spectrum antibiotics
   c. Febrile after 10–14 days of broad-spectrum antibiotics
   d. Should be started concurrently with broad-spectrum antibiotics

9. Identify the most appropriate time to discontinue antibiotics in BF. (EO-11)
   a. 1 week
   b. 24–48 hours after being afebrile and ANC >100
   c. 3–5 days after being afebrile and ANC >500
   d. 10–14 days for line infection and afebrile with ANC >500

10. Compare the advantages and disadvantages of using oral fluconazole instead of topical antifungal products (e.g., nystatin suspension) for oral candidiasis in BF. (EO-5, 8, 10)

11. BF complains of dysphagia and becomes nauseous from oral fluconazole. Select the most appropriate treatment for oral candidiasis. (EO-10, 11)
    a. Clotrimazole troches
    b. Fluconazole 200 mg IV QD
    c. Itraconazole 200 mg PO (with 12 ounces of Coca-Cola) QD
    d. Flucytosine 900 mg PO q6h

12. Based on pharmacoeconomic issues and disease state management of the current conditions in BF, characterize the appropriateness of starting granulocyte colony-stimulating factor in this patient. (EO-8, 12, 17, 18)

13. Outline the psychosocial factors that may affect BF's outcome. (EO-15)

14. Summarize pathophysiologic, therapeutic, and disease management concepts for infections in the immunosuppressed patient utilizing a key points format. (EO-18)

CASE 125
G. Christopher Wood
Topic: Bacteremia
Level 1
EDUCATIONAL MATERIALS
Chapter 82: Bacteremia and Sepsis (signs and symptoms, diagnosis, treatment, immunotherapy of sepsis); Chapter 67: Pneumonia (pathogen-specific treatment of CAP)

SCENARIO

Patient and Setting
SF, a 28-year-old male; intermediate care "step down" unit

Chief Complaint
New onset confusion

History of Present Illness
Received second- and third-degree burns on both hands and forearms in an industrial accident 1 week ago; transferred from the burn ICU 2 days ago; over the past 24 hours developed new-onset confusion and fever

Past Medical History
None

Past Surgical History
None

Family/Social History
Noncontributory

Medication History
Cimetidine, 300 mg IV q8h
Morphine, 2–4 mg IV q1–2h PRN pain
Sulfamylon cream, topical to burn wounds QID

Allergies
NKDA

Physical Examination

GEN: Well-developed, well-nourished man in no apparent distress

VS: BP 120/77, HR 95, RR 16, T 36.9°C, Wt 77 kg, Ht 178 cm

NEURO: Intermittently oriented to time, place, and person (previously was fully oriented); lethargic, claims to be a television sportscaster

EXT: Hands and forearms bandaged, burns healing appropriately

All other systems: WNL

Results of Pertinent Laboratory Tests, Serum Drug Concentrations, and Diagnostic Tests

Na 140 (140)　　BUN 5.4 (15)　　Lkcs 13.3 × 10^9

K 3.5 (3.5)　　Cr 100 (0.9)　　(13.3 × 10^3)

Cl 99 (99)　　Glu 6.4 (118)　　Baseline Lkcs 9.0 × 10^9

HCO$_3$ 24 (24)　　　　(9.0 × 10^3)

Lkc differential: Neutrophils 0.88 (88%), bands 0.12 (12%), lymphs 0.04 (4%)

Blood: Today Gram stain shows gram-negative rods in 3 of 4 bottles; cultures: pending

Urine and wound: No organisms on Gram stain; cultures pending

PROBLEM LIST

Identify principal problems from the scenario in priority order [completed Problem List and SOAP Note at end of casebook]

SOAP NOTE

To be completed by student

QUESTIONS

[Answers at end of casebook]

1. According to ACCP/SCCM guidelines, which of the following best describes SF's clinical condition? (EO-2)
   a. Bacteremia
   b. Sepsis
   c. Severe sepsis
   d. Septic shock

2. Which of the following would be the most appropriate empiric therapy for SF's infection? (EO-5, 11, 12)
   a. Ampicillin/sulbactam, gentamicin
   b. Ceftazidime, gentamicin, piperacillin
   c. Vancomycin, ceftriaxone, tobramycin
   d. Vancomycin, ceftazidime, tobramycin

3. SF did not receive prophylactic systemic antibiotics to prevent sepsis. Which of the following is the primary reason prophylactic antibiotics are not routinely used to prevent sepsis? (EO-8, 11, 12)
   a. Development of bacterial resistance
   b. High cost of antibiotics
   c. Renal toxicity of many antibiotics
   d. Prophylactic antibiotics have never been studied

4. Based on preliminary culture results, which of the following is the likely pathogen in SF? (EO-3)
   a. *Staphylococcus aureus*
   b. *Klebsiella pneumoniae*
   c. *Candida albicans*
   d. *Mycoplasma pneumoniae*

5. SF's final culture results are: *Enterobacter cloacae* from blood (3/4 bottles), no growth from urine, and no growth from wounds. The organism is sensitive to ceftazidime, ciprofloxacin, imipenem, gentamicin, and tobramycin. Which of the following should be used to treat SF's *Enterobacter* infection? (EO-5, 8, 11, 12)
   a. Vancomycin
   b. Ceftazidime
   c. Ciprofloxacin
   d. Tobramycin

6. Within 24 hours of initiation of antibiotic therapy, SF's clinical condition deteriorates somewhat, then improves over the next 48 hours. Which of the following is the most likely explanation of this phenomenon? (EO-1)
   a. Adverse reaction to vancomycin
   b. Empiric therapy with vancomycin, ceftazidime, and tobramycin is inappropriate
   c. SF most likely has fungal sepsis
   d. Temporary deterioration is thought to be due to the release of bacterial endotoxins as a result of the bactericidal effects of antibiotic therapy

7. When using aminoglycosides to treat infections, peak concentrations of how many times the minimum inhibitory concentration of the infecting organism have been associated with positive clinical outcomes? (EO-6)
   a. 1–2
   b. 8–12
   c. 4–6
   d. 18–20

8. Why might continuous infusion administration of cephalosporins be more beneficial than conventional intermittent dosing? (EO-6, 7)

9. How long should SF be treated for the *Enterobacter* infection? (EO-12)

10. If SF's condition progressively declines, should corticosteroids, HA1A, or E5 be used as adjunctive therapy? (EO-8, 11, 12)

11. If SF develops ARDS, which of the following may be useful for treatment of late (fibroproliferative stage) ARDS? (EO-8, 11, 12)
    a. Ibuprofen
    b. Ketoconazole
    c. Corticosteroids
    d. Pentoxifylline

12. The development of sepsis in a patient in a surgical intensive care unit increases his or her total hospitalization cost by: (EO-17)
    a. 10%
    b. 50%
    c. 100%
    d. 200%

13. Describe psychosocial issues related to SF's continuing care. (EO-16)

14. Summarize disease management concepts of bacteremia/sepsis utilizing a key points format. (EO-18)

CASE 126
G. Christopher Wood
Topic: Sepsis
Level 2
EDUCATIONAL MATERIALS
Chapter 82: Bacteremia and Sepsis (signs and symptoms, therapeutic plan); Chapter 67: Pneumonia (diagnosis, pneumococcal pneumonia, therapeutic plan for community acquired pneumonia)

SCENARIO

Patient and Setting

MA, a 62-year-old female; medical intensive care unit (MICU)

Chief Complaint

Shortness of breath, weakness, lethargy, increasing sputum production

History of Present Illness

Increasing shortness of breath, sputum production (thick, white), weakness, lethargy, fever, tachypnea over past 2–3 days; found by neighbors unconscious in kitchen; intubated and has been in the MICU for 1 day

Past Medical History

COPD × 10 years

Past Surgical History

None

Family/Social History

Family History: Noncontributory
Social History: Smokes 30 packs/year

Medication History

Cefepime, 1 g IV q12h

Ciprofloxacin, 400 mg IV q12h

Cimetidine, 300 mg IV q8h

Heparin, 5000 units SC q12h

Albuterol, nebulization treatment q4h

Albuterol MDI, 2 puffs PRN shortness of breath

Allergies

NKDA

Physical Examination

GEN: Ill-appearing woman, somewhat undernourished looking
VS: BP 90/65, HR 110, RR 12, T 40°C, Wt 60 kg, Ht 166 cm
HEENT: WNL
COR: WNL
CHEST: Bibasilar rales and crackles
ABD: WNL, positive bowel sounds
GU: WNL, catheter in place
RECT: WNL
EXT: 1+ edema in all extremities
NEURO: Intermittently oriented to time, person, and place; lethargic

Results of Pertinent Laboratory Tests, Serum Drug Concentrations, and Diagnostic Tests

Na 138 (138)	Cr 150 (1.4)	ALT 0.86 (52)
K 3.6 (3.6)	Glu 8 (144)	LDH 1.67 (100)
Cl 100 (100)	Lkcs 21.0 × 10⁹	Alb 34 (3.4)
HCO₃ 26 (26)	(21.0 × 10³)	Plts 125 × 10⁹
Hct 0.34 (34%)	Hgb 125 (12.5)	(125 × 10³)
BUN 5.4 (15)	AST 0.82 (49)	

Lkc differential: Neutrophils 0.90 (90%), bands 0.18 (18%), lymphs 0.02 (2%)

Chest x-ray: Bilateral lower lobe infiltrates consistent with pneumonia

Blood culture: Gram-positive cocci on preliminary results

Urine culture: Negative

Ventilator settings: SIMV rate 12/FiO_2 60%/PEEP 10

ABGs: pH 7.26/pCO_2 45/pO_2 98

Pulmonary artery catheter readings: Cardiac index 2.8, PAOP 6

Urine output: < 10 mL/hr

PROBLEM LIST

Identify principal problems from the scenario in priority order [completed Problem List and SOAP Note at end of casebook]

SOAP NOTE

To be completed by student

QUESTIONS

[*Answers at end of casebook*]

1. Identify organisms that should be covered empirically in MA and provide appropriate antibiotic recommendations. (EO-3, 8)

2. Which of the following therapies should MA receive immediately to help optimize her hemodynamic status? (EO-5, 8, 12)
   a. Epinephrine infusion
   b. Normal saline infusion
   c. D5W infusion
   d. Dobutamine infusion

3. Which of the following methods should be used to obtain quantitative cultures for diagnosis of pneumonia in MA? (EO-5, 12)
   a. Sputum collection
   b. Transthoracic needle aspiration
   c. Open lung biopsy
   d. Bronchoscopy with bronchoalveolar lavage or protected specimen brush

4. After initial therapy, MA's PAOP has improved to 16, BP is 140/78, but her CI has dropped to 1.9. What should be administered next? (EO-5, 8, 12)
   a. Dobutamine
   b. Low-dose dopamine
   c. Norepinephrine
   d. Furosemide

5. Which of the following may be used in an attempt to improve MA's poor urine output? (EO-5, 8, 12)
   a. Dobutamine
   b. Epinephrine
   c. Low-dose dopamine
   d. Norepinephrine

6. Final culture results show significant quantities of *Streptococcus pneumoniae* in MA's lungs and blood which is only intermediately sensitive to penicillin and ceftriaxone and is fully sensitive to vancomycin. Which of the following should be used as definitive therapy for MA's pneumonia? (EO-5, 8, 11, 12)
   a. Cefepime and ciprofloxacin
   b. Penicillin G
   c. Ceftriaxone
   d. Vancomycin

7. What is MA's PaO_2:FiO_2 ratio? (EO-5)
   a. 1.63
   b. 0.6
   c. 61
   d. 163

8. Does MA have ARDS? State rationale for answer. (EO-5)

9. In light of MA's existing lung disease, which of the following may help her pulmonary status? (EO-5, 8, 11, 12)
   a. Albuterol
   b. Corticosteroids
   c. Ipratropium
   d. Cromolyn

10. What would be expected to be the last sign/symptom of pneumonia to resolve in MA? (EO-5)
    a. Chest x-ray abnormalities
    b. Fever
    c. Leukocytosis
    d. Dyspnea

11. One week later, MA develops pneumonia caused by *Pseudomonas aeruginosa*. The organism is reported as sensitive to gentamicin with an MIC of 4 μg/mL. Should gentamicin be used in the treatment of this episode of pneumonia? State rationale for answer. (EO-5, 8, 12)

12. It is estimated that development of nosocomial pneumonia adds approximately how many days to the length of hospital stay? (EO-17)
    a. 0
    b. 3–4
    c. 7–9
    d. 14–17

13. Describe how common psychosocial factors may increase a patient's risk for developing pneumonia. (EO-16)

14. Summarize disease management concepts for sepsis in this patient using a key points format. (EO-18)

CASE 127
Dorthea Rudorf
Topic: Skin and Soft Tissue Infection—Cellulitis

EDUCATIONAL MATERIALS
Chapter 83: Skin and Soft Tissue Infections
(cellulitis, treatment, pressure sores, treatment)

SCENARIO

Patient and Setting

AA, a 48-year-old, morbidly obese male; ED

Chief Complaint

Swelling of left lower leg; redness and pain; open weepy sore on left calf; fever and chills

History of Present Illness

Gradually worsening leg pain, inflammation, and edema over the past 10 days; small skin break developed into open sore; low-grade fever for 2 days; recently treated for cellulitis

Past Medical History

Leg cellulitis—hospitalized 5 weeks ago, and several times in the past; morbid obesity; hypertension (HTN); past episodes of depression associated with weight gain and death of parents

Past Surgical History

None

Family/Social History

Family History: Father and mother died in 1996 (diabetes, myocardial infarct, respectively)

Social History: Lives with wife and 2 children; works as computer analyst; smokes ½ PPD × 15 years; no alcohol

Medication History

Furosemide, 20 mg PO BID

Diltiazem SR, 120 mg PO QD

Acetaminophen, 650 mg PO PRN (recently up to 4 doses/day)

Tolnaftate cream, 1% applied PRN to feet

Allergies

Cephalexin (itching, rash)

Oxacillin (hives, rash)

Physical Examination

GEN: Morbidly obese, pleasant middle-aged man in no acute distress

VS: BP 140/80, HR 96, RR 16, T 37.9°C, Wt 150 kg, Ht 173 cm

HEENT: PERRLA

COR: RRR, distant heart sounds

CHEST: Clear to auscultation; slight dyspnea on exertion; inflamed itching areas between skin folds on breast area

ABD: Obese, soft, nontender

GU: Deferred

RECT: Deferred

EXT: Coarse gray skin on both calves; extremely edematous left lower leg, warm and painful to touch; 5 cm superficial ulceration midway between ankle and knee on left calf; inflamed, itching areas between his toes

NEURO: A and O × 4

Results of Pertinent Laboratory Tests, Serum Drug Concentrations, and Diagnostic Tests

Na 139 (139)	HCO$_3$ 28 (28)	Lkcs 16.1 × 10^9
K 4.9 (4.9)	Hct 0.43 (43)	(16.1 × 10^3)
Cl 99 (99)	Hgb 137 (13.7)	Plts 231 × 10^9 (231 × 10^3)

Glu 8.44 (152) (random)	Ca 2.38 (9.5)	BUN 6.43 (18) Cr 97.24 (1.1)

Diff: 85 Neutrophils, 1 band, 9 lymphs, 5 monos, 0 eos, 0 basos

Wound: Gram stain results—gram-positive cocci in pairs, clusters, and chains; gram-negative rods, PMNs; cultures pending

Skin culture (toe areas; breast area): *Candida* spp.

PROBLEM LIST

Identify principal problems from the scenario in priority order [completed Problem List and SOAP Note at end of casebook]

SOAP NOTE

To be completed by student

QUESTIONS

[*Answers at end of casebook*]

1. The most probable cause for AA's cellulitis is: (EO-1)
   a. Hypertension
   b. Obesity
   c. Smoking
   d. Diabetes

2. Identify the signs and symptoms associated with cellulitis in AA's clinical presentation, and other possible signs and symptoms. (EO-2)

3. The most common organisms causing cellulitis in adults are: (EO-5)
   a. Streptococci and staphylococci
   b. *Haemophilus influenzae*
   c. Gram-negative organisms
   d. Fungi

4. Discuss the factors that should be considered in choosing pharmacologic and nonpharmacologic therapy for AA's cellulitis. (EO-8)

5. The rapid infusion of vancomycin has been associated with which of the following adverse effects: (EO-10)
   a. Gastrointestinal side effects
   b. Seizures
   c. "Red Man's syndrome"
   d. Peripheral neuropathy

6. Ciprofloxacin may interact with other drugs. Which of the following agents AA is currently taking or may consider taking should either be avoided or given at different times than ciprofloxacin? (EO-9)
   a. Diltiazem
   b. Furosemide
   c. Tylenol
   d. Antacids

7. The successful outcome of antimicrobial therapy is associated with differences in drug pharmacokinetic properties (AUC, Cmax) in relationship to the MIC. Which of the following concepts is thought to be responsible for successful eradication of organisms for quinolone antibiotics such as ciprofloxacin? (EO-6, 7, 8)
   a. Minimizing the ratio of Cmax or AUC to MIC
   b. Concentration-dependent activity
   c. Time-dependent activity
   d. Short postantibiotic effect

8. List the pharmacologic and nonpharmacologic treatment problem(s) present in AA's treatment plan. (EO-11)

9. Given AA's data, calculate the ideal body weight and creatinine clearance as parameters for dosing adjustments, and recommend an appropriate dose for vancomycin and ciprofloxacin. (EO-6, 12)

10. AA is receiving IV vancomycin as empiric therapy to cover for potential MRSA. The physician wants to check the serum concentration of vancomycin after the second dose (peak and trough level). Which recommendation should be given? (EO-5, 10)
    a. Yes, the level needs to be checked right away to avoid nephrotoxicity
    b. There is no need to check the level at all because the pharmacokinetic calculations and dosing adjustments are correct
    c. If vancomycin is continued, obtain serum concentration levels after the 4th dose because AA is obese
    d. The level should be checked after the patient has received at least 10 doses

11. Two days after starting the empiric treatment, the culture and sensitivity report shows predominant *Staphylococcus aureus* sensitive to cefazolin, oxacillin, clindamycin, vancomycin, and amoxicillin-clavulanate. Which of the following agents should AA receive as follow-up therapy? (EO-8, 12)
    a. Cephalexin
    b. Dicloxacillin
    c. Clindamycin
    d. Amoxicillin-clavulanate

12. IgE-mediated hypersensitivity reactions are not uncommon with beta-lactam antibiotics, and cross-reactivity between structurally related drugs can occur. Which of the following drugs most likely does *not* cross-react in penicillin-allergic patients? (EO-8, 10)
    a. Imipenem
    b. Cefotetan
    c. Meropenem
    d. Aztreonam

13. What psychosocial factors may affect AA's adherence to both pharmacologic and nonpharmacologic therapy? (EO-15)

14. Describe the health care provider's role relative to the proposed psychosocial factors identified. (EO-16)

15. Evaluate the pharmacoeconomic considerations relative to AA's care plan. (EO-17)

16. Summarize therapeutic, pathophysiologic, and disease management concepts for skin and soft tissue infections utilizing a key points format. (EO-18)

CASE 128
Donna L. Baxter, Bill McIntyre
Topic: Chronic Myelogenous Leukemia
Level 1
EDUCATIONAL MATERIALS
Chapter 85: Chronic Leukemias (therapeutic goals, clinical presentation and diagnosis, psychosocial issues, treatment)

SCENARIO

Patient and Setting
KC, a 50-year-old male; clinic

Chief Complaint
Three-day history of swelling of his right lower leg; complains of moderate to severe pain in his right calf, and right lower leg erythematous with positive Homans' sign; fatigue, 4.5-kg weight loss over 1 month, anorexia and abdominal fullness

History of Present Illness
Diagnosed 1 month ago with chronic myelogenous leukemia (CML); laboratory data included Lkcs 130 × 10^9 (130 × 10^3), Plts 100 × 10^9 (100 × 10^3), Hgb 70 (7), Hct 0.22 (22%), low leukocyte alkaline phosphatase (LAP) level [40 U/I], LDH 440, and uric acid 376 (6); bone marrow biopsy revealed hypercellular marrow with 80% myeloid cells; cytogenetics at that time positive for translocation of t(9,22) Philadelphia chromosome; treated with hydroxyurea to decrease WBC to <20 × 10^9 followed by interferon alpha-3 MU per day × 3 days, 5 MU per day × 3 days, then 10 MU

Past Medical History
Hypertension; gastroesophageal reflux (GERD)

Past Surgical History
None

Family/Social History
Family History: Married with two daughters
Social History: Negative alcohol or tobacco use

Medication History
Interferon alpha-2b, 10 × 10^6 units SC QD (started 1 month ago)

Hydrochlorothiazide, 25 mg PO QD
Famotidine, 20 mg PO BID

Allergies
Sulfa (rash)

Physical Examination
GEN: Pale, weak-appearing man
VS: BP 186/90, RR 22, HR 100, T 37°C, Ht 180 cm, Wt 90 kg
HEENT: PERRL, EOMI
COR: Normal S1 and S2, no murmurs
CHEST: Clear to auscultation and percussion
ABD: Soft, NT, splenomegaly, positive bowel sounds
GU: Normal
RECT: Normal
EXT: No clubbing, cyanosis, or edema
NEURO: A and O × 3

Results of Pertinent Laboratory Tests, Serum Drug Concentrations, and Diagnostic Tests

Na 143 (143)	Hgb 70 (7)	T Prot 68 (6.8)
K 4.5 (4.5)	Lkcs 22 × 10^9	T Bili 5.1 (0.5)
Cl 100 (100)	(22 × 10^3)	Glu 7.7 (138)
HCO$_3$ 22 (22)	Plts 150 × 10^9	Ca 2.35 (9.4)
BUN 3.9 (11)	(150 × 10^3)	PO$_4$ 1.32 (4.1)
Cr 106 (1.2)	AST 0.62 (37)	Mg 1.1 (2.2)
Uric Acid 286 (4.8)	ALT 0.5 (30)	PT 11.8
LAP 40 U/I	Alk Phos 1.5 (90)	PTT 22.0
Hct 0.22 (22%)	Alb 40 (4.0)	INR 1.1
	LDH 3.4 (204)	

Doppler studies: Extensive thrombosis in right popliteal vein

PROBLEM LIST
Identify principal problems from the scenario in priority order [completed Problem List and SOAP Note at end of casebook]

SOAP NOTE
To be completed by student

QUESTIONS
[Answers at end of casebook]
1. Which of the following therapies is curative for CML? (EO-8)
   a. Autologous bone marrow transplant

b. Treatment with interferon

c. Allogenic bone marrow transplant

d. Treatment with hydroxyurea

2. Risk factors for CML include: (EO-3)

a. Infection with the Epstein-Barr virus

b. First-degree relative with CML

c. Exposure to cigarette smoke

d. Exposure to large amounts of radiation

3. Allogenic bone marrow transplant has the best long-term survival benefit when it is performed in _____. (EO-8)

a. Blast crisis

b. Chronic phase

c. Accelerated phase

d. First complete remission following blast crisis

4. Which of the following statements concerning treatment for CML with interferon alpha is correct? (EO-8, 17)

a. It produces optimal results when initiated in the accelerated phase

b. It is capable of producing a complete cytogenetic response

c. It is clearly cost effective in terms of quality-adjusted life years saved

d. It is well tolerated with minimal side effects

5. Describe at least three psychosocial aspects of CML. (EO-15)

6. The medical resident is concerned that KC's aPTT has not been checked since initiation of his enoxaparin therapy. Explain why this is or is not a valid concern. (EO-5)

7. The primary reason to initiate enoxaparin prior to warfarin would be to: (EO-7, 10)

a. Decrease risk of pulmonary embolism

b. Prevent warfarin-induced skin necrosis

c. Increase warfarin's efficacy

d. Inhibit platelets

8. The mechanism of action of hydroxyurea is thought to be: (EO-7)

a. Inhibition of purine synthesis

b. Inhibition of protein synthesis

c. Inhibition of RNA synthesis

d. Inhibition of DNA synthesis

9. The dose-limiting effect of hydroxyurea is: (EO-10)

a. Uremia

b. Pulmonary fibrosis

c. Myelosuppression

d. Hepatotoxicity

10. List key counseling points that should be covered regarding KC's warfarin therapy. (EO-14)

11. Which of the following medications can increase the effect of warfarin? (EO-9)

a. Cimetidine

b. Phenobarbital

d. Rifampin

e. Phenytoin

12. Summarize therapeutic, pathophysiologic, and disease management concepts for chronic myelogenous leukemia utilizing a key points format. (EO-18)

CASE 129
Donna L. Baxter, Bill McIntyre
Topics: Acute Myelogenous Leukemia (AML), Nausea and Vomiting

 Level 3

EDUCATIONAL MATERIALS

Chapter 86: Acute Leukemias (classification of acute leukemias; treatment plan; AML: treatment, prognosis)

SCENARIO

Patient and Setting

EH, a 50-year-old female; hospitalized

Chief Complaint

Intractable nausea and vomiting, rigors, and severe mouth pain 1 week after chemotherapy initiated

History of Present Illness

3 weeks ago, presented to emergency room with progressive fatigue, decreased energy over several weeks, sore throat, nasal congestion, and gum swelling; lkcs 15.4×10^9 (15.4×10^3) and a peripheral smear with leukemic blasts; diagnosed with acute myelogenous leukemia (AML) through cytogenic testing; chemotherapy initiated: induction course of ARA-C (cytarabine) and daunorubicin

Past Medical History

Hot flashes secondary to a bilateral salpingo-oophorectomy performed 10 years ago

Past Surgical History

Oophorectomy

Central line placement

Family/Social History

Family History: Husband, 2 children

Social History: No alcohol or tobacco use

Medication History

Conjugated estrogens, 0.625 mg PO QD

Medroxyprogesterone, 10 mg PO QD

Allergies

NKDA

Physical Examination

GEN: Diaphoretic, weak-appearing woman
VS: BP 110/56, HR 100, RR 20, T 39.5°C, Wt 77.5 kg, Ht 167.5 cm
HEENT: NC/AT, PERRL, EOMI, + prominent gingival hyperplasia, erythematous buccal cavity
COR: NL S1 and S2, no murmurs
CHEST: CTA
ABD: Bowel sounds absent, soft, nontender, no masses
EXT: No clubbing, cyanosis, or edema
NEURO: A and O × 3, CN II-XII intact

Results of Pertinent Laboratory Tests, Serum Drug Concentrations, and Diagnostic Tests

Na 138 (138)	Hct 0.21 (21)	Ca 1.9 (8.0)
K 3.1 (3.1)	Hgb 80 (8)	PO_4 0.65 (2)
Cl 115 (115)	Lkcs 0.3 × 10^9	PT 24
HCO_3 22 (22)	(0.3 × 10^3)	PTT 46.2
BUN 3.2 (9)	Plts 134 × 10^9	Fib 1.06 (106)
Cr 88.4 (1.0)	(134 × 10^3)	INR 1.8

Bone marrow biopsy: Hypocellular marrow

Peripheral smear: No blasts

Blood cultures: Negative to date

Chest x-ray: WNL; no change from baseline

PROBLEM LIST

Identify principal problems from the scenario in priority order [completed Problem List and SOAP Note at end of casebook]

SOAP NOTE

To be completed by student

QUESTIONS

[Answers at end of casebook]

1. All-transretoinic acid, in combination with cytarabine and daunomycin, has been shown to improve disease-free survival in which FAB-classified leukemia? (EO-8, 11)
   a. ANLL, M4
   b. ANLL, M3
   c. ALL, childhood
   d. ALL, adult

2. All of the following are common causes of morbidity and mortality in ANLL, *except:* (EO-1)
   a. Liver failure
   b. Tumor lysis syndrome
   c. Infection
   d. Hemorrhage

3. Which of the following is a favorable prognostic factor for patients with ANLL? (EO-1, 5)
   a. Age >60 years
   b. Male gender
   c. M1 FAB with Auer Rods
   d. Monosomy 7

4. Tumor lysis syndrome is characterized by which of the following laboratory abnormalities: (EO-5)
   a. Hypercalcemia
   b. Hypophosphatemia
   c. Hypokalemia
   d. Hyperuricemia

5. EH is now 3 weeks out from the start of chemotherapy. The medical resident wants to start her on a colony-stimulating factor, but is concerned about safety. How would you answer the resident's concerns? (EO-8)

6. Transretinoic acid is indicated in patients with which chromosomal abnormality? (EO-8)
   a. 15:17 translocation
   b. Ph chromosome
   c. 9:22 translocation
   d. BCL2 mutation

7. Compared with other AML subgroups, patients with acute promyelocytic leukemia (APL) are at risk for: (EO-1)
   a. Relapse
   b. CNS involvement
   c. DIC
   d. Tumor lysis

8. All of the following are causes of anemia in cancer patients, *except:* (EO-1)
   a. Direct tumor invasion of the bone marrow
   b. Chemotherapy-induced myelosuppression
   c. Chemotherapy-induced renal damage
   d. Tumor-enhanced expression of interleukin-6

9. What are the pharmacoeconomic factors to be considered in utilizing recombinant erythropoietin (rh EPO) in cancer patients? (EO-17)

10. Retinoic acid syndrome in patients with APL treated with tretinoin can be fatal due to: (EO-1)
    a. Hypoxia
    b. Hypotension
    c. Hepatic failure
    d. Uremic syndrome

11. Retinoic acid syndrome should be treated with: (EO-8, 12)
    a. Serotonin antagonists
    b. Dexamethasone
    c. Antihistamines
    d. Bronchodilators

12. Describe psychosocial factors that EH and her family would experience if she needs a bone marrow transplant. (EO-15)

13. Summarize therapeutic, pathophysiologic, and disease management concepts for acute myelogenous leukemia utilizing a key points format. (EO-18)

CASE 130
Donna L. Baxter, Bill McIntyre
Topics: Non-Hodgkin's Lymphoma, Nausea and
Vomiting, Anemia

EDUCATIONAL MATERIALS
Chapter 87: Lymphomas (clinical presentation and
diagnosis, treatment, non-Hodgkin's lymphoma,
complications); Chapter 84: Supportive Care
Therapies for the Patient with Cancer

SCENARIO

Patient and Setting
CD, a 38-year-old male; hospitalized

Chief Complaint
Weakness, weight loss, night sweats, and fevers

History of Present Illness
In good health until 2 months ago, then began to experience night sweats, lymphadenopathy, and fever, 12-lb weight loss over 2 months; tuberculin skin test negative; chest x-ray showed marked lymphadenopathy

Past Medical History
None

Past Surgical History
Arthroscopic knee surgery

Family/Social History
Family History: Married; no children
Social History: 1–2 beers per week; no tobacco use

Medication History
Multivitamin PO QD
Milk of magnesia, 30 mL PO PRN

Allergies
NKDA

Physical Examination
GEN: Thin-appearing man in no apparent distress
VS: BP 150/78, HR 64, T 38°C, Ht 175 cm (5′9″), Wt 58 kg (64 kg 2 months ago)

CHEST: Clear to auscultation and percussion
ABD: Hepatosplenomegaly, enlarged inguinal lymph nodes; 3 × 5 cm mass in the lower right quadrant

Results of Pertinent Laboratory Tests, Serum Drug Concentrations, and Diagnostic Tests

Na 137 (137)	Lkcs 10.7 × 10⁹	T Prot 68 (6.8)
K 4.2 (4.2)	(10.7 × 10³)	T Bili 12 (0.7)
Cl 100 (100)	Plts 284 × 10⁹	Glu 4.7 (85)
HCO₃ 24 (24)	(284 × 10³)	Ca 2.35 (9.4)
BUN 3.9 (11)	AST 1.0 (60)	PO₄ 1.32 (4.1)
Cr 104 (1.1)	ALT 0.92 (55)	Mg 1.1 (2.2)
Uric Acid 250 (4.2)	Alk Phos 1.5 (90)	PT 11.8
Hct 0.304 (30.4)	Alb 40 (4.0)	PTT 22.0
Hgb 98 (9.8)	LDH 4.9 (190)	INR 0.9

Abdominal and chest CT: Extensive lymphadenopathy, two liver nodules consistent with metastatic disease, and a 2 × 4 cm right supraclavicular node

Inguinal node biopsy is consistent with follicular small-cleaved cell non-Hodgkin's lymphoma which was CD 20(+), CD 45 (−), and CD 19(+)

PROBLEM LIST

Identify principal problems from the scenario in priority order

SOAP NOTE

To be completed by student

QUESTIONS

1. Which of the following statements is correct? (EO-3)
   a. The incidence of lymphoma in the U.S. appears to be decreasing
   b. Patients with immunodeficiency disorders are at increased risk for developing non-Hodgkin's lymphoma
   c. The incidence of Hodgkin's lymphoma is inversely proportional to educational level
   d. The peak incidence of Hodgkin's lymphoma occurs before age 20

2. Rituximab is a chimeric, monoclonal antibody that binds to what cell surface antigen? (EO-7)
   a. CD 20
   b. CD 5
   c. CD 34
   d. CD 4

3. Early stage (Stage I and II) Hodgkin's lymphoma is generally treated with which of the following: (EO-12)
   a. Chemotherapy plus irradiation to the involved areas
   b. Subtotal nodal irradiation

   c. Combination chemotherapy with MOPP/ABVD
   d. Autologous bone marrow transplant

4. Which of the following statements is correct? (EO-1)
   a. Lymphoma is listed as an AIDS-defining illness
   b. Most NHL associated with AIDS is indolent, and presents at a limited stage
   c. There is a higher incidence of CNS involvement in HIV-infected patients with NHL than in non-HIV-infected patients with NHL
   d. HIV is believed to be directly responsible for the malignant transformation from normal lymphocytes to lymphoma

5. CD returned to the clinic on day 5 of the first course of rituximab complaining of fever for the past 8–12 hours. His Lkc is 1.2 with 68% neutrophils. Upon arrival in the clinic his temperature is 101.4°F, BP 140/80, and he feels fairly well. There are no obvious new clinical findings. What are the potential causes of the fever, and how should CD be managed? (EO-1)

6. CD received his first course of cyclophosphamide-doxorubicin-vincristine-prednisone (CHOP) for his lymphoma yesterday. Today his serum potassium is 5.1 (from 4.0), phosphate 1.6 (4.9) (from 1.13 [3.5]), uric acid 583 (9.8) (from 250 [4.2]), BUN 9.3 (26) (from 6.8 [19]), and creatinine is 141 (1.6) (from 80.4 [1.0]). What is the probable cause of these acute changes, and how should CD be managed at this time? (EO-1, 8, 12)

7. What agent is approved for prevention of doxorubicin-induced cardiac toxicity? (EO-8, 10)
   a. Thiamine
   b. Iron
   c. Dexrazoxane
   d. Mesna

8. All of the following are long-term complications of CHOP therapy, *except:* (EO-1)
   a. Secondary malignancies
   b. Sterility
   c. Cataracts
   d. Diabetes

9. The classic finding in Hodgkin's disease is: (EO-5)
   a. Sideroblasts
   b. Promyeloblasts
   c. Target cells
   d. Reed-Sternberg cells

10. Which of the following antineoplastics has a significant interaction with allopurinol? (EO-9)
   a. 6-mercaptopurine
   b. 6-thioguanine
   c. Cyclophosphamide
   d. Methotrexate

11. What psychosocial issue should be considered in a young male receiving CHOP? (EO-15)

12. Why should CD be given hydration prior to CHOP? (EO-8)

13. Summarize therapeutic, pathophysiologic, and disease management concepts for non-Hodgkin's lymphoma utilizing a key points format. (EO-18)

CASE 131
Donna L. Baxter, Bill McIntyre
Topics: Breast Cancer, Bone Pain
 Level 2
EDUCATIONAL MATERIALS
Chapter 88: Breast Cancer (clinical presentation and diagnosis, psychosocial aspects, therapeutic plan, locally advanced breast cancer)

SCENARIO

Patient and Setting
MF, a 54-year-old female; clinic

Chief Complaint
Presents 5 years after completion of adjuvant chemotherapy for stage IIIA breast carcinoma with a 2-week history of increasing shortness of breath and cough and mild/moderate pain in left side

History of Present Illness
Infiltrating intraductal adenocarcinoma of the left breast 5 years ago; at that time, ER(−) / PR(−); her-2/neu (+); p53 (+); staged as having T3N1M0, stage IIIA, high-risk breast cancer; underwent a modified radical mastectomy with axillary node dissection followed by 6 cycles of CMF chemotherapy

Past Medical History
Gravida 4, para 4; menses onset age 13; HTN × 10 years; Type 2 DM × 8 years; breast cancer as above; remained disease free until present follow-up

Past Surgical History
Left modified radical mastectomy 5 years ago; cholecystectomy 14 years ago

Family/Social History
Family History: Breast cancer—mother and sister
Social History: Noncontributory

Medication History
Glyburide, 5 mg PO BID
Verapamil SR, 240 mg PO QD
Furosemide, 40 mg PO QD

Allergies
NKDA

Physical Examination

GEN: Well-developed, obese woman in no acute distress

VS: BP 120/88, HR 80, RR 20, T 37°C, Ht 167.6 cm, Wt 92 kg

HEENT: PERRLA, no JVD, no lymphadenopathy

COR: Normal S1 and S2, no murmurs, rubs, or gallops

CHEST: Well-healed scar left breast area; dullness of percussion over left lung bases, decreased breath sounds

ABD: Obese, soft, nontender, no masses or organomegaly

GU: WNL

RECT: External hemorrhoids noted

EXT: No clubbing, cyanosis, or edema

NEURO: A and O × 3; cranial nerves intact, normal deep tendon reflexes

Results of Pertinent Laboratory Tests, Serum Drug Concentrations, and Diagnostic Tests

Na 143 (143)	Lkcs 6.8 × 10^9	T Prot 68 (6.8)
K 4.5 (4.5)	(6.8 × 10^3)	T Bili 5.1 (0.5)
Cl 100 (100)	Plts 372 × 10^9	Glu 7.7 (138)
HCO_3 22 (22)	(372 × 10^3)	Ca 2.35 (9.4)
BUN 3.9 (11)	AST 0.62 (37)	PO_4 1.32 (4.1)
Cr 106 (1.2)	ALT 0.5 (30)	Mg 1.1 (2.2)
Uric Acid 286 (4.8)	Alk Phos 1.5 (90)	INR 1.0
Hct 0.426 (42.6)	Alb 40 (4.0)	PTT 22.0
Hgb 130 (13)	LDH 204 (204)	

Lkc differential: Neut 0.7 (70%), lymph 0.20 (20%), mono 0.065 (6.5%), baso 0.013 (1.3%), eos 0.022 (2.2%)

Urinalysis: WNL

ECG: Normal sinus rhythm

CXR: Effusion in left lower lobe. Fluid layers out on lateral x-ray.

Bone scan: Multiple metastases to left lower ribs.

Pleural fluid: Thoracentesis: Glucose 5.3 (95), LDH 234 (234), pH 7.5, specific gravity 1.025, protein 50 g/L (5.0 g/dL), Lkcs 2.6 × 10^9, RBC 110 × 10^{12} (110 × 10^6); cytology: adenocarcinoma breast

PROBLEM LIST

Identify principal problems from the scenario in priority order [completed Problem List and SOAP Note at end of casebook]

SOAP NOTE

To be completed by student

QUESTIONS

[Answers at end of casebook]

1. Which of the following factors remains controversial as a potential cause of breast cancer? (EO-3)
   a. Alcohol consumption ≥2 drinks/day
   b. Mutations in the BRCA1 and BRCA2 genes
   c. Estrogen use
   d. Smoking

2. According to the American Cancer Society Guidelines, all of the following are correct, *except:* (EO-3, 5)
   a. Beginning at age 30, women should perform monthly breast self-exams
   b. Women over the age of 40 should have a breast exam conducted by their physician on a yearly basis
   c. All women should begin annual or biannual mammography screening at age 40
   d. Both physical examination and screening mammography should be conducted, starting at age 40

3. Which of the following psychosocial issues associated with women with breast cancer is *incorrect?* (EO-15)
   a. Transition in role from "support-giver" to "care-receiver"
   b. Increased financial burden
   c. Change in appearance due to breast removal and/or alopecia
   d. Improved QOL while receiving chemotherapy

4. Which of the following statements is correct? (EO-8)
   a. Early stage (Stage I and II) breast cancer is most often managed with radical mastectomy and radiation
   b. The goal of treatment of metastatic breast cancer is to provide disease-free survival in 90% of patients for up to 5 years
   c. Early stage (Stage I) breast cancer is easily controlled with surgery alone, or surgery and radiation
   d. Although new agents, including monoclonal antibodies and taxanes, have helped prolong survival in patients with metastatic disease, they are of no benefit in the treatment of early stage breast cancer

5. MF presents to the clinic 2 months later complaining of shortness of breath upon exertion, orthopnea requiring two pillows at night, and 2+ pitting edema bilaterally of her lower extremities. A MUGA scan indicated MF has an ejection fraction of 20%. What is the most likely cause of MF's congestive heart failure, and what would you recommend for treatment? (EO-10)

6. Which of the following is the mechanism of action of docetaxel? (EO-7)
   a. Inhibition of tubulin
   b. Enhanced microtubulin formation
   c. Adduct formation
   d. Inhibition of purine synthesis

7. Dexamethasone is administered with docetaxel to: (EO-7, 10)
   a. Prevent hypotension
   b. Prevent wheezing
   c. Prevent edema
   d. Prevent nausea

8. What would MF's expected response rate to hormonal therapy be? (EO-11)
   a. 10%
   b. 25%
   c. 60%
   d. 80%

9. MF's serum creatinine has increased to 2.0 mg/dL, and she appears to be adequately hydrated. What is the most likely cause for this change? (EO-10)

10. How would pleural effusion be expected to influence the pharmacokinetics of MF's chemotherapy? (EO-6)

11. If MF's blood glucose elevates during her chemotherapy, what would be the most probable cause? (EO-10)
    a. Trastuzumab
    b. Docetaxel
    c. Dexamethasone
    d. Ibuprofen

12. How might early detection of breast cancer affect pharmacoeconomic outcomes of disease? (EO-17)

13. Summarize the therapeutic, pathophysiologic, and disease management concepts for the treatment of breast cancer utilizing a key points format. (EO-18)

CASE 132
Donna L. Baxter, Bill McIntyre
Topics: Gastrointestinal Cancer, Chemotherapy-Induced Nausea and Vomiting

Level 1

EDUCATIONAL MATERIALS
Chapter 90: Gastrointestinal Cancers (chemotherapy-induced nausea and vomiting, clinical presentation and diagnosis, treatment); Chapter 84: Supportive Care Therapies for Patients with Cancer

---

SCENARIO

Patient and Setting
JS, a 45-year old man; emergency room

Chief Complaint
3-day history of diffuse abdominal pain, fatigue, malaise, pallor, dysphagia, nausea, and up to 3–4 episodes of vomiting per day; vomitus was usually watery except for two episodes of bloody emesis this morning; last ate 5 days ago; nasogastric (NG) aspirate in the ED positive for 60 mL of red bloody material; admitted for supportive measures and GI work-up

History of Present Illness
Experienced severe weight loss (18.2 kg) over the past 2 months and a change in eating habits; initially, experienced early satiety which was unnoticeable until began to lose weight; approximately 5 months ago, began having upper epigastric pain associated with food; took magnesium/aluminum antacids, which provided some relief; episodes of pain worsened about 1 week ago; pain is no longer epigastric but associated with stomach cramps, and occurs throughout the day

Past Medical History
Hypertension diagnosed 7 years ago

Past Surgical History
None

Family/Social History
Family History: Married with 2 adult children; father with prostate cancer diagnosed at age 50, and mother with hypertension diagnosed at age 45
Social History: Noncontributory

Medication History
Nifedipine, sustained-release (SR), 30 mg PO QD (last taken 3 days ago)

Magnesium/aluminum antacid, 30 mL PO q4h PRN, epigastric pain

Allergies
Penicillin (loss of consciousness age 5)

Physical Examination
GEN: Thin, pale-looking 45-year-old man in severe distress
VS: T 37.0°C, BP 150/95, HR 90, RR 20, Ht 175 cm, Wt 62 kg, BSA 1.74 m^2
HEENT: Head, neck adenopathy, PERRLA, EOMI
COR: Sinus tachycardia, no murmurs or gallops
CHEST: Clear to auscultation and percussion
ABD: Diffuse tenderness and distention, (−) bowel sounds
GU: Unremarkable
RECT: Guaiac positive
EXT: Unremarkable
NEURO: Lethargic, oriented × 3, NL gait

Results of Pertinent Laboratory Tests, Serum Drug Concentrations, and Diagnostic Tests

Na 133 (133)	BUN 12.9 (36)	Lkcs 9.5 × 10^9
K 4.6 (4.6)	SCr 141.4 (1.6)	(9.5 × 10^3)
Cl 104 (104)	Glu 5.28 (95)	Hgb 16 (10.0)
HCO$_3$ 26 (26)		Hct 0.38 (38)

Plts 110 × 10⁹   PO₄ 1.59 (4.8)   AST 5.7 (342)

$Plts\ 110 \times 10^9$ (110×10^3)
$PO_4\ 1.59\ (4.8)$
$AST\ 5.7\ (342)$
LDH 2.0 (120)
$Mg\ 1.25\ (2.5)$
$ALT\ 7.32\ (437)$
Ca 39.2 (9.8)
Alk Phos 18.7 (1120)
Amylase 72 (72)
Alb 23 (2.3)
INR 1.2
T Bili 32.7 (1.9)

Additional diagnostic findings: (obtained 2 days after admission to the medicine unit)

Abdominal CT scan: (+) multiple liver mass, about 2 × 4 × 3 cm in diameter;

Gastric biopsy results: Consistent with adenocarcinoma

Barium upper GI (BaGI): Small, discrete multiple ulcerative mass 2 cm in diameter with a central necrotic crater confined to the antrum mucosa; pathology result revealed a poorly differentiated adenocarcinoma of signet-ring cell types

Chest CT scan: Normal

Chest x-ray: Clear, (−) infiltrates, (−) metastasis

PROBLEM LIST

Identify principal problems from the scenario in priority order

SOAP NOTE

To be completed by student

QUESTIONS

1. The risk of gastric cancer in patients infected with *H. pylori* is increased:
   a. 1.5 fold
   b. 2 fold
   c. 4 fold
   d. 6 fold

2. What percent of patients with early gastric cancer demonstrate signs and symptoms? (EO-2, 3)
   a. 25%
   b. 50%
   c. 75%
   d. 100%

3. What best describes the use of carcinoembryonic antigen (CEA) screening for early detection of gastric adenocarcinoma? (EO-5)
   a. CEA is very useful since it is not elevated in patients with gastric ulcers
   b. Failure to detect CEA does not rule out gastric cancer because CEA is elevated in less than 30% of patients with gastric cancer
   c. CEA is elevated in most patients with gastric cancer
   d. CEA is elevated in colon cancer patients, but not in patients with gastric cancer

4. Which of the following has been shown to be a useful screening tool in countries where there is a high incidence of gastric cancer? (EO-5)
   a. Carcinoembryonic antigen (CEA)
   b. Stool guaiac
   c. Endoscopic ultrasound
   d. Esophagogastroduodenoscopy

5. Discuss the different surgical interventions between subtotal gastrectomy and radical total gastrectomy for management of gastric adenocarcinoma. (EO-8)

6. Dietary risk factors for gastric cancer include: (EO-3)
   a. Increased vitamin C intake
   b. Increased vitamin A intake
   c. High-fat diets
   d. High-salt diets

7. What toxicities would be expected with the chemotherapy regimen suggested for JS? (EO-10)

8. Based on NCCTG studies comparing single-agent 5-FU and combination regimens in advanced gastric cancer, _____. (EO-12)
   a. Single-agent 5-FU is less toxic, but less effective than combination regimens
   b. Single-agent 5-FU is less toxic, but as effective as combination regimens
   c. Single-agent 5-FU has equal toxicity and efficacy to combination regimens
   d. Single-agent 5-FU had a statistical survival advantage over combination regimens

9. What is the most common side effect of 5-HT antagonists? (EO-10)
   a. Extrapyramidal effects
   b. Headache
   c. Diarrhea
   d. Glucose intolerance

10. Describe how diarrhea associated with gastrointestinal carcinoma may affect JS's psychosocial functioning. (EO-15)

11. Address JS's future nutritional needs from a pharmacoeconomic standpoint. (EO-17)

12. Summarize therapeutic, pathophysiologic, and disease management concepts for gastric carcinoma utilizing a key points format. (EO-18)

CASE 133
Donna L. Baxter, Bill McIntyre
Topics: Pancreatic Cancer, Pain
Level 1

EDUCATIONAL MATERIALS

Chapter 90: Gastrointestinal Cancers (pancreatic cancer, clinical presentation and diagnosis, staging/prognosis, supportive care, localized, unresectable disease); Chapter 84: Supportive Care Therapies for Patients with Cancer

---

SCENARIO

Patient and Setting

ML, a 72-year-old male; hospitalized

Chief Complaint

Poor pain control; pain mainly in the epigastric area and right upper abdomen; progressive nausea with occasional vomiting and fatigue

History of Present Illness

Three months ago ML presented to his primary care physician with a history of 20-lb (9-kg) weight loss, abdominal discomfort, and lack of appetite; CT scan: large pancreatic mass; several liver masses; biopsy: consistent with adenocarcinoma

Past Medical History

Benign prostatic hypertrophy (BPH); peptic ulcer disease; HTN

Past Surgical History

TURP 4 years ago, appendectomy 40 years ago

Family/Social History

Family History: Widower

Social History: No alcohol or tobacco use

Medication History

Hydrochlorothiazide/triamterene 50/75 mg, 1 PO q AM

Acetaminophen with codeine, 60 mg 1–2 tablets PO q4–6h

Ibuprofen, 600 mg PO QID

Gemcitabine, 1000 mg/m² IV weekly × 7 weeks, second cycle finished 1 week ago

Allergies

Morphine (hives)

Sulfa (rash)

Physical Examination

GEN: Thin white male in mild distress
VS: BP supine: 120/80 [HR 82], standing: 96/60 [HR 105], T 38.1°C, Wt 74 kg (80 kg 1 month ago)
HEENT: Dry mucous membranes, slight oral erythema
COR: RRR
CHEST: Lungs clear to a/p
ABD: Tenderness in epigastrium and right upper abdomen
RECT: Guaiac positive
EXT: Poor skin turgor
NEURO: Oriented × 3

Results of Pertinent Laboratory Tests, Serum Drug Concentrations, and Diagnostic Tests

Na 148 (148)	Lkcs 6.7 × 10⁹	LDH 3.2 (190)
K 4.8 (4.8)	(6.7 × 10³)	Alk Phos 2.0 (122)
Cl 106 (106)	Hgb 139 (13.9)	Alb 30 (3.0)
HCO₃ 25 (25)	Hct 0.44 (44)	T Bili 18.8 (1.1)
BUN 13.6 (38)	Plts 167 × 10⁹	Ca 1.97 (7.9)
Cr 150 (1.7)	(167 × 10³)	PO₄ 0.8 (2.4)
Glu 5.6 (101)	AST 1.1 (65)	Mg 1.2 (2.4)
	ALT 0.7 (42)	

CT abdomen: 5-cm mass in head of pancreas, enlarged lymph nodes, multiple liver metastases, slightly dilated biliary ducts; impression: disease progression compared with pretreatment scan

Chest x-ray: WNL

KUB: No evidence of intestinal obstruction

Upper endoscopy: Diffuse erythema, small erosions, no definite ulcers

PROBLEM LIST

Identify principal problems from the scenario in priority order [completed Problem List and SOAP Note at end of casebook]

SOAP NOTE

To be completed by student

QUESTIONS

[Answers at end of casebook]

1. Which of the following is a risk factor for pancreatic cancer? (EO-1)
   a. Chewing tobacco
   b. High-fiber diets
   c. Diabetes
   d. Retinoic acid

2. The dose-limiting side effect of gemcitabine is: (EO-10)
   a. Myelosuppression
   b. Cardiomyopathy
   c. Mucositis
   d. Hepatotoxicity

3. For maximum effect, 5-FU should be given: (EO-7, 9)
   a. Before methotrexate
   b. After methotrexate
   c. Co-administered with methotrexate
   d. Within 7 days of methotrexate administration

4. What are the goals of ML's therapy? (EO-12, 14)

5. How does response of pancreatic cancer to gemcitabine compare with the response to 5-fluorouracil? (EO-8)

6. Which of the following would not be an appropriate laxative for ML? (EO-8)
   a. Docusate
   b. Metamucil

c. Bisacodyl
d. Senna

7. The risk of addiction in a patient with pain secondary to malignancy is: (EO-8, 11)
   a. Extremely high
   b. High
   c. Low
   d. Very low

8. What is the usual conversion from oral morphine to parenteral morphine? (EO-6)
   a. 1:1
   b. 2:1
   c. 3:1
   d. 10:1

9. Which of the following opiates should be avoided for chronic pain? (EO-8)
   a. Fentanyl
   b. Methadone
   c. Meperidine
   d. Codeine

10. Naloxone is indicated in a patient: (EO-8, 10)
    a. Having hallucinations
    b. Who is unarousable
    c. With respiratory rate less than 15 per minute
    d. Who is sleeping all day

11. What psychosocial considerations are present in ML's case? (EO-15)

12. Related to medication costs only, patients who are offered patient-controlled analgesia (PCA): (EO-17)
    a. Typically use less medication than those with scheduled pain medication administration
    b. Typically use more medication than those with scheduled pain medication administration
    c. Do not require any additional administration devices
    d. Are at greater risk for medication overuse

13. Summarize therapeutic, pathophysiologic, and disease management concepts for pancreatic cancer utilizing a key points format. (EO-18)

CASE 134
Donna L. Baxter, Bill McIntyre
Topic: Colon Cancer
Level 1
EDUCATIONAL MATERIALS
Chapter 90: Gastrointestinal Cancers (colorectal cancer, clinical presentation, staging and prognosis)

SCENARIO

Patient and Setting

HJ, a 67-year-old female; medical oncology clinic

Chief Complaint

Increased abdominal cramping and diarrhea

History of Present Illness

Diagnosed 2 years ago with adenocarcinoma of sigmoid colon, which was resected and found to be a Dukes B2 lesion; no adjuvant chemotherapy given; presented 3 months ago with occasional fevers and upper quadrant pain unresponsive to ibuprofen; was found to have hepatomegaly; was started on 5-fluorouracil and leucovorin for adenocarcinoma; LFTs and CEA continue to be elevated; subsequent CT scan of the abdomen and pelvis revealed new multiple abdominal masses and increased bilobar hepatic metastases; chemotherapy was changed to irinotecan; presents to clinic three days S/P irinotecan with the above complaints

Past Medical History

Congestive heart failure (CHF) since age 60
Colonic polyp removed at age 62

Past Surgical History

Sigmoid colectomy 2 years ago
Appendectomy at age 35

Family/Social History

Family History: Lives with husband who is healthy; has two grown healthy children; mother died of breast cancer at age 63; father died of lung cancer at age 62

Social History: Drinks 1–2 glasses of wine per day; no tobacco

Medication History

Chemotherapy: 4 cycles of 5-fluorouracil, 600 mg/m² IV days 1–5 (discontinued); leucovorin, 20 mg/m² IV days 1–5 (discontinued); irinotecan, 125 mg/m² IV over 90 min/week–started 3 days ago

Medications: Digoxin, 0.125 mg tab PO QD; acetaminophen with codeine, 30 mg PO q4–6h PRN

Allergies

Penicillin (rash)

Physical Examination

GEN: Well-developed, well-nourished, distressed woman
VS: BP 120/70 (sitting) 100/72 (standing), HR 88, RR 15, T 39°C, Wt 65 kg, Ht 177 cm
HEENT: Normal

COR: Normal
CHEST: Normal; no rales
ABD: Liver 6 cm below right costal margin
GU: Deferred
RECT: Normal
EXT: Normal
NEURO: Normal

Results of Pertinent Laboratory Tests, Serum Drug Concentrations, and Diagnostic Tests

Na 140 (140)   Lkcs 8.0 × 10⁹   Alb 40 (4.0)
K 2.5 (2.5)   (8 × 10³)   T Bili 10 (0.5)
Cl 104 (104)   Plts 125 × 10⁹   Ca 2.35 (9.4)
HCO₃ 26 (26)   (125 × 10³)   PO₄ 1.1 (3.4)
BUN 5 (40)   MCV 80 (80)   Mg 1.0 (2)
Cr 70.7 (1.2)   AST 0.73 (44)   Uric Acid 240 (4.0)
Glu 5.5 (100)   ALT 0.79 (47)   Digoxin level: 1.92
Hgb 140 (14)   LDH 4 (240)   mmol/L (1.5 mg/mL)
Hct 0.41 (41)   Alk Phos 3 (180)   CEA 91 mg/L

Chest x-ray: Normal

Abdominal CT scan: Multiple abdominal masses and bilobar liver metastases

ECG: Normal

PROBLEM LIST

Identify principal problems from the scenario in priority order

SOAP NOTE

To be completed by student

QUESTIONS

1. What is the role of leucovorin when combined with 5-fluorouracil? (EO-7, 9)
   a. Modulates immune response
   b. Rescues normal cells
   c. Modulates activity of 5-fluorouracil by stabilizing the ternary complex thymidylate synthase
   d. Enhances 5-fluorouracil's binding to dihydrofolate reductase

2. Changing 5-fluorouracil administration from infusion to bolus affects its toxicity by enhancing the: (EO-6)
   a. Overall toxicity of 5-fluorouracil
   b. Mucositis
   c. Diarrhea
   d. Myelosuppression

3. Colon cancer most often occurs in the _____. (EO-1)
   a. Ascending colon
   b. Anus
   c. Sigmoid colon

   d. Splenic flexure

4. What is the response rate of irinotecan for relapsed colon cancer? (EO-8)
   a. 10%
   b. 25%
   c. 40%
   d. 50%

5. What is the rationale for adjuvant chemotherapy in HJ's case? (EO-8)

6. What is the mechanism of action of irinotecan? (EO-7)
   a. Inhibition of topoisomerase I
   b. Inhibition of topoisomerase II
   c. Inhibition of microtubules
   d. Formation of DNA adducts

7. What psychosocial factors could influence HJ's therapy? (EO-15)

8. What pharmacoeconomic factors could influence the choice of irinotecan versus oral capecitabine? (EO-17)

9. What best describes the role of CEA in colon cancer? (EO-5)
   a. CEA is specific for colon cancer and is a useful screening test for colon cancer
   b. A low CEA guarantees a localized primary
   c. CEA is useful as the sole monitoring method
   d. An elevated CEA may indicate metastatic disease

10. Justify why HJ should or should not receive intrahepatic chemotherapy. (EO-6, 8)

11. Which of the following reduces a person's risk for colon cancer? (EO-2)
    a. Increased dietary fat
    b. High dietary fiber
    c. A first-degree relative with colon cancer
    d. Familial adenomatous polyposis

12. Of all diagnosed cancers in men and women, colon cancer accounts for _____. (EO-3)
    a. 5%
    b. 15%
    c. 25%
    d. 30%

13. Utilizing a key points format, describe the therapeutic, pathophysiologic, and disease management concepts for the treatment of colon cancer. (EO-18)

CASE 135
Donna L. Baxter, Bill McIntyre
Topics: Lung Cancer, Syndrome of Inappropriate Antidiuretic Hormone (SIADH)

Level 1

EDUCATIONAL MATERIALS

Chapter 91: Lung Cancer (clinical presentation, staging/treatment, small cell lung cancer, treatment complications, psychosocial, patient education)

SCENARIO

Patient and Setting

GC, a 61-year-old woman; hospitalized

Chief Complaint

Family states that GC is confused and difficult to awaken

History of Present Illness

At previous checkup 3 weeks prior, complained of intractable cough and undesired 12-lb weight loss; poor appetite; some episodes of hemoptysis, coughing, and SOB; chest x-ray consistent with lobular pneumonia with possible mass; bronchial biopsy, chest and brain CT completed; diagnosed with unresectable, extensive small cell lung cancer; currently admitted for chemotherapy with cisplatin/etoposide

Past Medical History

Benign gastric ulcer 2 years ago, menopause 13 years ago—taking estrogen and medroxyprogesterone, stopped smoking immediately upon diagnosis 3 weeks ago, began nicotine gum as part of a smoking cessation program

Past Surgical History

None

Family/Social History

Family History: Noncontributory

Social History: Smokes 2 PPD × 30 years; drinks 2 glasses wine per night

Medication History

Conjugated estrogens, 0.625 mg PO QD

Erythromycin, 500 mg PO QID

Magnesium oxide, 400 mg PO TID

Nicotine gum PO (was using 25 pieces/day at start of therapy, now using 4 pieces/day)

Cisapride, 10 mg PO QID

Etoposide, 100 mg/m² IV D1 (3 weeks ago)

Cisplatin, 75 mg/m² IV D1 (3 weeks ago)

Allergies

Sulfa (rash and hives)

Physical Examination

GEN: Pale, thin woman appearing slightly anxious
VS: BP 140/82, HR 82, RR 17, T 38.3°C, Wt 53 kg, Ht 152 cm

HEENT: PERRLA; oral cavity showing mild mucositis (Stage I)
COR: RRR; normal S1 and S2
CHEST: Mild expiratory wheezing; central line shows no redness or erythema
ABD: Rebound tenderness; no hepatosplenomegaly
RECT: Guaiac negative
EXT: Normal pulses, no bruising, no edema
NEURO: Oriented to person; cranial nerves intact

Results of Pertinent Laboratory Tests, Serum Drug Concentrations, and Diagnostic Tests:

Na 130 (130)	ANC 253	AST 0.5 (30)
K 3.5 (3.5)	Plts 70 × 10⁹	ALT 0.45 (27)
Cl 98 (98)	(70 × 10³)	Alk Phos 1.32 (79)
HCO₃ 25 (25)	Ca 2.1 (8.5)	LDH 1.65 (99)
BUN 7.5 (21)	PO₄ 0.872 (2.7)	Alb 30 (3.0)
Cr 97.2 (1.1)	Mg 0.65 (1.3)	T Bili 22.2 (1.3)
Glu 5.55 (100)	Hct 0.31 (31)	PT 14
Lkcs 1.5 × 10⁹	Hgb (10.0)	INR 1.2
(1.5 × 10³)		

PROBLEM LIST

Identify principal problems from the scenario in priority order [completed Problem List and SOAP Note at end of casebook]

SOAP NOTE

To be completed by student

QUESTIONS

[Answers at end of casebook]

1. What percentage of patients with lung cancer have a history of smoking? (EO-1, 3)
   a. 50%
   b. 75%
   c. 80%
   d. 95%

2. What is the most common histology of NSCLC found in nonsmokers? (EO-1)
   a. Squamous cell
   b. Large cell
   c. Clear cell
   d. Adenocarcinoma

3. Facial swelling may be a sign of what paraneoplastic syndrome associated with lung cancer? (EO-5)
   a. Superior vena cava
   b. Horner's
   c. SIADH
   d. Pancoast's

4. Patients with SCLC whose tumor can be treated with one radiotherapy port are considered to have: (EO-5)
   a. Stage I cancer

b. Stage II cancer
c. Limited disease
d. Extensive disease

5. What are alternatives to nicotine gum for smoking cessation? (EO-12)

6. For patients with stage IV NSCLC the 5-year survival rate is: (EO-11)
   a. 5%
   b. 7%
   c. 10%
   d. 25%

7. Is there a pharmacoeconomic justification to using chemotherapy in patients with stage IV NSCLC? (EO-17)

8. In limited SCLC, the EP (etoposide, cisplatin) regimen is preferred over the CAV (cyclophosphamide, doxorubicin [Adriamycin], vincristine) regimen because: (EO-8)
   a. It has superior survival rates
   b. It has superior response rates
   c. It produces less neurologic toxicity
   d. CAV is preferred over EP

9. Describe the response and survival rates to chemotherapy for patients with extensive SCLC. (EO-11, 12)

10. Describe the psychosocial impact of lung cancer on the patient. (EO-15)

11. Compare and contrast the toxicities of cisplatin and carboplatin. (EO-10)

12. Explain why GC should or should not receive prophylactic filgrastim therapy while receiving cisplatin/etoposide regimen. (EO-8)

13. Summarize therapeutic, pathophysiologic, and disease management concepts for small cell lung cancer utilizing a key points format. (EO-18)

CASE 136
R. Michelle Sanders
Topics: Pediatric Oncology, Osteosarcoma
Level 2
EDUCATIONAL MATERIALS
Chapter 93: Pediatric Tumors (osteosarcoma: therapeutic goals, clinical presentation and diagnosis, surgery, chemotherapy, patient education)

SCENARIO

Patient and Setting
RT, a 16-year-old white male; oncology clinic

Chief Complaint
Fever, nausea & vomiting, diarrhea, abdominal discomfort, decreased urination, and line-site irritation

History of Present illness
Diagnosed 8 months ago with osteosarcoma; chemotherapy: received 3 courses of ifosfamide, cisplatin/doxorubicin and 6 courses of high-dose methotrexate (HDMTX). Surgical: Limb salvage

Past Medical History
Healthy and active in a number of sports until 4–5 months prior to diagnosis when pain in right arm noticed; assumed result of an injury, so did not seek treatment; 8 months ago, seen by orthopedic surgeon for an unrelated injury; MD noticed mass in proximal humerus; diagnosis of osteosarcoma confirmed; schedule of chemotherapy altered due to missing clinic appointments for past 2 months of therapy; 2 courses of chemotherapy required admission for IV antibiotics

Past Surgical History
Central line placement; limb salvage surgical procedure

Family/Social History
Family History: Lives with parents; makes average grades
Social History: Denies tobacco or alcohol use

Medication History
Three courses of ifosfamide, cisplatin/doxorubicin, and six courses of high-dose methotrexate

Last course of HDMTX given 1 day ago; HDMTX course includes oral bicarbonate & oral hydration the night before sulfamethoxazole/trimethoprim 2 tablets PO BID Monday, Tuesday, Wednesday

Magnesium oxide, 1200 mg PO TID

Naproxen (nonprescription), 220 mg PO PRN–received one dose last evening and one dose this morning

Allergies
NKDA

Physical examination
GEN: Well-nourished adolescent with fatigue, pallor, generally not feeling well
VS: BP 108/66, HR 80, RR 20, T 39°C, Wt 76 kg, Ht 168 cm
HEENT: Redness with 2 lesions in mucosa of mouth
COR: Clear
CHEST: Mild redness & erythema over line site
ABD: Slight tenderness without guarding
RECTAL: Normal
NEURO: Normal

Results of Pertinent Laboratory Tests, Serum Drug Concentrations, and Diagnostic Tests

Na 140 (140)   Lkcs 1 × 10^9 Ca 4.0 (8.0)
K 4.2 (4.2)   (1 × 10^3)   PO$_4$ 1.55 (4.8)
Cl 102 (102)   ANC 680   Alb 32 (3.2)
HCO$_3$ 28 (28)   Hgb 82 (8.2)   AST 1345 (1345)
BUN 16.1 (45)   Plts 75 × 10^9 ALT 989 (989)
SCr 159 (1.8)   (75 × 10^3)   T Bili 23.9 (1.4)
               Mg 0.41 (1.0)

Differential: Segs 68, bands 0, lymphs 21, monos 11

Prior to HDMTX: Lkcs 2.5 × 10^9 (2.5 × 10^3), ANC 1500, Hgb 92 (9.2), Plts 110 × 10^9 (110 × 10^3)

Urinalysis: Clear

Urine pH (before & during HDMTX) 5.0, 5.5, 5.0

MTX serum concentration at 20 hours post HDMTX: 50 μM (normal < 10 μM)

PROBLEM LIST

Identify principal problems from the scenario in priority order

SOAP NOTE

To be completed by student

QUESTIONS

1. Which of the following best describes osteosarcoma? (EO-1, 8)
   a. Small round cell neoplasm with neural histogenesis
   b. Radiation is an effective treatment option
   c. Most common site of metastatic disease is in the lung
   d. May originate in bone or soft tissue

2. Which of the following regarding osteosarcoma is true? (EO-1)
   a. The damage done to the bones by osteosarcoma occurs between the diaphysis and metaphysis and is known as "onion skinning"
   b. The deregulation of the p53 tumor suppressor gene appears to be important in the development of osteosarcoma
   c. The African-American child has a significantly lower incidence of osteosarcoma than does the Caucasian child
   d. Dactinomycin is an effective agent against osteosarcoma

3. What diagnostic test is the least helpful in the diagnosis of osteosarcoma? (EO-5)
   a. Biopsy
   b. CT and MRI
   c. Serum alkaline phosphatase
   d. Thallium bone scan

4. The expected overall survival rate for a patient like RT is: (EO-3)
   a. 70%
   b. 50%
   c. 20%
   d. 90%

5. Summarize the treatment goals and plan of therapy for the treatment of osteosarcoma. (EO-12)

6. What are the advantages of neoadjuvant chemotherapy in osteosarcoma? (EO-12)

7. RT has an elevated serum MTX concentration: (a) List 5 possible causes for the delay in MTX clearance from the body, and (b) list 5 possible side effects that RT has experienced that are most likely due to MTX. (EO-1, 10)

8. Suggest a treatment plan to reduce the toxicity of HDMTX for RT now and for future courses. (EO-8)

9. List the side effects that may occur and monitoring required while RT is receiving the following chemotherapeutic regimen: ifosfamide, cisplatin, doxorubicin. (EO-5, 8, 10)

10. The possible causes of RT's hypomagnesemia include:
    a. Cisplatin therapy, nonadherence with oral magnesium, and ifosfamide therapy
    b. Hypoalbuminemia: low albumin level reflects low serum magnesium level but the ionized fraction of the serum magnesium is normal; and cisplatin therapy
    c. Ifosfamide therapy and inability to take oral medication due to nausea and vomiting
    d. Cisplatin therapy and possible nonadherence with oral magnesium

11. Describe Fanconi's syndrome and 3 predisposing factors to developing Fanconi's syndrome. (EO-1, 2)

12. What are the risk factors for this patient with fever and neutropenia? (EO-1)

13. Describe psychosocial issues affecting RT directly related to cancer therapy. (EO-15)

14. Which of the following interventions is important in optimizing pharmacoeconomic outcomes of filgrastim therapy? (EO-17)
    a. Adjusting initial dosage to 15 μg/kg/day
    b. Ensuring the dose is administered within 90 minutes following chemotherapy
    c. Diluting filgrastim in saline solution
    d. Adjusting dose by monitoring for increases in the CBC

15. Summarize therapeutic, pathophysiologic, and disease management concepts for osteosarcoma utilizing a key points format. (EO-18)

CASE 137
Donna L. Baxter, Bill McIntyre
Topics: Ovarian Cancer, Anemia

Level 1

EDUCATIONAL MATERIALS

Chapter 94: Gynecologic Cancers (ovarian cancer: histology, prognosis, treatment, salvage therapy)

SCENARIO

Patient and Setting

LL, a 55-year-old woman; gynecology/oncology clinic

Chief Complaint

Abdominal discomfort and bloating

History of Present Illness

Diagnosed 10 months ago with ovarian carcinoma; underwent debulking and completed 6 cycles of cisplatin/cyclophosphamide

Past Medical History

Ovarian carcinoma; mitral valve prolapse; P0, G0

Past Surgical History

Exploratory laparotomy and debulking

Family/Social History

Family History: Married, no children

Social History: Quit smoking last year, had smoked 2 PPD × 25 years; drinks 1–2 times per month, 2–3 glasses of red wine

Medication History

Cisplatin/cyclophosphamide, 6 cycles (completed 6 months ago)

Ferrous sulfate, 325 mg PO TID

Allergies

NKDA

Physical Examination

GEN: Well-nourished woman with slight abdominal discomfort

VS: BP 110/60, HR 88, RR 18, T 37.2°C, Wt 73 kg, Ht 165 cm

HEENT: WNL

COR: Clear

CHEST: Lungs clear

ABD: Distended with ascites and gas; firm irregular mass approximately 15 cm

GU: Vagina smooth, narrow cervix small, smooth; uterus anteverted 5–6 cm with decreased mobility with tumor extension to midline

RECT: Normal

EXT: Normal

NEURO: Normal

Results of Pertinent Laboratory Tests, Serum Drug Concentrations, and Diagnostic Tests

Na 143 (143)	BUN 3.2 (9)	Lkcs 6.8 × 10⁹
K 4.3 (4.3)	Cr 53 (0.6)	(6.8 × 10³)
Cl 100 (100)	Hct 0.33 (33)	Plts 375 × 10⁹
HCO₃ 25 (25)	Hgb 108 (10.8)	(375 × 10³)

Na 143 (143)   BUN 3.2 (9)   Lkcs 6.8×10^9
K 4.3 (4.3)   Cr 53 (0.6) (6.8×10^3)
Cl 100 (100)   Hct 0.33 (33)   Plts 375×10^9
HCO_3 25 (25)   Hgb 108 (10.8) (375×10^3)

PROBLEM LIST

Identify principal problems from the scenario in priority order [completed Problem List and SOAP Note at end of casebook]

SOAP NOTE

To be completed by student

QUESTIONS

[Answers at end of casebook]

1. Which of the following is a risk factor for ovarian cancer? (EO-3)
   a. Multiple pregnancies
   b. Oral contraceptives
   c. Nulliparity
   d. Decreased ovulation

2. The lifetime risk for females for the development of ovarian cancer is: (EO-1)
   a. 10%
   b. 15%
   c. 5%
   d. 1.5%

3. The most common histology of ovarian cancer is: (EO-1)
   a. Epithelial
   b. Sarcoma
   c. Stromal
   d. Germ cell

4. In patients with ovarian carcinoma, which of the following is the most common site of distant metastasis? (EO-1)
   a. Lung
   b. Liver
   c. Kidney
   d. Bladder

5. What is the limitation of the tumor marker CA-125 as a screening tool? (EO-5)

6. What is the expected 5-year survival for a patient like LL with initial stage III disease? (EO-5, 11)
   a. 90%
   b. 60%
   c. 45%
   d. 20%

7. Which of the following histologies are associated with a worse prognosis? (EO-5)
   a. Cystic
   b. Borderline

c. Mucinous

d. Histocytic

8. How does cytoreductive therapy enhance the response of ovarian cancer to chemotherapy? (EO-7)

9. The usual target AUC for carboplatin is: (EO-6)

a. 2

b. 4

c. 5

d. 6

10. LL is scheduled to receive paclitaxel as a second-line regimen. What premedication would you recommend? (EO-10, 11)

11. What is the percentage of patients with chemotherapy who are likely to achieve a 2 g/dL rise in hemoglobin? (EO-8)

a. 5–10%

b. 15–25%

c. 25–30%

d. 40–70%

12. What are the pharmacoeconomic and psychosocial considerations that must be observed when using erythropoietin? (EO-15, 17)

13. Summarize the therapeutic, pathophysiologic, and disease management concepts for the treatment of ovarian carcinoma utilizing a key points format. (EO-18)

CASE 138
Donna L. Baxter, Bill McIntyre
Topics: Melanoma, Biotherapy
Level 3
EDUCATIONAL MATERIALS
Chapter 95: Skin Cancers and Melanomas (clinical presentation, chemotherapy, metastatic melanoma, combination chemotherapy)

SCENARIO

Patient and Setting

MB, a 48-year-old male; hospitalized

Chief Complaint

Admitted for treatment of metastatic melanoma; severe chills, shortness of breath, swelling in legs; lethargy

History of Present Illness

Diagnosed 2 years ago with malignant melanoma; presented with 5-mm nevi on his right forearm that changed in appearance; referred to dermatologist who performed an excisional biopsy that was positive for 4-mm-thick Stage 3 $T_3N_0M_0$; underwent 6 months of adjuvant high-dose interferon alpha-2b; discontinued therapy secondary to severe fatigue; 1 month ago, noted enlarged axillary lymph node (biopsy consistent with malignant melanoma); chest CT consistent with multiple metastatic lesions; presents for his first cycle of biochemotherapy, 10.5-kg (23-lb) weight gain since admission

Past Medical History

No significant illness

Past Surgical History

Excision and biopsy right forearm; axillary lymph node dissection

Family/Social History

Family History: Noncontributory

Social History: Occasional alcohol intake; smokes 1 PPD cigarettes × 27 years

Medication History

Ranitidine, 50 mg IVPB q8h

Naproxen, 250 mg PO q6h PRN fever

Meperidine, 25 mg IV q3–4h PRN rigors

Diltiazem sustained release, 240 mg PO QD

Aldesleukin (interleukin-2), 15 MU IV q8h

Interferon alpha-2b, 9 MU/M2 subcutaneous d1–5 IV

Allergies

NKDA

Physical Examination

GEN: Lethargic male in moderate distress

VS: BP 104/64 (lying), HR 88, RR 16, T 39°C, Wt 78.5 kg (admission 68 kg), Tmax 39°C

HEENT: Mild flushing, supple, no nodes

COR: RRR

CHEST: Rales, labored breathing

ABD: Nontender, nondistended

GU: WNL

RECT: WNL

EXT: 2+ edema bilaterally lower extremities

NEURO: Lethargic, disoriented to place

Results of Pertinent Laboratory Tests, Serum Drug Concentrations, and Diagnostic Tests:

Na 140 (140)	SCr 265 (3.0)	Hct 32 (32)
K 3.6 (3.6)	Glu 11.8 (214)	Plts 117 × 10⁹
Cl 114 (114)	Lkcs 4.4 × 10⁹	(117 × 10³)
HCO₃ 17 (17)	(4.4 × 10³)	Mg 1.9 (1.9)
BUN 14.9 (42)	Hgb 6.2 (10)	

PROBLEM LIST

Identify principal problems from the scenario in priority order [completed Problem List and SOAP Note at end of casebook]

SOAP NOTE

To be completed by student

QUESTIONS

[Answers at end of casebook]

1. What is the typical response rate of melanoma to immunotherapy? (EO-8)
   a. 20%
   b. 35%
   c. 45%
   d. 50%

2. What is the role of adjuvant interferon alpha in high-risk melanoma? (EO-11)

3. Interferon alpha has been reported to increase the concentration of: (EO-9)
   a. Theophylline
   b. Diltiazem
   c. Cimetidine
   d. Erythromycin

4. Which of the following should be monitored in patients receiving interferon alpha? (EO-10)
   a. Prothrombin time
   b. Liver transaminases
   c. Creatinine
   d. Ejection fraction

5. In order to reduce risk of developing melanoma, the minimal recommended SPF in sunscreen products is: (EO-12)
   a. 4
   b. 8
   c. 15
   d. 35

6. Adjuvant high-dose interferon is indicated in patients with: (EO-8)
   a. Node involvement
   b. Lesions < 3 mm deep
   c. Lung involvement
   d. CNS involvement

7. Risk factors for melanoma include all of the following *except:* (EO-1)
   a. Immunosuppression
   b. Fair skin
   c. Intermittent sun exposure before the age of 20
   d. Female gender

8. Antineoplastic effects of interleukin-2 are thought to be primarily through: (EO-7)
   a. Direct inhibition of tumor protein production
   b. Inhibition of BCL2 expression
   c. Stimulation of cytotoxic cells
   d. Stimulation of other cytokines

9. What factors affect patient adherence with interferon therapy? (EO-8, 15)

10. What recommendations can be made to increase the tolerability of interferon therapy? (EO-10, 12)

11. Patients receiving interleukin-2 should not be given: (EO-9)
    a. Opiates
    b. Loperamide
    c. Albumin
    d. Dexamethasone

12. Address psychosocial factors patients suffering from melanoma may experience as a result of the length of therapy for this disease. (EO-15)

13. Summarize therapeutic, pathophysiologic, and disease management concepts for melanoma utilizing a key points format. (EO-18)

CASE 139
Catherine M. Crill
Topic: Neonatology
Level 1
EDUCATIONAL MATERIALS
Chapter 96: Pediatric and Neonatal Therapy; Chapter 65: Immunization Therapy; Chapter 75: Sexually Transmitted Diseases

---

SCENARIO

Patient and Setting

GJ, a 1-day-old female; NICU

Chief Complaint

Admitted to neonatal intensive care unit secondary to high-risk pregnancy

History of Present Illness

High-risk pregnancy, status post cesarean section

Past Medical History

Delivered via cesarean section due to mother's prolonged labor at 38 weeks gestation

Past Surgical History

None

Family/Social History

Family History: Mother: 19 years old; first pregnancy; no prenatal care; RPR (+); FTA-abs (+) (denies past history of syphilis infection)

Social History: Mother: IV drug abuse; HBsAg (+), HIV (−)

GJ: mother's history as above; no paternal history

Medication History

None

Allergies

NKDA

Physical Examination

GEN: Vigorous newborn, yellow tint to skin
VS: BP 61/38, HR 142, RR 36, T 37.4°C, Wt 2.885 kg, length 48 cm
HEENT: Open anterior fontanel, EOMI, (+) red reflex, purulent nasal discharge, TM visualized
COR: RRR, no murmur, nl S_1 and S_2
CHEST: CTA
ABD: (+) BS, soft, NTND, no hepatosplenomegaly
RECT: Patent
EXT: Pulses 2+ deep tendon reflexes (DTR)–patella (2+ is a normal finding)
NEURO: (+) Grasp, good thumb suck

Results of Pertinent Laboratory Tests, Serum Drug Concentrations, and Diagnostic Tests

GJ's laboratory results:

Na 137 (137)
K 3.8 (3.8)
Cl 102 (102)
HCO_3 22 (22)
BUN 3.9 (11)
Cr 97.2 (1.1)
Hct 0.5 (50)
Hgb 169 (16.9)

Lkcs 13.1 × 10⁹
  (13.1 × 10³)
Plts 271 × 10⁹
  (271 × 10³)
MCV 72 (72)
T Bili 136.8 (8.0)
AST 1.00 (60)
ALT 0.08 (5)

LDH 7.4 (446)
Alk Phos 3.03 (182)
Alb 28 (2.8)
D Bili 0.0 (0.0)
Glu 4.4 (79)
Ca 2.4 (9.4)
PO_4 1.74 (5.4)
Mg 0.6 (1.1)

CBC with differential: Neut 35%, bands 3%, lymphs 50%, monos 9%, eos 3%

Serologic tests for syphilis: RPR (+), FTA-abs (+)

Lumbar puncture: RBC 10, WBC 6, Glu 51, Prot 163, VDRL pending

EEG: WNL

Toxicology screen: Negative

Chest x-ray: WNL

PROBLEM LIST

Identify principal problems from the scenario in priority order [completed Problem List and SOAP Note at end of casebook]

SOAP NOTE

To be completed by student

QUESTIONS

[Answers at end of casebook]

1. This infant acquired syphilis through which of the following mechanisms: (EO-1)
   a. Congenital inheritance from maternal DNA
   b. Transcervical infection to the fetus in utero
   c. Transplacental transmission of spirochetes to the fetus in utero
   d. Exposure to infected maternal blood during cesarean section

2. Which one of the following objective evidence is a primary manifestation of syphilis infection in this neonate? (EO-2)
   a. Yellow tint to the skin
   b. Purulent nasal discharge
   c. Abnormal LP
   d. Hyperbilirubinemia

3. The mother's history is significant for which of the following major risk factors for hepatitis B infection: (EO-3)
   a. Young age
   b. No prenatal care
   c. Prior syphilis infection
   d. IVDA

4. The anterolateral thigh is the preferred site for IM injections in neonates because it: (EO-8)
   a. Is less painful to the neonate
   b. Receives a greater percentage of blood flow in the neonate
   c. Has a greater amount of muscle mass in the neonate
   d. Allows for decreased drug toxicity in the neonate

5. Which of the following is an explanation for the development of hyperbilirubinemia and jaundice during the neonatal period? (EO-1)
   a. Immature liver conjugation of bilirubin
   b. Decreased renal excretion of bilirubin
   c. Decreased protein status
   d. Hepatotoxicity from congenital infections

6. Explain the rationale for using UV light therapy to prevent kernicterus in the neonatal period. (EO-7)

7. Which of the following agents might be contraindicated in this neonate with hyperbilirubinemia? (EO-9)
   a. Acetaminophen
   b. Aspirin
   c. Phenobarbital
   d. Pseudoephedrine

8. Which of the following should be monitored in this neonate to observe adverse drug effects with penicillin therapy: (EO-5, 10)
   a. Renal function and urine output
   b. Thrombophlebitis at injection site
   c. Allergic reactions
   d. The incidence of febrile occurrences

9. Why is it necessary to increase the schedule of penicillin dosing in this neonate after 7 days of treatment? (EO-4, 6)
   a. Syphilis infection will be more virile as maternal antibodies decrease
   b. Increased renal tubular capacity after 7 days of life
   c. Increased liver metabolism of penicillin after 7 days of life
   d. Increased protein status allowing for less free drug concentration

10. List counseling topics that should be discussed with the mother regarding the use of HBIG and hepatitis B vaccine in this patient. (EO-14, 16)

11. List 3 risk management steps that a health care provider could use in this case to reduce medication errors. (EO-8, 10, 14, 15)

12. Summarize pathophysiologic, therapeutic, and disease management concepts for this neonate's condition utilizing a key points format. (EO-18)

CASE 140
Catherine M. Crill
Topic: Pediatric and Neonatal Therapy

EDUCATIONAL MATERIALS
Chapter 96: Pediatric and Neonatal Therapy;
Chapter 49: Common Ear Disorders;
Chapter 52: Seizure Disorders;
Chapter 73: Central Nervous System Infections

SCENARIO

Patient and Setting
JD, a 5-month-old male; ED

Chief Complaint
Fever, vomiting, decreased urine output, and seizure activity

History of Present Illness
Two days ago, mother noticed JD was "not himself"; not breastfeeding as usual and sleeping more than usual; had only two wet diapers; today had a fever of 39°C and began to vomit, then began to have seizures

Past Medical History
First case of otitis media (OM) 2 weeks prior to arrival (prescribed 10-day course of amoxicillin); mother discontinued amoxicillin after 3 days secondary to diarrhea and because symptoms disappeared

Past Surgical History
None

Family/Social History
Family History: Lives at home with mother, father, and 2 sisters (age 2 and 3 years) who both attend daycare centers

Social History: Noncontributory

Medication History

Acetaminophen drops, 15 mg/kg/dose q4–6h PRN fever

Allergies

NKDA

Physical Examination

GEN: Lethargic infant with generalized seizure activity

VS: BP 93/55, HR 175, RR 35, T 40°C, Wt 6 kg (previously 7 kg), Ht 65 cm

HEENT: PERRLA, dry mucous membranes, red, bulging TM bilaterally, bulging fontanel

COR: Normal S_1 and S_2

CHEST: Clear to auscultation and percussion

ABD: Soft, no masses

GU: WNL

RECT: Guaiac negative

EXT: Skin tenting noted

NEURO: Generalized seizures, lethargic, nuchal rigidity

Results of Pertinent Laboratory Tests, Serum Drug Concentrations, and Diagnostic Tests

Na 135 (135)	Hgb 105 (10.5)	CSF appearance
K 5.5 (5.5)	Hct 0.35 (35)	xanthochromic
Cl 100 (100)	WBC 21 × 10⁹	WBC 600
HCO₃ 26 (26)	(21 × 10³)	Glu 1.6 (28)
BUN 10.7 (30)	Plts 300 × 10⁹	Protein 0.75 (75)
SCr 61.9 (0.7)–	(300 × 10³)	Gram stain:
normal at visit 2	Alb 39 (3.9)	Gram-negative bacilli
weeks earlier	Glu 4.4 (80)	Bld Cx's pending

PROBLEM LIST

Identify principal problems from the scenario in priority order

SOAP NOTE

To be completed by student

QUESTIONS

1. What is the most likely cause for JD's acute meningitis? (EO-1)
   a. Hematogenous infection of CSF from the middle ear
   b. Inhalation of bacteria from siblings
   c. Bacterial passage through breastmilk
   d. Viral infection transmitted at delivery

2. JD exhibits which of the following signs or symptoms of dehydration: (EO-2)
   a. Bulging fontanel
   b. Skin tenting
   c. Decreased BUN
   d. Elevated WBC

3. All of the following are risk factors for JD's current OM infection, *except:* (EO-3)
   a. Age
   b. Previous OM infection
   c. Male gender
   d. Meningitis infection

4. All of the following in JD are predictors of success of antimicrobial therapy for meningitis, *except:* (EO-4, 6)
   a. Inflamed meninges
   b. Immature blood brain barrier
   c. Choice of antibiotic
   d. Ability to measure serum drug concentrations

5. Describe the importance of and parameters involved in physical assessment to diagnose JD's dehydration. (EO-5)

6. If JD's continues to be symptomatic after cefotaxime therapy for OM (bilateral bulging TM), what would be the best approach to therapy? (EO-12)
   a. Begin amoxicillin/clavulanate therapy for 10 days
   b. Begin cephalexin therapy for 14 days
   c. Observe patient for 24–48 hours for resolution of symptoms
   d. Perform tympanocentesis to isolate the organism

7. Discuss maternal traits that have been found to improve compliance with drug therapy. (EO-15)

8. Describe how the health care provider should counsel a parent who expressed noncompliance with drug regimens because the child was unwilling to take the medication. (EO-15, 16)

9. The mother expresses a desire to stop breastfeeding JD because it is becoming inconvenient and cumbersome. Which of the following is an advantage to continue breastfeeding JD? (EO-12, 14)
   a. Decreased incidence of OM
   b. Decreased immunologic factors
   c. Decreased risk of recurrent meningitis
   d. Decreased risk of dehydration

10. The mother insists on discontinuing breastfeeding. The best source of nutrition in JD at this time is: (EO-8)
    a. Baby food alone
    b. Baby food plus cow's milk formula
    c. 20 cal/oz cow's milk formula
    d. 16 cal/oz cow's milk formula

11. What is the most important patient factor that should be considered when choosing a replacement IV fluid to treat JD's dehydration? (EO-8, 12)
    a. Availability of central venous access
    b. Electrolyte content of the fluid
    d. Dextrose content of the fluid
    d. Length of time needed for volume replacement

12. Lorazepam is the drug of choice in treating JD's seizure activity because it: (EO-6, 8, 12)
    a. Has a long duration of action
    b. Penetrates the blood-brain barrier

c. Has a longer time to onset of action

d. Has less side effects than other benzodiazepines

13. Summarize pathophysiologic, therapeutic, and disease management concepts for JD's OM utilizing a key points format. (EO-18)

CASE 141
Catherine M. Crill
Topic: Pediatric Nutrition Support
Level 2
EDUCATIONAL MATERIALS
Chapter 97: Pediatric Nutrition Support

SCENARIO

Patient and Setting

SR, a 13-month-old female; pediatric hospital

Chief Complaint

Fever

History of Present Illness

Admitted today after GI clinic visit when mother described SR's spiking temperatures for the past 3 days "like she does when her line is infected"

Past Medical History

Born at 34 weeks gestational age with malrotation/mid-gut volvulus; had almost complete bowel resection; now with short gut syndrome secondary to bowel resection; chronic total parenteral nutrition (TPN) for nutritional needs; receives small amount of oral feedings (infant formula); otherwise stable except for 3 central line infections (IV antibiotics given)

Past Surgical History

Intestinal resection of bowel at 3 weeks of age + ileostomy; central venous line (CVL) placement at 3 weeks of age and again at 8 months of age (current CVL is tunneled catheter)

Family/Social History

Family History: Lives at home with mother and older brother, age 5, and sister, age 3

Social History: Home health agency expressed concerns over SR's history of CVL infections and possibility mother may not be practicing proper line care; mother with little support other than home health nurses that provide some assistance with TPN

Medication History

Diphenhydramine cream to skin PRN itching

Acetaminophen drops PRN fever

TPN + lipids nightly (4-hour off cycle from 1200–1600)

Total daily volume: 900 mL

Composition:

3% crystalline amino acid formulation (changed from 2.4% pediatric amino acid formulation 1 month prior at 1 year of age by the home health care provider)

25% dextrose

20% lipids (2 g/kg/day)

1/4 NS

20 mEq/L K

40 mEq/L Cl

12 mEq/L acetate

6 mmol/ L PO4

15 mEq/L Ca

4 mEq/L Mg

Standard trace elements (combination product)

Standard vitamins (combination product)

Allergies

NKDA

Physical Examination

GEN: lethargic child, cheeks appear rounded

VS: BP 100/60, HR 117, RR 30, T 39.5°C, Wt 9 kg, Ht 65 cm

HEENT: PERRLA, sclera icteric

COR: Normal S_1 and S_2

CHEST: Clear to auscultation and percussion

ABD: No masses, slight hepatomegaly, large amount of ostomy output

GU: WNL

RECT: WNL

EXT: Flaking skin, eczematous appearance (mother reports patient continually scratching skin)

NEURO: Alert with a strong cry and normal muscle tone, reflexes

Results of Pertinent Laboratory Tests, Serum Drug Concentrations, and Diagnostic Tests

Na 136 (136)	Mg 1.0 (2.0)	T Bili 41 (2.4)
K 4.3 (4.3)	Trig 1.4 (125)	D Bili 37.6 (2.2)
Cl 103 (103)	Glu 3.3 (60)	Plts 300 × 10⁹
HCO₃ 23 (23)	Alb 38 (3.8)	(300 × 10³)
BUN 50 (18)	AST 112 (112)	WBC 21 × 10⁹
SCr 38 (0.5)	ALT 92 (92)	(21 × 10³)
Ca 2.5 (10)	GGT 120 (120)	Hgb 1.1 (11)
PO₄ 1.45 (4.5)		Hct 0.36 (36)

CVL culture (catheter tip): Gram-positive cocci in chains and clusters

Urinalysis: Negative

LFTs at last clinic visit (2 months ago): WNL

PROBLEM LIST

Identify principal problems from the scenario in priority order

SOAP NOTE

To be completed by student

QUESTIONS

1. List the problems with SR's home parenteral nutrition solution. (EO-11)

2. The probable cause for SR developing cholestasis is: (EO-1)
   a. Long-term parenteral nutrition therapy
   b. Initiation of 3% amino acid formulation
   c. Recurrent infectious insults
   d. Lack of enteral nutrient absorption

3. SR exhibits all of the following signs and symptoms of cholestasis, *except:* (EO-2)
   a. Icteric sclera
   b. Increased AST
   c. Increased BUN
   d. Increased GGT

4. What are the mechanisms of action of cycling TPN and giving trophic feedings for the treatment and prevention of cholestasis? (EO-7)

5. Which of the following is most important for evaluating SR's nutrition therapy? (EO-8, 5)
   a. Functionality of the gastrointestinal tract
   b. Weight history
   c. Visceral protein status
   d. Anthropometric measurements

6. All of the following may be contributing to SR's CVL infections, *except:* (EO-3)
   a. Ostomy placement near CVL site
   b. Lack of proper line care by mother
   c. SR continually scratching skin
   d. Use of heparin flushes in the line

7. Identify factors that may affect the care of SR's CVL by her mother. (EO-15)

8. Describe how the health care provider might have an impact on the quality of CVL care provided by SR's mother. (EO-14, 16)

9. Which of the following might be appropriate to enhance SR's nutrition therapy? (EO-12)
   a. Increasing IV lipids to provide additional fat calories
   b. Decreasing dextrose concentration to 15%
   c. Initiating phenobarbital therapy for cholestasis
   d. Evaluating SR for metabolic bone disease

10. All of the following are factors that should be considered when choosing a drug therapy for SR's skin condition, *except:* (EO-8, 9)
    a. Underlying cause of the skin condition
    b. Drug distribution within the body
    c. Drug elimination from the body
    d. Drug interactions with vancomycin

11. If SR is found to be zinc deficient, what other abnormality might be expected in SR? (EO-1)
    a. Impaired immune function
    b. Increased hair growth
    c. Decreased copper concentrations
    d. Decreased chromium concentrations

12. All of the following should be considered when initiating antibiotic therapy to treat SR's CVL infection, *except:* (EO-8, 9)
    a. Absorption from GI tract
    b. Antimicrobial spectrum of activity
    c. Culture and sensitivity results
    d. Compatibility with TPN

13. Calculate SR's fluid requirements at 9 kg, 15 kg, and 29 kg. (EO-8)

14. Summarize pathophysiologic, therapeutic, and disease management concepts for SR's nutrition therapy utilizing a key points format. (EO-18)

CASE 142
Catherine M. Crill
Topic: Pediatric Nutrition Support

EDUCATIONAL MATERIALS
Chapter 97: Pediatric Nutrition Support

SCENARIO

Patient and Setting

CD, a 6-week-old male; special care nursery, pediatric hospital

Chief Complaint

Weight loss of 1.5 kg since birth and vomiting/diarrhea/dehydration

History of Present Illness

Admitted 2 weeks ago and appropriately rehydrated; continued to have emesis and diarrhea with feedings; made NPO and an NG tube placed; receiving total parenteral nutrition (TPN) through a percutaneously inserted central catheter (PICC); flushing the line for the past several days has been difficult and now does not allow infusion; IVF (D10 ¼ NS + 20 mEq/L KCl) started in a peripheral line (placed in his foot) and central TPN stopped; physician wants to give peripheral TPN and reattempt feeding; bloody NG tube aspirates

Past Medical History

Born at 40 weeks gestational age, birth weight 3.4 kg; discharged from the hospital on DOL 3 on standard cow's milk formula; mother reports CD disinterested in feedings at home; vomited frequently (occasionally blood-tinged) and had diarrhea; evaluated since admission for all possible causes of failure to thrive or gastrointestinal abnormalities (findings for these negative up to this point)

Past Surgical History

None

Family/Social History

Family History: Lived at home for 1 month after delivery; born to 31-year-old mother who had prenatal care; no family history of congenital or medical problems

Medication History

Ranitidine, 3 mg/kg/day (given continuously via TPN)

Mylanta, 3 mL q4h PRN bloody NG tube aspirates

Multivitamin with iron (oral liquid preparation), 1 mL QD

Heparin flushes, 10 U/mL per PICC care protocol

TPN composition (total daily volume: 312 mL + 45.6 mL lipids):

    2.4% pediatric crystalline amino acid formulation

    40 mg cysteine/g amino acid

    25% dextrose

    20% lipids (3 g/kg/day)

    1/4 NS

    30 mEq/L K

    40 mEq/L Cl

    12 mEq/L acetate

    8 mmol/L PO_4

    25 mEq/L Ca

    4 mEq/L Mg

    Standard trace elements (combination product)

    Standard vitamins (combination product)

Allergies

NKDA

Physical Examination

GEN: small infant in NAD

VS: BP 105/65, HR 145, RR 30, T 37.0°C, Wt 3.0 kg, Ht 65 cm

HEENT: NC/AT, EOMI, PERRLA, nl conjunctiva, TM clear bilaterally

COR: Normal S_1 and S_2

CHEST: Clear to auscultation and percussion

ABD: Soft, NTND, (+) BS, bloody appearance of NG tube aspirates

GU: WNL

RECT: Stool guaiac positive

EXT: WNL

NEURO: Alert infant, normal muscle tone and reflexes

Results of Pertinent Laboratory Tests, Serum Drug Concentrations, and Diagnostic Tests

Na 142 (142)	PO_4 1.9 (6.0)	ALT 35 (35)
K 4.0 (4.0)	Mg 1.23 (3.0)	GGT 68 (68)
Cl 106 (106)	Trig 2.8 (250)	T Bili 17.7 (1.0)
HCO_3 22 (22)	Glu 4.9 (88)	D Bili 3.4 (0.2)
BUN 5.4 (15)	Alb 18 (1.8)	Hgb 130 (13)
SCr 53 (0.6)	AST 46 (46)	Hct 0.37 (37)
Ca 2.2 (8.9)		

Stool cultures: No infectious organisms

Blood cultures: No growth for 5 days (final)

Urinalysis/culture: Negative/no growth (final)

PROBLEM LIST

Identify principal problems from the scenario in priority order [completed Problem List and SOAP Note at end of casebook]

SOAP NOTE

To be completed by student

QUESTIONS

[Answers at end of casebook]

1. The probable cause of CD's clotted catheter include all of the following *except:* (EO-1)
   a. Fibrin deposition
   b. Heparin deposition
   c. Calcium phosphorus precipitation
   d. Calcium lipid saponification

2. Signs and symptoms of a clotted catheter include all of the following *except:* (EO-2)
   a. Difficulty withdrawing from the line
   b. Low IV infusion pump pressures
   c. Inability to infuse into the line
   d. Cardiac dysrhythmias

3. What are the advantages of using lipid emulsions in parenteral nutrition? (EO-8)

4. Which of the following TPN components is least likely to increase the risk of infiltration in a peripheral line? (EO-3, 8)

a. Carbohydrate
b. Lipid
c. Potassium
d. Calcium

5. All of the following can be utilized to increase caloric content of peripheral parenteral nutrition, *except:* (EO-8)
   a. Increasing maintenance volume
   b. Increasing dextrose concentration
   c. Increasing lipid infusion
   d. Giving IV medications in D10W

6. List the benefits of adding cysteine to CD's TPN? (EO-8)

7. Which of the following is inappropriate therapy in conjunction with CD's TPN? (EO-11)
   a. Ranitidine
   b. Mylanta
   c. Multivitamin with iron
   d. Heparin

8. The most likely cause of CD's feeding intolerance is: (EO-1, 3)
   a. Disacharidase deficiency
   b. Soy protein allergy
   c. Triglyceride intolerance
   d. Immature GI tract

9. All of the following are signs and symptoms of feeding intolerance, *except:* (EO-2)

a. Abdominal distention
b. Emesis
c. Diarrhea
d. Bloody aspirates

10. List advantages of using calcium carbonate over Mylanta for antacid therapy in CD. (EO-8, 9, 10)

11. What is the mechanism of action of carnitine in the treatment of hypertriglyceridemia? (EO-7)

12. Which of the following is the most appropriate way to limit the expense of CD's TPN solution? (EO-17)
    a. Discontinue cysteine
    b. Discontinue lipid emulsion
    c. Eliminate overfill when providing albumin
    d. Provide TPN for 5 days per week

13. Which of the following should be a flag to the health care provider to review CD's medication profile and TPN solution to avoid drug-related complications: (EO-5, 9, 11)
    a. Low albumin concentration
    b. High triglyceride concentration
    c. Decreased renal function
    d. Decreased hepatic function

14. Summarize therapeutic, pathophysiologic, and disease management concepts for CD's nutrition therapy using a key points format. (EO-18)

CASE 143
Nicole G. Parker
Topic: Gynecologic Disorders
Level 2
EDUCATIONAL MATERIALS
Chapter 98: Gynecologic Disorders

CASE SCENARIO

Patient and Setting

SK, a 32-year-old female; OB-GYN clinic

Chief Complaint

Moderately severe menstruation, dysuria, and thick, gray malodorous vaginal discharge

History of Present Illness

Pelvic cramping occurring 2 days before each menses, heavy flow, dysmenorrhea; vaginal discharge; euphoric, flight of ideas, hyperactivity escalating rapidly for a few days to a few months followed by depressive episodes lasting for a week

Past Medical History

Bipolar disorder for 2 years; facial acne for 19 years

OB-GYN History

LMP 1 week ago; heavy menstrual bleeding; dysmenorrhea helped only by acetaminophen/codeine (failed with both ibuprofen and naproxen); pelvic cramping first 2 days of menses; anovulatory cycles; pelvic inflammatory disease (PID) at ages 19 and 23; contraception: intrauterine device (IUD) removed 3 months ago (aggravated dysmenorrhea); diaphragm discontinued (caused urinary tract infections); combination oral contraceptive (COC) discontinued (triggered depressive episodes)

Past Surgical History

None

Family/Social History

Family History: Mother cyclothymic with history of substance abuse

Social History: Sexually active with multiple sex partners; single; waitress; social drinker

Medication History

Nortriptyline, 10 mg 2 capsules PO QHS

Acetaminophen 325 mg with codeine, 30 mg PO q3–4h PRN dysmenorrhea

Tetracycline, 500 mg PO BID

Allergies

Clotrimazole vaginal cream

Physical Examination

GEN: Well-nourished, well-developed female
VS: BP 126/85, HR 74, RR 20, T 37°C, Wt 58 kg, Ht 163 cm
HEENT: Facial skin clear of acne
COR: WNL
CHEST: Bilateral fibrocystic breast densities
ABD: WNL
GU: Thick, gray, malodorous vaginal discharge: "strawberry cervix"; meatal erythema
RECT: WNL
EXT: WNL
NEURO: WNL

Results of Pertinent Laboratory Tests, Serum Drug Concentrations, and Diagnostic Tests

Na 143 (143)	BUN 6.4 (18)	AST 0.17 (10)
K 4.4 (4.4)	Cr 88 (1.0)	ALT 0.2 (12)
Cl 99 (99)	Hct 0.33 (33)	T Bili 9 (0.5)
HCO₃ 26 (26)	Hgb 120 (12)	Glu (fasting) 5.3 (95)

Protriptyline: 380 nmol/L (100 ng/mL)

Stool: Guaiac negative

Vaginal fluid: Normal saline slide: highly motile, pear-shaped, unicellular *Trichomonas vaginalis*

Pregnancy test: Negative

PROBLEM LIST

Identify principal problems from the scenario in priority order [completed Problem List and SOAP Note at end of casebook]

SOAP NOTE

To be completed by student

QUESTIONS

[Answers at end of casebook]

1. The probable cause of SK's dysmenorrhea includes all of the following *except:* (EO-1)
   a. Adhesions on the reproductive organs
   b. IUD
   c. PID
   d. Endometriosis

2. The signs and symptoms associated with *Trichomonas* vaginitis include which of the following: (EO-2)
   a. Clear vaginal discharge
   b. Presence of hyphae
   c. Pain and itching
   d. Malodorous vaginal discharge

3. A disulfiram-like reaction may occur with administration of which of the following agents: (EO-9, 10)
   a. Metronidazole and oral contraceptives
   b. Oral contraceptives and NSAIDs
   c. Metronidazole and alcohol-containing products
   d. NSAIDs and alcohol-containing products

4. Symptoms associated with dysmenorrhea are related to the pharmacologic actions of which of the following: (EO-2)
   a. Prostaglandin E2
   b. Prostaglandin A2
   c. Prostaglandin E1
   d. Prostaglandin F1

5. When selecting a NSAID for dysmenorrhea, which of the following statements is true? (EO-8)
   a. If SK does not respond to mefenamic acid, ibuprofen should be tried
   b. The initial selection of NSAIDs should be tried for at least one menstrual cycle
   c. SK should be instructed to take NSAIDs prior to the onset of symptoms to reduce the intensity of pain
   d. Clonidine may be used for patients with dysmenorrhea that fail NSAIDs

6. Although oral contraceptives (OCs) are effective agents for the treatment of dysmenorrhea, SK should avoid OCs because of the potential to trigger a depressive episode. Describe the mechanism by which OCs trigger a depressive episode. (EO-10)

7. Factors placing SK at risk for bipolar symptoms include all of the following *except:* (EO-3, 4)
   a. Oral contraceptives
   b. NSAIDs
   c. Family history of depression or related illnesses
   d. Nortriptyline

8. The onset of dysmenorrhea usually occurs _____ and may last _____ (EO-2)
   a. A few days prior to menses; 48–72 hours
   b. A few hours prior to menses; 48–72 hours
   c. A few hours prior to menses; 6–12 hours
   d. A few days prior to menses; 48–72 hours

9. GU on physical exam reveals a strawberry cervix. This finding suggests: (EO-5)
   a. Condyloma
   b. Swollen papillae projecting through vaginal secretions
   c. Bacterial vaginosis
   d. Yeast

10. List the pharmacologic and nonpharmacologic treatment problem(s) present in SK's treatment plan. (EO-11)

11. Evaluate the mechanism of action of the pharmacologic and nonpharmacologic interventions in this case. (EO-7)

12. What psychosocial factors may affect SK's adherence to both pharmacologic and nonpharmacologic therapy? (EO-15)

13. Describe the health care provider's role relative to the proposed psychosocial factors identified. (EO-16)

14. Evaluate the pharmacoeconomic considerations relative to SK's plan of care. (EO-17)

15. Summarize pathophysiologic, therapeutic, and disease management concepts for gynecologic disorders utilizing a key points format (EO-18)

CASE 144
Nicole G. Parker
Topic: Gynecologic Disorders
Level 2
EDUCATIONAL MATERIALS
Chapter 98: Gynecologic Disorders

SCENARIO

Patient and Setting
HD, a 26-year-old female; clinic

Chief Complaint
Follow-up for a UTI; has noticed vaginal discharge and "fishy" odor occurring primarily after intercourse; desires contraception

History of Present Illness
Treated with 10 days of cotrimoxazole for an *Escherichia coli* UTI; previously treated 6 months ago for a UTI

Past Medical History
Stage IIB Hodgkin's disease in remission for 1 year: treated with radical radiation (5000 rads over 4–6 weeks 11 months ago) therapy and chemotherapy not necessary at that time

OB-GYN History
G1P1, LMP 21 days ago; regular 28-day cycle; combination oral contraceptive (COC) for 5 years; currently uses diaphragm with spermicide; recurrent UTI

Past Surgical History
Appendectomy at age 14

Family/Social History

Family History: Spouse works as a mechanic; 1 child (4-year-old daughter)

Social History: Nonsmoker, nondrinker; vegetarian; works as an x-ray technician

Medication History

Vinegar douches after intercourse (self-initiated)

Clotrimazole vaginal cream, 1 applicatorful QD × 7 days (self-initiated)

Acetaminophen, 2 tablets PO PRN

Allergies

NKDA

Physical Examination

GEN: Well-developed, well-nourished woman
VS: BP 106/65, HR 50, RR 18, Wt 62 kg, Ht 165 cm
HEENT: WNL
COR: WNL
ABD: Nontender, no masses
GU: Gray, homogeneous vaginal discharge, ovaries were palpable, normal-sized uterus, no tenderness, cervix normal
RECT: Small hemorrhoids
EXT: WNL
NEURO: WNL

Results of Pertinent Laboratory Tests, Serum Drug Concentrations, and Diagnostic Tests

Na 140 (140)	Cr 61.9 (0.7)	Plts 220 × 10^9 (220 × 10^3)
K 4.1 (4.1)	Hct 0.34 (34)	Glu 4.4 (80)
Cl 100 (100)	Hgb 110 (11)	Chol 4.14 (160)
HCO_3 (24) 24	Lkcs 7.8 × 10^9 (7.8 × 10^3)	Trig 0.98 (87)
BUN 5.36 (15)		

Vaginal discharge: Normal saline wet mount "clue cells": pH 5, positive KOH sniff test

Urine culture: Negative

Pregnancy test: Negative

PROBLEM LIST

Identify principal problems from the scenario in priority order

SOAP NOTES

To be completed by student

QUESTIONS

1. HD has presented previously with which of the following symptoms associated with UTIs: (EO-2)
   a. Fever
   b. Suprapubic pain
   c. Burning on urination
   d. Malodorous vaginal discharge
2. The foul "fishy" odor associated with HD's bacterial vaginosis is due to: (EO-1)
   a. A shift to an acidic pH in the vagina
   b. A shift to an alkaline pH in the vagina
   c. A shift to a neutral pH in the uterus
   d. A shift from an alkaline pH in the uterus
3. The probable cause of HD's reinfection: (EO-1)
   a. Stage II Hodgkin's disease
   b. Use of oral contraceptives
   c. Irritation of the urethra at time of intercourse
   d. Chronic use of acetaminophen
4. Women of childbearing age have a thick protective epithelium that is maintained by all of the following *except:* (EO-3)
   a. Estrogen
   b. Progesterone
   c. Aerobic bacteria
   d. Anaerobic bacteria
5. Physical assessment findings apparent in HD that point to vaginosis include all of the following *except:* (EO-5)
   a. The presence of clue cells
   b. A negative KOH test
   c. A positive sniff test
   d. A pH of 5
6. Describe the mechanism of action of the pharmacologic and nonpharmacologic interventions in this case. (EO-7)
7. Several factors predispose HD to complications with OC use. All of the following may increase her risk for complications, *except:* (EO-4, 6, 8)
   a. Stage III hypertension
   b. Thromboembolic disease
   c. Stage II Hodgkin's disease
   d. Hyperlipidemia
8. Another form of birth control would be indicated in HD when which of the following occurs: (EO-4, 6, 8, 12)
   a. 3 consecutive readings of high blood pressure
   b. Reduction in menstrual cramping
   c. Reduction in menstrual flow
   d. Increased vaginal discharge
9. Which microorganism is responsible for maintaining normal flora in the vagina? (EO-2)
   a. *Corynebacterium*
   b. Aerobic streptococci
   c. Lactobacilli
   d. Anaerobic group D hemolytic streptococci
10. HD is placed on COC for contraception and has missed 2 pills during the third week of OC. What advice should be given to her? (EO-14)
11. If HD required chronic treatment for UTIs, what effect would it have on her COC use? (EO-9)

12. Develop a detailed education plan for HD including necessary lifestyle changes, medication counseling, and adherence strategies to both pharmacologic and nonpharmacologic therapy. (EO-14, 15)

13. Evaluate the pharmacoeconomic considerations relative to the proposed psychosocial factors identified. (EO-17)

14. Summarize therapeutic, pathophysiologic, and disease management concepts for gynecologic disorders utilizing a key points format. (EO-18)

CASE 145
Nicole G. Parker
Topic: Contraception
Level 3
EDUCATIONAL MATERIALS
Chapter 99: Infertility and Contraception

SCENARIO

Patient and Setting
KK, a 45-year-old female; OB-GYN clinic

Chief Complaint
Severe itching of the vulva and vagina, and painful burning during urination; seeking method of birth control; premenstrual syndrome (PMS) symptoms including mood swings, forgetfulness, migraines, and phobia of being replaced by a younger employee

History of Present Illness
Vaginal itching and painful urination; treated 1 week ago for profuse vaginal discharge with no itching or burning; discontinued combination oral contraceptive (COC) several weeks ago; now with complaints of PMS symptoms and hairy chin

Past Medical History
Episodic migraine for 22 years (since her menarche at age 13); symptoms include frontal unilateral dull aches that progress to throbbing pain with nausea, vomiting, diarrhea, and vertigo; rectal soreness and flatulence intermittently

OB-GYN History
G4P1Mis2Ectopic1; LMP 2 weeks ago; recurrent vulvovaginal candidal infections for 4 years; PMS for 4 years, only symptom free for several days after onset of menses until near ovulation; discontinued COC 2 weeks ago, now using vaginal contraceptive suppositories, which irritate spouse's genitals

Past Surgical History
Left salpingo-oophorectomy resulting from an ectopic pregnancy at age 23

Family/Social History
Family History: Mother has "common" migraines; mother and father with HTN
Social History: Smokes 1.75 PPD × 18 years

Medication History
Progesterone suppositories, 200 mg PR BID × 4 years
COC, 1 tablet PO QD for 6 months (discontinued 2 weeks ago)
Hydrocodone bitartrate 5 mg/acetaminophen 500 mg PO PRN
Clotrimazole, 500 mg vaginal tablets; 1 PRN
Contraceptive vaginal suppositories PRN

Allergies
Latex

Physical Examination
GEN: Well-developed, well-nourished female
VS: BP 124/83 LA (sitting), HR 76, RR 18, T 37.1°C, Wt 61 kg, Ht 168 cm
HEENT: Chin many short, coarse, dark hair follicles
COR: WNL
CHEST: Breasts swollen and tender to palpation
ABD: WNL, except for bikini scar
GU: Vulvar erythema with white patches; intertrigo with satellite lesions; thick, white, curd-like secretions
RECT: Perianal erythema, flatulence, no hemorrhoids; guaiac positive
EXT: WNL
NEURO: WNL

Results of Pertinent Laboratory Tests, Serum Drug Concentrations, and Diagnostic Tests
Na 141 (141)   BUN 5.0 (14)   Hgb 130 (13)
K 4.1 (4.1)   Cr 71 (0.8)   Glu (fasting) 4.9 (89)
Cl 101 (101)   Hct 0.39 (39%)

Oral glucose tolerance test: Normal
Vaginal fluid: KOH slide—long threadlike fibers of mycelia with tiny buds of conidia attached

PROBLEM LIST
Identify principal problems from the scenario in priority order

SOAP NOTES

To be completed by student

QUESTIONS

1. Which of the following statements is true? (EO-1)
   a. PMS is a cyclic recurrence of a group of symptoms that peak during the follicular phase and disappear during the luteal phase
   b. The cause of PMS is thought to be due to pyridoxine (vitamin B_6) excess
   c. An estrogen/progestin imbalance may contribute to PMS
   d. PMS may be triggered by increases in serotonin levels

2. KK presents with all of the following signs and symptoms of PMS *except:* (EO-2)
   a. Somatic symptoms
   b. Cognitive symptoms
   c. Mood swings
   d. Personality disorder

3. The incidence of women experiencing unintended pregnancy during the first year of typical use of contraception is greatest with which method of birth control? (EO-1)
   a. Diaphragm
   b. Periodic abstinence
   c. Progestin-only contraceptives
   d. Withdrawal

4. The risk of cardiovascular complications with oral contraceptives may be increased by all of the following *except:* (EO-4, 6, 8)
   a. Using a COC with 50 µg/mL of ethinyl estradiol
   b. Using DMPA for a method of contraception
   c. Tobacco use × 18 years
   d. Using a COC with 50 µg/mL copper T380A

5. Physical assessment findings apparent in KK that point to vulvovaginal candidiasis include: (EO-7)
   a. Thick, white curd-like secretions
   b. pH 5.0–6.0
   c. pH 6.0–7.0
   d. Positive guaiac test

6. The probable cause of KK's recurrent vulvovaginal candidiasis may include all of the following *except:* (EO -2)
   a. Intestinal reservoir for microorganisms
   b. Sexual transmission
   c. Toxic shock syndrome
   d. Therapeutic failure

7. Which of the following medications should be avoided to prevent hirsutism in KK? (EO-10)
   a. Desogestrel
   b. Norgestrel + ethinyl estradiol
   c. Norgestimate
   d. Norgestrel + tartrazine

8. Vulvovaginal candidiasis occurs in what percentage of women? (EO-3)
   a. <5 %
   b. >5 %
   c. >10 %
   c. >15 %

9. Describe the mechanism of action of the pharmacologic interventions in this case. (EO-7)

10. What factors should be considered when choosing an appropriate method of birth control for KK? (EO-8, 15)

11. Provide recommendations to optimize pharmacologic and nonpharmacologic treatment of KK's PMS. (EO-11)

12. Adverse effects associated with COC are either due to the estrogen or the progesterone component. Hirsutism would result from which of the following: (EO-10)
    a. Androgen excess
    b. Progesterone deficiency
    c. Estrogen excess
    d. Estrogen deficiency

13. Noncontraceptive benefits of oral contraceptives include all of the following *except:* (EO-8)
    a. Decrease risk of ovarian cancer
    b. Decrease risk of chlamydia
    c. Decrease risk of breast cancer
    d. Decrease risk of endometrial cancer

14. All of the following can lead to contraceptive failure in KK, *except:* (EO-9)
    a. Poor compliance with oral contraceptives
    b. Concomitant use with broad-spectrum antibiotics
    c. Concomitant use with stimulant laxatives
    d. Concomitant use with agents that decrease GI motility

15. Evaluate the pharmacoeconomic considerations relative to KK's plan of care. (EO-17)

16. Summarize pathophysiologic, therapeutic, and disease management concepts for contraception utilizing a key points format. (EO-18)

CASE 146
Nicole G. Parker
Topic: Pregnancy

EDUCATIONAL MATERIALS
Chapter 100: Drug Use in Pregnancy and Lactation

SCENARIO

Patient and Setting

CC, a 33-year-old pregnant female; OB-GYN clinic

Chief Complaint

8 weeks gestation with severe vaginal and vulvar itching, burning, and nonmalodorous discharge

History of Present Illness

Vaginal discomfort; Type 1 diabetes mellitus (DM) poorly controlled over the past several weeks; HTN, epilepsy, asthma, and impaired renal function

Past Medical History

Type 1 DM for 19 years; history of epilepsy: last seizure 1 year ago; mild HTN for 6 years controlled with methyldopa and taken during pregnancy with no complaints; asthma controlled with metaproterenol PRN; given prednisone after last attack; and impaired renal function

OB-GYN History

G2P2; 8 weeks pregnant

Past Surgical History

None

Family/Social History

Family History: Lives with dependent children

Social History: Smokes 1 PPD × 8 years; occasional use of alcohol

Medication History

Phenytoin, 100 mg PO QHS

Metaproterenol, 1–2 puffs QID PRN

Prednisone, 12 mg PO q AM

Methyldopa, 250 mg PO BID

Insulin ultralente, 14 U SC before breakfast

Insulin reg, 7 U SC before breakfast, lunch, and evening meal

Allergies

NKDA

Physical Examination

GEN: 33-year-old female in acute distress, with complaints of severe vaginal itching and burning and a nonmalodorous vaginal discharge; recently found to be 8 weeks pregnant

VS: BP 150/100, HR 85, RR 20, T 37°C, Wt 65 kg, Ht 168 cm

HEENT: Pale mucous membranes and skin, no nystagmus, no retinopathy

COR: Normal sinus rhythm, no murmurs, rubs, gallops

CHEST: Clear to auscultation

ABD: No pain, tenderness, guarding

GU: Positive vaginal, "cottage cheese," curd-like discharge, nonmalodorous

EXT: Cool to touch, dry skin; full range of motion of all extremities; no bruises

NEURO: No noticeable neuropathies, peripheral tingling, or numbness; no ataxia, dizziness

Results of Pertinent Laboratory Tests, Serum Drug Concentrations, and Diagnostic Tests

BUN 8.9 (25)	MCV 90 (90)	Glu (fasting)
Cr 123 (1.4)	MCHC 330 (33)	16 (290)
Hct 0.38 (38)	Alb 55 (5.5)	HbA$_{1C}$ 8%
Hgb 120 (12)		Phenytoin 47.6 (12)

Urinalysis: Protein 1+; glucose 3+ to 4+

ABGs: pO$_2$ 90, pCO$_2$ 22

Pulmonary function tests: FEV$_1$ 800 mL

PROBLEM LIST

Identify principal problems from the scenario in priority order [completed Problem List and SOAP Note at end of casebook]

SOAP NOTES

To be completed by student

QUESTIONS

[Answers at end of casebook]

1. The probable cause for CC's yeast infection could be due to which of the following: (EO-1)
   a. Impaired renal function
   b. Phenytoin use
   c. Diabetes mellitus
   d. Use of metaproterenol

2. Pharmacokinetic changes that may occur in CC during pregnancy include all of the following *except:* (EO-4, 6, 8)
   a. Increased renal and hepatic clearance
   b. Decreased protein binding capacity
   c. Decreased volume of distribution
   d. Increased volume of distribution

3. Which of the following antifungals for the treatment of vulvovaginal candidiasis should be avoided in CC? (EO-2)
   a. Ketoconazole
   b. Nystatin oral tablets
   c. Miconazole cream
   d. Clotrimazole

4. All of the following physical assessment findings would determine phenytoin toxicity in CC, *except:* (EO-5)
   a. HEENT–nystagmus
   b. NEURO–ataxia
   c. EXT–peripheral tingling
   d. NEURO–dizziness

5. Which of the following disease processes listed in CC's medical history probably contributed to her seizures? (EO-1)
   a. Impaired renal function
   b. Her asthma
   c. Her HbA$_{1C}$
   d. Her arterial blood gases

6. Which of the following may increase CC's risk for phenytoin toxicity? (EO-4, 6, 8)
   a. Corticosteroid use
   b. Acute alcohol ingestion
   c. Chronic alcohol ingestion
   d. Impaired renal function

7. CC may be at risk for pregnancy-induced hypertension or preeclampsia. Identify the risk factors. (EO-1, 3)

8. Pregnancy Category D is described by the Food and Drug Administration as positive evidence of human fetal risk, but the benefits from use in pregnancy may be acceptable despite the risk. Which of CC's medications is Pregnancy Category D?
   a. Methyldopa
   b. Phenytoin
   c. Insulin
   d. Prednisone

9. Factors which influence teratogenicity of a drug include all of the following *except:* (EO-4, 8)
   a. The embryonic stage at exposure
   b. The duration of exposure
   c. The phenotype of the mother and fetus
   d. Maternal and fetal metabolism of the drug

10. What psychosocial factors may affect CC's pharmacologic and nonpharmacologic therapy? (EO-15)

11. Describe the health care provider's role relative to CC's plan of care. (EO-16)

12. CC's use of phenytoin during pregnancy increases the risk of which of the following birth defects: (EO-10)
    a. Fetal hydantoin syndrome
    b. Polydactyly
    c. Gray baby syndrome
    d. Cleft palate

13. Evaluate the pharmacoeconomic considerations relative to CC's plan of care. (EO-17)

14. Summarize pathophysiologic, therapeutic, and disease management concepts of drugs in pregnancy utilizing a key points format. (EO-18)

CASE 147
Nicole G. Parker
Topic: Infertility
`Level 1`
EDUCATIONAL MATERIALS
Chapter 99: Infertility and Contraception

SCENARIO

Patient and Setting
BB, a 32-year-old female; gynecology clinic

Chief Complaint
Concerns of infertility; bumps around rectum for 6 months

History of Present Illness
Hyperthyroidism previously treated successfully with propylthiouracil (PTU)–euthyroid; inability to conceive

Past Medical History
Hyperthyroidism for 4 years

OB-GYN History
G0P0, LMP 10 days ago, regular 31-day cycle except for decreased menstrual flow during hyperthyroid state; no history of endometriosis or pelvic inflammatory disease (PID)

Family/Social History
Family History: Mother has Graves' disease; no family history of other endocrine abnormalities; BB is an only child; spouse is a lawyer with two children by a previous marriage

Social History: Master's degree in library science, currently works at the public library; denies tobacco use and drinks socially (1–2 drinks/weekend)

Medication History
PTU therapy was completed 3 years ago; currently takes no medications

Allergies
Iodine

Physical Examination
GEN: Well-developed, well-nourished female
VS: BP 110/72, HR 60, T 37°C, Wt 59 kg, Ht 168 cm
HEENT: Mild proptosis that has remained unchanged for past 4 years; thyroid not enlarged
COR: WNL
ABD: Nontender, no masses
GU: 5–6 pink-white warts with fine fingerlike fronds on the vulva and perineum; no apparent cervical involvement; cervix appeared normal; ovaries were palpated; normal-sized uterus; no adnexal tenderness noted on examination
RECT: 2–3 small condyloma acuminatum around anus
EXT: No pretibial myxedema
NEURO: No hyperreflexia; no fine resting tremor

Results of Pertinent Laboratory tests, Serum Drug Concentrations and Diagnostic Tests

Na 138 (138)
K 4.5 (4.5)
Cl 100 (100)
HCO_3 23 (23)
BUN 4.28 (12)
Cr 79.56 (0.9)
Hct 0.41 (41)
Hgb 138 (13.8)

Lkcs 6.6×10^9
    (6.6×10^3)
Plts 298×10^9
    $(298 \times 10_9)$
MCV 91.4 (91.4)
MCHC 335 (33.5)
AST 0.33 (20)
ALT 0.27 (16)
LDH 1.92 (115)

Alk Phos 0.85 (51)
Alb 47 (4.7)
T Bili 8.55 (0.5)
Glu 5.0 (90)
Ca 2.37 (9.5)
PO_4 0.9 (2.8)
Chol 4.42 (171)
Trig 0.79 (70)

Thyroid function tests: T4: 102.96 (8.0) (RIA); RT3 U: 0.3 (30%); FTI: 30.9 (2.4)

Ultrasensitive TSH: 2.1 (2.1)

UA: Glucose, ketones, and protein: negative; pH 6.5

PAP: Koilocytosis with mild inflammation

PROBLEM LIST

Identify principal problems from the scenario in priority order [completed Problem List and SOAP Note at end of casebook]

SOAP NOTES

To be completed by student

QUESTIONS

[Answers at end of casebook]

1. All of the following are true of condyloma acuminata, *except:* (EO-1)
   a. Caused by human papilloma virus (HPV)
   b. May be documented by a Pap smear
   c. Average incubation period usually 10–14 days
   d. A sexually transmitted disease

2. Signs and symptoms of hyperthyroidism include all of the following *except:* (EO-2)
   a. Heat intolerance
   b. Irritability
   c. Tremor
   d. Systolic hypotension

3. Which of the following statements is true? (EO-5)
   a. A TSH level of <0.01 U/mL excludes hyperthyroidism
   b. A TSH level of >0.01 U/mL excludes hyperthyroidism
   c. An elevated T_4 level may indicate hypothyroidism
   d. A normal TSH level and an elevated T_4 level may indicate hyperthyroidism

4. Choose the correct statement: (EO-7, 10)
   a. PTU is a thioamide that may safely be used by BB if she wishes to become pregnant
   b. Methimazole is a thioamide that may safely be used by BB is she wishes to become pregnant

   c. Methimazole inhibits both thyroid hormone synthesis and extrathyroidal conversion of T_4 to T_3
   d. PTU inhibits both thyroid hormone synthesis and extrathyroidal conversion of T_3 to T_4

5. Which of the following are risk factors of BB's infertility? (EO-4)
   a. Endometriosis
   b. Tubal damage
   c. Cervical mucus abnormalities
   d. STD

6. Which of the following diagnostic tools provide valuable information regarding both the presence and timing of ovulation? (EO-5)
   a. A postcoital test
   b. Basal body temperature
   c. Daily axillary temperatures
   d. A hysterosalpingogram

7. The most common adverse effects associated with trichloroacetic acid include: (EO-10)
   a. Headaches
   b. Burning
   c. Rash
   d. Fever

8. Which of the following medications may be continued (if needed) for condyloma acuminata if BB becomes pregnant? (EO-8)
   a. Trichloroacetic acid
   b. Imiquimod
   c. Podophyllin
   d. Podofilox

9. Describe the mechanism of action of the pharmacologic and nonpharmacologic interventions in this case. (EO-7)

10. Evaluate the pharmacoeconomic considerations relative to BB's plan of care. (EO-17)

11. If BB's hyperthyroidism remains stabilized and her genital warts have been successfully managed, what medications may be used for infertility? (EO-8)

12. If BB is started on clomiphene, what recommended dose regimen would be suggested to optimize pharmacologic treatment to achieve fertility? (EO-14)
    a. Clomiphene 50 mg PO QD on day 5 of menses; repeat same dose if ovulation occurs without conception
    b. Clomiphene 50 mg PO QD × 2 cycles
    c. Clomiphene 100 mg PO QD on day 5 of menses; repeat for 6 months until conception
    d. Clomiphene 100 mg PO QD × 2 cycles

13. What psychosocial factors may affect SK's adherence to both pharmacologic and nonpharmacologic therapy? (EO-15)

14. Summarize pathophysiologic, therapeutic, and disease management concepts for infertility utilizing a key points format. (EO-18)

CASE 148
Nicole G. Parker
Topic: Drugs in Lactation

EDUCATIONAL MATERIALS
Chapter 100: Drug Use in Pregnancy and Lactation

SCENARIO

Patient and Setting
MW, a 20-year-old female; OB-GYN clinic

Chief Complaint
Genital pain and newly formed genital vesicles; depression

History of Present Illness
Herpes simplex virus (HSV) 2; depressed mood, symptoms include sleep disturbances, fatigue, anhedonia, poor hygiene, and feeling that life is not worth living

Past Medical History
HSV 2 since age 18 with 3 recurrences since diagnosis; 6 days postpartum, infant born without complications; depression 3 years ago with symptoms of decreased sleep, decreased appetite, and anhedonia; treated with amitriptyline but discontinued during pregnancy

OB-GYN History
G1P1AB0; 6 days postpartum; HSV 2 with newly formed genital vesiculopustules

Allergies
Yeast

Family/Social History
Family History: Single, unemployed
Social History: Smokes 2 PPD ×10 years; frequent alcohol use

Medication History
Docusate sodium, 100 mg PO q AM
Acetaminophen/codeine, 15 mg PO q4–6h PRN

Physical Examination
GEN: Thin, 20-year-old, depressed woman 6 days postpartum with painful genital vesicles

VS: BP: 110/85, HR 85, RR 18, T 37°C, Wt 50 kg, Ht 155 cm
HEENT: WNL; no apparent oropharynx or mucosal vesicle formation; normal sclerae
COR: Regular sinus rhythm, no murmurs
CHEST: Clear to auscultation and percussion; tender, full breasts
ABD: No masses or guarding, tenderness from recent delivery
GU: Grossly visible vesiculopustules on labia, urethra, and vulva; some with a slight erythematous zone
RECT: Normal, no vesicles, no hemorrhoids
EXT: Normal-appearing skin color and range of motion
NEURO: A and O × 3, CNI-12 intact, normal tendon reflexes

Results of Pertinent Laboratory Tests, Serum Drug Concentrations, and Diagnostic Tests

BUN 3.2 (9)	Hct 0.33 (33)	Alb 40 (4.0)
Cr 79 (0.9)	Hgb 110 (11)	Glu 5 (90)

Antibody to HSV: Positive
Pap smear/Giemsa: Giant cells
Lkc differential: WNL

PROBLEM LIST
Identify principal problems from the scenario in priority order [completed Problem List and SOAP Note at end of casebook]

SOAP NOTES
To be completed by student

QUESTIONS
[Answers at end of casebook]

1. MW's Pap smear reveals Giemsa: Giant cells. Which of the following statements is true with regard to this Pap smear finding? (EO-5)
   a. Giemsa is a test to determine vesicle size in order to distinguish between varicella-zoster and HSV
   b. Giemsa are multinucleated giant cells that form the vesicles
   c. Giemsa is a type of smear that shows multinucleated giant cells, which does not distinguish between varicella-zoster and HSV
   d. Giemsa is a type of smear that shows multinucleated giant cells that can distinguish between varicella-zoster and HSV

2. Which of the following drugs should be avoided in MW to reduce the risk of exposure to the infant through breast milk? (EO-4)
   a. Nonionized drugs
   b. Highly water soluble drugs
   c. Highly protein bound drugs
   d. Ionized drugs

3. All of the following factors influence drug concentration in breast-fed infants, *except:* (EO-4, 8)
   a. The molecular weight of the drug
   b. Maternal drug metabolism
   c. Prolonged GI transit time in the mother
   d. Altered GI flora in the infant

4. Which of the following statements is *false* regarding breast-feeding? (EO-4)
   a. Breast-feeding may protect the infant against infection for at least 3 months
   b. Breast-fed infants have a measurable increase in intellectual development scores compared with those in bottle-fed infants
   c. Breast milk is equally nutritious as formula supplements and is high in vitamin D
   d. Breast-feeding decreases the risk for subsequent breast cancer in the nursing mother

5. Fluoxetine would be indicated in MW if the following occurs: (EO-4, 6, 8, 12)
   a. Suicidal ideation (infant no longer worth living for)
   b. Increased alcohol consumption
   c. MW wishes to breast-feed
   d. MW needs continuous acyclovir therapy

6. List the pharmacologic and nonpharmacologic treatment problems present in MW's treatment plan. (EO-11)

7. The appropriate regimen for MW's infant if she develops lesions on the mouth is: (EO-6, 8)
   a. Acyclovir 30 mg/kg/d PO in 3 divided doses $\times$ 14–21 days
   b. Acyclovir 30 mg/d PO $\times$ 14–21 days
   c. Indinavir 30 mg/d PO $\times$ 14–21 days
   d. Acyclovir 30 mg/kg/d PO $\times$ 10 days

8. The potentiation of hypothrombinemic bleeding, a pseudo-Cushing's syndrome, has been reported in nursing mothers using: (EO-10)
   a. Caffeine
   b. Nicotine
   c. Alcohol
   d. Docusate sodium

9. Drug-free intervals and dose adjustments may be needed for which of MW's medications: (EO-8)
   a. Acetaminophen/codeine
   b. Valacyclovir
   c. Docusate sodium
   d. Amitriptyline

10. What psychosocial factors may affect MW's adherence to both pharmacologic and nonpharmacologic therapy? (EO-15)

11. Describe the health care provider's role relative to proposed psychosocial factors identified. (EO-16)

12. Evaluate the pharmacoeconomic considerations relative to MW's plan of care. (EO-17)

13. Summarize therapeutic, pathophysiologic, and disease management concepts for drugs used in lactation utilizing a keys point format. (EO-18)

CASE 149
Susan W. Miller
Topic: Alzheimer's Disease
Level 3
EDUCATIONAL MATERIALS

Chapter 101: Alzheimer's Disease (clinical presentation and diagnosis, psychosocial, therapeutic plan, treatment); Chapter 61: Alcoholism (therapeutic goals, chronic alcohol abuse/alcoholism, psychosocial); Chapter 42: Ischemic Heart Disease (therapeutic goals, psychosocial, pharmacotherapy); Chapter 40: Congestive Heart Failure (therapeutic goals, therapy, prognosis)

SCENARIO

Patient and Setting

LB, a 79-year-old male; physician's office

Chief Complaint

Forgetful, nervous; irritable; 12-lb weight loss over 3 months

History of Present Illness

Increasing irritability with wife; problems grooming; refuses to bathe; episodes of agitation, with anger, and verbal abuse; daytime naps; early to bed, early AM awakening; suspicious; paranoid; daughter has seen steady decline in LB's memory over the past 4–5 years

Past Medical History

Nontransmural myocardial infarction (MI) 13 months ago; arrhythmias; angina; congestive heart failure (CHF); confused, agitated, and hallucinations while hospitalized

Past Surgical History

Gallbladder removed 20 years prior

Family/Social History

Family History: Noncontributory

Social History: Tobacco: 75 pack/year history, quit 3 years ago; history of chronic alcohol use (heavy in the past, averaging 2–5 drinks per day). Currently drinks 2–3 drinks per day (per daughter)

Medication History

Digoxin, 0.25 mg PO QD

Furosemide, 40 mg PO QD

KCl 10%, 15 mL (20 mEq) PO QD

Verapamil, 80 mg PO q8h

Diphenhydramine, 50 mg PO QHS

Nitroglycerin, 0.4 mg 1 tablet SL PRN chest pain

Allergies

NKDA

Physical Examination

GEN: Well-developed, well-nourished male, unkempt appearance

VS: BP 150/90, HR 71, T 37.0°C, Wt 71.4 kg, Ht 172 cm

HEENT: WNL

COR: Regular rate and rhythm with frequent ectopic beats

CHEST: Inspiratory crackles at both bases

ABD: Mild left lower quadrant tenderness

GU: WNL

RECT: Slightly enlarged prostate

EXT: 2+ pitting edema of feet and ankles

NEURO: Oriented × 1; Mini-Mental Status Examination: 11/30

Results of Pertinent Laboratory Tests, Serum Drug Concentrations, and Diagnostic Tests

Na 140 (140)	HCO$_3$ 25 (25)	AST 0.65 (39)
K 4.0 (4.0)	BUN 7.5 (21)	ALT 0.58 (35)
Cl 102 (102)	Cr 105 (1.2)	Glu 5.3 (95)

Digoxin: 2.2 nmol/L (1.7 ng/mL)

ECG: NSR with frequent (greater than 30/hr), multifocal PVCs; left axis deviation

Echocardiogram: Normal chamber size; mild aortic stenosis

PROBLEM LIST

Identify principal problems from the scenario in priority order

SOAP NOTE

To be completed by student

QUESTIONS

1. All of the following are signs and symptoms of dementia exhibited by LB, *except:* (EO-2)
   a. Memory loss
   b. Problems grooming
   c. Daily consumption of alcohol
   d. Confusion

2. Which of the following is a probable cause of LB's dementia? (EO-1)
   a. Advanced age
   b. Previous alcohol abuse
   c. Previous tobacco use
   d. Digoxin use

3. Which of the following would *not* be a good choice for treatment of LB's memory loss due to its adverse effects on the liver and liver function tests? (EO-8, 10)
   a. Tacrine
   b. Haloperidol
   c. Donepezil
   d. Risperidone

4. Which of the following medications in LB's regimen could be contributing to his memory loss? (EO-10)
   a. Digoxin
   b. Furosemide
   c. Diphenhydramine
   d. Verapamil

5. Which of the following is a good alternative to the current regimen and doses of digoxin, furosemide, and nitroglycerin to treat the CHF exacerbation in LB? (EO-12)
   a. Discontinue digoxin and furosemide and start fosinopril 10 mg PO QD
   b. Discontinue current regimen and start atenolol 50 mg PO BID
   c. Increase dose of digoxin to 0.25 mg PO QD
   d. Decrease the dose of furosemide to 40 mg PO QOD

6. The probable cause for the CHF exacerbation in LB is: (EO-1)
   a. Verapamil use
   b. Renal dysfunction
   c. Nitroglycerin use
   d. KCl use

7. Which of the following is a reasonable alternative for management of the agitation, anger, and paranoia reported by LB's wife: (EO-12)
   a. Lorazepam 0.5 mg PO BID
   b. Haloperidol 0.25 mg PO BID
   c. Nortriptyline 25 mg PO BID
   d. Donepezil 5 mg PO HS

8. The nitroglycerin should remain in LB's drug regimen to control which of the following: (EO-8, 12)
   a. CHF
   b. Arrhythmia
   c. Angina
   d. Elevated heart rate

9. All of the following can contribute to the recent weight loss experienced by LB, *except:* (EO-1, 10)
   a. Digoxin
   b. Memory loss
   c. KCl use
   d. Diphenhydramine

10. Evaluate the pharmacoeconomic considerations relative to LM's plan of care. (EO-17)

11. All of the following are possible etiologies of arrhythmias in LM *except:* (EO-1)
    a. History of MI
    b. Exacerbation of CHF
    c. Multifocal PVCs
    d. History of tobacco use

12. LB's family wants to maintain his care at home. What caregiver resources can be offered? (EO-16)

13. Describe the mechanisms of the medications used to treat the cognitive symptoms of Alzheimer's disease. (EO-7)

14. Describe the characteristics of a drug or drug class that can contribute to cognitive dysfunction. (EO-10)

15. Identify possible psychosocial effects that caregivers of patients with Alzheimer's disease must overcome. (EO-15)

16. Summarize therapeutic, pathophysiologic, and disease management concepts for geriatric disease states present in this case utilizing a key points format. (EO-18)

CASE 150
Susan W. Miller
Topic: Alzheimer's Disease

EDUCATIONAL MATERIALS

Chapter 101: Alzheimer's Disease (therapeutic plan, treatment, psychosocial aspects); Chapter 53: Parkinsonism (psychosocial aspects, therapeutic plan, pharmacotherapy, nonpharmacologic management); Chapter 39: Hypertension (complications, treatment, patient education); Chapter 27: Constipation and Diarrhea (therapeutic goals, psychosocial, therapeutic plan, pharmacotherapy)

SCENARIO

Patient and Setting
SP, a 68-year-old male; ED

Chief Complaint
Has become disoriented; unable to recognize familiar people

History of Present Illness
Daughter reports a mental status decline over the past 2 weeks, drowsy most of the day, frequent periods of severe agitation

Past Medical History

Parkinson's disease for 10 years; hypertension (HTN) for 30 years; depression for 35 years; chronic constipation with frequent impactions

Past Surgical History

Noncontributory

Family/Social History

Family History: Unknown

Social History: No tobacco products; occasional social drinker; no additional information available

Medication History

Levodopa/carbidopa 25/250, 2 tabs PO TID

Benztropine, 2 mg PO TID

Hydrochlorothiazide (HCTZ), 50 mg PO q AM

KCl, 20 mEq PO BID

Thioridazine, 50 mg PO BID

Phenolphthalein, 60 mg 2 tabs PO q AM PRN

Alprazolam, 1 mg PO QID agitation

Flurazepam, 15 mg PO HS PRN sleep, may repeat × 1

Allergies

NKDA

Physical Examination

GEN: Well-developed, overweight, confused male in no acute distress who appears extremely drowsy

VS: BP 150/94, HR 85, RR 20, T 38.4°C, Wt 72 kg, Ht 185.42 cm

HEENT: WNL; wears corrective lenses

COR: Normal S1 and S2; no murmurs, rubs, or gallops

CHEST: Clear, no rales present

ABD: Flat, nontender

GU: Prostatic hypertrophy

RECT: Hard stool in rectum

EXT: No skin tears or lesions; slightly pale

NEURO: Bilateral rigidity; slight tremor present, oriented to person only

Results of Pertinent Laboratory Tests, Serum Drug Concentrations, and Diagnostic Tests

Na 137 (137)	BUN 8.6 (24)	ALT 0.47 (28)
K 4.8 (4.8)	Glu 7.1 (128)	LDH 2.5 (150)
Cl 102 (102)	Cr 97 (1.1)	Alk Phos 1.75 (1105)
HCO_3 28 (28)	AST 0.40 (24)	Alb 41 (4.1)

T Protein 72 (7.2)	PO_4 1.4 (4.2)	Chol 6.47 (250)
T Bili 14 (0.82)	Uric Acid 420 (7.0)	Iron 15 (85)
Ca 2.3 (9.2)		

Urinalysis: Negative for glucose and microorganisms

Chest x-ray: WNL

ECG: WNL

PROBLEM LIST

Identify principal problems from the scenario in priority order [completed Problem List and SOAP Note at end of casebook]

SOAP NOTE

To be completed by student

QUESTIONS

[Answers at end of casebook]

1. Which of the following medications in SP's drug regimen is *least* likely to be contributing to his mental status decline? (EO-10)
   a. Levodopa/carbidopa
   b. Benztropine
   c. Thioridazine
   d. Alprazolam

2. Which of the following is *not* an option in the management of Parkinson's disease drug therapy for SP? (EO-8, 12)
   a. Double the dose of levodopa/carbidopa to 25/250 4 tablets PO TID
   b. Add a dopamine agonist to the regimen
   c. Add selegiline to the regimen
   d. Change to levodopa/carbidopa in the extended release form

3. Which of the following is least likely to contribute to SP's constipation? (EO-10)
   a. Benztropine
   b. Parkinson's disease
   c. Phenolphthalein
   d. Reduction in activity level

4. Describe management strategies for treatment of constipation in SP. (EO-12)

5. Which of the following signs or symptoms of advancing Parkinson's disease are present in SP? (EO-2)
   a. Increased blood pressure
   b. Drowsiness
   c. Prostatic hypertrophy
   d. Problems with balance

6. Hydrochlorothiazide is not useful in many geriatric patients because it: (EO-4, 8)
   a. Is not effective in creatinine clearance < 30 mL/min
   b. Causes excessive sedation
   c. Exerts potent anticholinergic activity
   d. Decreases cardiac output

7. Agitation in demented geriatric patients is best treated initially with which of the following: (EO-8, 12)
   a. Lorazepam
   b. Risperidone
   c. Hydroxyzine
   d. Carbamazepine

8. Which of the following is correct when converting from levodopa/carbidopa immediate release to levodopa/carbidopa sustained release? (EO-6)
   a. Base new dose on creatinine clearance
   b. Use equivalent levodopa doses
   c. Use 10–30% increase in levodopa dose
   d. Use 10–30% decrease in levodopa dose

9. Which of the following antipsychotic agents is most useful in patients with concomitant Parkinson's disease? (EO-12)
   a. Thioridazine
   b. Haloperidol
   c. Risperidone
   d. Molindone

10. Evaluate the pharmacoeconomic considerations relevant to the therapy for Parkinson's disease in SP. (EO-17)

11. All of the following are complications or adverse effects of levodopa, *except:* (EO-10)
    a. Urinary retention
    b. Hallucinations
    c. Wearing-off effect
    d. Muscle dystonias

12. What monitoring parameters are appropriate for SP's drug therapy? (EO-8)

13. Describe caregiver issues important to SP's case. (EO-14, 15)

14. Summarize therapeutic, pathophysiologic, and disease management concepts for Parkinson's disease utilizing a key points format. (EO-18)

CASE 151
Susan W. Miller
Topic: Geriatric Drug Therapy
Level 3

EDUCATIONAL MATERIALS
Chapter 102: Geriatric Drug Therapy (psychosocial, medication-related problems, effect of aging on drug actions); Chapter 17: Thyroid Disorders (clinical presentation and diagnosis, therapeutic plan, treatment, pharmacotherapy); Chapter 19: Diabetes (monitoring, therapy); Chapter 98: Gynecologic Disorders (estrogen replacement therapy, the role of the pharmacist as menopause counsellor); Chapter 32: Osteoarthritis (pharmacotherapy, nonpharmacologic therapy, psychosocial)

SCENARIO

Patient and Setting
JM, a 72-year-old female; ambulatory clinic

Chief Complaint
No chief complaint; patient presents to clinic for annual physical examination

History of Present Illness
Home blood glucose readings in the range of 180–230 mg/dL, heartburn, easy fatigability, urinary frequency, persistent pains in hips and knees; requests a vitamin supplement

Past Medical History
History of type 2 diabetes mellitus (DM): no menopausal vasomotor symptoms for 5 years; no history of vaginal bleeding or discharge; negative mammogram 5 years previous; last visit (12 months ago) lipid profile normal; hyperthyroidism currently controlled

Past Surgical History
Thyroidectomy for treatment of hyperthyroidism

Family/Social History
Family History: Both parents died of lung cancer
Social History: Moderate alcohol use; no history of smoking

Medication History
Levothyroxine, 0.05 mg PO q AM
Conjugated estrogens, 1.25 mg PO QD
Medroxyprogesterone, 10 mg PO as directed
Glyburide, 2.5 mg PO BID
Piroxicam, 20 mg PO q AM (started 3 months ago)
Ibuprofen, 200 mg 2 tabs PO q8h PRN

Allergies
Codeine, sulfa

Physical Examination
GEN: Pale, overweight woman with no acute distress or symptoms
VS: BP 160/80 (lying), HR 60, RR 16, T 38.2°C, Wt 70 kg (increased from 65 kg on last visit), Ht 162.5 cm (164 cm on prior visit)
HEENT: Hair coarse, arteriole-venule nicking in the eye, thyroid slightly enlarged, mild lid lag

COR: WNL
CHEST: Lungs clear, breast examination normal
ABD: WNL
GU: Atrophic changes present on pelvic examination
RECT: No hemorrhoids present
EXT: Skin warm and dry to touch, grooved nails and decrease in deep tendon reflexes, with no edema present, bilateral varicose veins
NEURO: WNL

Results of Pertinent Laboratory Tests, Serum Drug Concentrations, and Diagnostic Tests

Cr 120 (1.4) Hgb 117 (11.7) TSH 5.2 (5.2)
Glu (fasting) 13 (234) RBC 3.7×10^{12} T_3 uptake 0.39 (39)
K 4.7 (4.7) (3.7×10^6) Iron 9.2 (51.4)
Hct 0.34 (34) T_4 54 (4.2) HbA_{1C} 12%

Urinalysis: Negative for Lkcs, bacteria, ketones; 1+ protein, 2+glucose

Pap smear: Atypical cells present (normal 2 years ago)

Occult blood: Guaiac positive

PROBLEM LIST

Identify principal problems from the scenario in priority order

SOAP NOTE

To be completed by student

QUESTIONS

1. All of the following are signs and symptoms of hypothyroidism exhibited by JM *except:* (EO-2, 5)
   a. Fatigue
   b. Elevated TSH
   c. Urinary frequency
   d. Coarse hair and skin

2. Describe methods to adjust thyroid medication. (EO-8)

3. Which of the following monitoring parameters is the *least important* for thyroid replacement therapy? (EO-8)
   a. TSH, T_4
   b. Heart rate
   c. Potassium level
   d. Excessive sweating

4. Nutritional advice would benefit all of the following problems present in JM *except:* (EO-11)
   a. Type 2 diabetes mellitus
   b. Degenerative joint disease
   c. Fatigue
   d. Hypothyroidism

5. The guaiac-positive occult blood test in JM is most likely due to: (EO-10)
   a. Levothyroxine
   b. Piroxicam
   c. Conjugated estrogens
   d. Glyburide

6. JM's reported sulfa allergy is a potential problem with which of the following: (EO-8, 9)
   a. Levothyroxine
   b. Piroxicam
   c. Conjugated estrogens
   d. Glyburide

7. Which of the following NSAIDs would be a better choice for JM due to the guaiac-positive occult blood test? (EO-8, 10)
   a. Ibuprofen
   b. Salsalate
   c. Nabumetone
   d. Naproxen

8. What therapies other than NSAIDs are available for the management of the pain due to degenerative joint disease? (EO-12)

9. Which of the following is most appropriate concerning the dose of conjugated estrogens prescribed for JM? (EO-8, 11)
   a. Leave at current level of 1.25 mg PO QD
   b. Increase to 2.5 mg PO QD
   c. Decrease to 0.625 mg PO QD
   d. Change to 1.25 mg PO QOD

10. The urinary frequency reported by JM is most likely a result of which of the following? (EO-1, 2)
    a. Piroxicam
    b. Levothyroxine
    c. Status post thyroidectomy
    d. Vaginal atrophy

11. Discuss pharmacoeconomic considerations important to the selection of a thyroid supplementation product. (EO-17)

12. What psychosocial factors may affect EM's adherence to the nonpharmacologic and pharmacologic therapies? (EO-15)

13. Summarize therapeutic, pathophysiologic, and disease management concepts for the treatment of common geriatric problems present in this case utilizing a key points format. (EO-18)

CASE 152
Susan W. Miller
Topic: Geriatric Drug Therapy
Level 1

EDUCATIONAL MATERIALS
Chapter 102: Geriatric Drug Therapy (psychosocial, medication-related problems, effect of aging on drug actions); Chapter 44: Thromboembolic Disease (psychosocial, therapeutic plan, pharmacologic therapy, patient education)

SCENARIO

Patient and Setting

EM, an 81-year-old female; nursing home resident

Chief Complaint

Stroke rehabilitation; no specific complaints

History of Present Illness

Requires assistance in all activities of daily living (dressing, bathing, eating); spends most of day in a wheelchair; often disoriented and slumps in wheelchair; responds poorly to commands; noted to be lethargic, and sleeping most of the day for the past week; 6-lb weight loss over past 30 days

Past Medical History

Left-sided weakness and unsteady gait following CVA; chronic atrial fibrillation

Past Surgical History

Noncontributory

Family/Social History

Family History: Mother died age 65 with CVA

Social History: No history of smoking; light alcohol intake × 40 years; no alcohol since admission to nursing home

Medication History

Digoxin, 0.125 mg PO QD

Furosemide, 40 mg PO QD

KCl 10%, 20 mEq PO QD

Dipyridamole, 25 mg PO BID

Multivitamin with minerals tablet PO QD

Psyllium, 15 mL in fluids PO BID

Allergies

Penicillin

Physical Examination

GEN: EM is a very thin, pale female

VS: BP 110/70, HR 120 (irregular), T 37.0°C, Wt 42.5 kg, Ht 155 cm

HEENT: Cerumen in both ears, blocking canal

COR: Irregularly, irregular heart rate (120 bpm)

CHEST: Clear to auscultation

ABD: Hypoactive bowel sounds

BACK: Kyphotic

GU: Deferred

RECT: Occult blood–negative

EXT: Skin tear on right forearm; 1+ pitting ankle edema

NEURO: Lethargic, arousable to name; left upper extremity weakness; hyperactive reflexes left elbow and knee; upgoing toe (positive Babinski sign); oriented to person

SKIN: Dry mucous membranes, poor skin turgor

Results of Pertinent Laboratory Tests, Serum Drug Concentrations, and Diagnostic Tests

Na 148 (148)	Glu (fasting) 7.8	Lkcs 10.8 × 10⁹
K 3.3 (3.3)	(140)	(10.8 × 10³)
Cl 115 (115)	Hct 0.32 (32)	Ca 2.4 (9.6)
HCO₃ 28 (28)	Hgb 108 (10.8)	Mg 1.0 (2.0)
BUN 10.5 (30)	Plts 240 × 10⁹	
Cr 120 (1.4)	(240 × 10³)	

Lkcs differential: WNL

Digoxin 3 months prior: 2.3 nmol/L (1.8 ng/dL)

ECG shows atrial fibrillation, ST-T wave changes

PROBLEM LIST

Identify principal problems from the scenario in priority order [completed Problem List and SOAP Note at end of casebook]

SOAP NOTE

To be completed by student

QUESTIONS

[Answers at end of casebook]

1. Which of the following physical findings/lab values is indicative of dehydration? (EO-2)
   a. Low sodium level
   b. Elevated creatinine clearance
   c. Poor skin turgor
   d. Weight loss of 10% from usual weight

2. All of the following can contribute to anorexia and weight loss in this patient, *except:* (EO-10)
   a. Digoxin
   b. Lethargy
   c. Dipyridamole
   d. Upper extremity weakness

3. EM presents with all of the following signs and symptoms of atrial fibrillation *except:* (EO-2)
   a. Irregular heart rate
   b. Lack p-waves on ECG
   c. Periods of lethargy
   d. Weight loss

4. List pharmacologic and nonpharmacologic therapeutic options for treatment of a post-CVA patient. (EO-11)

5. What future health care decisions should be anticipated for EM? (EO-1)

6. All of the following are usual doses of aspirin for CVA prophylaxis *except:* (EO-12)
   a. 325 mg PO QD
   b. 325 mg PO QOD
   c. 81 mg PO QD
   d. 81 mg PO QOD

7. By itself, which of the following is an important consideration in determining the maintenance dose of digoxin? (EO-5, 6)
   a. Renal function
   b. Hepatic function
   c. Mental status
   d. Serum albumin level

8. Based on adverse effects and relative expense, which of the following antiplatelet agents should be reserved for patients intolerant to aspirin? (EO-8, 17)
   a. Dipyridamole
   b. Warfarin
   c. Clopidogrel
   d. Salsalate

9. Should medications be prescribed for EM's deteriorated mental status? (EO-14)

10. What is the prognosis for this patient? (EO-12)

11. What is the most likely cause of EM's deteriorated mental status? (EO-1)

12. What psychosocial factors may affect EM's adherence to both pharmacologic and nonpharmacologic therapy? (EO-15)

13. Summarize therapeutic, pathophysiologic, and disease management concepts for dementia utilizing a key points format. (EO-18)

CASE 153
Scott D. Hanes
Topic: Neurotrauma

Level 1

EDUCATIONAL MATERIALS
Chapter 103: Critical Care Therapy (neurotrauma, pharmacokinetic and pharmacodynamic considerations, seizure treatment and prophylaxis)

SCENARIO

Patient and Setting
FF, a 36-year-old male; ED

Chief Complaint
Decreased level of consciousness, inability to move extremities

History of Present Illness
Involved in a head-on collision motor vehicle accident; unrestrained driver, thrown approximately 90 feet upon impact

Past Medical History
Unremarkable

Past Surgical History
Unremarkable

Family/Social History
Family History: Father died of MI at 67

Social History: No alcohol, tobacco, or recreational drug use

Medication History
Heparin, 5000 U SC q12h

Cimetidine, 300 mg IV q8h

Cefazolin, 1 g IV q8h

Gentamicin, 100 mg IV

Phenytoin, 150 mg IV q12h

Allergies
NKDA

Physical Examination
GEN: Well-developed, well-nourished male, unresponsive (Glasgow Coma Score = 6)
VS: BP 160/72, HR 95, RR 14 (mechanically ventilated), T 37°C (rectal), Wt 80 kg, Ht 185 cm
HEENT: Both pupils sluggishly reactive to light; no blood or CSF otorrhea/otorhonorrhea
COR: S1 and S2 normal; no murmurs or gallops
CHEST: Clear to auscultation
ABD: Soft, no masses or rigidity
GU: Normal male genitalia; no blood in urine
RECT: Weakly positive anal sphincter tone; hemoccult negative
EXT: Multiple scrapes and lacerations; open right femur fracture
NEURO: No eye opening or verbal response to painful stimulus; withdraws with painful stimulus in upper extremities, no movement in lower extremities. Lower extremity reflexes absent

Results of Pertinent Laboratory Tests, Serum Drug Concentrations, and Diagnostic Tests

Na 139 (139)	T Bili 94 (5.5)	Uric Acid WNL
K 3.9 (3.9)	AST WNL	CBC with differential
Cl 100 (100)	ALT WNL	Hct 0.40 (40%)
CO_2 24 (24)	LDH WNL	Hgb 155 (15.5)
BUN 4.3 (12)	Alk Phos WNL	Lkcs 7.8 × 10^9 (7.8 × 10^3)
Cr 70.7 (0.8)	Ca 2.6 (10.0)	Plts 220 × 10^9 (220
Glu 6.4 (115)	PO_4 1.1 (3.4)	× 10^3)
Alb WNL	Mg 1.05 (2.1)	MCV 82 (82)

Lkc differential: Normal

Alcohol: Negative

Urine drug screen: Negative

Urinalysis: Normal

Chest x-ray: Clear

ECG: Normal

ICP: 25–35 mm Hg

CT head: Multiple cerebral contusions; cisterns absent; brain swelling noted

Spinal x-rays: Complete subluxation at C6–C7

PROBLEM LIST

Identify principal problems from the scenario in priority order

SOAP NOTE

To be completed by student

QUESTIONS

1. What other pharmacologic and nonpharmacologic therapies can be used to decrease ICP if mannitol fails? (EO-12)

2. Which of the following findings is consistent with the diagnosis of severe head injury? (EO-2)
   a. Weak anal sphincter tone
   b. ICP > 20 mm Hg
   c. GCS > 8
   d. Lower extremity paralysis

3. What is the recommended duration of phenytoin therapy in the absence of head injury-related seizures? (EO-11)
   a. One month
   b. One week
   c. One day
   d. One year

4. If FF began the methylprednisolone-dosing regimen between 3 and 8 hours from the time of injury, how long should the infusion last? (EO-8)
   a. 23 hours
   b. 24 hours
   c. 72 hours
   d. 48 hours

5. What is a potential complication of methylprednisolone therapy in this patient? (EO-10)
   a. Urinary tract infection
   b. Bronchospasm
   c. Diabetes
   d. Pneumonia

6. Which of the following statements is true regarding phenytoin concentrations in the presence of decreased serum albumin concentrations? (EO-8)
   a. Total concentration increases, free concentration is unchanged
   b. Total concentration decreases, free concentration is unchanged
   c. Total concentration is unchanged, free concentration decreases
   d. Total concentration decreases, free concentration increases

7. Which of the following drugs alters the pharmacokinetics of phenytoin? (EO-9)
   a. Cimetidine
   b. Heparin
   c. Cefazolin
   d. Mannitol

8. After mannitol therapy is given, the ICP falls to 12 mm Hg with a MAP of 75 mm Hg. What therapy (if any) should be given to optimize cerebral hemodynamics in this patient? (EO-8)
   a. Phenylephrine infusion
   b. Hyperventilate to a pCO_2 < 30 mm Hg
   c. A second dose of mannitol
   d. Furosemide IV bolus

9. Why is the duration of time elapsed between time of injury and the start of methylprednisolone therapy important for the treatment of spinal cord injury? (EO-6)

10. Describe the potential pharmacoeconomic benefits of receiving methylprednisolone therapy for spinal cord injury. (EO-17)

11. Identify the psychosocial issues that may occur following severe head injuries. (EO-15)

12. Summarize therapeutic, pathophysiologic, and disease management concepts for neurotrauma utilizing a key points format. (EO-18)

CASE 154

Scott D. Hanes

Topics: Heart Failure, Type 1 Diabetes Mellitus (DM)

 Level 1

EDUCATIONAL MATERIALS

Chapter 103: Critical Care Therapy
(cardiogenic shock)

SCENARIO

Patient and Setting

DK, a 58-year-old male; intensive care unit

Chief Complaint

N/A

History of Present Illness

Three-vessel coronary artery bypass graft surgery (CABG); became hypotensive (90/50 mm Hg) when removed from bypass machine

Past Medical History

Unstable angina × 10 years; myocardial infarction 5 years prior to admission; hypertension × 15 years; Type 1 diabetes mellitus (DM) since age 15

Past Surgical History

Unremarkable

Family/Social History

Family History: Noncontributory

Social History: Smoked 1½ PPD × 30 years; no alcohol or recreational drug use

Medication History

Hydrochlorothiazide, 25 mg PO q AM

ASA, 325 mg PO q AM

Isosorbide dinitrate, 30 mg PO TID

Verapamil, 120 mg PO TID

Nitroglycerin, 0.4 mg SL PRN chest pain

Insulin NPH (human), 26 units SC q AM/12 units SC q PM plus 5 units regular insulin 30 minutes before meals

Cimetidine, 300 mg PO q8h

Allergies

NKDA

Physical Examination

GEN: Well-developed, well-nourished male, intubated and appearing drowsy post-CABG

VS: BP 90/50/63, HR 110, RR 18 (controlled ventilation), T 37.0°C (rectal), Wt 85 kg, Ht 183 cm

HEENT: WNL

COR: Tachycardic with normal S1, S2; grade III/VI SEM at LLSB

CHEST: Bibasilar rales

ABD: Soft, no masses or rigidity

GU: WNL

RECT: Deferred

EXT: Slightly cool

NEURO: Responsive to verbal stimuli, reflexes normal

Results of Pertinent Laboratory Tests, Serum Drug Concentrations, and Diagnostic Tests

Na 136 (136)	PO_4 1.29 (4.0)	Uric Acid WNL
K 4.0 (3.5)	Mg 1.0 (2.0)	HbA_{1C} 9.0%
Cl 105 (105)	AST WNL	Hct 0.38 (38%)
CO_2 24 (24)	ALT WNL	Hgb 140 (14.0)
BUN 7.14 (20)	LDH WNL	Lkcs 8.2×10^9 (8.2×10^3)
Cr 150 (1.7)	Alk Phos WNL	Plts 220×10^9 (220×10^3)
Glu 6.7 (120)	Alb WNL	MCV 82 (82)
Ca 2.6 (10.0)	T Bili WNL	

Lkc differential: Normal

Urinalysis: Normal

Chest x-ray: Cardiomegaly; mild pulmonary edema

ECG: NSR, rate 110–120, evidence of LVH

Urine output of 20 mL/hr

BP 90/50/63 mm Hg (S/D/M)

HR 110 beats/min

Right atrial pressure (RAP) 10 mm Hg (mean)

Pulmonary artery pressure (PAP) 38/24/29 mm Hg (S/D/M)

Pulmonary capillary wedge pressure (PCWP) 21 mm Hg

Cardiac index (CI) 1.2 L/min/m^2

Systemic vascular resistance (SVR) 2080 dynes-sec-cm^5

SaO_2 0.95

PROBLEM LIST

Identify principal problems from the scenario in priority order [completed Problem List and SOAP Note at end of casebook]

SOAP NOTE

To be completed by student

QUESTIONS

[Answers at end of casebook]

1. The administration of dopamine (current rate 10 µg/kg/min) resulted in the following hemodynamic parameters:
   CI 2.0 L/min/m^2
   SVR 1900 dynes-sec-cm^5
   PCWP 19 mm Hg
   Mild pulmonary edema persists and urine output remains at 20 mL/hr

   What drug therapy should be initiated next in the treatment of cardiogenic shock? (EO-12)
   a. Furosemide 60 mg IV push
   b. Increase dopamine to 20 µg/kg/min
   c. Start dobutamine at 5 µg/kg/min
   d. Give 500 mL of 0.9% NaCl

2. What signs of hypoperfusion are present in this patient? (EO-2)

3. Dobutamine's mechanism of action is primarily as a: (EO-7)
   a. β_1-Agonist
   b. β_2-Antagonist
   c. α_1-Agonist
   d. α_1-Antagonist

4. What intervention will produce the greatest oxygen delivery increase? (EO-12)
   a. Fraction of inspired oxygen
   b. Mean arterial pressure
   c. Hemoglobin
   d. Cardiac output

5. The patient develops sustained ventricular tachycardia. A lidocaine infusion is started at 4 mg/min. The serum concentration obtained at steady state is 8.1 mg/L. What is the most likely explanation for this abnormal lidocaine level? (EO-9)
   a. Concomitant cimetidine administration
   b. History of heavy tobacco use
   c. Decreased cardiac output
   d. Decreased renal function

6. Why is the determination of creatinine clearance using the Cockroft and Gault method inaccurate in DK's clinical scenario? (EO-5)

7. What is the etiology of this patient's acute renal failure? (EO-1)

8. What is the most life-threatening electrolyte abnormality that may occur in patients with acute renal failure? (EO-1)
   a. Hypokalemia
   b. Hyperkalemia

c. Hyponatremia

d. Hypernatremia

9. Aggressive insulin dosing should be implemented to prevent what acute diabetic complication? (EO-1)

a. Peripheral neuropathy

b. Osmotic diuresis

c. Hyperlipidemia

d. Diabetic ketoacidosis

10. Cardiogenic shock is most frequently a complication of: (EO-1)

a. Nonsustained ventricular tachycardia

b. Acute myocardial infarction

c. Verapamil therapy

d. Compensated heart failure

11. Describe the impact of diuretic therapy on mortality in patients with acute renal failure. (EO-17)

12. Calculate the clearance of lidocaine using information provided in question 5. It would be: (EO-6)

a. 500 mL/min

b. 30 mL/hr

c. 500 mL/hr

d. 2 L/min

13. Prior to discharge from the hospital, what other test should be performed in DK? (EO-5)

a. Electrocardiogram

b. Echocardiogram

c. Serum troponin, creatine kinase

d. Serum lipids

14. What are the pharmacoeconomic benefits of using intensive insulin therapy for Type 1 diabetics? (EO-17)

15. Describe the psychosocial issues that must be addressed during a period of life-threatening illness. (EO-15)

16. Summarize therapeutic, pathophysiologic, and disease management concepts for treating critically ill patients with heart failure and diabetes mellitus utilizing a key points format. (EO-18)

CASE 155
Scott D. Hanes
Topic: Solid Organ Transplantation
Level 2
EDUCATIONAL MATERIALS
Chapter 104: Transplantation (clinical presentation and diagnosis, therapeutic strategies to prevent rejection, infection, cardiovascular complications, alternative medicine, pharmacoeconomic considerations, patient education)

SCENARIO

Patient and Setting
CL, a 49-year-old male; hospital

Chief Complaint
Inability to sleep at night due to having to urinate, extreme thirst for several weeks; painful rash

History of Present Illness
Blood sugar has been progressively increasing over several months; fasting blood sugar (FBS) level from this morning was 23.3 mmol/L (420 mg/dL), and 26.4 mmol/L (475 mg/dL) 2 hours after breakfast; urine has been negative for ketones; hospitalized for hyperglycemia and glucose management

Past Medical History
Orthotopic heart transplantation (OHT) 7 months ago secondary to severe dilated cardiomyopathy; over the past 3 months, CL has developed hypertension; treatment with diltiazem initiated 1 month ago

Past Surgical History
OHT 7 months ago

Family/Social History
Family History: Father AMI

Social History: Noncontributory

Medication History
Cyclosporine liquid, 200 mg PO BID

Prednisone, 5 mg PO BID

Azathioprine, 200 mg PO QD

Trimethoprim 80 mg/sulfamethoxazole 400 mg PO QOD

Digoxin, 0.25 mg PO QD

Ethacrynic acid, 25 mg PO QOD

Diltiazem, sustained-release, 90 mg PO QD

Magnesium complex, 600 mg PO BID

Multivitamins, 1 PO q AM

Aspirin, enteric-coated, 80 mg PO QD

Allergies
Penicillin—rash

Physical Examination
GEN: Thin-appearing male with painful, macular, weeping rash that follows the 10th thoracic dermatome

S: BP 130/100, HR 80 reg, RR 22, T 37.4°C, Wt 77 kg (68 kg 7 months ago, IBW 81 kg)

HEENT: PERRLA

COR: (−) JVP, (+) S4
CHEST: Lungs clear
ABD: Soft, nondistended, nontender
GU: WNL
RECT: Deferred
EXT: No edema
NEURO: A and O × 3

Results of Pertinent Laboratory Tests, Serum Drug Concentrations, and Diagnostic Tests

Na 132 (132)   Mg 0.75 (1.5)   TG 1.9 (168)
K 4.9 (4.9)   AST 0.55 (33)   Hct 0.43 (43.2)
Cl 104 (104)   ALT 0.3 (18)   Hgb 131 (13.1)
HCO₃ 22 (22)   Alk Phos 1.1 (68)   Lkcs 4.8 × 10⁹
BUN 9.6 (27)   Alb 32 (3.2)   (4.8 × 10³)
Cr 115 (1.3)   T Bili 17 (1.0)   Plts 251 × 10⁹
Glu 23.3 (420)   Chol 7.3 (275)   (251 × 10³)
Ca 2.3 (9.3)   LDL 5.8 (225)   MCV 98 (98)

Cyclosporine (CSA): 375 ng/mL
Digoxin: 1.2 nmol/L (0.9 μg/L)

PROBLEM LIST

Identify principal problems from the scenario in priority order

SOAP NOTE

To be completed by student

QUESTIONS

1. What common opportunistic infection is this patient at risk of developing secondary to immunosuppression? (EO-10)
   a. Legionella
   b. Cytomegalovirus
   c. Tuberculosis
   d. HIV

2. In the clinic 2 weeks after discharge from the hospital, the patient says that his serum glucose levels have been fine except that his bedtime level is always high, usually around 18.2 mmol/L (325 mg/dL). What change should be made to his insulin therapy? (EO-11)
   a. Increase AM (before breakfast) NPH insulin dose
   b. Increase PM (before dinner) NPH insulin dose
   c. Add regular insulin to PM (before dinner) dose
   d. Change PM (before dinner) NPH dose to "at bedtime"

3. Which of the following combinations of drugs results in a significant medication cost savings to the patient as a result of a pharmacokinetic interaction? (EO-17)
   a. Diltiazem and digoxin
   b. TMP-SMZ and digoxin
   c. Diltiazem and azathioprine
   d. Diltiazem and cyclosporine

4. Following an increase in diltiazem dose, what is the expected effect on the steady-state digoxin concentration and why? (EO-9)

5. Calculate the estimated steady-state digoxin concentration given the following information: (EO-6)

   Bioavailability/salt factor = 0.7

   Volume of distribution = 250 L

   Half-life = 46.2 hr

   Dose = 0.25 mg QD

6. Describe the pharmacist's role in counseling CL about his therapy. (EO-14)

7. What is the mechanism of cyclosporine's immunosuppressive effects? (EO-7)
   a. Inhibition of calcineurin
   b. IL-2 receptor antagonism
   c. Suppressor T-cell activation
   d. Inactivation of mature cytotoxic T cells

8. CL has been stabilized on cyclosporine USP (non-microemulsion formula) 350 mg PO q12h. He is now hospitalized and unable to take oral medications. What is the recommended IV dose for this patient? (EO-8)
   a. 230 mg q12h
   b. 175 mg q12h
   c. 350 mg q12h
   d. 115 mg q12h

9. Which of the following symptoms would be consistent with the development of rhabdomyolysis in this patient? Skeletal muscle: (EO-10)
   a. Atrophy
   b. Pain
   c. Weakness
   d. Paralysis

10. Describe why atropine does not have pharmacologic activity in a heart transplant patient. (EO-1)

11. Which of the following drugs would have the most dramatic effects on the pharmacokinetics of azathioprine if taken concomitantly? (EO-9)
    a. Erythromycin
    b. Cimetidine
    c. Allopurinol
    d. Rifampin

12. Given that cyclosporine microemulsion (CSA-micro) generally has a higher Cmax and AUC compared with the nonmicroemulsion formulation (CSA), a rational pharmacokinetic explanation is that CSA-micro has a _____ compared to CSA. (EO-6)
    a. Decreased V
    b. Increased K_a
    c. Decreased $t_{1/2}$
    d. Increased F

13. What psychosocial issues should be addressed with this patient regarding his newly diagnosed hyperglycemia? (EO-15)

14. Summarize the therapeutic, pathophysiologic, and disease management concepts for solid organ transplantation utilizing a key points format. (EO-18)

CASE 156
Scott D. Hanes
Topics: Critical Care, Gastrointestinal Bleed,
Liver Failure
Level 3
EDUCATIONAL MATERIALS
Chapter103: Critical Care Therapy (pharmacokinetic
and pharmacodynamic considerations, drug
administration in the ICU, liver dysfunction,
hematologic system); Chapter 29: Cirrhosis (clinical
presentation and diagnosis, pharmacotherapy)

SCENARIO

Patient and Setting

DD, a 45-year-old male; intensive care unit

Chief Complaint

Vomiting bright red blood; abdominal pain; productive
cough

History of Present Illness

Nasogastric (NG) lavage performed, active bleeding noted;
esophageal gastroduodenoscopy (EGD) revealed actively
bleeding large esophageal varices; transfused 8 units of
packed red blood cells; varices sclerosed and bleeding controlled with vasopressin 0.8 units/min infusion

Past Medical History

Alcoholic cirrhosis and hepatitis; chronic obstructive pulmonary disease; gastrointestinal bleed secondary to esophageal varices (4 episodes in past year); alcohol withdrawal;
last drink 4 days ago

Past Surgical History

None

Family/Social History

Family History: Noncontributory

Social History: Alcohol abuse for 20 years–6 pack
beer/day; smokes 2 PPD × 22 years; no recreational
drug use

Medication History

Sucralfate, 1 g PO q6h since admission

Cefotaxime, 2 g IV q8h since admission

Lactulose, 30 mL PO q6h since admission

Diazepam, 5 mg PO q6h begun day 2 of admission

Multivitamin, 1 PO QD begun day 3 of admission

Folic acid, 1 mg PO QD begun day 3 of admission

Thiamine, 100 mg PO QD since admission

Aspirin, 325 mg PO q6h PRN headache

Allergies

Penicillin (hives)

Physical Examination

GEN: Thin male, arousable to voice, oriented to
person only

VS: BP 120/85, HR 110, RR 20-unlabored, T
39.4°C (rectal), Wt 64 kg, Ht 170 cm

HEENT: Icteric sclera, EOM intact, PERRLA, throat
clear, poor dentition, no nuchal rigidity

COR: S_1 and S_2 normal; no murmurs or gallops

CHEST: Clear to auscultation and percussion, spider
angiomas seen on chest

ABD: Protuberant abdomen, diffuse tenderness, no
rebound, could not palpate liver or spleen,
hypoactive bowel sounds, fluid wave present,
shifting dullness present

GU: Bilateral testicular atrophy, no penile or scrotal
lesions

RECT: No stool in rectal vault, no masses, normal
prostate

EXT: No clubbing, cyanosis, or edema; palmar
erythema, no asterixis, IV catheter insertion
sites are clean

NEURO: Drowsy but answers to name, no focal
neurologic signs, all reflexes present and equal,
cranial nerves II–XII intact

Results of Pertinent Laboratory Tests, Serum Drug Concentrations, and Diagnostic Tests

Na 136 (136)	Mg 1.0 (2.0)	Uric Acid 387 (6.5)
K 3.5 (3.5)	GGT 60 (60)	Hct 0.30 (30%)
Cl 98 (98)	AST 4.5 (270)	Hgb 102 (10.2)
CO_2 22 (22)	ALT 3.7 (220)	Lkcs 17 × 10⁹
BUN 4.3 (12)	LDH 3.33 (200)	(17 × 10³)
Cr 70.7 (0.8)	Alk Phos 2.0 (118)	Plts 220 × 10⁹
Glu 4.4 (80)	Alb 20 (2.0)	(220 × 10³)
Ca 2.00 (8.0)	T Bili 94 (5.5)	MCV 82 (82)
PO_4 1.29 (4.0)		

Lkcs differential: 0.79 (79%) polys, 0.14 (14%) bands, 0.04
(4%) lymphs, 0.02 (2%) monos

Urinalysis: Bilirubin positive

INR 2.1

Arterial blood gas: pH 7.41, pCO_2 42 mm Hg, pO_2 92
mm Hg, room air

Chest x-ray: Clear

Pulmonary function tests: FEV_1 65% predicted, FVC 72% predicted

ECG: Normal

Paracentesis: Cloudy fluid; lkcs 500/mm^3 with 96% polys; Gram stain reveals many lkcs and gram-negative rods; culture pending

PROBLEM LIST

Identify principal problems from the scenario in priority order [completed Problem List and SOAP Note at end of casebook]

SOAP NOTE

To be completed by student

QUESTIONS

[Answers at end of casebook]

1. Defend the decision to change the antibiotic regimen from cefoxitin to gentamicin plus metronidazole. (EO-8)

2. Decreased cytochrome P450 activity associated with liver failure would be expected to: (EO-6)
   a. Increase bioavailability for low extraction drugs
   b. Increase bioavailability for high extraction drugs
   c. Decrease bioavailability for low extraction drugs
   d. Decrease bioavailability for high extraction drugs

3. Which of the following should be started for long-term treatment of portal hypertension? (EO-12)
   a. Octreotide
   b. Vasopressin
   c. Spironolactone
   d. Propranolol

4. On day 8, the patient is recovering well and in good spirits when he develops severe nausea and vomiting. Upon questioning the patient's brother, he admitted to bringing in a bottle of whiskey for his brother that morning. What is most likely the cause of the patient's nausea and vomiting? (EO-9)

5. Provide recommendations for the treatment of this patient's ascites. (EO-7, 12)

6. The gentamicin levels obtained at the third dose are 6.5 mg/L (drawn at 13:00) and 2.1 mg/L (drawn at 10:30). The dose was given at 12:00 over 30 minutes. The patient's WBC count remains elevated, and he is febrile. Please provide recommendations to achieve peak level of 9 mg/L and a trough level of 1.0 mg/L. (EO-5, 6)

7. In the event of a major gastrointestinal bleed in this patient, what therapy would correct the coagulopathy in the shortest period of time? (EO-8)
   a. Vitamin K 20 mg SC
   b. Packed red blood cell infusion

   c. Fresh frozen plasma infusion
   d. Platelets infusion

8. Based on DD's paracentesis Gram-stain results, which of the following organisms is most likely to grow in the culture? (EO-5)
   a. *Escherichia coli*
   b. *Staphylococcus aureus*
   c. *Bacteroides fragilis*
   d. *Candida albicans*

9. What pharmacokinetic alteration would be expected in DD with regards to gentamicin therapy? (EO-4)
   a. Increased k_{el}
   b. Decreased k_{el}
   c. Increased V
   d. Decreased V

10. Identify the signs and symptoms of peritonitis in DD. (EO-2)

11. Which cephalosporins should be avoided in this patient and why? (EO-10)

12. Identify the psychosocial factors that are important to this patient's treatment plan. (EO-15)

13. Which of the following is the correct order of chronological events, from earliest to latest, for this patient? (EO-1)
    a. Portal hypertension, ascites, cirrhosis
    b. Cirrhosis, portal hypertension, ascites
    c. Ascites, portal hypertension, cirrhosis
    d. Portal hypertension, cirrhosis, ascites

14. Summarize the nonpharmacologic therapies that should be instituted in this patient. (EO-12)

15. What route of drug administration should be avoided in this patient at this time? (EO-15)
    a. IV
    b. SC
    c. PO
    d. IM

16. What changes could be made to this patient's antibiotic regimen to decrease the overall cost of therapy? (EO-17)

17. Summarize therapeutic, pathophysiologic, and disease management concepts for the critically ill patient with liver failure utilizing a key points format. (EO-18)

CASE 157
Scott D. Hanes
Topics: Solid Organ Transplantation, Critical Care, Infectious Disease

 Level 3

EDUCATIONAL MATERIALS

Chapter 104: Transplantation (therapeutic strategies to prevent rejection, cytomegalovirus, *Pneumocystis carinii* pneumonia); Chapter 103; Critical Care Therapy (pain and anxiety)

SCENARIO

Patient and Setting

DM, a 40-year-old male; hospital

Chief Complaint

Two-day history of fever, chills, malaise, decreased appetite, abdominal pain, loose stools, and purulent discharge from abdominal wound site

History of Present Illness

As above

Past Medical History

Orthotopic liver transplant (OLT) 2 months ago for chronic active hepatitis secondary to IV drug abuse and alcoholic cirrhosis; postoperative course complicated by ascites leak, *Staphylococcus aureus* wound infection and bacteremia; treated for acute rejection 1 week ago; peptic ulcer disease and upper GI bleeding with encephalopathy

Past Surgical History

OLT 2 months ago

Family/Social History

Family History: Noncontributory

Social History: Quit alcohol and cigarettes 1 year ago; occasionally smokes cigars; no recreational drug abuse

Medication History

Cyclosporine (CSA) capsules, 400 mg PO BID

Prednisone, 7.5 mg PO QD

Azathioprine (AZA), 50 mg PO QHS

Trimethoprim 80 mg/sulfamethoxazole (TMP-SMX) 400 mg PO QOD

Magnesium complex, 300 mg PO QD

Acyclovir, 800 mg PO QD

Multivitamins, 1 PO q AM

Allergies

NKDA

Physical Examination

GEN: Thin, ill-appearing male in no apparent distress

VS: BP 130/70, HR 100 regular, RR 16, T 37.7°C, Wt 54.3 kg

HEENT: Normocephalic; no JVD, thyromegaly, or nodules noted

COR: NL S1 and S2; soft I/IV systolic murmur

CHEST: Lungs clear to auscultation

ABD: Soft, thin, positive bowel sounds; liver and spleen not appreciated, abdominal scar with multiple areas of pinkish material and raised areas of skin

GU: WNL

RECT: Guaiac negative

EXT: WNL

NEURO: A and O × 3

Results of Pertinent Laboratory Tests, Serum Drug Concentrations, and Diagnostic Tests

Na 134 (134)	Mg 0.6 (1.2)	Hgb 73 (7.3)
K 4.5 (4.5)	AST 0.95 (57)	Lkcs 2.7 × 10^9
Cl 109 (109)	ALT 1.15 (69)	(2.7 × 10^3)
HCO$_3$ 26 (26)	Alk Phos 1.18 (71)	Plts 164 × 10^9
BUN 11.1 (31)	Alb 18 (1.8)	(164 × 10^3)
Cr 150 (1.7)	T Bili 39.3 (2.3)	MCV 102 (102)
Glu 5.3 (96)	Hct 0.24 (24.4)	

Lkcs differential: 0.62 (62%) N, 0.3 (30%) L, 0.05 (5%) M, 0.02 (2%) E, 0.01 (1%) B

Urinalysis: WNL

Blood culture: CMV positive

Liver biopsy: Areas of focal cellular necrosis consistent with CMV hepatitis with viral inclusions

Cyclosporine: 295 ng/mL, whole blood HPLC

PROBLEM LIST

Identify principal problems from the scenario in priority order

SOAP NOTE

To be completed by student

QUESTIONS

1. The blood cultures return with methicillin-resistant *Staphylococcus aureus* (MRSA) and *Pseudomonas aeruginosa.* How should the patient's antibiotic regimen be modified? (EO-5, 8)

2. The *Clostridium difficile* stool culture is positive. The physician orders vancomycin 250 mg PO q6h. Please provide recommendations for alternative therapy. (EO-8, 12)

3. Which of the following stress ulcer prophylactic regimens would be most appropriate for this patient as an alternative to sucralfate? (EO-8, 12)
   a. Cimetidine 300 mg IV q8h
   b. Milk of magnesia 30 mL PO q2h

   c. Ranitidine 150 mg IV q2h

   d. Omeprazole 30 mg PO q12h

4. Which of the following is a common adverse effect of ganciclovir? (EO-10)

   a. Neutropenia

   b. Pulmonary fibrosis

   c. Seizures

   d. Bradycardia

5. What type of acid-base disorder would be expected as a result of persistent diarrhea? (EO-1)

   a. Anion-gap metabolic acidosis

   b. Non-anion-gap metabolic acidosis

   c. Metabolic alkalosis

   d. Respiratory acidosis

6. After 5 days of antibiotic therapy, *Pseudomonas aeruginosa* is again cultured from the blood. Based on the following sensitivities, which aminoglycoside would be the best pharmacologic choice for therapy? (EO-5, 12)

   a. Gentamicin MIC 4

   b. Tobramycin MIC 0.5

   c. Amikacin MIC 16

   d. Neomycin MIC 4

7. Which of the following is a therapeutic alternative for PCP prophylaxis in patients who are intolerant to TMP-SMX therapy? (EO-8, 12)

   a. Chloroquine

   b. Mebendazole

   c. Ciprofloxacin

   d. Dapsone

8. Describe how diarrhea may alter the pharmacokinetics of orally administered medications. (EO-4)

9. Which of the following is a common side effect from oral iron supplementation therapy? (EO-10)

   a. Skin rash

   b. Headache

   c. GI upset

   d. Dizziness

10. Given DM's past social and medical history, comment on the likelihood of this patient being HIV positive. (EO-1, 5)

11. Vancomycin trough serum level is obtained on the third day of therapy. The patient's vancomycin dose is normally given at 12:00; however, at the time of the levels being drawn, the dose was given at 14:00 because the patient was in x-ray. The trough was 4 mg/L (drawn at 13:59). Recommend any changes, if needed, to this patient's vancomycin therapy. (EO-6)

12. DM complains of persistent abdominal pain that is moderate in intensity. Which of the following medications would be the best choice for analgesia in this patient? (EO-11, 12)

   a. Ketorolac

   b. Meperidine

   c. Acetaminophen

   d. Lorazepam

13. Comment on how the pharmacist can assist in preventing hospital-induced sleep deprivation in this patient. (EO-16)

14. Describe the indirect and direct nonmedical costs for this patient and his family. (EO-17)

15. Summarize therapeutic, pathophysiologic, and disease management concepts for the critically ill patient following OLT utilizing a key points format. (EO-18)

CASE 158
Scott D. Hanes
Topic: Solid Organ Transplantation

EDUCATIONAL MATERIALS
Chapter 104: Transplantation (rejection, pancreas, therapeutic strategies to prevent rejection, monoclonal antibodies, infection, cardiovascular complications, osteoporosis, malignancy, pharmacoeconomic considerations, patient education)

SCENARIO

Patient and Setting

30-year-old male; transplant unit

Chief Complaint

Urinating less than normal, confusion, hands shaking more during last few days

History of Present Illness

Cadaveric pancreas-renal transplantation 14 days ago; currently managed with cyclosporine, azathioprine, and prednisone; uneventful postoperative course with Cr decreasing to 97.2 μmol/L (1.1) by post-op day 6 and serum and urine amylase levels stabilizing at 0.90 μkat/L (54) and 2.2 μkat/L (134.8), and fasting blood sugars averaging 5.6 mmol/L (102); since surgery, has not required insulin; now experiencing sudden change in renal and pancreatic function with increasing serum Cr and amylase; renal biopsy reveals 1+ vasculitis and 1+ interstitial rejection

Past Medical History

Type 1 diabetes mellitus since age 2, diabetic nephropathy, peripheral neuropathy, hypertension, and anemia; hemodialysis prior to transplant

Past Surgical History

S/P renal-pancreas transplant 14 days ago

Family/Social History

Family History: Father has hypertension

Social History: Drinks 1–2 beers or glasses of wine per week), no cigarette or illicit drug use

Medication History

Cyclosporine, 300 mg PO BID

Prednisone, 40 mg PO QD

Azathioprine, 50 mg PO QD

Nifedipine XL, 30 mg PO q AM

Clonidine patch #2 per week

Ranitidine, 150 mg PO BID

Acyclovir, 800 mg PO QID

Clotrimazole troches, 10 mg dissolved in mouth QID

Allergies

NKDA

Physical Examination

GEN: Well-developed male in no acute distress

VS: BP 142/96, HR 82, RR 18, T 37.8°C, Wt 75 kg, Ht 162 cm

HEENT: Normocephalic, fundal examination shows laser scarring; no evidence of oral thrush

COR: WNL

CHEST: Lungs clear

ABD: WNL except for allograft incision scar

GU: WNL

RECT: Guaiac negative

EXT: No clubbing, cyanosis, or edema

NEURO: Slightly confused, not oriented to time; fine hand tremor present

Results of Pertinent Laboratory Tests, Serum Drug Concentrations, and Diagnostic Tests

Na 131 (131)	PO_4 1.1 (3.4)	T Bili 34.2 (2)
K 5.0 (5.0)	Mg 1.05 (2.1)	Hct 0.3 (30)
Cl 100 (100)	Uric Acid 188 (3.1)	Hgb 94 (9.4)
HCO_3 25 (25)	AST 0.17 (10)	Reticulocyte count 2%
BUN 12.5 (35)	ALT 0.25 (15)	Lkcs 18×10^9 (18×10^3)
Cr 239 (2.7)	LDH 1.7 (100)	Plts 431×10^9 (431×10^3)
Glu 6.1 (111)	Alk Phos 0.9 (53)	MCV 88 (88)
Ca 2.5 (10.1)	Alb 33 (3.3)	

Serum amylase: 2.7 μkat/L (162)

Urine amylase: 1095 μkat/L (65,700)

CSA level: 398 (whole blood HPLC)

Anti-OKT3 antibodies: Negative

Urinalysis: pH 6.2, specific gravity 1.0, color yellow, appearance cloudy

Lkcs: Esterase positive, protein negative, glucose negative, ketones negative, occult blood negative

CMV blood culture: Negative

Renal biopsy: 1+ vasculitis, 1+ interstitial changes

PROBLEM LIST

Identify principal problems from the scenario in priority order [completed Problem List and SOAP Note at end of casebook]

SOAP NOTE

To be completed by student

QUESTIONS

[Answers at end of casebook]

1. Provide dosing recommendations for acyclovir and ranitidine in this patient. (EO-5, 6)

2. What counseling information should be provided for the treatment of this patient's hypertension? (EO-14)

3. Which of the following is a common adverse effect of nifedipine? (EO-10)
   a. Rash
   b. Nausea
   c. Headache
   d. Bradycardia

4. Which laboratory parameter shows that this patient's anemia is neither macrocytic nor microcytic? (EO-5)
   a. MCV
   b. HCT
   c. Reticulocyte count
   d. Ferritin

5. Assuming a cyclosporine serum half-life of 18 hours, how long will it take for the level to decrease from 398 ng/mL to 150 ng/mL with no further cyclosporine doses? (EO-6)
   a. 12 hours
   b. 57 hours
   c. 48 hours
   d. 25 hours

6. Comment on the influence of erythromycin and rifampin therapy on the metabolism of cyclosporine and potential consequences of such therapy. (EO-6, 9)

7. Discuss the role of beta-blocker therapy for the treatment of this patient's hypertension. (EO-8)

8. What is the therapeutic indication for acyclovir therapy in this patient? (EO-11)
   a. Varicella virus prophylaxis
   b. Cytomegalovirus prophylaxis
   c. PCP treatment
   d. No appropriate indication exists

9. During the health care provider's discussions with the patient, he states that he is worried he won't be able to afford the medications prescribed. What interventions could result in a pharmacoeconomic benefit for this patient? (EO-16, 17)

10. Which of the following cancers is most likely to occur in this patient? (EO-10)
    a. Lung cancer
    b. Prostate cancer
    c. Brain cancer
    d. Skin cancer

11. Osteoporosis associated with immunosuppression therapy is mostly due to which of the following drugs: (EO-10)
    a. Prednisone
    b. Cyclosporine
    c. Azathioprine
    d. OKT3

12. Identify additional pharmacologic therapy that should be considered in this patient. (EO-12)

13. Summarize therapeutic, pathophysiologic, and disease management concepts for immunosuppression following solid organ transplantation utilizing a key points format. (EO-18)

CASE 159
Scott D. Hanes
Topics: Critical Care, Septic Shock, Acute Respiratory Distress Syndrome, Renal Failure, Hematology

Level 2

EDUCATIONAL MATERIALS
Chapter 103; Critical Care Therapy (pharmacokinetic and pharmacodynamic considerations, pain and anxiety, mechanical ventilation, acute respiratory distress syndrome, principles of oxygen delivery and consumption, renal system, colonization of the GI tract and nosocomial infections, platelet disorders, deep venous thrombosis, systemic inflammatory response syndrome [SIRS], compensatory anti-inflammatory response syndrome [CARS], and multiorgan dysfunction syndrome [MODS])

SCENARIO

Patient and Setting
CE, a 45-year-old male; ICU

Chief Complaint
Tired; sore throat for 1 week

History of Present Illness
WBC revealed 43×10^9/L (43×10^3/mL) with 0.4 (40%) blasts; bone marrow biopsy–acute myelocytic leukemia (AML); received induction regimen of daunorubicin 45 mg/m^2 on days 1–3 and cytarabine 100 mg/m^2 on days 1–7, completed 8 days ago; Lkc count has fallen since chemotherapy; now has temperature of 39.4°C, a change in mental status, blood pressure of 80/50 mm Hg, and a urine output of 100 mL over the past 8 hr

Past Medical History
None

Past Surgical History
None

Family/Social History
Noncontributory

Medication History
No medications prior to admission

Allergies
NKDA

Physical Examination
GEN: Well-developed, well-nourished male, obtunded but arousable
VS: BP 80/50, HR 136, RR 40, T 39.4°C (rectal), Wt 80 kg, Ht 183 cm
HEENT: Mouth ulcerations, no evidence of oral thrush, EOM intact, PERRLA, funduscopic examination is normal
COR: S_1 and S_2 normal; no murmurs or gallops heard
CHEST: Diffuse rales throughout both lung fields
ABD: Soft. Liver and spleen enlarged and palpable, no tenderness to palpation, active bowel sounds, no rebound tenderness
GU: Normal male genitalia
RECT: Guaiac negative
EXT: Extremities warm bilaterally, no petechiae, IV sites clean and without tenderness
NEURO: Reflexes normal and symmetrical, no nuchal rigidity, CN II–XII intact

Results of Pertinent Laboratory Tests, Serum Drug Concentrations, and Diagnostic Tests

Na 136 (136)	Ca 2.27 (9.1)	Hct 0.31 (31%)
K 4.7 (4.7)	PO$_4$ 1.58 (4.9)	Hgb 100 (10.0)
Cl 101 (101)	Mg 1.05 (2.1)	Lkcs 0.2×10^9
CO$_2$ 12 (12)	Uric Acid: WNL	(0.2×10^3)
BUN 21 (60)	AST 0.58 (35)	Plts 20×10^9 (20×10^3)
Cr 185 (2.1)	ALT 0.50 (30)	MCV 82 (82)
Glu 6.1 (120)	Alk Phos 1.8 (110)	

Lkcs differential: Cannot be done due to low Lkcs count

INR 1.6

Fibrinogen: 3.3 (330)

Fibrinogen split products: negative

Urinalysis: Specific gravity 1.033; (+) granular casts; 0 RBC; 0 Lkcs; Gram stain: no organisms seen

Chest x-ray: Diffuse infiltrates throughout both lung fields

Arterial blood gases: pH 7.24, pCO$_2$ 25 mm Hg, pO$_2$ 55 mm Hg; 82% hemoglobin saturation on 50% oxygen via face mask

Sputum Gram stain: Few Lkcs, many gram-negative rods; culture pending

Blood cultures: Pending

PROBLEM LIST

Identify principal problems from the scenario in priority order [*completed Problem List and SOAP Note at end of casebook*]

SOAP NOTE

To be completed by student

QUESTIONS

[*Answers at end of casebook*]

1. Which of the following cytokines is responsible for inducing the inflammatory response seen in sepsis and septic shock? (EO-1)
   a. IL-10
   b. IL-1
   c. IL-4
   d. IL-13

2. Which of the following measurements from the pulmonary artery catheter confirms the diagnosis of ARDS? (EO-5)
   a. Cardiac output: 8.1 L/min
   b. Systemic vascular resistance: 541
   c. Pulmonary capillary wedge pressure: 16 mm Hg
   d. Pulmonary artery pressure: 43/21 mm Hg

3. Describe the complications associated with mechanical ventilation. (EO-8)

4. The patient requires a high amount of positive end-expiratory pressure (PEEP) for adequate oxygenation. How can this affect the pharmacokinetics of drugs requiring either hepatic metabolism or renal elimination? (EO-6)

5. Comment on the accuracy of the Cockcroft and Gault formula for estimated creatinine clearance in this patient. (EO-5, 6)

6. Which of the following are the risk factors for stress ulcer formation in this patient? (EO-8)
   a. Mechanical ventilation and coagulopathy
   b. Mechanical ventilation and neutropenia
   c. Acute renal insufficiency and neutropenia
   d. Coagulopathy and pneumonia

7. Despite thrombocytopenia, a decision has been made to place the patient on deep venous thrombosis prevention. What potentially fatal event is being prevented with this therapy? (EO-1)
   a. Cerebral infarction
   b. Acute myocardial infarction
   c. Lower limb ischemia
   d. Pulmonary embolism

8. Which of the following economic consequences would most greatly offset advantages of giving stress ulcer prophylaxis? (EO-17)
   a. Cost of IV preparation
   b. Cost of treating pneumonia
   c. Cost of treating thrombocytopenia
   d. Cost of doses prepared but not given

9. The decision is made to start G-CSF therapy to treat this patient's neutropenia. What is a common side effect with this therapy? (EO-10)
   a. Emesis
   b. Skin necrosis
   c. Anaphylaxis
   d. Bone pain

10. Which of the following best describes the bactericidal effects of ceftazidime? (EO-7)
    a. Bacterial cell wall synthesis inhibitor; concentration-independent bacterial killing
    b. Protein synthesis inhibitor; concentration-independent bacterial killing
    c. Bacterial cell wall synthesis inhibitor; concentration-dependent bacterial killing
    d. Protein synthesis inhibitor; concentration-dependent bacterial killing

11. A decision is made to start sucralfate for stress ulcer prophylaxis. Describe how sucralfate could potentially decrease respiratory muscle function. (EO-1, 9, 10)

12. What therapeutic intervention would result in the greatest increase in oxygen delivery to the tissues? (EO-8)
    a. Increase oxygen consumption
    b. Increase arterial pH
    c. Increase cardiac output
    d. Increase arterial oxygen content

13. Identify signs of renal insufficiency in this patient. (EO-2)

14. Describe the pharmacist's psychosocial role in this patient's care. (EO-15)

15. Summarize therapeutic, pathophysiologic, and disease management concepts for the critically ill patient with septic shock utilizing a key points format. (EO-18)

CASE 160
Scott D. Hanes
Topics: Solid Organ Transplantation, Hypertension, Urinary Tract Infection

Level 2

EDUCATIONAL MATERIALS
Chapter 104: Transplantation
(therapeutic strategies to prevent rejection, monoclonal antibodies, cytomegalovirus)

SCENARIO

Patient and Setting

RH, a 36-year-old male; admitted to kidney transplant floor

Chief Complaint

Pain at transplant site, low-grade fever, pain on urination

History of Present Illness

Admitted to the hospital to rule out allograft rejection. Differential diagnosis—rejection, CMV infection, cyclosporine toxicity, and drug-induced increase in Cr; CMV cultures negative; cyclosporine trough level is 78 ng/mL; biopsy results include 2+ vascular and 2+ interstitial changes consistent with acute rejection; methylprednisolone 500 mg IV × 3 days with no response; also complains of pain on urination

Past Medical History

End-stage renal disease (ESRD) secondary to glomerulonephritis; cadaveric renal transplant 3 months ago, managed postoperatively with sequential immunosuppression including prednisone, azathioprine, and antilymphocyte globulin (ALG) followed by cyclosporine (CSA). HLA tissue typing for donor and recipient revealed 4/6 HLA antigen match. RH experienced one episode of mild allograft rejection, which responded to high-dose methylprednisolone (500 mg IV QD × 3 days); baseline Cr level since this episode has been 123.8 mmol/L (1.4). Other medical problems include hypertension, currently controlled with nifedipine and a clonidine patch.

Past Surgical History

Cadaveric renal transplant 3 months ago

Family/Social History

Noncontributory

Medication History

Cyclosporine, 200 mg PO BID

Prednisone, 200 mg PO QD

Azathioprine, 50 mg PO QD

Nifedipine, 10 mg PO q6h

Clonidine patch #1 per week

Trimethoprim/sulfamethoxazole DS, 1 tab PO 3 times weekly

Allergies

NKDA

Physical Examination

GEN: Well-developed male in mild distress; cushingoid appearance

VS: BP 126/86, HR 92, RR 16, T 38.5°C, Wt 71 kg, Ht 176 cm

HEENT: Normocephalic, cushingoid facial features

COR: WNL

CHEST: Lungs clear

ABD: Pain at allograft site upon palpation

GU: WNL

RECT: Guaiac negative

EXT: Some muscle wasting; no clubbing, cyanosis, or edema; defined area of skin irritation on shoulder

Results of Pertinent Laboratory Tests, Serum Drug Concentrations, and Diagnostic Tests

Na 136 (136)	PO$_4$ 0.84 (2.6)	T Bili 10.3 (0.6)
K 4.2 (4.2)	Mg 1.0 (2.0)	Hct 0.36 (36)
Cl 101 (101)	Uric Acid 184 (3.1)	Hgb 132 (13.2)
HCO$_3$ 26 (26)	AST 0.3 (18)	Lkcs 1.5 × 10^9
BUN 12.5 (35)	ALT 0.27 (16)	(1.5 × 10^3)
Cr 221 (2.5)	LDH 1.3 (78)	Plts 155 × 10^9
Glu 6.1 (110)	Alk Phos 1.0 (62)	(155 × 10^3)
Ca 2.5 (10.1)	Alb 35 (3.5)	MCV 88 (88)

Urinalysis: pH 6.2, specific gravity 1.0, color yellow, appearance cloudy

Leukocyte esterase positive, protein negative, glucose negative, ketones negative, occult blood negative, bacterial smear positive, many WBC seen, nitrate positive

Culture: 100,000 colonies *Escherichia coli;* sensitivity: resistance to ampicillin but sensitive to cefazolin, gentamicin, tobramycin, ceftizoxime, and ciprofloxacin

CMV culture: Negative

Renal biopsy: 2+ vasculitis, 2+ interstitial rejection

CSA 78 ng/mL

PROBLEM LIST

Identify principal problems from the scenario in priority order [completed Problem List and SOAP Note at end of casebook]

SOAP NOTE

To be completed by student

QUESTIONS

[Answers at end of casebook]

1. What are the expected side effects of OKT3 therapy? (EO-10)

2. Four days after starting OKT3 therapy, RH's CD3 counts are still elevated. What action should be taken? (EO-11)

3. Assuming the patient responds to OKT3 therapy for this rejection episode, how should a future rejection episode be managed? (EO-8)

4. What components of this patient's urinalysis are consistent with a urinary tract infection? (EO-2)

5. Which of the following is a common complication of poly- and monoclonal antibody therapy? (EO-10)
   a. Cytomegalovirus infection
   b. Liver dysfunction
   c. Neurotoxicity
   d. Parasitic infection

6. Which of the following options should be considered if RH does not respond to OKT3 therapy? (EO-12)
   a. Increase methylprednisolone dose
   b. Repeat biopsy
   c. Change from cyclosporine to tacrolimus
   d. Extend OKT3 dosing to 30 days

7. What is the therapeutic indication for sulfamethoxazole/trimethoprim in this patient? (EO-11)
   a. Urinary tract infection prophylaxis
   b. Cytomegalovirus infection prophylaxis
   c. Urinary tract infection treatment
   d. *Pneumocystis carinii* pneumonia prophylaxis

8. What factors may be contributing to RH's hypertension? (EO-9, 10)

9. What is the mechanism of OKT3 immunosuppressive effects? (EO-7)

10. What is the equivalent oral prednisone dose of 80 mg methylprednisolone? (EO-8)
    a. 100 mg
    b. 64 mg
    c. 320 mg
    d. 32 mg

11. Due to the high immunosuppressive effects of OKT3, prophylaxis against cytomegalovirus infection is started. What is the preferred agent and route of administration for this indication? (EO-12)
    a. Acyclovir PO
    b. Acyclovir IV
    c. Ganciclovir PO
    d. Ganciclovir IV

12. What is a probable mechanism for this patient's allograft rejection? (EO-1)
    a. Preformed donor cytotoxic antibodies
    b. Anti-class I antibodies
    c. T-helper and cytotoxic T-cell hypersensitivity
    d. T-lymphocyte antibodies to allograft vasculature

13. Detail the factors that affect the pharmacoeconomic impact of acute rejection therapies. (EO-17)

14. Which of the following is a common psychosocial consequence of chronic and severe illness such as in this patient's case? (EO-15)
    a. Paranoia
    b. Depression
    c. Delirium
    d. Obsessive-compulsive disorder

15. Summarize therapeutic, pathophysiologic, and disease management concepts for patients receiving renal transplantation utilizing a key points format. (EO-18)

SECTION 2 / FLUID AND ELECTROLYTES AND NUTRITION

CASE 1

PROBLEM LIST

1. Impending Malnutrition
2. High Gastric Residuals
3. Hyperglycemia
4. Hypophosphatemia
5. Severe TBI
6. Post-traumatic Seizures
7. Suspected Nosocomial Pneumonia
8. Sedation While Mechanically Ventilated

SOAP NOTE

S: Currently comatose (Glasgow coma score 7) and mechanically ventilated S/P TBI from MVA; complications include post-traumatic seizure, enteral feeding intolerance, hyperglycemia, hypophosphatemia, and suspected nosocomial pneumonia

O: Severe TBI (GCS 7, eye 1, verbal 1, motor 5); febrile; enteral intake = 125 mL/day for 4 days; gastric residuals >150 mL; no seizures reported since admission; intubated; Wt 90 kg (IBW 87 kg) Serum glucose 13.3 (240); urine dipstick shows 2+ glucose; serum phosphorus 0.9; phenytoin level 8.0; albumin 26 (2.6) Bronchoalveolar lavage culture results pending

A: **Problem 1:** Impending malnutrition due to enteral feeding intolerance and hypermetabolic state

Problem 2: Intolerance of gastric feedings due to severe head injury and underlying mild diabetic gastroparesis

Problem 3: Hyperglycemia due to type 1 DM, trauma, and possibly pneumonia

Problem 4: Hypophosphatemia due to low nutritional intake and trauma

Problem 5: Severe TBI; currently the ICP monitor has been removed

Problem 6: Post-traumatic seizures

Problem 7: Suspected nosocomial pneumonia; currently receiving empiric therapy for late, severe nosocomial pneumonia

Problem 8: Sedation while mechanically ventilated

P: **Problem 1: Impending Malnutrition**
- AW's nonprotein calorie and protein goals while in a critically ill, hypermetabolic state are as follows:
  - Total calorie goal: 30 kcal/kg/day × 90 kg = 2700 kcal/day
  - Protein goal: 1.8 g/kg/day × 90 kg = 162 g protein/day
- Begin feeding with a high-fat "diabetic" formula (e.g., Glucerna), since AW has had high accuchecks on a standard formula which provide approximately 1 kcal/mL and 44 g protein/L
- Starting rate should be 25 mL/hr; history of feeding intolerance
- Add 20 g/L of a powdered protein supplement to the formula in order to provide adequate protein
- Goal feeding rate: 115 mL/hr, which will provide 31 kcal/kg/day and 2.0 g/kg/day of protein
- Increase rate by 25 mL/hr/day as tolerated until goal rate achieved
- Decrease IVF rate (mL per mL) as enteral feeding rate increased
- Routine monitoring:
  - Raise head of bed 30° at all times
  - Check gastric residuals q6h. If >150 mL, replace residual and hold feedings for 4 hours and recheck. If <150 mL restart feedings, if still >150 mL, hold feedings
  - Perform physical exam of abdomen daily
  - Monitor for diarrhea/constipation
  - q6h accuchecks with sliding scale insulin
  - Draw metabolic labs as indicated by severity of illness
  - Draw weekly prealbumin or transferrin and perform weekly nitrogen balance

Problem 2: High Gastric Residuals
- Begin metoclopramide 10 mg IV q6h
- Clamp nasogastric tube and monitor gastric residuals q6h
- When residuals are <150 mL, replace NG tube with a small bore feeding tube
- Increase metoclopramide to 20 mg IV q6h if necessary
- Monitor for possible side effects of metoclopramide which include extrapyramidal symptoms

Problem 3: Hyperglycemia

- Administer IV piggybacks in NS instead of D5W
- Change to q4h accuchecks
- "Tighten" the sliding scale; current insulin doses are inadequate (example: if 150–175 give 4 units, 176–200 give 6 units, 201–225 give 8 units, etc.)
- Titrate sliding scale daily based on recent accuchecks to ensure blood glucose <200 and no glucosuria

Problem 4: Hypophosphatemia

- Give 30 mmol of sodium phosphate over 4–6 hours IV
- Recheck phosphorus 4–6 hours after the end of the phosphorus infusion
- Do not start feedings until phosphorus replaced

Problem 5: Severe TBI

- Pharmacologic therapy limited now that ICP monitoring ended
- Eliminate dextrose from IV fluids when possible

Problem 6: Post-traumatic Seizures

- Hold enteral feedings for at least 1 hour before and after phenytoin doses
- Adjust enteral feeding rate to account for phenytoin administration (2760 mL/day over 18 total hours of feeding = 150 mL/hr)
- Phenytoin is currently therapeutic after correcting for hypoalbuminemia, but not at steady state
- Monitor level again in 4–5 days; AW on the low end of dosing range (5 mg/kg/day) and may require increased dosing

Problem 7: Suspected Nosocomial Pneumonia

- Continue broad-spectrum therapy until BAL culture and sensitivity results are known
- Once results obtained, narrow antibiotic therapy accordingly or discontinue antibiotics if culture results negative and clinical symptoms resolve

Problem 8: Sedation

- Monitor amount and effectiveness of morphine use daily
- Titrate to light sedation and keep from being a danger by pulling out lines/tubes
- May use an infusion or combine with short-acting benzodiazepine (midazolam) if higher doses required
- Morphine is a good choice because inexpensive, short acting to allow neurologic examination, and provides analgesia for rib fractures

ANSWERS

1. b. Enteral feedings may decrease serum phenytoin concentrations if administered to AW concurrently

2. d. Change to IV phenytoin
3. a. Dextrose from feedings may induce intracellular shift of phosphorus and result in dangerously low serum level
4. c. Diabetic retinopathy and microvascular disease
5. b. + 1
6. d. No change, nitrogen balance is acceptable for now
7. a. Decreased risk of aspiration pneumonia
8. c. Diarrhea
9. Fluid restrict by changing to a concentrated formula (2 kcal/mL)
   Will need to add protein 20 g/L
   Adding 40 g/L would be needed to equal current EN regimen but >20 g/L of protein increases viscosity too much
   New goal rate will be 60 mL/hr and will provide 32 kcal/kg/day and 1.7 g/kg/day protein
10. Clinical data for this indication are very sparse; no large comparative trials exist
    Metoclopramide—first line since available IV push and inexpensive
    Cisapride—only available orally; may not be absorbed due to gastroparesis; drug interaction potential (torsade de pointes) exists, especially with fluconazole and erythromycin; more expensive than metoclopramide
    Erythromycin—available IV; limit use to 48–72 hours in order to avoid selection/development of resistant bacteria; oral erythromycin may not be absorbed due to gastroparesis; IV piggyback administration more expensive than other options
11. No; the long duration of action of NPH insulin may cause hypoglycemia if feedings are stopped (high residuals, surgery/procedure, pulls out feeding tube); also, home regimen may be inadequate due to many factors affecting glucose (hypermetabolic state, sepsis, continuous feedings rather than separate meals)
    Scheduled NPH insulin—only consider after feedings have been tolerated at goal for several days and patient more metabolically stable
12. a. Devise administration schedule compatible with patient lifestyle (e.g., one that allows employment; usually requires cycled feedings overnight or bolus feedings)
    b. Coordinate schedule with home health care to ensure proper therapy
    c. Train patient/family to recognize metabolic adverse effects of enteral nutrition (e.g., hyperglycemia, dehydration)
    d. Train patient/family to store and administer nutrition support properly
    e. Follow-up clinic visits as needed
13. Key points are:
    a. Enteral nutrition can be delivered safely and effectively in the majority of patients by nasogastric tube, nasoenteric tube, gastrostomy, or jejunostomy. Numerous enteral products are marketed in the U.S. and may be administered as a continuous infusion, intermittent infusion, or as a bolus.
    b. Factors involved in selection of an EN regimen include body weight, level of metabolic stress, presence of normal

kidney and liver dysfunction, previous intolerance, hyperglycemia, and hypophosphatemia.

c. Patients receiving EN require frequent monitoring to ensure safety and efficacy and prevent potential complications. Complications of EN may be broadly categorized as pulmonary, gastrointestinal, mechanical, and metabolic.

CASE 2

PROBLEM LIST

1. Dehydration
2. Electrolyte Abnormalities
3. Fever and GI Disturbances
4. Chronic Renal Insufficiency
5. Malnutrition

SOAP NOTE

S: "I've been so tired and weak feeling for the past few days and I haven't been able to keep anything down in my stomach. I'm thirsty but I don't think I can drink anything because I'm so nauseated."

O: Decreased food/fluid intake (only orange juice, ice cream, antacid), cool extremities, dry lips and skin, sunken eyes, history of chronic renal insufficiency, has not taken meds in 3 days, few rales, no rhonchi on chest exam, moderate lethargy, mild tachycardia, some peripheral muscle wasting, 2 kg weight loss
Na 128, K 5.2, Cl 90, PO_4 1.8 (5.6), Mg 2 (4), Cr 280 (3.1), BUN 20 (57), T 38.2°C, Alb 34 (3.4)
Urine output 20 mL/hr (normal per history), urinalysis WNL, no bacteria, urine and sputum cultures negative to date

A: **Problem 1:** Dehydration secondary to poor oral intake, nausea and vomiting

Problem 2: Electrolyte abnormalities secondary to dehydration/poor oral intake and discontinuation of medications:
Hypermagnesemia–from antacids, contributes to lethargy
Hyperkalemia–from fruit juices
Hypercalcemia–from ice cream and fruit juices
Hyponatremia–from vomiting/poor oral intake, contributes to lethargy
Hypochloremia–from vomiting/poor oral intake

Problem 3: Fever and GI disturbances of unknown origin; most likely etiology is a viral infection, which was contracted from co-workers; no evidence of profound hypovolemia since (urine output similar to baseline); tachycardia, skin turgor, and temperature suggest systemic sequelae

Problem 4: Chronic renal insufficiency secondary to polycystic kidney disease; renal function stable (Cr and urine output are similar to baseline)

Problem 5: Malnutrition possibly secondary to hypermetabolism caused by chronic disease (polycystic kidney disease) coupled with a restricted protein "renal" diet; body weight approximately 10 kg under ideal body weight; serum albumin of 34 (3.4) suggests moderate malnutrition

P: **Problem 1: Dehydration**

- Sodium deficit (mmol) = [140–128] × 53 × 0.6 = 380 mmol
- Administer 2–3 L of NS IV over the next 24 hours (85–125 mL/hr; provides approximately 300–450 mmol of Na) if admitted to hospital or held for observation in ED
- Fluid/sodium replacement relatively quickly (over 24 hours) as mildly/moderately symptomatic
- Monitor for correction of signs and symptoms of dehydration
- Counsel to drink Gatorade or water rather than fruit juices in order to avoid excess potassium
- Recommend return to ED if unable to keep down 1500–2000 mL of fluid over the next 24 hours

Problem 2: Electrolyte Abnormalities

- Check serum electrolytes 12 and 24 hours after NS infusion starts
- Do not allow sodium to increase by more than 12 mmol/L during a 24-hour period to avoid possible neurologic sequelae (central pontine myelinolysis or osmotic demyelination syndrome)
- Ca × Phos product of >5 increases risk of calcium phosphate precipitation in organs and soft tissue
- Ca (mmol) × Phos (mmol) product = 1.8 × 2.6 = 4.7 (no immediate risk of precipitation)
- Discontinue aluminum hydroxide/magnesium hydroxide and aluminum hydroxide antacids
- Once fluid and electrolytes are stabilized, resume calcium carbonate and calcitriol
- If Ca/Phos product <5, then bind PO_4 with calcium carbonate only (discontinue aluminum antacids); if Ca/Phos product >5, then add aluminum hydroxide for additional phosphate binding
- Electrolyte abnormalities indicate the impact that minor changes in intake and output of fluids and electrolytes can have on CB due to kidney disease

Problem 3: Fever and GI Disturbances of Unknown Origin

- Antibiotic therapy not indicated at this time
- Discontinue antacids, as not providing relief of GI symptoms and contributing to electrolyte abnormalities

- Recommend acetaminophen 650 mg q4–6h PRN fever
- Recommend obtain an influenza vaccine before the next flu season

Problem 4: Chronic Renal Insufficiency

- Emphasize importance of keeping well-hydrated to prevent acute renal failure
- Monitor BUN following fluid therapy

Problem 5: Malnutrition

- Renal failure diets that restrict to 1 g/kg/day of protein may not be adequate to avoid protein malnutrition
- Protein intake should be increased to 1.2–1.5 g/kg/day as tolerated in addition to increasing caloric intake to at least 30 kcal/kg/day
- Weight gain goal: 0.5–1 kg/week as close to IBW as possible
- Provide appropriate counseling for diet with follow-up

ANSWERS

1. b. Sodium polystyrene sulfonate 30 g PO
2. d. Vitamin D is not hydroxylated to its most active form in patients with renal dysfunction
3. a. Calcium phosphate precipitation in soft tissue
4. c. Dehydration
5. c. NS at 65 mL/hr
6. c. Central nervous system dysfunction from aluminum toxicity
7. b. Causes intracellular shift of potassium
8. a. Contraction metabolic alkalosis
9. Fluid choice: NS was chosen over D5W or hypotonic saline in order to correct hyponatremia; also, a greater proportion of NS stays in the vasculature compared to D5W or hypotonic saline

   Amount of fluid: need to determine sodium and water deficits

   Water deficit (L) = [1 − 140/serum Na (mmol/L)] × body wt. (kg) × 0.6 (only useful when patients have dehydration with hypernatremia; will show a water "excess" in patients with hyponatremia)

   Sodium deficit (mmol) = [140 − serum Na (mmol/L)] × body wt. (kg) × 0.6

   Sodium deficit = 380 mmol (3 L of NS provides 462 mmol Na)

10. Increasing protein intake will not automatically increase serum BUN

    CB has evidence of protein malnutrition; therefore, a moderate increase in protein intake should be utilized for repletion of lean body mass

    Patients with chronic renal dysfunction have difficulty with urea excretion when protein intake is too high or in the setting of hypovolemia (decreased kidney perfusion)

    Cautious elevation of dietary protein should not compromise CB's renal function

11. Must use actual body weight and not ideal body weight in underweight patients to avoid overfeeding

    This is especially true in CB to avoid excessive protein intake

    As CB gains weight, protein and calorie goals can be adjusted accordingly

    Protein goal (1.25 g/kg/day) = 66 g/day

    Calorie goal (30 kcal/kg/day) = 1600 kcal/day

12. Standard crystalloid solutions (NS, Lactated Ringer's) are very inexpensive

    Hetastarch is moderately expensive

    Albumin and plasma protein fraction are very expensive

13. Key points are:
    a. Advocate the principles of a healthful diet rich in fruits and vegetables and low in saturated fat.
    b. Encourage achievement and maintenance of an appropriate body weight through dietary modification and exercise.
    c. Encourage optimal calcium intake to reduce the risk of osteoporosis.
    d. Be aware of the often unsubstantiated claim for nutritional supplements, especially in the areas of sports medicine and immune enhancement.

CASE 3

PROBLEM LIST

1. Acute Flank Pain
2. Dermatitis
3. Diarrhea

SOAP NOTE

S: "My right side has been hurting pretty bad for the past couple of days. Also I've got dry, scaly spots on both of my arms that have been getting worse over the past month or so; I've had some diarrhea lately too."

O: Dry, scaly skin; right side pain, ascorbic acid >3 g/day; multivitamin providing 20,000 IU/day vitamin A; afebrile; VS stable
Urinalysis normal

A: **Problem 1:** Acute flank pain caused by kidney stone formation from hypervitaminosis C

Problem 2: Dermatitis due to hypervitaminosis A

Problem 3: Diarrhea due to hypervitaminosis C

P: **Problem 1: Kidney Stones**

- Discontinue ascorbic acid and multivitamin supplements; after symptoms resolve, counsel to take only one multivitamin/day
- Keep well hydrated, avoid alcohol until kidney stones pass

- Provide analgesia as necessary for pain

Problem 2: Dermatitis

- Discontinue multivitamin supplements
- After symptoms resolve, counsel to take only one multivitamin/day
- Treat topically with lotion of choice

Problem 3: Diarrhea

- Discontinue ascorbic acid supplements

ANSWERS

1. a. Bleeding gums
2. Adequate dietary intake should provide essential vitamins. Use caution with vitamin supplements because of potential for toxicity.
3. b. Zinc lozenges
4. c. Natural vitamins are more expensive
5. c. 10,000 IU
6. a. Increased oxalic acid concentrations as a result of ascorbic acid metabolism
7. d. Iron
8. b. Vitamin C
9. c. Daily value
10. No, a likely explanation (ascorbic acid toxicity) already exists.
    GM has no other signs/symptoms of systemic infection such as fever, leukocytosis, dysuria, and has stable vital signs; also, no bacteria were seen on the UA.
11. Medical evidence is inconclusive at this time regarding the use of ascorbic acid for the prevention or treatment of common colds. Some studies have shown a benefit, while others have not; well designed, conclusive studies have not been conducted. Ascorbic acid is inexpensive, may benefit some patients, and ingestion of up to 1 g/day is safe in most patients. GM should be educated regarding recommended dosages and toxic doses of vitamins and minerals.
12. No, a likely explanation (ascorbic acid toxicity) already exists; GM doesn't have a recent history of taking antibiotics—the most important risk factor for *Clostridium difficile* colitis; diarrhea is mild; GM is not dehydrated and does not have electrolyte abnormalities; GM has no other signs/symptoms of systemic infection such as fever, leukocytosis, dysuria, and has stable vital signs.
13. Key points are:
    a. Consumers should be encouraged to maintain an adequate dietary intake in order to obtain vitamins that are essential for the body's biochemical processes. Caution should be exercised with use of vitamin supplements since vitamin toxicity may occur with intake of moderately high dose or megadose vitamin supplements.
    b. Food product labels contain daily values, which are nutrient references that have replaced the Recommended Dietary Allowances (RDA).
    c. The pharmacist is vital in dissemination of accurate information to consumers and other health care professionals regarding safe and efficacious administration of vitamins and minerals.

CASE 5

PROBLEM LIST

1. Malnutrition
2. Esophagitis
3. Osteoporosis Prevention

SOAP NOTE

S: "It really hurts when I swallow anything and it's been getting worse. I've lost a lot of weight. I usually take my 'fosphomax' with my oral supplement before bedtime."

O: 10 kg wt. loss in 6 months (approx. 20% below IBW)
Alb 28 (2.8)
Esophagitis on endoscopy, mild osteopenia on bone density scan

A: **Problem 1:** Moderate to severe malnutrition; inadequate protein and caloric intake secondary to esophagitis

Problem 2: New onset esophagitis secondary to alendronate, which was not taken properly

Problem 3: Osteoporosis prevention; receiving alendronate and calcium carbonate therapy

P: **Problem 1: Malnutrition**

- Enteral access may be required if esophagitis not quickly controlled and oral intake not improved
- Sleep with head of bed elevated to avoid aspiration
- Suggest follow-up in clinic to ensure weight gain

Problem 2: Esophagitis

- Discontinue alendronate and initiate proton-pump inhibitor therapy
- Follow-up to ensure that symptoms improve with therapy

Problem 3: Osteoporosis Prevention

- Discontinue alendronate
- Discontinue calcium carbonate until esophagitis healed
- Long-term therapy should include calcium and vitamin D supplementation with possible addition of estrogen replacement therapy or calcitonin

ANSWERS

1. d. 60 mL/hr
2. a. Switch to a fiber-containing enteral feeding

3. b. 100 mL/hr from 8 PM to 10 AM

4. c. 2 cans TID

5. b. 3750 mg

6. d. Take with a full glass of plain water and remain in an upright position for 30 min.

7. b. Administration with breakfast

8. a. Lower calcium and magnesium intake seems to be associated with a higher prevalence of hypertension

9. a. Gastrointestinal–vomiting, diarrhea, abdominal distention

   b. Pulmonary–aspiration

   c. Mechanical–feeding tube occlusion

   d. Metabolic–hyperglycemia, electrolyte abnormalities

10. CM has no clinical manifestations of hypoalbuminemia (i.e., third-spacing fluid from decreased oncotic pressure).

    At this time albumin will probably be metabolized by CM's body as a protein source.

    Albumin has not consistently demonstrated improvement in outcomes in malnourished patients.

    Albumin is very expensive.

11. Refeeding syndrome: Providing glucose causes insulin production, which will shift potassium intracellularly; magnesium and phosphorus will also shift into cells to participate in metabolism of nutrients; hypokalemia, hypophosphatemia, and hypomagnesemia may occur.

    Management: Advance feedings slowly, monitor electrolytes, supplement as needed.

12. Low income; illiteracy; unwillingness to read nutrition information; perception that preparing meals high in fruits and vegetables is more costly and time consuming than high-fat meals; dietary patterns instilled in childhood.

13. Key points are:

    a. Clinicians play an important role in optimizing the nutritional intake of patients. In this case, the clinician should work closely with the patient to develop an acceptable enteral regimen, educate the patient on monitoring therapy, and transition the patient back to oral nutrition when possible.

    b. Some medications have the potential to adversely affect the nutritional status of patients because of gastrointestinal side effects. Appropriate medication counseling and monitoring of drug therapy is key to avoiding such outcomes.

    c. Clinicians should be aware of the special nutritional needs of high risk groups including patients with diabetes, hypertension, and the elderly.

    d. Optimal calcium and vitamin D intake are important in the prevention of osteoporosis.

CASE 6

PROBLEM LIST

1. Loss of Taste and Smell

2. Urinary Tract Infection

3. Poorly Controlled DM

4. Inappropriate Chromium Use

5. Moderate/Heavy Alcohol Use

SOAP NOTE

S: 2–3 month history of increasing loss of taste and smell, 2 day history of dysuria

O: Dysuria; loss of taste and smell, Hx of type 1 DM, chromium picolinate 1 mg/day, moderate to heavy alcohol use, recent use of oral contraceptives

Accucheck 11.3 (203), HbA$_{1C}$ 8.4

UA: glucosuria, 10 leukocytes, 3+ bacteria

A: **Problem 1:** Loss of taste and smell most likely due to zinc deficiency; recent initiation of estrogen therapy, alcohol use, and DM are factors which may have contributed to increased zinc excretion

Problem 2: UTI; no previous history of UTI; uncomplicated; *E. coli* most likely pathogen; probably due to poorly controlled DM

Problem 3: Hyperglycemia–inadequate management of DM; increasing HbA$_{1C}$ indicates worsening of DM, UTI may contribute to acute hyperglycemia

Problem 4: Inappropriate chromium use–high dose taken unsupervised by health care provider

Problem 5: Moderate/heavy alcohol use

P: **Problem 1: Loss of Taste and Smell**

- Begin oral zinc sulfate 220 mg TID and monitor for symptomatic improvement

- Educate regarding likely causes of zinc deficiency including ethanol use

Problem 2: Urinary Tract Infection

- Start ciprofloxacin 200 mg PO q12h × 3 days

- Monitor for improvement in symptoms

- Improve diabetic control

Problem 3: Hyperglycemia

- Instruct to perform 4–6 Accuchecks daily and keep a record of them (per standards from DCCT trial)

- Adjust insulin appropriately based during this admission; once UTI resolves, assess the amount of insulin required to manage DM adequately and adjust accordingly

- Assess current diet since loss of taste and smell may cause to eat more flavored foods high in sugar

Problem 4: Inappropriate Chromium Use

- Counsel on current state of medical knowledge regarding chromium use in DM

- Discontinue chromium since it has not been studied adequately in type 1 DM

- Explain that DM can be controlled with conventional therapy

Problem 5: Moderate/Heavy Alcohol Use

- Counsel regarding the importance of reducing alcohol intake; only consume alcohol with meals to reduce risk of hypoglycemia
- Address psychosocial issues and refer to a specialist if necessary
- Refer to specialist to assist in treatment of alcohol abuse and suggest support system that is most suitable for RB

ANSWERS

1. b. Dermatitis
2. d. 90%
3. Chromium increases insulin receptor sensitivity and lowers blood glucose

    Clinical trials have shown 2-hour postprandial glucose, fasting glucose, and HbA$_{1C}$ to be lowered by chromium supplements in type 2 diabetics.

    Large trials confirming efficacy and long-term effects need to be performed before its use can be widely accepted.

    Mechanism of action may help type 2 patients more than type 1 due to high rate of impaired insulin receptor sensitivity in type 2 DM.

    Reports of serious side effects (e.g., renal dysfunction) make unsupervised use dangerous.
4. a. Gastrointestinal irritation
5. b. 3500 mg
6. b. Calcium citrate
7. d. 100 mmol (1.8 g)
8. d. Vegetarians
9. a. Magnesium
10. Take ciprofloxacin as far away in time from zinc as possible (at least 30 min before or 2 hours after zinc dose)

    Another option is to wait until ciprofloxacin course is over in 3 days to start zinc

    Divalent cations (i.e., zinc, magnesium, calcium) bind quinolones in the GI tract and impair absorption

    The same advice should be given for calcium carbonate
11. Advise against taking calcium supplements made from bone meal or dolomite due to possibility of lead contamination

    Help RB choose a calcium carbonate or acetate supplement that does not contain artificial colors or preservatives

    Generic supplements will likely be less expensive than brand name products
12. Signs/symptoms include sweating, tachycardia, tremor, syncope, confusion, visual disturbances, headache

    Immediately give oral sugar (e.g., candy, soft drink, fruit)

    Call for help if unconscious

    May train to inject SC glucagon
13. Key points are:

    a. Minerals are important to good health, but the consumer must be cautioned that with all minerals, a narrow therapeutic index exists between general requirements and toxic levels. RB became zinc deficient due to a combination of lifestyle, disease, and drug therapy factors.

    b. Consumers should rely on adequate dietary intake of minerals rather than supplements to support good health. Due to the popularity of dietary supplements, health care providers must be knowledgeable regarding the safe and appropriate use of these agents.

SECTION 3 / DISEASES OF THE BLOOD

CASE 8

PROBLEM LIST

1. Ulcerative Colitis (UC) Exacerbation
2. Iron Deficiency Anemia
3. Anorexia
4. Depression

SOAP NOTE

S: Complains of bloody diarrhea with severe abdominal pain, arthritic pain in both knees (tender and warm), increased fatigue, and decreased appetite; also complains of increased headaches, intermittent nausea and vomiting, malaise, and anorexia since sulfasalazine dose increased; patient also reports heavy menses for 4 days

O: PE: HR 104; T 99.8°F; lower abdomen tender to palpation; bloody diarrhea per rectum; tenderness and warmth in both knees

Laboratory: ESR 60 (60), AST 0.75 (45), ALT 0.58 (35), Alk Phos 3.0 (180), WBC 16×10^9 (16×10^3) K 3.3 (3.3), Hct 0.28 (28), Hgb 87 (8.7), MCV 60 (60), transferrin saturation 14 (14), ferritin 11 (11)

Diagnostic: Stool examination: numerous RBCs and WBCs, culture negative

Sigmoidoscopy: edematous and friable mucosa, with extent of disease to 23 cm

A: Problem 1: Ulcerative colitis (UC) exacerbation

Problem 2: Iron deficiency anemia secondary to rectal and menstrual blood loss

Problem 3: Anorexia secondary to increased dose of sulfasalazine

Problem 4: Depression currently managed by fluoxetine

P: Problem 1: Ulcerative Colitis (UC) Exacerbation

- GI consult to rule out Crohn's disease and misdiagnosis of UC
- Discontinue sulfasalazine
- Admit for high-dose parenteral corticosteroid; methylprednisolone 40 mg IV QD for 7–10 days
- Monitor number of stools q24h
- Monitor electrolytes (potassium)
- Switch to oral prednisone 40 mg QD once a satisfactory initial response to IV corticosteroids. Taper steroids slowly over 6–8 weeks
- Restart sulfasalazine at lower dose (500 mg PO QID) or olsalazine 500 mg PO BID
- Avoid excessive use of antimotility agents (diphenoxylate/atropine) due to increased risk of toxic megacolon
- Consider surgery consult if no improvement with IV corticosteroids

Problem 2: Iron Deficiency Anemia

- Initiate ferrous sulfate 300 mg PO TID
- Monitor reticulocyte count, Hct, Hgb, MCV, ferritin, iron saturation
- Discuss use of oral contraceptives long term to minimize menstrual blood loss
- If deficiency does not correct with oral iron replacement, consider parenteral replacement with iron dextran

Problem 3: Anorexia

- Consider lower dose of sulfasalazine or switch to olsalazine when oral therapy restarted
- Consider discontinuing fluoxetine, or switching to agent without anorexic side effects

Problem 4: Depression

- Consider discontinuing fluoxetine and/or switching to tricyclic antidepressant less likely to cause anorexia or diarrhea
- Recommend involvement with UC support group
- Consider referring to biofeedback or stress management as indicated

ANSWERS

1. c. Increased fatigue
2. b. T 99.8°F
3. b. Sulfasalazine
4. a. Heavy menstruation
5. The mechanism of action of pharmacologic and nonpharmacologic interventions are:
   1. Pharmacologic interventions
      a. Corticosteroids—anti-inflammatory agent; used to treat active UC and induce remission
      b. Ferrous sulfate—an iron salt used for prevention and treatment of iron deficiency anemia
      c. Iron dextran—a complex of ferric hydroxide and dextran used for parenteral iron replacement
      d. Olsalazine—converted to 5-ASA (mesalamine) in the colon; anti-inflammatory agent activity appears to be due to blocking of cyclooxygenase and inhibition of colon prostaglandin production in bowel mucosa.
      e. Fluoxetine—selective serotonin reuptake inhibitor; inhibits CNS neuronal uptake of serotonin
      f. Oral contraceptives—inhibit ovulation by inhibiting gonadotropins, FSH, and LH; use results in decreased menstrual blood loss
   2. Nonpharmacologic interventions
      a. UC support group—allows patient to speak with others with the disease state; may improve patient's ability to cope with her symptoms/disease
      b. Biofeedback/stress management—decreases depression, stress, and tension; increases coping mechanisms
6. Pharmacologic treatment problems present in AM's case:
   a. Decreased appetite, anorexia, and weight loss due to elevated sulfasalazine dose
   b. Increased fatigue due to elevated sulfasalazine dose
   c. Potential anorexia effect from chronic fluoxetine therapy
7. The equation used to calculate the amount of iron needed to replenish stores and correct hemoglobin levels is:

$$\text{Dose (mg)} = 0.66 \times \text{wt (kg)} \times \left[100 - \frac{\text{Hgb(g/dL)} \times 100}{14.8} \right]$$

$$\text{Dose (mg)} = 0.66 \times 43 \times \left[100 - \frac{8.7 \times 100}{14.8} \right]$$

Dose = 1170 mg iron dextran

8. c. Anaphylaxis
9. a. Lower total dose required, so less expensive
10. d. Anorexia
11. Discuss lifestyle changes and medication counseling for ferrous sulfate therapy in AM:
    a. For maximal absorption, best to take before meals or between meals
    b. GI side effects common—stomach upset, abdominal cramping, nausea, constipation
    c. Iron therapy can also cause black stools; need to educate on difference between iron stools and changes seen with GI bleeding

d. If GI side effects intolerable, can minimize by taking iron with food

e. Avoid use of enteric coated iron products, as the coating does not allow for good dissolution and thus minimizes absorption

f. Make aware that other medicines can bind the iron and reduce absorption; dosing of these medicines should be separated from iron: antacids, tetracycline, fluoroquinolones

g. Make aware that certain food items may form complexes with iron and reduce absorption: coffee, tea, milk, eggs, whole grain breads, cereals

h. Counsel on medication adherence strategies

12. Psychosocial factors that may affect AM's adherence to therapy:
    1. Issues patient must address:
       a. QOL affected, some restrictions of activities due to symptoms of a chronic illness
       b. Chronic medications with multiple daily dosing and sometimes intolerable side effects
    2. Common emotional disorders associated with chronic diseases:
       a. Depression
    3. Other:
       a. Presence/absence of family and social support
       b. Financial hardship associated with management of chronic illness

13. Key points are:
    a. Nutritional anemias may be prevented by early identification of "at risk" patients, monitoring for vitamin deficiency and providing supplementation.
    b. Iron deficiency is common during pregnancy and early childhood, and the CDC now recommends supplementation in both populations.
    c. Based on elemental iron content and absorption, the usual dose of ferrous sulfate to treat iron deficiency is 300 mg taken three times daily.
    d. If parenteral iron therapy is required, the total dose infusion method offers the advantage of fewer office visits, less needle sticks, and less local side effects than IM or bolus IV dosing.
    e. Response to therapy generally occurs with the first week, although correction of the anemia may not be seen for 2–3 months.

CASE 9

PROBLEM LIST

1. Peptic Ulcer Disease
2. Folate Deficiency (Megaloblastic) Anemia
3. Alcohol Abuse

SOAP NOTE

S: Complains of stomach pain, and loose, tarry stool; also reports dizziness, weakness, and a "painful tongue"; admits to drinking alcohol on a daily basis and two DUIs

O: PE: BP 120/75, HR 80, RR 12, T 37.5°C, Wt 55 kg; abdomen tender to palpation; pale nail beds; bruising; guaiac-positive stool
Laboratory: Hct 25; Hgb 10; MCV 104; serum folate 2 (1.2)
Diagnostic: Endoscopy: 0.5 cm ulcer in the duodenum, no active bleeding

A: **Problem 1:** Duodenal ulcer secondary to alcohol abuse, smoking, or ulcerogenic medication; *Helicobacter pylori* status unknown

Problem 2: Folate deficiency anemia due to malnutrition and chronic alcohol use

Problem 3: Alcohol abuse

P: **Problem 1: Peptic Ulcer Disease**
- Start H2 antagonist therapy–ranitidine 150 mg BID for 8 weeks, then re-evaluate
- Discontinue ibuprofen
- Encourage patient to discontinue alcohol use
- Encourage smoking cessation, discuss trial of bupropion or nicotine replacement patches
- Consider evaluation of *Helicobacter pylori* status

Problem 2: Megaloblastic Anemia
- Start folic acid 1-mg tablet PO daily
- Increase amount of folate-rich foods in diet (suggest: legumes, green leafy vegetables, citrus fruits, lentils, black-eyed peas, soy nuts, pinto beans, chickpeas, kidney beans, green soybeans, pinto beans, spinach, asparagus, split peas, avocado, orange juice from concentrate, soybeans, collards, peanuts, wheat germ)
- Recheck Hct, Hgb, and MCV in 2 months
- If hematologic parameters WNL and abstaining from alcohol, consider discontinuing folate therapy

Problem 3: Alcohol Abuse
- Encourage discontinuation of alcohol
- Refer to support and counseling program, Alcoholics Anonymous
- Discuss option of disulfiram therapy (500 mg daily for 2 weeks, then 250 mg a day)

ANSWERS

1. d. GI blood loss
2. a. Digoxin
3. c. Depression
4. a. Pale nail beds
5. The mechanism of action of pharmacologic and nonpharmacologic interventions in this case are:
   1. Pharmacologic interventions

a. Ranitidine–a reversible competitive blocker of histamine at the H2 receptors on the gastric parietal cells, resulting in inhibition of all phases of gastric acid secretion.

b. Acetaminophen–mechanism of analgesic effect is unclear; inhibits prostaglandin synthetase in CNS similar to aspirin, but minimal inhibition in the peripheral system.

c. Folic acid–a vitamin required for nucleoprotein synthesis and maintenance of erythropoiesis.

d. Disulfiram–blocks oxidation of alcohol by inhibiting aldehyde dehydroxygenase, resulting in accumulation of acetaldehyde.

e. Bupropion–a weak inhibitor of neuronal uptake of norepinephrine, dopamine and serotonin. The mechanism by how it enhances smoking cessation is unknown, but thought to be mediated by noradrenergic and dopaminergic mechanisms.

2. Nonpharmacologic interventions
   a. Discontinuing alcohol
   b. Smoking cessation
   c. Folate-rich diet
   d. Alcoholics Anonymous
6. d. Post gastric resection
7. Discuss classes of pharmacologic agents to treat peptic ulcer disease:
   a. Antacids:
   Advantages:
   • Available OTC, in different dosage forms and flavors
   • Relatively inexpensive
   Disadvantages:
   • Require frequent dosing (6–8 doses/day)
   • Must dose on an empty stomach
   • Potential for drug interactions (binds other drugs in gut and decreases absorption)
   b. Sucralfate:
   Advantages:
   • Equally effective to H2 blockers
   Disadvantages:
   • Requires multiple daily dosing
   • Drug interactions (due to decrease in drug bioavailability)
   • GI side effects (constipation, etc.)
   • More costly than other available agents
   c. H2 antagonists:
   Advantages:
   • Well studied, have been the mainstay of therapy
   • Very effective
   • Low toxicity/side effect profile
   • Can be dosed once daily
   • Can be taken without regard to meals
   • Available in generic and OTC
   Disadvantages:
   • Therapy with some agents still can be costly
   • Drug interaction potential (especially with cimetidine)
   d. Proton pump inhibitors:
   Advantages:
   • Very efficacious
   • Once daily dosing
   Disadvantages:

• Lacks long-term safety data
• Very costly
• Drug interaction potential (via cytochrome P450 system)
8. a. Evaluation for *H. pylori*
9. Education plan for disulfiram use:
   a. Lifestyle changes to be instituted prior to initiating therapy:
   • Ensure patient is committed to stop abusing alcohol
   • Ensure patient is involved with a support group, such as Alcoholics Anonymous
   • Educate patient on the risk of a disulfiram-alcohol reaction, and that it can be fatal
   • Educate patient and family to avoid alcohol of all forms, including alcohol contained in food items (vinegar, cooking sherry, etc.) and cosmetic items (aftershave lotions, colognes, and liniments). These can also cause a reaction with disulfiram.
   b. Medication counseling when therapy is initiated:
   • Patient must be free of alcohol for at least 12 hours prior to starting therapy
   • Initiate therapy at 500 mg daily for 1–2 weeks, then decrease dose to 250 mg daily (maintenance dosing). Maintenance therapy may be required for weeks to months depending on the patient's recovery.
   • Educate on side effects. Most common is drowsiness. May take at bedtime.
   • Recommend patient minimize caffeine intake, since disulfiram may increase CNS and cardiovascular stimulation effects of caffeine
   • Recommend patient obtain a medic alert bracelet stating that he is an alcoholic and taking disulfiram therapy
   • Educate patient and family about OTC medicines (to become a label reader to ensure product contains no alcohol, especially cough and cold liquid products)
   • Educate patient and family on the symptoms of a disulfiram-alcohol reaction. If patient does drink and develops reaction, educate family to get medical attention immediately.
   • Educate patient that reaction can occur up to 2 weeks after discontinuing disulfiram therapy.
10. Psychosocial factors that may affect KL's adherence to both pharmacologic and nonpharmacologic therapy are:
   1. Issues the patient must address
      a. Chronic addictions to alcohol and tobacco
      b. Motivation to participate and continue with a support group
      c. adherence with medications to correct diseases caused by his addictions (PUD, megaloblastic anemia)
      d. lifestyle changes, including dietary habits
   2. Common emotional disorders presenting in patients with addictions
      a. Anxiety
      b. Depression
      c. Suicide
   3. Other barriers
      a. Family and friend support
      b. Other stressors in life (work, etc.)
      c. Second DUI, patient may lose driving privileges and need to rely on other forms of transportation

11. Pharmacoeconomic considerations relative to KL's plan of care may include:
    1. Costs of disease management by patient at home
       a. Pharmacotherapy costs
       b. Transportation costs (to work, support groups, etc.)
    2. Costs of disease uncontrolled by patient to patient and family
       a. Direct medical
          • Hospitalization
          • Treatment and complications
    3. Direct nonmedical
       • Lost wages
       • Litigation/attorney fees
    4. Indirect personal
       • Decreased productivity
       • Quality of life
12. Key points are:
    a. Nutritional anemias may be prevented by early identification of "at risk" patients, monitoring for vitamin deficiency, and providing supplementation and/or replacement therapy.
    b. The nutritional deficiencies develop in stages, with anemia occurring in the final stage. Other hematological and biochemical changes occur first, allowing the diagnosis to be made prior to the development of anemia.
    c. Responses to therapy generally occur within the first week, though correction of the anemia may take 2–3 months.
    d. For patients requiring long-term vitamin supplementation, compliance should be monitored, as patients may discontinue use once symptoms improve.

CASE 12

PROBLEM LIST

1. Painful Sickle Cell Crisis
2. Dehydration
3. Viral Gastroenteritis
4. Sickle Cell Anemia
5. Narcotic Addiction
6. Need for Preventative Care

SOAP NOTE

S: Pain in abdomen, arms and legs refractory to oral hydromorphone; reports dizziness on standing × 1 day and malaise, fever and diarrhea × 3–4 days

O: PE: BP 100/60, HR 104, RR 18, T 38.0°C, Wt 46 kg, Ht 160 cm (usual weight 48 kg); icteric sclera; dry mucous membranes and skin; systolic ejection murmur; hyperactive bowel sounds
Laboratory: Lkcs 13.6, differential with 45% lymphocytes; Hgb 81 (8.1), Hct 0.243 (24.3); iron 16 (88), TIBC 68 (380)
Diagnostic: Peripheral blood smear: sickled cells and schistocytes
CXR and ECG: left ventricular hypertrophy; h/o pneumococcal pneumonia

A: **Problem 1:** Painful sickle cell crisis precipitated by acute infection and dehydration

Problem 2: Dehydration due to fever, diarrhea, and lack of oral intake

Problem 3: Viral gastroenteritis

Problem 4: Sickle cell anemia

Problem 5: Narcotic addiction

Problem 6: Need for preventative care

P: **Problem 1: Painful Sickle Cell Crisis**
• Initiate hydration: 500 cc bolus of 0.9% NS, followed by 150 cc/hr 0.9% NS with 20 mEq/L KCl
• Oxygen 2 L by nasal cannula
• Morphine sulfate 1 mg/1 mL D5W by PCA pump
  • Loading dose: 2 mg (2 mL)
  • Maintenance dose: 1 mg (1 mL)
  • Lockout: 10 minutes
  • 4-Hour limit: 15 mg (15 mL)
• Evaluate control q hour; once controlled, switch to morphine sulfate IV bolus q4–6h
• Convert to oral analgesics prior to discharge

Problem 2: Dehydration
• Initiate hydration as noted above
• Encourage liquids by mouth; reduce IV fluid infusion rate as oral intake increases
• Monitor input and output daily
• Monitor weight daily
• Monitor vital signs q8h
• Monitor electrolytes daily

Problem 3: Viral Gastroenteritis
• Initiate hydration as noted above
• Encourage liquids by mouth
• As diarrhea improves, initiate solids slowly
• Acetaminophen 1 g q4h PRN, T >38°C
• Monitor CBC and differential

Problem 4: Sickle Cell Anemia
• Continue folic acid 1 mg QD
• Educate on factors that may precipitate painful crisis
• Encourage high oral fluid intake (3–5 L/day) on an outpatient basis
• Discuss the option of initiating hydroxyurea once outpatient to increase fetal hemoglobin (Hb F) levels and decrease incidence of painful crisis

Problem 5: Narcotic Addiction

- Educate about the role of narcotic analgesics in sickle cell anemia and probable addiction; provide referral for counseling and support
- Develop a mutual plan regarding management of pain that includes continuity of care and close follow up
- Taper narcotic dose outpatient; counsel to use only as needed for pain, and when NSAID therapy has failed

Problem 6: Need for Preventative Care

- Give polyvalent pneumococcal vaccine outpatient
- Give *H. influenzae* vaccination outpatient
- Consider meningococcus vaccine outpatient

ANSWERS

1. a. United States
2. d. Malaise
3. c. Systolic ejection murmur
4. c. Tenderness to palpation in legs and arms
5. b. Aplastic crisis
6. The mechanism of action of the pharmacologic and nonpharmacologic interventions in this case are:
   1. Pharmacologic interventions:
      a. Morphine sulfate–acts as agonist to the mu, kappa, and sigma receptors in the CNS resulting in analgesia, euphoria, sedation, and respiratory depression.
      b. Acetaminophen–acts directly on the hypothalamic heat-regulating centers in the CNS, which increases dissipation of body heat and inhibits endogenous pyrogens.
      c. Folic acid–a vitamin required for nucleoprotein synthesis and maintenance of normal erythropoiesis.
      d. Hydroxyurea–increases the production of hemoglobin F, but the exact mechanism is unknown. Also causes increases in red blood cell water content and deformability of sickle cells. All these actions result in prolonged red blood survival.
      e. 0.9% NS–fluid rehydration
      f. Pneumococcal vaccination–stimulates antipneumococcal antibody production to prevent pneumococcal disease.
      g. *H. influenzae* vaccination–stimulates antibody production to provide protection against *H. influenzae* type b infections.
   2. Nonpharmacologic interventions:
      a. High oral fluid intake–prevents/minimizes the incidence of painful crisis
      b. Education on precipitating factors–prevents/minimizes the incidence of painful crisis
      c. Counseling for narcotic addiction–provides support so patient may learn to confront and live with the addiction
7. d. *C. difficile*
8. c. Meperidine
9. a. Increases production of hemoglobin F

10. Provide medication counseling on the following:
    1. Folic acid
       - Used to prevent folate deficiency and to decrease risk of an aplastic crisis
       - No special precautions
       - Take as directed daily by physician
    2. Ibuprofen
       - First line analgesic for sickle cell pain
       - Take with food or milk to minimize GI upset; notify MD if GI upset severe
       - May cause some drowsiness; know how it affects you before driving your car, etc.
       - Avoid taking additional OTC aspirin or NSAIDs–increases risk of GI toxicity
       - Avoid alcohol–increases risk of GI toxicity
       - Watch for and report black tarry stools
       - Notify physician of weight gain, edema
    3. Hydromorphone
       - Use only if pain relief not adequate with ibuprofen
       - Counsel on the potential for narcotic addiction
       - Avoid combining with alcohol and other CNS depressant medications
       - Common side effects includes drowsiness, dizziness, GI upset
       - Take with food if experience GI upset
       - Notify physician if experience any difficulty breathing or difficulty in staying awake when taking this medication
    4. Hydroxyurea
       - Used to decrease the frequency and severity of painful crisis
       - Take exactly as directed by physician
       - Follow up closely with physician for required monitoring (CBC, SCr, LFTs) due to increased risk of toxicity
       - Most common adverse effects are hematologic: leukopenia and anemia; notify physician if have fever, chills, sore throat, unusual tiredness, bruising, or bleeding
       - Report sores on mouth or lips
       - Increase fluid intake to avoid any renal toxicities
       - Can be teratogenic; use contraceptive measures
11. Psychosocial factors that may affect AB's adherence to both pharmacologic and nonpharmacologic therapy are:
    1. Issues the patient must address
       a. Limited activity/decreased quality of life due to disease complications (anemia, painful crisis, LVH)
       b. Required to take medications on chronic basis at young age
       c. Potential for narcotic addiction/dependence
    2. Common emotional disorders presenting in patients with sickle cell disease
       a. Depression
       b. Anxiety
    3. Other barriers
       a. Family and friend support
       b. Relation with healthcare providers
12. The health care provider's role relative to the proposed psychosocial factors identified include:
    a. Maintain close follow up/contact with the patient; develop a good relationship based on trust and respect for one another

b. Educate patient–on the disease, factors that may precipitate painful crises, importance of hydration, etc.

c. Counsel on medications–how and when to take, importance of adherence, how to minimize side effects, etc.

13. Pharmacoeconomics considerations relative to AB's plan of care may include:

1. Costs of sickle cell anemia controlled at home
   a. Pharmacotherapy costs
      • Traditional therapy
      • New/experimental therapy
      • Vaccinations
2. Costs of painful sickle cell crisis to patients and families
   a. Direct medical
      • Hospitalization expenses
      • Treatment and complications
   b. Direct nonmedical
      • Travel, hotels, meals
      • Lost wages (patient & family)
   c. Indirect Personal
      • Decreased productivity
      • Quality of life
      • Emotional stress (patient & family)

14. Key points are:
   a. Sickle cell anemia is a genetic disorder subject to inter-individual variability, but may include vaso-occlusive crises, CVA, aplastic crisis, splenic dysfunction, infectious complications, and recurrent, debilitating pain.
   b. In addition to managing complications, definitive therapy for sickle cell anemia may now include hydroxyurea and bone marrow transplantation.

CASE 13

PROBLEM LIST

1. Epistaxis
2. Thrombocytopenia
3. Rheumatoid Arthritis

SOAP NOTE

S: Concerned and upset patient with 4-day history of epistaxis; admits being quite frustrated about this unpredictable epistaxis

O: Mild petechiae and purpura on upper arms; irritated and reddened skin near nasal areas; tachycardic; agitated, concerned, and upset male
BP 142/88, RR 22, HR 116, T 39°C
Hct 0.29 (29), Plts 55×10^9 (55×10^3)

A: **Problem 1:** Epistaxis–secondary to drug-induced thrombocytopenia

Problem 2: Thrombocytopenia–possibly indomethacin-induced

Problem 3: Rheumatoid arthritis–stable; however, need to re-evaluate due to problem 2

P: **Problem 1: Epistaxis**
• Stop indomethacin
• Inform that the epistaxis seems to be the result of indomethacin-induced thrombocytopenia
• Inform PA if the epistaxis returns, to continue to handle it as previously (leaning his head back, using tissues to absorb the bleeding, etc.); if unable to control bleeding in this manner, PA should contact physician or go to ED
• Monitor cessation of indomethacin in terms of epistaxis; should expect improvement in 1–3 days; call if episodes of epistaxis have not ceased within 3 days

Problem 2: Thrombocytopenia
• Stop indomethacin
• Educate patient on drug-induced thrombocytopenia
• Recommend follow-up appointment in 2 weeks to assess thrombocytopenia; obtain CBC and check for improvement in rash at this time

Problem 3: Rheumatoid Arthritis (RA)
• Start salsalate 1500 mg PO BID for RA
• Recommend regular follow-up appointments to assess disease state and to make sure that salsalate controls symptoms
• Obtain x-rays of joints to monitor for disease progression
• Educate patient on benefits and limitations of salsalate so PA may better detect adverse drug effects
• Stress adequate rest and exercise, if possible, to better improve symptoms of RA

ANSWERS

1. c. Acetylcholine activity
2. a. Vomiting
3. d. Celecoxib
4. b. Prevents thromboxane A_2 generation by inhibiting cyclooxygenase
5. b. Correction with platelet transfusions for all patients
6. c. Increased production of white blood cells
7. d. 20,000–50,000
8. a. Dose-related
9. The rationale for using salsalate is:
   a. Experiencing epistaxis, petechiae, and purpura all likely due to indomethacin-induced thrombocytopenia
   b. Decreased doses of indomethacin will not affect the thrombocytopenia status, nor will it be effective for RA
   c. Salsalate does not inhibit platelet aggregation.

10. The pharmacoeconomic considerations are:
    a. Direct cost of salsalate compared to indomethacin
    b. Direct cost of follow-up appointment concerning thrombocytopenia and RA
    c. Direct cost of labs used to monitor the thrombocytopenia
    d. Indirect cost involved with lost work time/productivity
11. The psychosocial aspects are:
    a. Embarrassment experienced when epistaxis occurs in public places
    b. Anxiety, frustration, and concern experienced when epistaxis occurs with unknown cause
    c. Lack of understanding of risk of drug-induced thrombocytopenia
12. Key points are:
    a. Thrombocytopenia is defined as a decrease in the number of blood platelets and is one of the most common causes of abnormal bleeding. A decrease in platelets may occur from (1) a decrease in production, (2) altered distribution (sequestration), or (3) increased destruction of platelets.
    b. Drug-induced platelet disorders include those that alter platelet function and those that cause thrombocytopenia by decreased production or increased destruction of platelets.
    c. Platelet function disorders may cause bleeding or thrombosis independent of the platelet count and are commonly associated with uremia, cardiac bypass, liver disease, dysproteinemias, and myeloproliferative disorders. The underlying disorder should be corrected or treated when possible.
    d. Drug-induced immune thrombocytopenia can be caused by the formation of an immunoglobulin-drug immune complex that attaches to and destroys the platelet or the binding of the drug to the platelet membrane, creating a hapten that ultimately results in the formation of antiplatelet antibodies.

CASE 14

PROBLEM LIST

1. Pulmonary embolism (PE)
2. Bilateral DVT
3. Acquired Protein C Deficiency
4. Hypertension
5. Lifestyle–Obesity, Tobacco

SOAP NOTE

S: Pain and swelling of LLE × 2 days; sudden SOB, cough, dyspnea, chest pain × 20 min

O: HR 110, RR 30, Wt 109 kg, O_2 sat 88% INR 1.7, pO_2 9.2

Protein C 13% (65–130%), pCO_2 4.0, HCO_3 22

Physical findings: Obese male; LLE–erythematous, 2+ pitting edema, tenderness, +Homan's sign; RLE–mild edema, tachycardic, tachypneic, coarse breath sounds

Diagnostic tests: Doppler ultrasound consistent with DVT; V/Q scan: high probability PE

A: **Problem 1:** PE–supported by V/Q scan, physical exam, laboratory, and symptoms; no evidence of MI

Problem 2: Bilateral DVT–evidenced by Doppler and symptoms, probably due to improper management of 1st DVT; anticoagulated with warfarin only, not heparinized first

Problem 3: Inherited protein C deficiency; protein C level 13%; positive family history of protein C deficiency

Problem 4: Hypertension well controlled with HCTZ 25 mg PO daily

Problem 5: Obesity and tobacco smoking additional risk factors for thrombosis

P: **Problem 1: PE**
- Stop warfarin temporarily
- Start heparin: 8500 U bolus and 1800 U/hr infusion; check aPTT q6h and adjust infusion to keep aPTT 1.5x control; monitor for signs and symptoms of bleeding
- Restart warfarin 5 mg PO once therapeutic aPTT achieved; continue heparin infusion until INR is therapeutic; monitor for signs and symptoms of bleeding
- Educate regarding proper adherence to warfarin therapy including dietary and drug interaction effects
- Discuss the possibility of surgical placement of IVC interruption (Greenfield Filter) if anticoagulation fails

Problem 2: DVT
- Treat with heparin and warfarin as above

Problem 3: Protein C Deficiency
- Long-term management with warfarin, titrated to therapeutic INR.

Problem 4: HTN
- Continue HCTZ 25 mg QD

Problem 5: Lifestyle–Obesity and Tobacco Use
- Counsel on need for proper diet modification
- Assist with smoking cessation program
- Begin exercise program

ANSWERS

1. d. Autosomal–dominant, homozygous
2. c. 65–130%
3. a. DVT and/or PE
4. b. Affected by warfarin
5. b. Until therapeutic INR is achieved
6. a. 2.0–3.0
7. d. Skin necrosis
8. b. Inhibiting hepatic synthesis of vitamin K-dependent clotting factors
9. c. Low-molecular-weight heparin
10. DVT management in patients with known protein C deficiency includes:
    a. Begin heparin first to achieve therapeutic aPTT
    b. Begin warfarin at low dose and titrate to therapeutic INR, while continuing heparin infusion
    c. Discontinue heparin after warfarin is at steady-state with therapeutic INR
11. Start low-molecular weight heparin as an outpatient and instruct to start taking warfarin in 2–3 days, thus avoiding costs of hospital stay and aPTT monitoring
12. Protein C deficiency in JD is identified by:
    a. First thrombotic episode before age 40
    b. Presents with DVT/PE
    c. Positive family history of protein C deficiency in father
    d. Protein C level 18%
13. DVT prevention in high-risk situations can also be accomplished using:
    a. Fresh frozen plasma
    b. Protein C concentrate

    c. Compression stockings
14. Key points are:
    a. Protein C-deficient patients are at high risk for venous and arterial thromboembolic disease. Disruption of coagulation may occur on an inherited (primary) or acquired (secondary) basis.
    b. Treatments for acute thromboembolism for patients with protein C deficiency are heparin or LMWH with or without warfarin. Heparin or LMWH should be given before warfarin is initiated.
    c. Patients with protein C deficiency should receive short-term prophylaxis during exposure to situations with a high risk of thrombosis, with heparin or LMWH with or without warfarin regardless of thromboembolic history.
    d. Because of the high risk of recurrence of thromboembolism, prophylaxis after the first event should be considered in patients with protein C deficiency. Warfarin is generally the drug of choice.
    e. Pregnancy increases the risk of thromboembolism in patients with inherited protein C deficiency. Patients who become pregnant should receive anticoagulation with heparin or LMWH, regardless of history.
    f. Oral contraceptives can increase the risk of thrombosis in protein C-deficient patients and should be avoided.
    g. Warfarin-induced skin necrosis can occur in patients with inherited protein C deficiency when large warfarin loading doses are given. It is caused by a transient hypercoagulable state due to short half-life of protein C.
    h. Other acute complications of protein C deficiency include neonatal purpura fulminans and acute thromboembolism.

SECTION 4 / ENDOCRINE AND METABOLIC DISEASES

CASE 15

PROBLEM LIST

1. Respiratory Infection
2. DM Type 2
3. Insomnia

SOAP NOTE

S: Ill-appearing and complaining of an acute onset of fever, chills, pleuritic chest pain, productive cough, and fatigue; has not been sleeping well for the last week secondary to restlessness, anxiousness, cough, and nocturia; experienced toe numbness and burning leg pain for the last 2 months, unrelieved by opioid analgesics; not following a diabetic diet consistently

O: BP 140/90, RR 28, HR 125, Temp 39.5°C
HbA$_{1C}$ 12%, fasting glucose 12.2 (220), proteinuria, glucosuria
Yellow purulent sputum with gram (−) coccobacilli, chest x-ray with LLL consolidation, leukocytosis with left shift

A: **Problem 1:** Respiratory infection–community acquired pneumonia, possibly due to *Haemophilus influenzae*

Problem 2: DM Type 2 with peripheral neuropathy—poorly controlled due to current infection, inadequate therapy, and poor adherence to diet; pain poorly controlled with opioids

Problem 3: Insomnia secondary to jet lag, use of caffeine, and pseudoephedrine

P: Problem 1: Pneumonia

- Treat on outpatient basis; severity does not necessitate inpatient treatment (does not have serious comorbid conditions, physical exam reveals RR <30, HR =125, Temp <40°C, SBP >90 mmHg); recommend azithromycin 500 mg × 1 day followed by 250 mg QD × 4 days.
- Monitor response to treatment; expect subjective improvement by 3–5 days
- Check results of cultures/sensitivities; adjust therapy if needed
- Encourage smoking cessation
- Discuss importance of taking antibiotics as directed for the entire course of treatment

Problem 2: Type 2 Diabetes

- Add metformin 500 mg BID after acute illness is resolved
- Begin home blood glucose monitoring
- Adjust metformin dose after several weeks based on response
- Emphasize importance of healthy diet and exercise; refer for diabetes education
- Check HbA$_{1C}$ in 3 months
- Discontinue opioid analgesics; begin tricyclic antidepressant (i.e., amitriptyline 25 mg PO QHS) for peripheral neuropathy. Assess response after several weeks.
- Educate on importance of good foot care
- Educate on use of new medications; review use of glipizide

Problem 3: Insomnia

- Advise to reduce use of caffeine and pseudoephedrine
- Tricyclic antidepressant for neuropathy may also improve insomnia
- Try relaxation techniques
- Improvement in diabetes control should reduce nocturia

ANSWERS TO QUESTIONS

1. a. *Streptococcus pneumoniae*
2. c. Nocturia
3. a. Cephalexin
4. d. Proteinuria

5. a. Decreased hepatic glucose production
6. b. Frequency of testing is dependent on patient variables
7. d. Serum creatinine >124 (1.4)
8. b. Decrease the metformin
9. c. ACE inhibitors
10. a. Experiencing secondary failure of the sulfonylurea most likely due to progression of disease; increased doses are unlikely to improve control enough to achieve goals
    b. Metformin has a different mechanism of action (decreases hepatic glucose production) which may improve insulin sensitivity and have additive effects in combination with the sulfonylurea
    c. Single agent therapy is unlikely to be effective at this point.
11. a. Decrease total caloric intake to achieve weight loss
    b. 10 to 20% total calories from protein
    c. 50 to 60% total calories from carbohydrate
    d. <30% total calories from fat
    e. Increase fiber intake
12. a. Involve in developing a plan specific to needs
    b. Offer encouragement and support
    c. Educate on how to read food labels
    d. Demonstrate how home blood glucose monitoring is helpful in assessing response to food choices and activity level
    e. Offer resources/referral for further help
13. Consider:
    a. Direct costs of frequent medical office visits
    b. Direct costs of drug therapy
    c. Direct costs of home blood glucose monitoring
    d. Indirect costs with time involved adhering to treatment plan (taking medications, monitoring blood glucose, planning meals, exercising, etc.)
    e. Costs involved with lost work time/productivity
14. a. Increases uptake of glucose into muscle cells
    b. Improves circulation, breathing, digestion, and metabolism
    c. Helps people to lose weight and/or maintain ideal body weight
15. a. Infections commonly lead to loss of control of diabetes due to stimulation of counter-regulatory hormones
    b. Combination therapy with sulfonylureas and metformin may be necessary when monotherapy with one class fails to achieve adequate control
    c. Patients should be assessed for risk factors for lactic acidosis before using metformin
    d. People with diabetes have high direct and indirect costs of treatment
    e. Pharmacists may be instrumental in assisting patients in managing their diabetes

CASE 17

PROBLEM LIST

1. DM Type 1 with Neuropathy and Proteinuria
2. Hyperlipidemia

3. Hypertension
4. Gastroesophageal Reflux Disease

SOAP NOTE

S: Has not taken benazepril, ranitidine, and amitriptyline for 3 days due to difficulty getting them refilled; presents with heartburn symptoms and painful burning feet; has been adhering to a diabetic diet and checks blood glucose regularly

O: BP 164/100, HR 85, RR 14, Wt 68 kg,
BUN 7.1 (20), Cr 132.9 (1.5), Glu 13.3 (240), HbA$_{1C}$ 8.2%
Chol 6.2 (240), TG 2.1 (186), HDL 1.34 (52), LDL 3.9 (151)
UA: +protein, +glucose
ECG: LVH

A: **Problem 1:** Type 1 DM: Not adequately controlled with no signs/symptoms of hypoglycemia or hyperglycemia; neuropathy symptoms now present after stopping amitriptyline; proteinuria; on ACE inhibitor

Problem 2: Hyperlipidemia: Not controlled; with multiple risk factors and goal LDL cholesterol <100 mg/dl as stated by the American Diabetes Association

Problem 3: Hypertension: Stage 2 with LVH. Off benazepril × 3 days

Problem 4: GERD: Not controlled, off ranitidine × 3 days

P: **Problem 1: Type 1 DM**

• Increase NPH insulin dose to 22 U every morning and 18 U every evening; maintain same regular insulin dose
• Ask to check blood glucose QID (AC and HS) × 2 weeks to assess for further insulin adjustments
• Restart amitriptyline 25 mg QHS; monitor for relief of symptoms and for side effects

Problem 2: Hyperlipidemia

• Increase simvastatin to 20 mg q PM
• Review low-cholesterol, low-fat diet, and need for regular exercise
• Recheck fasting lipids and liver function tests in 6 weeks

Problem 3: Hypertension

• Restart benazepril 10 mg BID
• Educate on importance of taking medications daily
• Assess if could check BP at home
• Follow up in ~2 weeks

Problem 4: GERD

• Restart ranitidine 150 mg BID

ANSWERS

1. b. Two
2. c. Diabetes
3. a. Increase HDL, increase triglycerides
4. d. Niacin
5. a. Renal impairment
6. c. Secondary prevention in those with established CHD
7. d. Cholesterol synthesis peaks at night
8. b. No other routine tests are necessary
9. c. Delayed progression of nephropathy
10. a. Echocardiography
11. a. Decrease cholesterol intake to <300 mg/day
    b. Decrease total fat consumption to <30% of calories
    c. Decrease saturated fat consumption to <10% of calories
    d. Total calories should be based on need for weight loss or maintenance
12. a. Financial difficulty obtaining medications
    b. Transportation difficulties
    c. May not understand connection between cholesterol and increased risk for heart disease
    d. May not understand purpose of each medicine
    e. May be experiencing side effects from drug therapy
    f. May feel doesn't have enough time to accomplish all tasks
13. a. Suggest less expensive alternatives to prescriber when appropriate
    b. Use reminder system for refills
    c. Offer delivery service
    d. Provide education on proper uses of medications, purpose, common side effects, and dosing
    e. Provide information or resources for low-cholesterol-diet information
    f. Devise schedule for medicines to assist with keeping dosing simple
14. *Advantages*
    Decreases triglycerides by 20 to 50%
    Decreases LDL by 10 to 25%
    Increases HDL by 15 to 35%
    Inexpensive
    Shown to decrease mortality
    Disadvantages
    Frequent side effects
    Dose titration necessary
    Must be cautious in patients with DM, PUD, gout, or liver disease
    LFT monitoring recommended
15. Key points are:
    a. Risk factor assessment is an important part of managing hyperlipidemia and determining goals of therapy
    b. A low fat, low cholesterol diet is the foundation of cholesterol reduction
    c. Several factors are involved in the decision of which lipid lowering drug to use such as, type of hyperlipidemia,

concurrent conditions, goals of therapy, and cost of therapy

   d. Statin type drugs are cost effective in secondary prevention in patients with established CHD

   e. Monitoring of drug therapy with statins includes obtaining liver function tests periodically

CASE 18

PROBLEM LIST

1. Type 1 Diabetes, with Diabetic Ketoacidosis
2. Possible Infection
3. Depression
4. Allergic Rhinitis

SOAP NOTE

S: Pale and ill looking; 2 day history of nausea, vomiting, myalgia, polydipsia and polyuria; fruity breath and breathing quickly; has not taken any insulin since unable to eat; has a headache but denies chest pain, cough, fever, upper respiratory symptoms, or abdominal pain

O: BP 100/84, HR 120 (supine); BP 98/60, HR 140 (sitting)
RR 34, T 37.0°C
Glu 30 (541)
Na 130 (130), K 6.0 (6.0), Cl 96 (96), HCO_3 14 (14), PO_4 1.5 (4.8)
BUN 14.2 (40), Cr 141 (1.6)
ABG: pH 7.2, pCO_2 26
UA: trace protein, +glucose, +ketones
Lungs are clear, mucous membranes are dry, skin turgor is poor

A: **Problem 1:** Type I DM with diabetic ketoacidosis, moderate dehydration, hyperglycemia, hyperkalemia, and hyponatremia; off insulin × 2 days; appears to have a poor understanding of appropriate treatment of diabetes

Problem 2: Elevated white count and no clinical signs of infection

Problem 3: Depression on sertraline; needs further evaluation of effectiveness

Problem 4: Allergic rhinitis on nasal corticosteroid and oral antihistamine

P: **Problem 1: Type 1 DM with DKA**

- Begin normal saline at 1 L/hr for 2–3 hours
- Monitor BP and HR, check blood glucose and serum potassium hourly

- Give 0.1 U/kg insulin IV, followed by constant infusion of 0.1 U/kg/hr
- Change fluids to 0.45% sodium chloride when vascular status is stabilized
- As blood glucose approaches 13.8 (250), change fluids to dextrose 5%/0.45% sodium chloride and decrease insulin infusion
- Add potassium to fluids if serum potassium is <5.0
- Monitor input and output, electrolytes, BUN, and creatinine
- As ketoacidosis improves, switch to PO fluids and sliding scale insulin
- When alert, educate on insulin dosing, sick day management, short- and long-term complications of diabetes

Problem 2: Possible Infection

- Continue to monitor temperature, white blood cells, and blood and urine cultures
- Begin levofloxacin 500 mg IV QD, modify therapy per cultures, switch to PO as soon as possible if further antibiotic treatment is indicated by cultures

Problem 3: Depression

- Evaluate compliance and effectiveness of sertraline; adjust therapy if needed; offer counseling

Problem 4: Allergic Rhinitis

- Evaluate compliance and effectiveness of loratidine and fluticazone; advise to use inhaled corticosteroid on a regular basis

ANSWERS

1. b. Lack of insulin
2. d. Headache
3. a. Compensation for metabolic acidosis
4. c. It should be given if his pH is <7.0
5. a. Double the infusion rate
6. b. Intensive control of Type 1 diabetes will decrease risk of long-term complications
7. d. Use of alcohol should be kept to a minimum and taken with food
8. d. Add 3 U 70/30 at suppertime
9. c. Humalog has a quicker onset of action and shorter duration
10. b. His NPH dose should be moved to bedtime
11. a. Continue taking insulin even if not eating
    b. Monitor blood sugars more frequently (every 3–4 hours)
    c. Test urine for ketones
    d. Drink plenty of fluids
    e. Keep in touch with health care provider (may need supplemental insulin)
12. Insulin has to be continued to reduce acidosis and ketonemia–so dextrose is added to prevent hypoglycemia while the insulin infusion continues until the acidosis is resolved.

13. a. Sick-day management
    b. Appropriate use of alcohol
    c. Insulin dosing (review)
    d. Blood glucose monitoring (review)
14. a. Concurrent depression
    b. Knowledge and acceptance of diabetes and its management
    c. Lifestyle–balancing work and social life, consistency of routine
    d. Family support
15. a. Assess depression/use of antidepressant medication; refer for counseling if needed
    b. Offer education and support to improve understanding of diabetes
    c. Discuss other alternatives/compromises to agree on a treatment plan that will fit patient's lifestyle
    d. Enlist help of family members/friends; offer educational materials
16. Direct costs of hospitalization and outpatient treatment, direct costs of medications/supplies, indirect costs of lost work time and time involved with monitoring and planning
17. Key points are:
    a. Diabetic ketoacidosis is a life-threatening complication of diabetes and must be managed carefully
    b. DKA in patients with Type 1 diabetes may be caused by many different factors such as nonadherence with insulin, infection, acute illness, etc.
    c. Appropriate fluid and electrolyte replacement as well as insulin infusions are necessary to resolve DKA
    d. Patients with diabetes should be taught correct sick-day management
    e. Understanding the peak, onset and duration of different types of insulin allows the clinician to make rational adjustments to insulin therapy

CASE 19

PROBLEM LIST

1. Acute Adrenal Insufficiency
2. Anemia
3. Rheumatoid Arthritis
4. GERD
5. Osteoporosis
6. History of Hypertension

SOAP NOTE

S: Pale and semiconscious; per husband prior to becoming semiconscious has complained of weakness, dizziness, diarrhea, and severe vomiting and then experienced progressive confusion; her husband also states she ran out of her prednisone ~1 week ago while they were on vacation

O: BP 100/52, P 112, RR 28, T 37.3°C, Wt 65 kg

Na 119, K 5.8, Cl 92, HCO$_3$ 26, BUN 17.8, Cr 150
Hct 0.38, Hgb 110
Glu 2.8
Stool: Guaiac positive
UA: SG 1.025
ECG: tachycardia, regular rhythm

A: **Problem 1:** Acute adrenal insufficiency with dehydration, hyponatremia, hyperkalemia, and hypoglycemia due to running out of prednisone resulting in abrupt discontinuation of chronic corticosteroid therapy

Problem 2: Anemia possibly due to gastric irritation and blood loss from chronic prednisone use and exacerbated by recent ibuprofen use

Problem 3: Rheumatoid arthritis off corticosteroid therapy currently due to running out of medication

Problem 4: GERD on famotidine; possibly exacerbated by prednisone use

Problem 5: Osteoporosis secondary to estrogen deficiency and chronic prednisone use

Problem 6: History of hypertension: currently hypotensive

P: **Problem 1: Acute Adrenal Insufficiency**

- Start hydrocortisone sodium succinate 100 mg IV stat, followed by 100 mg IV q6h × 24 hours. As condition stabilizes, decrease dose to 50 mg IV q6h, and continue to taper
- Give 50 ml 50% dextrose IV stat, followed by dextrose 5%/normal saline 1000 ml over 1 hour
- Give a second 1000 mL D5/NS at 125 mL/hr × 8 hours, then change to D5/0.45% NaCl at 125 mL/hr
- Monitor mental status, BP, serum electrolytes, glucose, intake and output frequently

Problem 2: Anemia

- Discontinue ibuprofen
- Give famotidine 20 mg IV q12h until able to eat, then change to oral
- Monitor Hgb, Hct, and stool guaiac
- Evaluate source of blood loss when stable

Problem 3: Rheumatoid Arthritis

- Restart prednisone when oral therapy tolerated
- Educate on prednisone use
- Investigate other treatment options with the goal of tapering prednisone after stable and starting a disease-modifying treatment such as methotrexate

Problem 4: GERD

- Continue famotidine on discharge

Problem 5: Osteoporosis

- Stop magnesium hydroxide/aluminum hydroxide antacid

- Start calcium carbonate 500 mg BID
- Start conjugated estrogens 0.625 mg QD after baseline mammogram
- Educate on risks/benefits of estrogen replacement therapy
- Encourage weight-bearing exercise when able

Problem 6: History of Hypertension

- Hold atenolol
- Monitor BP; restart atenolol if hypertensive

ANSWERS

1. c. Moon facies
2. a. Hyperglycemia
3. b. 7.5 mg/day
4. d. Mitral valve prolapse
5. a. Hypotonic
6. b. Osmotic brain injury
7. c. Weight
8. d. If ECG changes occur
9. d. Celecoxib
10. a. She is not at risk for uterine cancer
11. b. Increase famotidine to 20 mg BID
12. Acute GI bleed–could worsen anemia and hypovolemia with increased confusion, tachycardia, hypoxia, hypotension, and shock
    Treatment–plasma expanders, oxygen, and medication to decrease gastric acidity to prevent further erosion
13. a. Do not stop taking prednisone without consulting physician
    b. Carry ID card with medication names and doses and physicians' names and telephone numbers
    c. Take prednisone at same time each morning with food or milk
    d. Avoid taking with other irritating medications such as aspirin, NSAIDs, or alcohol
    e. Get refills on time; do not run out
    f. As dose is decreased, follow schedule carefully and notify physician if weakness, fatigue, nausea, or fever occurs
14. Hypertension, gastropathy, immunosuppression, impaired wound healing, osteoporosis, myopathy, insomnia, psychosis, cataracts, glaucoma, amenorrhea, adrenal suppression, diabetes, impotence, hyperlipidemia
15. Alternate day therapy might reduce the HPA axis suppression potential and might be a reasonable method to start trying to decrease her dose, but her arthritis symptoms may worsen on the "off" days and become intolerable. The dosing regimen is also likely to be confusing.
16. Key points are:
    a. Acute adrenal insufficiency can present with nonspecific signs and symptoms
    b. Acute adrenal insufficiency is life-threatening; treatment should be initiated quickly
    c. Electrolyte disturbances are common in patients with acute adrenal insufficiency and must be managed carefully

d. Corticosteroids are associated with many adverse effects; use of corticosteroids should be monitored closely
e. Patient education regarding the chronic use of prednisone is necessary to avoid serious problems

CASE 21

PROBLEM LIST

1. Hyperlipidemia
2. Type 2 Diabetes
3. Hypothyroidism

SOAP NOTE

S: Appears healthy; no apparent distress; follows good diabetic diet; exercises occasionally; does not smoke; does drink alcohol regularly; recently told his cholesterol was elevated

O: BP 138/88, HR 85, RR 18, Wt 83 kg
Total cholesterol 6.03, HDL cholesterol 0.83, LDL cholesterol 4.14
Triglycerides 2.3, TSH 4.2, Glu 7.5, HbA$_{1C}$ 7.0%
No proteinuria

A: **Problem 1:** Hyperlipidemia with elevated LDL cholesterol and numerous cardiovascular risk factors. Following a consistent diabetic diet; goal for LDL reduction is <2.6 (<100 mg/dL) as stated by the American Diabetes Association

Problem 2: Type 2 diabetes in fair control on glyburide and diet

Problem 3: Hypothyroidism stable on levothyroxine replacement

P: **Problem 1: Hyperlipidemia**

- Reinforce dietary principles to keep total cholesterol consumption <300 mg/day and total fat consumption to <30% of total calories
- Encourage regular exercise, at least 20 minutes 3 times a week to start
- Obtain baseline liver function tests
- Begin atorvastatin 10 mg every day
- Counsel on possible adverse effects of atorvastatin and need for monitoring
- Recheck fasting lipids and liver function tests in 6 weeks
- Recommend using alcohol in moderation

Problem 2: Type 2 DM

- Continue glyburide at present dose
- Repeat HbA$_{1C}$ in 6 months
- Monitor for microalbuminuria yearly

- Reinforce dietary principles to provide well balanced, low calorie, low fat diet
- Counsel on need for regular eye exams and routine foot care

Problem 3: Hypothyroidism

- Continue levothyroxine at present dose
- Repeat TSH in 1 year

ANSWERS TO QUESTIONS

1. c. Four
2. b. Congestive heart failure
3. a. Elevated blood pressure
4. d. Every 5 years starting now
5. d. High consumption of fish
6. a. May interfere with absorption of levothyroxine
7. b. Decreases cholesterol production and upregulates LDL receptors
8. b. fluvastatin 40 mg QD
9. Overuse of alcohol may worsen his lipid profile, especially triglycerides, as well as other concerns with possible alcohol abuse. If he wishes to continue to drink alcohol he should do so in moderation (i.e., no more than 8 ounces of wine per day). This may have some benefit in improving his HDL cholesterol levels. He should also be made aware of possible negative effects of alcohol on his diabetes.
10. Further dietary reductions in cholesterol and fat intake may be difficult to accomplish.
    Frequent travelling may mean he eats out often and may have trouble choosing low cholesterol options and he may find it hard to exercise.
    Atorvastatin may cause headaches, GI disturbances, and muscle aches.
    Follow-up is necessary every 3 to 6 months until goals are achieved and to monitor for toxicity.
    He will probably need lifetime therapy, which will be expensive.
11. Provide resources or referral for dietary counseling; give examples of menu selections that are good choices; offer ideas for exercising away from home (walking, hotel gyms, exercise videos, etc.)
    Monitor for side effects to therapy; adjust as needed
    Review risk factors with patient and discuss goals of therapy
    Review risks versus benefits of treatment (compare to costs for treatment of coronary heart disease)
12. Costs of treatment would include indirect costs of lost work time for appointments and lab tests, direct costs of office visits, lab tests, and prescription drug costs, as well as possible costs for reading materials for diet counseling and exercise equipment
13. Key points are:
    a. Conditions such as hypothyroidism and diabetes may complicate treatment of hyperlipidemia
    b. Treatment of hyperlipidemia lowers the risk of cardiovascular events
    c. Moderate alcohol use may improve HDL cholesterol; excessive alcohol use may worsen triglyceride levels

d. Statin drugs differ in their ability to decrease LDL cholesterol levels

CASE 22

PROBLEM LIST

1. Hypothyroidism
2. Iron Deficiency Anemia
3. Constipation

SOAP NOTE

S: Appears lethargic but otherwise in no apparent distress; reports weight gain, increasing fatigue, decreased concentration, and constipation; reports heavier menses; frequently feels cold; also states has difficulty swallowing due to a "lump" in throat; stopped taking iron pills due to the constipation; reports taking kelp tablets from the health food store

O: BP 138/82, HR 78, RR 10, T 37.8°C, Wt 60 kg (increase of 5 kg)
Hct 0.30, Hgb 120, MCV 78, MCHC 260, Fe 9, TIBC 75
Skin and scalp are dry and scaly; mucous membranes are pale; diffusely enlarged goiter without nodules; nail beds are pale, DTRs are delayed; heart is RRR

A: Problem 1: Hypothyroidism with associated signs and symptoms, decreased FT_4I, increased TSH, and positive thyroid antibodies; most likely due to Hashimoto's thyroiditis

Problem 2: Iron deficiency anemia most likely due to menstrual blood loss and hypothyroidism; nonadherent with iron therapy

Problem 3: Constipation most likely due to hypothyroidism

P: Problem 1: Hypothyroidism

- Stop kelp tablets
- Begin levothyroxine 0.1 mg QD
- Check TSH in 6 weeks
- Counsel on condition and treatment

Problem 2: Iron Deficiency Anemia

- Restart ferrous sulfate at 325 mg QD; increase as tolerated to TID
- Check Hct/Hgb after 1 month
- Recommend increasing intake of foods rich in iron
- Reduce alcohol consumption

Problem 3: Constipation

- Recommend increasing fiber and fluid intake
- May use bulk-forming laxatives (dosed separately from iron)

ANSWERS TO QUESTIONS

1. a. Headaches
2. d. Estrogen may falsely elevate total TT_4 levels due to alterations in TBG
3. b. Iodide in kelp causes an inability to escape the Wolff-Chaikoff block in PJ
4. b. Her family history of thyroid disease
5. c. Hashimoto's thyroiditis
6. d. Correct hypothyroidism first before implementing lipid-lowering treatment
7. b. Increase levothyroxine to 0.112 mg every day
8. a. She may require a 20–30% increase in dose
9. c. Ferrous sulfate
10. a. Signs/symptoms of hypothyroidism and hyperthyroidism (overreplacement)
    b. Need for adherence with daily dose and regular laboratory monitoring
    c. Symptoms such as weight gain, skin and hair changes will be slow to resolve
    d. Take levothyroxine on an empty stomach, separate from iron
11. a. Poorly standardized doses with variable hormone content
    b. Deteriorates with improper storage
    c. May result in supraphysiologic T_3 levels
12. a. Cardiac patients may be more sensitive to levothyroxine–replacement may precipitate chest pain, shortness of breath, and palpitations
    b. Levothyroxine should be started only when cardiac disease is stable
    c. Starting doses should be kept low and slowly increased as tolerated
13. a. Cost of drug therapy–consider cost difference between brand and generic products
    b. Cost of regular laboratory monitoring of thyroid function tests
    c. Cost of appointments for follow-up
    d. Indirect costs for lost work time
14. a. Signs and symptoms of hypothyroidism can be nonspecific and may mimic other conditions
    b. Certain medications may interfere with the interpretation of thyroid function tests
    c. Hashimoto's thyroiditis is a common cause of hypothyroidism
    d. Monitoring TSH levels is the most appropriate method for assessing levothyroxine replacement therapy
    e. Levothyroxine is the preferred product for thyroid replacement

CASE 24

PROBLEM LIST

1. Anemia
2. DM Type 1
3. Hypothyroidism
4. Impotence
5. ESRD on Hemodialysis

SOAP NOTE

S: Well-developed, well-nourished male in no apparent distress; complains of increasing fatigue, occasional shortness of breath with exertion and impotence; monitors blood glucose 3–4 times a day; follows a low protein diabetic diet

O: BP 124/84, HR 84, RR 12, T 37.9°C, Wt 75 kg
BUN 14, Cr 318, HbA_{1C} 9.2%, Glu 7.5
Hct 0.28, Hgb 90, Fe 13.4, Ferritin 160, TIBC 300, Transferrin Saturation 25%
TSH < 0.4
Home BGM averages: AM 6.4, noon 6.7, 5 PM 10.8, 11 PM 6.6

A: **Problem 1:** Anemia most likely related to renal disease with normal iron and transferrin saturation and no signs of acute or occult bleeding

Problem 2: DM Type 1 with good adherence to diet and monitoring but not in adequate control with HbA_{1C} of 9.2% and elevated predinner blood glucose

Problem 3: Hypothyroidism with symptoms of fatigue and shortness of breath, but suppressed TSH indicating overreplacement with levothyroxine

Problem 4: Impotence complicated by anemia and inadequate diabetes control

Problem 5: ESRD on hemodialysis with stable BUN and CR

P: **Problem 1: Anemia**
- Continue ferrous sulfate 325 mg every day
- Start erythropoietin 4000 units SC 3 times a week
- Monitor Hgb, Hct, and retic count weekly; adjust dose to attain target Hct of ~33%
- Monitor BP, serum ferritin, and transferrin saturation monthly

Problem 2: Type 1 DM
- Increase morning NPH dose to 24 U
- Continue checking blood glucose QID
- Follow up in 2–4 weeks for further adjustment

Problem 3: Overreplacement of Levothyroxine
- Decrease levothyroxine to 0.125 mg every day
- Recheck TSH in 6 weeks

Problem 4: Impotence
- Determine nature/severity of dysfunction–differentiate between change in libido versus erectile dysfunction versus ejaculatory dysfunction

- Check serum testosterone level and fasting lipids
- Counsel on role of good diabetes control and treatment of anemia on sexual function
- Consider use of sildenafil if no resolution with improvement in DM and anemia

Problem 5: ESRD on Hemodialysis

- Continue current treatment plan of hemodialysis three times a week
- Continue current medications
- Advise not to use more than 150 mg ranitidine per day

ANSWERS TO QUESTIONS

1. b. Replace lost nutrients from hemodialysis
2. d. Decrease his caloric intake at lunch
3. a. Varicella
4. b. 11.6 (210)
5. c. Serum fructosamine
6. a. The injection must be taken within 10 minutes of mixing
7. c. Binding phosphate in the GI tract
8. d. Quick-acting insulin before meals with long-acting insulin once or twice daily
9. d. Reduces the risk of lipohypertrophy
10. a. Increases blood glucose by causing glycogenolysis
    b. Give 0.5–1.0 mg IM or SC
    c. Patient should respond within 10 to 20 minutes
    d. May cause nausea/vomiting
11. KJ should check his blood glucose QID and supplement his usual insulin dose with regular insulin depending on the results, using this scale:

BG <140	no extra insulin
BG 141–200	+2 U
BG 201–300	+5 U
BG 301–400	+10 U
BG >400	+12 U

Adjustments to the scale would be based on response; adjustment to usual daily dose would be made based on amount of extra insulin needed

12. a. Do not skip pills; if doses missed, take as soon as remembered
    b. Separate iron pill from all others by at least 2 hours; take on empty stomach
    c. All others may by taken together
    d. May take calcium with meals
13. a. Diabetes, anemia, and hypothyroidism may all cause fatigue and decreased energy which may mimic depression
    b. Serious and chronic illness may lead to depression; patient may have difficulty coping with chronic problems and frequent need for health care
    c. Impotence may cause depression and problems with relationships
14. Key points are:
    a. Patients with end-stage renal disease may develop numerous complications that must be monitored carefully
    b. Erythropoietin is used to treat the anemia associated with ESRD
    c. Patients with diabetes should understand how to mix and administer insulin correctly
    d. Many insulin regimens may be used and should be designed based on the patient's lifestyle and individual needs

CASE 25

PROBLEM LIST

1. Hyperparathyroidism with Acute Hypercalcemia and Hypophosphatemia
2. Dehydration
3. Hyperglycemia
4. Hypertension
5. Constipation
6. Hyperlipidemia

SOAP NOTE

S: Ill-appearing male in moderate distress; complains of dehydration, nausea and vomiting, increased confusion and memory loss; recently has felt dizzy, fatigued, thirsty, and has had increased urination and constipation; worsening bone and joint pain; not able to work; missing doses of medications due to forgetfulness; drinks alcohol (binging on weekends); smokes 2 packs a day

O: BP 170/100, HR 96 (sitting), BP 130/60, HR 120 (standing) (+) tilt test
RR 22, T 37.0°C, Wt 85 kg
(+) arteriolar narrowing; dry mucous membranes
Positive bowel sounds; lower quadrant tenderness with impacted stool (guaiac negative)
(+) bone tenderness; poor skin turgor
3+ DTRs; (+) ataxia; unable to do serial 7's
Na 150, K 3.6, Cl 110, HCO_3 19, BUN 23.2, Cr 221
Glu 20.3, Ca 3.99, PO_4 0.58, Uric Acid 714
Alk Phos 3.3, Alb 3.6
Chol 6.3, TG 3.6, HDL 0.93, LDL 3.8
PTH 95
UA: SG 1.002, (+) glucose, (−) ketones, (−) protein, (−) nitrates, 0–2 RBCs
Ultrasound: (+) parathyroid mass
ECG: sinus tachycardia with shortened QT interval

A: Problem 1: Hyperparathyroidism with hypercalcemia and hypophosphatemia with evidence of increased PTH and mass on parathyroid gland; symptoms of hypercalcemia include nausea, vomiting, constipation, bone and joint pain, poor memory, and ataxia; dehydration and thiazide diuretic may be contributing to elevated calcium levels; hypercalcemia should be corrected before parathyroid surgery

Problem 2: Dehydration with signs and symptoms of hypovolemia; secondary to hypercalcemia, hyperglycemia, vomiting, sun exposure, and overuse of laxatives; need to increase intravascular volume and maintain vital tissue perfusion

Problem 3: Hyperglycemia with dehydration, but without ketonuria or proteinuria, possibly exacerbated by use of thiazide diuretics; need to reduce glucose and maintain euglycemia to reduce symptoms and prevent long-term complications

Problem 4: Hypertension with a history of missing doses of medications and signs of end organ damage; aggravated by hypercalcemia

Problem 5: Constipation with stool impaction worsened by dehydration, hypercalcemia, and possibly by use of verapamil

Problem 6: Hyperlipidemia with elevations in both cholesterol and triglycerides, exacerbated by uncontrolled diabetes; also has numerous cardiovascular risk factors including: being a male >45 years, hypertension, current smoking, family history, and new diagnosis of diabetes

P: **Problem 1: Hyperparathyroidism with Hypercalcemia and Hypophosphatemia**

- Stop hydrochlorothiazide/triamterene
- Stop aluminum sodium carbonate
- Begin rehydration with intravenous normal saline 100 to 150 mL/hr
- Monitor serum calcium, electrolytes, BUN/Cr, and urine output hourly
- When adequately rehydrated, begin furosemide 10 mg IV q6h with continued fluids; continue to monitor labs frequently
- If serum calcium still elevated above 3 mmol/L in 24 hours, begin pamidronate 60 to 90 mg IV infusion over 24 hours and monitor temperature, serum calcium, and phosphate
- When symptoms resolved and stable, discuss need for parathyroid surgery to prevent further complications
- Advise to avoid calcium-containing supplements or antacids unless advised to use them by physician

Problem 2: Dehydration

- Replace fluids (as per problem 1) with IV normal saline; add electrolytes as needed

- Monitor electrolytes, BUN/Cr, urine output, BP, and HR (sitting and standing)
- Do not use stimulant laxatives

Problem 3: Hyperglycemia

- Treat dehydration (as per problems 1 & 2); add regular insulin 10 U L of fluid to slowly reduce glucose
- Monitor fluid status, electrolytes and serum glucose frequently
- Check HbA$_{1C}$ to establish baseline level
- If hyperglycemia continues despite rehydration, start glipizide 5 mg q AM
- When acute illness resolved, begin diabetic teaching

Problem 4: Hypertension

- Stop verapamil due to constipation and poor adherence with TID dosing
- Reevaluate BP after rehydration and resolution of electrolyte imbalance
- If BP remains elevated and serum potassium and creatinine improve, begin benazepril 10 mg every morning
- Encourage to stop smoking and binge drinking
- Check BP, potassium, and creatinine 2 weeks after starting benazepril

Problem 5: Constipation

- May resolve with rehydration and correction of hypercalcemia
- May need manual disimpaction
- Encourage to maintain adequate fluid and fiber intake

Problem 6: Hyperlipidemia

- Improvement in diabetes control may improve lipid profile
- Educate on low fat/low cholesterol diet and risk factor reduction
- Continue gemfibrozil for now
- Recheck fasting lipids and liver function tests in 6 weeks

ANSWERS

1. d. Hyperuricemia
2. b. Parathyroid adenoma
3. b. Low serum albumin
4. c. Cause a decrease in calcium excretion
5. a. Can often be given orally
6. d. Has the most rapid onset of action
7. c. He is likely to progress to malignancy
8. b. More data to support use for delaying nephropathy
9. a. Less likely to cause hypoglycemia with renal impairment
10. a. Change to pravastatin 20 mg every evening
11. a. Monitor levels daily until levels are stabilized

b. Keep levels >8 mg/dL using calcium supplements or dietary sources

c. If symptomatic, give calcium gluconate IV

12. PTH increases the:

   a. Release of calcium and phosphate from osteoclastic bone resorption

   b. Reabsorption of calcium and magnesium from renal tubule

   c. Intestinal absorption of calcium

   d. Activation of vitamin D_3

   e. Renal excretion of bicarbonate and phosphate

13. Plicamycin inhibits bone resorption to lower serum calcium. Should be reserved for patients who fail bisphosphonates or who cannot tolerate bisphosphonates. Should not be used in patients with hepatic or renal dysfunction, bone marrow suppression, or coagulation disorders

14. a. Saline hydration with furosemide is inexpensive and effective

   b. Calcitonin is rapid acting but tolerance develops and is relatively expensive; reserve for those who need rapid reduction

   c. Pamidronate is more effective and may be given as an IV infusion at home, which is less expensive than a 3-day course of etidronate in the hospital

   d. Plicamycin is less expensive than pamidronate but has more significant toxicity

15. Key points are:

   a. Hyperparathyroidism results in hypercalcemia and hypophosphatemia.

   b. Treatment of hypercalcemia includes identifying sources of extra calcium and discontinuing them.

   c. Reduction of hypercalcemia begins with IV hydration with normal saline followed by furosemide.

   d. Other treatments for hypercalcemia include calcitonin, bisphosphonates, and plicamycin.

   e. Pamidronate is the preferred agent for lowering calcium after IV fluids and furosemide.

SECTION 5 / RENAL DISEASES

CASE 26

PROBLEM LIST

1. Dehydration
2. Acute Renal Failure
3. Diabetes Mellitus (Inadequate Monitoring & Control)

SOAP NOTE

S: Nausea, vomiting, fever, chills, orthostasis demonstrated with dizziness when going from sitting to standing position; appears ill & lethargic upon examination

O: BP 103/56, HR 125
Dry mucous membranes, dry skin
BUN (49), Cr (2.4), Glu (160), HgA$_{1c}$ (8.2), Hct (47), WBC 15,000
Urinalysis & Urine Chemistries: 1+ proteinuria, SG 1.035, Na 10 (10), FE$_{Na}$ 0.6%, osmolality 480 mmol/kg, volume 350 mL in 24 hrs

A: **Problem 1:** Dehydration secondary to vomiting and decreased intake of fluids

Problem 2: Acute renal failure likely secondary to dehydration and renal hypoperfusion; may also be exacerbated by ibuprofen use

Problem 3: Inadequate monitoring & control of diabetes mellitus: long-term complications of poor control evident, including peripheral neuropathy and possible diabetic nephropathy; blood glucose currently controlled but question compliance with regular glucose monitoring and long-term control

P: **Problem 1: Dehydration**

- Admit to hospital to correct hypovolemia and assess underlying cause of recent symptoms
- Administer IV fluids to replace volume and correct hypovolemia; normal saline at an initial rate of 250 mL/hr
- Once volume corrected, decrease IV infusion rate to maintain perfusion
- Monitor BP, HR, temperature, and urine output every 1–2 hours
- Monitor serum electrolytes at least daily while admitted
- Assess cause of underlying symptoms (nausea, vomiting, fever) and treat appropriately (i.e., antibiotics, antiemetics)
- Continue IV fluids until able to tolerate PO intake to maintain volume status
- Goal: Replace fluids and correct volume status while preventing volume overload and electrolyte abnormalities consistent with acute renal failure

Problem 2: Acute Renal Failure

- Correct volume status (see Problem 1) to maintain renal perfusion
- Monitor renal function (BUN, Cr, urine output) at least daily while admitted

- Discontinue use of ibuprofen
- Instruct to avoid use of ibuprofen due to potential effect on renal hemodynamics considering her baseline renal function
- Recommend acetaminophen use in the future for fever and pain management
- Explain factors that may have led to the current changes in renal function (hypovolemia, ibuprofen use)
- Schedule follow-up appointment with renal clinic to assess renal function and risk of progression to chronic renal failure; evaluate urine for microalbuminuria and protein loss (consider angiotensin-converting enzyme inhibitor as renal-sparing agent)
- Goal: Reverse renal impairment through return of renal perfusion, prevent future events that may precipitate renal failure

Problem 3: Inadequate Monitoring & Control of Diabetes Mellitus

- Monitor blood glucose every 4–6 hours
- Administer NPH insulin according to prescribed dosing regimen and give regular insulin PRN for elevated blood glucose while admitted
- Counsel on the importance of frequent blood glucose monitoring at home and the long-term effects of uncontrolled diabetes; encourage regular self-monitoring of blood glucose (SMBG), at least two times per day, and design a sliding scale regular insulin regimen
- Educate regarding the signs of hypo- and hyperglycemia and insulin use during acute illness
- Determine if regular follow-up appointments are scheduled in the diabetes clinic to assess diabetes management and long-term complications (i.e., peripheral neuropathy, nephropathy, retinopathy); obtain HbA_{1C} at follow-up exam and quarterly thereafter
- Goal: Provide education to ensure appropriate management of diabetes and prevent short-term and long-term complications

ANSWERS

1. c. Hematocrit
2. d. Fluid overload
3. c. Fever
4. c. Hyperkalemia
5. b. Oliguric
6. a. Urine pH
7. a. Furosemide
8. d. Efferent arteriole
9. c. Provide IV fluid replacement
10. a. Dehydration: Decreased renal perfusion

b. Ibuprofen use: Prostaglandins work to maintain intraglomerular pressure through vasodilation of the afferent arteriole, NSAIDs prevent this compensation

c. Enalapril use: Angiotensin II works to maintain intraglomerular pressure through vasoconstriction of the efferent arteriole. ACE inhibitors prevent production of angiotensin II.

d. Preexisting renal insufficiency: Baseline creatinine elevated at 1.8 mg/dL

11. a. Mechanisms of action of pharmacologic interventions:

(1) IV fluids: Replace intravascular volume resulting in increased perfusion to the kidney and symptomatic relief

(2) DC ibuprofen: Prevents inhibition of prostaglandin synthesis, allowing compensatory mechanisms to occur (i.e., vasodilation of afferent arteriole)

(3) Long-term glucose control with insulin: Tight glucose control will help to prevent or delay progression to chronic renal failure

b. Mechanisms of action of nonpharmacologic interventions:

(1) Regular blood glucose monitoring: Consistent monitoring and follow-up action (i.e., administration of insulin, intake of glucose for hypoglycemia, adjustments in diet, etc.) will provide information on patterns of glucose control and help determine a more appropriate plan for long-term control of diabetes mellitus

(2) Support network: Provide an arena for voicing concerns about chronic disease and learning from experiences of others

12. Educational intervention:

a. Provide diabetes education, including importance of long-term tight glucose control, potential for end organ damage, signs of hypo- and hyperglycemia, compliance with insulin therapy and diet, compliance with glucose monitoring and follow-up appointments

b. Educate on appropriate use of insulin, including use of syringes, rotation of injection sites, adjustments during hypo- and hyperglycemic episodes

c. Discuss current complications and precipitating factors, such as hypovolemia, use of NSAIDs, illness

d. Educate regarding medications to avoid

e. Stress importance of follow-up in outpatient clinics for diabetes management

f. Discuss potential involvement in a support group

g. Include sister and any other available family members in this intervention; consider who will provide sick day care and administer insulin or glucose if patient unable

13. Psychosocial factors that may affect CL's adherence include:

a. Support network of family/friends (encourage good health, assist with insulin regimen during illness, etc.)

b. Scheduling regular glucose monitoring into daily routine

c. Adherence to prescribed insulin regimen, particularly sliding scale use

d. Life stressors (work, social, family)

e. Financial resources—must purchase test strips for measuring blood glucose & medications

f. Anxiety from current episode of acute renal failure and

the potential long-term consequences of diabetes (e.g., end-stage renal disease, dialysis)

14. Treatment goals are to:
    a. Reverse underlying cause (infection, hypovolemia)
    b. Correct volume status and any electrolyte disturbances
    c. Provide supportive measures until recovery has occurred
    d. Educate on factors that may precipitate renal failure
    e. Maintain appropriate glucose control
    f. Provide education on long-term glucose control
    g. Provide follow-up for diabetes control
    h. Educate on availability of a support group
    i. Involve sister in patient care; educate about diabetes and instruct on treatment strategies, complications, etc.

15. Pharmacoeconomic considerations relative to CL's plan of care may include:
    a. Cost of regular medications
    b. Cost of glucose monitoring supplies
    c. Hospitalization cost
    d. Missed work time and subsequent loss of wages during acute treatment
    e. Cost of current treatment versus cost of treatment for end-stage renal disease (i.e., dialysis, chronic medications, etc.)

16. Key points are:
    a. Prerenal azotemia is the result of a decrease in effective circulating volume and subsequent hypoperfusion to the kidney. Conditions leading to decreased cardiac output, hypovolemia, increased renal vascular resistance, systemic vasodilation, or renovascular obstruction are possible causes of prerenal acute renal failure.
    b. The kidney compensates for acute declines in renal function by increasing glomerular filtration pressure through vasodilation of the afferent arteriole, mediated predominantly by prostaglandins, and vasoconstriction of the efferent arteriole, mediated by angiotensin II.
    c. Prerenal azotemia is generally reversible with correction of volume status (i.e., the effective circulating volume). If uncorrected, prolonged hypoperfusion from prerenal causes may result in structural damage to the kidney and an extended course of acute renal failure.
    d. Avoidance of agents that alter renal hemodynamics, primarily NSAIDs and ACE inhibitors, and nephrotoxic agents is advocated in patients at risk for renal impairment.

CASE 28

PROBLEM LIST

1. Type 2 Diabetes
2. Chronic Renal Insufficiency
3. Retinopathy

SOAP NOTE

S: Complaints of restlessness and anxiety over last week, weight gain 2 kg (5 lb), missed last 2 scheduled appointments

O: BP 148/84, Wt 70.3 kg (68 kg at last visit); HEENT: Retinal edema, punctate hemorrhages
Blood glucose 150 mg/dL 9 months ago, current blood glucose 180 mg/dL, reported blood glucose readings at home 130–180 mg/dL, HgA$_{1C}$ (8.4), Ca (8.3) − Ca corrected for albumin (9.2), PO$_4$ (5.0), Alb 29 (2.9), BUN 14 (38), Cr 176 (2.0), Cr (1.8) 9 months ago
UA: Protein 260 mg in 24 hr (100 mg 9 months ago), (1+) glucose

Medications:
Glipizide 20 mg PO BID
Sumatriptan 1 injection SC PRN migraine
Conjugated estrogens 0.625 mg PO QD

A: Problem 1: Type 2 diabetes mellitus currently uncontrolled with diet and medication

Problem 2: Chronic renal insufficiency most likely secondary to poorly controlled diabetes; secondary complications of renal insufficiency are not currently present (i.e., anemia, metabolic acidosis); current creatinine clearance is 34 mL/min (Cockroft-Gault)

$$CL_{CR}(mL/min) = \frac{(140 - 58)\ 70.3\ kg}{2.0\ mg/dL \times 72\ kg} \times 0.85 = 34\ mL/min$$

Problem 3: Retinopathy secondary to poorly controlled diabetes supported by findings of HEENT exam

P: Problem 1: Type 2 Diabetes

- Assess adherence to current medication regimen (glipizide), diet, and regular blood glucose monitoring
- Confirm ability to accurately perform home blood glucose monitoring and reiterate necessity of continued monitoring
- Add 10 units NPH insulin SC QHS
- Educate about insulin administration (syringe preparation, rotation of injection site, dose adjustment, etc.); consider pen device as an aid if unable to self-administer dose
- Instruct to monitor blood glucose multiple times a day to determine optimal insulin regimen
- Educate on signs of hyperglycemia and hypoglycemia
- Determine home environment and options for assistance with drug therapy and lifestyle modifications
- Continue glipizide 20 mg BID–counsel to take 30 minutes before meals for optimal effect
- Counsel on compliance diet and exercise
- Attempt to achieve ideal body weight of 55 kg [IBW = 45.5 + 2.3 kg for each inch above 60 inches]

- Provide information on smoking cessation programs
- Continue with regular follow-up appointments
- Monitor for progression/development of secondary complications with each evaluation (retinopathy, nephropathy, neuropathy, vascular disease)
- Discuss long-term consequences of uncontrolled diabetes
- Include daughter/caregiver in all educational efforts
- Goal: Achieve and maintain fasting glucose 70–140 mg/dL, minimize risk of developing secondary complications and prevent hypoglycemia and adverse events through dietary and lifestyle modification and pharmacological therapy

Problem 2: Chronic Renal Insufficiency

- Refer to a nephrologist to assess renal function and monitor appropriately for progression to end-stage renal disease
- Start an ACEI such as enalapril 5 mg PO QD to reduce proteinuria and delay progression to end-stage renal disease; monitor BP tolerance
- Achieve and maintain fasting blood glucose 70–140 mg/dL as above
- Restrict protein to 0.8 g/kg/day (dietitian counseling warranted)
- Monitor diabetes management and renal function at regular follow-up visits
- Evaluate insulin requirements with change in renal function (insulin requirements may decrease as renal function deteriorates)
- Consider potential time course to progression of end-stage renal disease
- Monitor BP, goal BP <130/85
- Monitor K^+ (particularly with ACEI therapy), Cr, BUN, weight, signs of fluid overload
- Assess development of secondary complications of chronic renal failure: Anemia (Hgb, Hct, iron indices), renal osteodystrophy (PO_4, Ca, PTH), metabolic acidosis (HCO_3)
- Limit phosphorus intake to prevent hyperphosphatemia (consider addition of a phosphate binder if phosphorus elevated >5.5–6.0)
- Educate on long-term consequences of end-stage renal disease (dialysis therapy, secondary complications)
- Goal: Delay/prevent progression to end-stage renal disease, address secondary complications of renal insufficiency

Problem 3: Retinopathy

- Achieve and maintain fasting blood glucose <140 mg/dL as above
- Consult ophthalmology to assess extent of microvascular involvement
- Evaluate at each follow-up appointment

- Promote smoking cessation
- Goal: Limit further microvascular damage to prevent vision impairment

ANSWERS

1. c. Chronic renal insufficiency secondary to diabetes mellitus
2. b. Continue glipizide and add NPH insulin
3. d. Urine glucose
4. b. Enalapril
5. Cockroft-Gault: $\dfrac{(140 - 58)\, 70.3 \text{ kg}}{2.0 \text{ mg/dL} \times 72 \text{ kg}} \times 0.85 = 34 \text{ mL/min}$

   This is compared to 36.6 mL/min 9 months ago; current rate of decline in GFR is approximately 3.5 mL/min/year; expect secondary complications (anemia of renal disease, altered calcium-phosphorus regulation, metabolic acidosis, etc.) as GFR <25–30 mL/min.
6. b. 5–<10 years
7. d. Anemia
8. b. Ca 7.8 mg/dL, P 7.2 mg/dL
9. a. Pharmacologic:

   ACEI: Reduce intraglomerular pressure by limiting efferent arteriolar vasoconstriction mediated by angiotensin II and activation of the renin-angiotensin-aldosterone system. Used to prevent/slow progression to chronic renal disease, particularly in diabetics.

   NPH insulin: Optimize glucose utilization in patients with Type 2 diabetes unresponsive to treatment with diet and oral hypoglycemics (maximum dose glipizide for HP).

   b. Nonpharmacologic:

   Lifestyle modification: Weight loss, smoking cessation, diet, exercise—reduce likelihood of insulin resistance and secondary complications
10. c. Acetaminophen
11. a. Decrease in total insulin dose
12. Psychosocial factors include:

   a. Home environment: Limited options for assistance with medications, blood glucose monitoring, lifestyle modifications (i.e., living alone)

   b. Absence of interaction with spouse & peer group: Less motivation to care for self, more prone to depression, etc.

   c. Understanding of long-term consequences of diabetes: Less motivation to care for self and follow lifestyle modifications and changes in therapy

   d. Financial: Ability to pay for additional medications prescribed

   e. Stressors: Loss of spouse, disease process, and secondary complications, etc.

   f. Vision changes: Affects ability to comply with insulin therapy & glucose monitoring

   g. Fear of hypoglycemia with addition of insulin

   h. Fear concerning ability to administer insulin injections

   i. Potential for depression due to recent loss of family member and chronic diseases
13. The health care provider should:

a. Discuss current home, social, and financial situation with HP and daughter to determine possible influence on adherence to prescribed therapy

b. Consider changes in regimen based on assessment and/or determine options for assistance with care

c. Educate HP on long-term outcome of end-stage renal disease (dialysis, drug therapies)

d. Provide information on diabetes support groups

14. Pharmacoeconomic issues include:

a. Cost effectiveness of additional therapy with ACEI (e.g., delay progression of end-stage renal disease and start of dialysis treatment)

b. Potential cost of missed follow-up appointments (i.e., increased likelihood of complications from poor blood sugar control, potential delay in initiation of ACEI therapy)

c. Cost of therapy: Medications, special food requirements due to dietary restrictions, eye examinations, and care

d. Financial resources with loss of spouse

15. Key points are:

a. Microalbuminuria is an early clinical manifestation of glomerular damage.

b. Early intervention is essential in efforts to delay progression of renal disease.

c. "Tight" control of glucose has been shown to slow the onset of diabetic nephropathy in Type 1 and Type 2 diabetics and pancreas transplant recipients.

d. Interventions to improve glycemic control, systemic hypertension, and protein intake help delay progression to end-stage renal disease.

e. ACEIs have been shown to prevent/delay the progression to end-stage renal disease, particularly in diabetics.

f. As renal function declines, intervention is necessary to treat secondary complications of chronic renal disease and adjust drug regimens based on changes in drug disposition.

CASE 29

PROBLEM LIST

1. Chronic CHF/Digoxin Toxicity
2. Chronic Renal Disease
3. Anemia
4. Hyperphosphatemia
5. Metabolic Acidosis
6. Hypertension

SOAP NOTE

S: Fatigue, weakness, nausea/vomiting, decreased appetite (new onset) unrelieved by antacids, "funny" heart beat; smokes 1 cigar per week

O: BP 135/80, HR 54; HEENT: Pale mucous membranes and skin; COR: early S3; CHEST: Few rales and dullness over bases of lungs
EXT: Pale nail beds; Na (133), K (5.5), HCO$_3$ (17),

BUN (56), Cr (3.5)–baseline Cr (3.3–3.5), Hct (28.0), Hgb (9.3), Ca (8.9), PO$_4$ (6.1)
Peripheral smear: Normochromic, normocytic
Chest radiography: Enlarged heart
ECG: Prolonged P-R interval with occasional PVCs
Digoxin level: 2.8 ng/mL

A: **Problem 1:** Chronic CHF/digoxin toxicity
CHF currently managed with digoxin and enalapril
Current digoxin dose of 0.25 mg QD may be excessive due to chronic renal insufficiency; expected parameters include the following:

$$CL_{CR} = \frac{(140 - 67)}{3.5 \text{ mg/dL} \times 72 \text{ kg}} = 0.29 \text{ mL/min/kg (73kg)} = 21 \text{ mL/min}$$

$$CL_{Dig} = 0.9(CL_{CR}) + 0.33 \text{ mL/min/kg (Wt)}$$

$$CL_{Dig} = 0.9(21 \text{ mL/min}) + (0.33 \text{ mL/min/kg}) \, 73 \text{ kg}$$

$$CL_{Dig} = 43 \text{ mL/min} = 2.6 \text{ L/hr}$$

$$Vd_{Dig} = 3.8 + 3.1 \, (Cl_{CR})$$

$$Vd_{Dig} = 3.8 + 3.1 \, (0.29 \text{ mL/min/kg})$$

$$Vd_{Dig} = 4.7 \text{ L/kg (73 kg)} = 343 \text{ L}$$

$$Kel = \frac{CL}{Vd} = \frac{2.6 \text{ L/hr}}{343 \text{ L}} = 0.0076 \text{ hr}^{-1}$$

$$T_{1/2} = \frac{0.693}{Kel} = \frac{0.693}{0.0076 \text{ hr}^{-1}} = 91.2 \text{ hr} = 3.8 \text{ days}$$

$$Cpssavg = \frac{SFD/\tau}{CL}$$

$$Cpssavg = \frac{0.75 \, (250 \, \mu g/24 \text{ hr})}{26 \text{ L/hr}} = 3.0 \, \mu g/L = 3.0 \text{ ng/mL}$$

A more appropriate dose is required based on renal function and digoxin pharmacokinetics to achieve a desired concentration of 1.5 µg/L:

$$Dose = \frac{CL \, (Cpssavg)(\tau)}{SF} = \frac{2.6 \text{ L/hr} \, (1.5 \, \mu g/L)(24 \text{ hr})}{0.75} = 125 \, \mu g$$

Problem 2: Chronic renal disease secondary to analgesic abuse indicated by history and possible contribution from longstanding hypertension Creatinine clearance is 21 mL/min; secondary complications of chronic renal disease include metabolic acidosis, anemia, and changes in calcium and phosphorus homeostasis

Problem 3: Anemia secondary to chronic renal disease and decreased production of erythropoietin by the kidney with decreased renal function

Problem 4: Hyperphosphatemia secondary to chronic renal disease

Problem 5: Metabolic acidosis due to advanced renal disease and diminished ability of the kidney to secrete H^+ and reabsorb bicarbonate

Problem 6: Hypertension for past 20 years; currently controlled with lisinopril and triamterene/HCTZ; requires close evaluation and follow-up if current diuretic therapy discontinued as recommendation based on chronic renal disease

P: **Problem 1: Chronic CHF/Digoxin Toxicity**

- Hold digoxin until symptoms of toxicity resolve and digoxin regimen reevaluated
- Schedule follow-up appointment in 3–4 days (one half-life for digoxin) to measure digoxin level and assess symptoms
- Educate on signs of digoxin toxicity and need for medical attention if symptoms worsen
- Monitor ECG, K^+, Mg^{2+}, Ca^{2+}, HR
- Avoid hypokalemia (predisposes digoxin toxicity)
- Administer either 0.125 mg per day or 0.250 mg every other day once symptoms of digoxin toxicity resolve and digoxin in therapeutic range of 1–2 ng/mL
- Continue to evaluate for signs of worsening CHF (orthopnea, shortness of breath, edema, weight gain, dyspnea on exertion)
- Correct anemia
- Encourage smoking cessation
- Consider use of furosemide if CHF symptoms worsen (cautious use to avoid hypotension and induce acute renal failure)
- Goal: Resolve digoxin toxicity and determine the optimal regimen to provide control of CHF and maintain therapeutic levels

Problem 2: Chronic Renal Disease

- Refer to a nephrologist for evaluation of renal involvement and discussion of potential long-term consequences (end-stage renal disease, dialysis)
- Further evaluate renal disease to determine rate of progression and cause (analgesic agents)
- Counsel on limiting use of acetaminophen
- Discontinue triamterene/HCTZ
- Address secondary complications (metabolic acidosis, anemia, calcium-phosphorus)
- Educate on extent of renal impairment and risk of acute renal failure with uncontrolled CHF in conjunction with ACEI therapy
- Stress importance of BP control to prevent progression of renal disease
- Avoid use of NSAIDs due to risk of acute renal failure and analgesic-associated nephropathy (give list of all agents to avoid)
- Discontinue use of Mg/Al antacid
- Monitor BUN, Cr, K^+, and other electrolytes
- Goal: Prevent additional renal insult and prevent/manage secondary complications

Problem 3: Anemia

- Assess for GI bleed
- Question regarding any notable blood loss
- Obtain iron indices: iron, ferritin, TIBC
- Consider iron supplementation based on iron indices (ferritin and % transferrin saturation)
- Start erythropoietin (EPO) 100 U/kg/wk (100 U/kg × 73 kg = 7300 U/wk) administered as 3600 U SC BIW
- Counsel on use of EPO (syringe preparation, injection method)
- Monitor BP
- Monitor Hct, Hgb at 1–2 week intervals until stable dose determined to achieve target Hct/Hgb
- Adjust doses at 2–4 week intervals based on Hct/Hgb response
- Decrease dose if Hct increase is >4% in a 2-week period
- Monitor iron indices every 3–4 months
- Evaluate for resistance if inadequate response to appropriate EPO dosing regimens
- Goal: Achieve target Hct/Hgb (33–36%/11–12 g/dL) and prevent contribution to cardiac disease (i.e., CHF)

Problem 4: Hyperphosphatemia

- Counsel on restriction of phosphorus (≤10 mg/kg/day) and appropriate food intake (consult dietitian)
- Measure PTH to evaluate for hyperparathyroidism—start PO calcitriol if PTH >2–3 times normal
- Start calcium carbonate at an initial dosage of 0.5–1.0 g elemental calcium PO TID with meals
- Counsel to separate phosphate binder and oral iron supplements (e.g., ferrous salts) by at least 2 hours to avoid interaction
- Correct metabolic acidosis
- Evaluate phosphorus, calcium, & PTH at follow-up visits
- Adjust phosphate binder based on phosphorus levels (goal 4.5–6.0 mg/dL)
- Goal: Maintain serum phosphorus and calcium levels near normal, suppress secondary PTH release, and correct calcitriol deficiency to prevent long-term manifestations of renal bone disease

Problem 5: Metabolic Acidosis

- Administer sodium bicarbonate 40 mEq/day (approximately 0.5 mEq/kg/day)–4 mEq in each 325 mg tablet

- Counsel on adverse effects (belching)
- Monitor K^+ and other electrolytes
- Monitor HCO_3 with each follow-up evaluation
- Consider sodium content administered given patient has CHF (4 mEq sodium in each 325 mg tablet)
- Goal: Achieve and maintain serum bicarbonate levels near 20 mEq/L

Problem 6: Hypertension

- Discontinue triamterene/HCTZ
- Monitor BP with each evaluation
- Continue lisinopril at current dose
- Goal blood pressure <135/85
- Goal: Maintain BP at <135/85 to prevent HTN as a contributor of cardiac morbidity and progression of renal disease

ANSWERS

1. a. Decreased digoxin tissue binding
2. c. Hold digoxin until level in therapeutic range
3. a. Mg/Al Antacid
4. Factors adding to risk of renal failure include:
   a. CHF—An exacerbation of CHF may result in decreased effective circulating volume and a prerenal azotemia (prerenal acute renal failure)
   b. Lisinopril use—Alter compensatory mechanism of kidney to increase intraglomerular pressure during states of hypoperfusion to the kidney (i.e., CHF, dehydration)—prevent vasoconstriction at efferent arteriole by angiotensin II
   c. Diuretic use—Potential for volume depletion if HJ is started on a diuretic (e.g., furosemide) for CHF exacerbation
   d. Analgesic use—If use NSAID may prevent compensatory vasodilation of the afferent arteriole mediated by prostaglandins
   e. Chronic renal disease
5. a. Pharmacologic problems include:
   Digoxin—Toxicity related to excessive dose in patient with renal insufficiency
   Triamterene/HCTZ—Diminished effect at CL_{CR} <30 mL/min, increased K^+
   Lisinopril—Increased K^+
   Mg/Al Antacid—Potential for accumulation in renal disease, interaction with digoxin (decreased absorption)
   Acetaminophen—Question indication with history of analgesic abuse and associated nephropathy
   b. Nonpharmacologic problems include:
   Diet—Requires evaluation for phosphorus, sodium, potassium, protein content
6. c. Congestive heart failure
7. d. Calcium carbonate
8. a. With meals to promote phosphorus elimination
9. b. Ferrous sulfate 300 mg PO TID
10. d. Hypertension
11. b. Vitamin D

Table 1 • Continuum of Progression: Pre-ESRD to End-Stage Renal Disease

Stage	Diminished Renal Reserve	Renal Insufficiency	Chronic Renal Failure	Uremia	End-Stage Renal Disease
Percent of function	50–75%	20–50%	10–25%	<10%	<5–10%
Usual SCr* (mg/dL)	1.4–2	1.8–4.5	4–10	8–12+	>8 (variable)
Creatinine clearance (mL/min)	60–90	30–60	10–30	<10	<5–10
Clinical signs, laboratory findings, and symptoms	↑BUN, ↑SCr Asymptomatic ↓Hematocrit (mild)	Nocturia Hypertension ↑iPTH (mild) Proteinuria	Urine volume ↓or → Mild hypervolemia ↑Hypertension ↓Hematocrit ↑↑iPTH ↑ Po_4^{2-}, ↓Ca^{2+} ↑K^+ (mild) Acidosis (mild) ↓Calcitriol Anorexia, dysgeusia Fatigue, malaise	↓Urine volume Hypervolemia Hypertension ↓↓Hematocrit ↑↑iPTH ↑↑Po_4^{2-}, ↓↓Ca^{2+} ↑↑K^+ ↑Acidosis ↓↓Calcitriol Severe nausea or vomiting ↑↑Malaise Pruritis ↓Mental status Neuropathy	Dialysis needed to control signs and symptoms of uremia Emergent indications for dialysis: seizures, pericarditis, hypervolemia, acidosis, or hyperkalemia (severe) Uremic signs and symptoms, to left, generally present

BUN, blood urea nitrogen; iPTH, intact parathyroid hormone; SCr, serum creatinine.
*Conversion to International System of Units: SCr in μmol/L = 88.4 × (SCr in mg/dL).

12. Factors to consider include:
    a. Type of pain (psychosomatic vs. true pain)
    b. History of abuse of pain medications
    c. History of analgesic nephropathy
    d. Strategies to minimize risk of further insult: limit total dose, avoid combination of two or more analgesics, maintain hydration to prevent renal ischemia
13. Refer to Table 1.
14. Psychosocial factors include:
    a. Home situation: Living alone versus with family or friend
    b. Ability to take responsibility for own health care (e.g., adherence to medication regimen, clinic appointments, diet, etc.)
    c. Potential addiction to analgesic agents
    d. Support network (family, friends, neighbors)
    e. Future planning (procedures for help in emergency situations, advanced directives)
    f. Stressors: Worry about health and self-care, finances
15. b. Determine need for iron supplementation
16. Key points include:
    a. Drug disposition and response to many agents can be altered by conditions present in renal failure.
    b. Plasma protein binding of acidic drugs is generally decreased in uremia.
    c. Measurement of "free" drug concentrations may be warranted to best determine the likelihood of drug efficacy or toxicity.
    d. Hepatic metabolism of drug may be altered in the presence of renal disease.
    e. The extent of renal elimination of metabolites must be considered when assessing potential for drug accumulation and toxicity.
    f. Changes in drug dosing most likely warranted in renal disease for drugs with $> 30\%$ renal elimination.
    g. The uremic state may alter the pharmacodynamic response to some agents.

CASE 31

PROBLEM LIST

1. Peritonitis
2. Hyperglycemia
3. Inadequate Dialysis
4. Hypercholesterolemia
5. Hyperphosphatemia

SOAP NOTE

S: Painful CAPD exchanges $\times$ 4 days; "hazy" dialysate fluid, abdominal tenderness, fatigued, fever $\times$ 2 days, decreased appetite, "I cannot do all my exchanges—I feel too bad," ankle edema, decreased motivation to continue peritoneal dialysis per wife

O: T 38°C; CHEST: Few rales in lower third of lung fields; EXT:1+ edema in ankles

BUN (98), Cr (6.8), Glu (190), HbA$_{1C}$ 0.062 (6.2), Ca (9.8), PO$_4$ (6.9), aluminum (75), total cholesterol (240), LDL cholesterol (184), HDL cholesterol (28), triglycerides (140), PTH (4 times normal); dialysate effluent: WBC 200/mm^3, neutrophils 110 /mm^3; measured Kt/V = 1.1; weekly creatinine clearance = 45 L/1.73 m^2; urine volume in 24 hr = 300 mL; dextrose content for CAPD increased to 4.25% 2 weeks ago

A: **Problem 1:** Peritonitis possibly secondary to nonadherence with aseptic technique during CAPD exchanges–two episodes of peritonitis per year; current symptoms preventing exchanges as prescribed and contributing to inadequate dialysis.

Problem 2: Hyperglycemia in a Type 2 diabetic despite scheduled NPH insulin; absorption of glucose from dialysate solution a contributing factor

Problem 3: Inadequate dialysis therapy as assessed by weekly Kt/V <2.0, creatinine clearance <60 L/ 1.73 m^2, and symptoms consistent with fluid accumulation; noncompliance with dialysis prescription a contributing factor

Problem 4: Hypercholesterolemia with total cholesterol 240 mg/dL

Problem 5: Hyperphosphatemia as secondary complication of ESRD; aluminum hydroxide is current phosphate binder used to minimize calcium and phosphorus absorption–aluminum concentration (75) places patient at risk for aluminum toxicity with prolonged use of aluminum-containing phosphate binder; PTH elevated, however, vitamin D therapy would put patient at increased risk for metastatic calcifications; corrected Ca = 10.1 mg/dL, Ca $\times$ P = 70; warrants need of noncalcium- and nonaluminum-containing phosphate binder

P: **Problem 1: Peritonitis**
- Perform 2–3 rapid dialysis exchanges (20 min each)
- Start empiric antibiotics: 1 g cefazolin in one 2-L bag of dialysate solution QD (500 mg/L) AND gentamicin 50 mg in one 2-L bag QD (0.6 mg/kg)
- Adjust antibiotics based on culture and sensitivity results
- Monitor temperature, WBCs, color of effluent, pain during exchanges, abdominal pain
- Consider switching to hemodialysis if peritoneal dialysis technique deemed inappropriate (i.e., true lack of motivation, nonadherence with aseptic technique)
- If continuing CAPD, educate about strategies to prevent infections (aseptic technique with demonstration by patient)
- Determine prior sources of infection in FK–if

multiple *S. aureus* consider intranasal mupirocin 2% ointment BID × 5 days every month
- If hemodialysis initiated, educate FK and family about process
- Goal: Treat peritonitis with appropriate antibiotics, minimize the risk of subsequent infections, provide most appropriate dialytic therapy

Problem 2: Hyperglycemia

- Determine history of glucose control (home monitoring, glucose during prior visits) & dietary intake
- Assess the need for 4.25% dialysate solution vs. solutions with lower amount of glucose
- Determine if dwell times are prolonged
- Add 4 units of regular insulin to each 2-L dialysate bag
- Monitor glucose several times daily (every 4–6 hours) to determine need for alteration in insulin regimen
- Educate about importance of regular glucose monitoring, hyperglycemia and hypoglycemia, insulin use during sick days, and appropriate adjustments in insulin doses
- Consider adjustments in insulin requirements with changes in dialysis prescription
- Goal: Prevent hyperglycemia and hypoglycemia (fasting glucose <60 mg/dL)

Problem 3: Inadequate Dialysis

- Discuss technique of peritoneal dialysis exchanges
- Evaluate all factors contributing to decreased Kt/V and creatinine clearance (decrease in residual renal function, noncompliance with exchanges, change in permeability of peritoneal membrane)
- Educate on the consequences of nonadherence with peritoneal exchanges (inadequate dialysis, possible need to switch to hemodialysis)
- Present hemodialysis as an alternative if a viable candidate
- Goal: Determine the optimal modality of renal replacement therapy consistent with management of ESRD and lifestyle

Problem 4: Hypercholesterolemia

- Educate on diet modification as appropriate in patient with ESRD to minimize intake of saturated fats and cholesterol
- LDL >130 mg/dL, begin drug therapy with an HMG-CoA reductase inhibitor such as simvastatin 5–10 mg PO QHS or lovastatin 20 mg PO QHS; monitor hepatic function
- Monitor total cholesterol and lipid profile every 3–6 months
- Goal: Lower LDL <100 mg/dL with use of diet

and drug therapy, reduce risk of cardiovascular events, minimize adverse effects of therapy

Problem 5: Hyperphosphatemia

- Discontinue aluminum hydroxide
- Begin sevelamer 2 capsules TID with meals
- Monitor phosphorus, calcium, PTH, alkaline phosphatase, aluminum
- Educate on importance of adherence with medications and use of phosphate binder with meals
- Goal: Phosphorus <6.0 mg/dL, Ca × P <65, minimize serum Al concentrations, minimize side effects of drug therapy, prevent manifestations of renal bone disease

ANSWERS

1. Findings consistent with peritonitis:
   a. Subjective: Painful CAPD exchanges × 4 days; "hazy" dialysate fluid, fatigued, fever × 2 days
   b. Objective: T 38°C; abdominal tenderness and guarding
   Dialysate effluent: WBC 200/mm^3, neutrophils 110/mm^3
   Dialysate culture (if positive)
2. a. Cefazolin + gentamicin
3. d. Is the preferred method of administration
4. c. Ceftazidime + gentamicin
5. Options for prevention of CAPD infections in FK include:
   a. Strict adherence to aseptic technique when performing PD exchanges
   b. Regular patient and family education regarding technique of PD exchanges
   c. Pharmacological: Intranasal mupirocin 2% ointment BID × 5 days every month to reduce risk of nasal carriage of *S. aureus* or rifampin 300 mg BID × 5 days every 12 weeks based on potential causative organism
6. b. Urine output
7. d. Increased glucose absorption from the dialysate solution
8. a. <100 mg/dL
9. a. Change the phosphate binder to sevelamer
10. c. Protein binding
11. FK's current regimen for management of the anemia of chronic renal failure:
    a. Current dose of erythropoietin appropriate–Hgb/Hct in target range (Hgb 11–12 g/dL, Hct 33–36%)
    b. Subcutaneous administration ideal compared to IV in PD population
    c. Oral administration of iron requires monitoring for potential drug interactions (i.e., oral antibiotics, phosphate binders)
    d. Periodic assessment of iron status warranted
12. Pharmacoeconomic factors to consider include:
    a. Influence of PD schedule on potential work schedule
    b. Financial burden if unable to work
    c. Increased cost associated with peritonitis
    d. Cost effectiveness of adequate training for peritoneal dialysis exchanges to minimize risk of infection (decrease cost of hospitalization and drug therapy for treatment of peritonitis)

e. Cost associated with change from PD to HD if peritonitis episodes prohibit continuation of PD as dialysis modality

13. Psychosocial factors that may influence FK's adherence with his PD exchanges include:

a. Social activities–may find PD restrictive to lifestyle

b. Family network–time and effort of strict adherence requires strong family support

c. Education–requires an understanding of the importance of adherence with PD prescription and adherence to aseptic technique

d. Demanding PD schedule

e. Acceptance by others–may view PD dialysis as less acceptable

f. Attitude–if depressed, motivation to adhere to all aspects of PD may decrease

14. Key points are:

a. Approximately 9.7% of all ESRD patients receive peritoneal dialysis (1996 data)

b. Peritonitis occurs at a rate of 1–2 episodes per patient-year and is the predominant reason patients switch from PD to HD

c. Prevention of peritonitis is dependent on strict adherence to aseptic technique during PD exchanges

d. Peritonitis is diagnosed based on the presence of two of the following: abdominal pain, >100 WBCs/mm^3 of peritoneal fluid (with >50% neutrophils), and a positive dialysate culture

e. Common organisms associated with peritonitis include *Staphylococcus* spp. (gram-positive) and Enterobacteriaceae, *Pseudomonas* spp., and *Acinetobacter* spp. (gram-negative)

f. Treatment is initially empiric with use of more appropriate antibiotics once the organism is identified

g. Strategies to prevent CAPD infection are essential for successful therapy and reduction in risk of CAPD-related morbidity

SECTION 6 / GASTROINTESTINAL DISEASES

CASE 32

PROBLEM LIST

1. Peptic Ulcer Disease (PUD)
2. IBS
3. Chronic Renal Dysfunction
4. Graves' Disease
5. Iron Deficiency Anemia

SOAP NOTE

S: "Over the past 3 weeks I have experienced stomach pains which wake me up at night. The pain goes away when I eat and use an antacid."

O: Intermittent, crampy, lower abdominal pain relieved by passage of flatus; point tenderness between xiphoid and umbilicus; guaiac-positive; pruritic pretibial myxedema; Na 128 (128); HCO$_3$ 20 (20); BUN 28.6 (80); Cr 283 (3.2); Hct 0.29 (29%); Hgb 100 (10); Mg 1.35 (2.7); uric acid 535 (9); urinalysis: hematuria, proteinuria; endoscopy: 2 small duodenal ulcers; peripheral blood smear: microcytic anemia; medications: propylthiouracil, magnesium hydroxide/aluminum hydroxide; propranolol; cigarette smoking; alcohol and caffeine consumption

A: **Problem 1:** Active PUD exacerbated by cigarette smoking, caffeine and alcohol consumption

Problem 2: IBS worsening over the past 2 months, although diarrhea still mild; worsening diarrhea may be secondary to propylthiouracil (PTU) and magnesium-containing antacid

Problem 3: Chronic renal dysfunction secondary to polycystic renal disease

Problem 4: Pruritic pretibial myxedema, a manifestation of Graves' disease

Problem 5: Iron deficiency anemia secondary to active PUD and menstruation

P: **Problem 1: Active PUD**

• Initiate H$_2$-antagonist for treatment of duodenal ulcers; renal dysfunction (calculated creatinine clearance of 21 mL/min) present so start ranitidine 150 mg PO QHS, which is one-half the usual recommended dose for treatment of PUD; continue ranitidine for 6 weeks with monitoring of renal function; assess the need for maintenance therapy of duodenal ulcers, which is one-half the treatment dose

• Counsel to avoid foods and beverages that aggravate her symptoms of ulcer disease, including caffeine; avoidance of aspirin and other NSAIDs should be emphasized

- Educate on the importance of smoking cessation and discontinuing ethanol; provide options for smoking cessation and support groups
- Monitor stool guaiac tests, Hgb, Hct, BUN, and Cr

Problem 2: IBS

- Discontinue magnesium-containing antacid, which is likely contributing to worsening diarrhea
- Adjust dose of PTU, which is also contributing to worsening diarrhea
- Since IBS for 20 years, techniques that she utilized to minimize stress and promote relaxing should be discussed; offer other relaxation techniques or biofeedback that may be helpful in managing this chronic and relatively benign syndrome
- If diarrhea continues to worsen after trial with medication adjustments, recommend a high-fiber diet
- Educate to monitor number of stools per day and contact physician if diarrhea persists or worsens
- Obtain serum electrolytes and check body weight at follow-up visit in 4 weeks

Problem 3: Chronic Renal Dysfunction

- Since renal dysfunction is secondary to polycystic renal disease, management is aimed at minimizing further damage to renal function
- Counsel to avoid OTC medications that can worsen kidney function such as NSAIDs; consult a pharmacist before taking any OTC medications including herbal and homeopathic products
- Since patient has low sodium and bicarbonate levels, initiate oral sodium bicarbonate, 650 mg PO TID; titrate based on response
- Currently, thrombocytopenia does not require management. Monitor platelets at follow-up visit
- Hyperuricemia (asymptomatic) secondary to renal failure requires no treatment
- Discontinue magnesium-containing antacid since patient has elevated magnesium level; monitor magnesium level at follow-up visit
- Monitor calcium and phosphate levels; can result in osteopenia, osteoporosis

Problem 4: Graves' Disease

- Has completed 2 months of treatment with high-dose PTU and currently has a normal TSH with no objective symptoms; decrease PTU dose to 50–100 mg PO QD for maintenance for 6 months and reevaluate
- No longer tachycardic because of Graves' disease; recommend taper propranolol; decrease dose to 20 mg PO TID and continue the taper until discontinuation; monitor HR and BP

- Pretibial myxedema self-limiting; recommend hydrocortisone 1% cream to be applied QID for symptomatic relief of pruritis
- Monitor TSH, WBC, and cholesterol periodically

Problem 5: Iron Deficiency Anemia

- Initiate ferrous sulfate, 325 mg PO TID for 6 months
- Instruct to take ferrous sulfate between meals for maximum absorption; review adverse effects of iron therapy, such as nausea, constipation, and diarrhea; since IBS, carefully monitor for these effects; she may take ferrous sulfate with food if GI upset occurs; assess tolerability of iron supplementation at follow-up visit
- Counsel regarding the dark stools that iron therapy may cause versus the black tarry stools due to blood in the stools.
- Repeat Hgb/Hct value in 4 weeks; false positive for blood in the stool by the guaiac test can occur with iron therapy

ANSWERS

1. c. Eat after the evening meal to prevent acid secretion during the night
2. b. Abdominal pain, relieved by food and antacids
3. b. CrCl:

$$\frac{(140-35) \times 55}{72 \times 3.2} \times (0.85) = 21 \text{ mL/min}$$

4. d. 150 mg PO QHS
5. c. 20 mg PO BID
6. a. Propylthiouracil and magnesium hydroxide
7. a. Small, symmetric goiter
8. b. On an empty stomach
9. c. The patient is no longer tachycardic because of Graves' disease
10. a. Rapid gastric epithelial cell turnover
11. Pharmacologic and nonpharmacologic treatment problem(s) present in AJ's treatment plan are:
    1. Pharmacologic
       a. Diarrhea related to PTU therapy and magnesium-containing antacid
       b. Patient needs to discontinue the antacid due to renal dysfunction and diarrhea. Start H_2-antagonist.
       c. Needs treatment for pruritis associated with pretibial myxedema
       d. Needs treatment for iron deficiency anemia
       e. Decrease dose of PTU therapy—normal TSH, no symptoms
       f. Taper propranolol—patient no longer tachycardic
    2. Nonpharmacologic
       a. Smoking cessation
       b. Avoid alcohol and caffeine consumption
       c. Avoid substances irritating to stomach
12. Factors to consider for AJ's treatment plan to make a pharmacoeconomic decision:

a. Assess therapeutic efficacy
b. Safety
c. Tolerance
d. Reduction in recurrence of PUD
These factors are considered because a regimen that is clinically less effective has the potential to result in PUD recurrence; therefore, more costly overall.

13. Psychosocial factors that may affect AJ's adherence to both pharmacologic and nonpharmacologic therapy are:
    1. Issues the patient must address
       a. Pain associated with PUD
       b. Potential need for chronic medications
       c. Alteration in diet and lifestyle modifications
    2. Other barriers
       a. Financial constraint (cost of medications)
       b. Other stressors

14. Key points are:
    a. Peptic ulcer disease is a chronic, recurrent inflammatory condition involving a group of disorders characterized by ulceration in regions of the upper gastrointestinal tract.
    b. Duodenal ulcers occur in the wall of the duodenum, and its cause is unknown, but it is thought to occur due to excess acid secretion.
    c. Cigarette smoking, use of NSAIDs, and alcohol use contribute to increased risk of ulcer development.
    d. Lifestyle modifications (i.e., avoidance of alcohol) play an integral role in the treatment of duodenal ulcers.
    e. H$_2$-antagonists are used in the treatment of duodenal ulcers. Selection is based upon potential for adverse effects, drug interactions, and cost.
    f. Sucralfate may be an alternative to H$_2$-antagonists. Proton pump inhibitors, such as omeprazole and lansoprazole, have also been shown to improve healing of duodenal ulcers compared to conventional therapy.

CASE 34

PROBLEM LIST

1. GERD
2. HTN
3. DVT
4. Motion Sickness

SOAP NOTE

S: "I feel as if the heartburn has gotten worse. My voice is hoarse in the morning and my throat is sore. It hurts to swallow and the antacid is not helping; this started 3 days ago when I started the medicine for the motion sickness."

O: Heartburn, dysphagia, laryngitis, odynophagia; BP 130/85, HR 80, RR 16, T 37°C; esophagoscopy shows: moderate esophagitis, friable mucosa; current medication for GERD: antacid without relief

A: **Problem 1:** Moderate GERD secondary to scopolamine transdermal system; symptoms appeared after start of this new therapy; verapamil, nicotine, and ethanol may also potentiate symptoms

Problem 2: HTN controlled on propranolol and verapamil; however, evaluate for potential therapeutic adjustment due to potentiation of GERD symptoms by verapamil

Problem 3: DVT–INR and PT therapeutic; evaluate for drug interactions

Problem 4: Motion sickness: nausea due to motion sickness; receiving scopolamine transdermal system; medication adjustment to avoid adverse drug reaction

P: **Problem 1: GERD**

- Discontinue antacid, scopolamine transdermal system, and verapamil
- Initiate ranitidine, 150 mg PO BID
- Encourage patient to initiate lifestyle modifications:
  - Limit alcohol intake
  - Lose weight
  - Stop smoking
  - Elevate head of bed 6 inches for toe to head incline, reduces reflux
  - Eat smaller meals during day
  - Eliminate meals before bedtime
- Offer positive reinforcement for lifestyle modification adherence
- Follow-up in 1 week for efficacy, adverse effects of ranitidine and other medications

Problem 2: HTN

- Discontinue verapamil
- Continue propranolol therapy; increase dosage to 60 mg PO BID; check BP in 1 week
- Encourage lifestyle modification adherence

Problem 3: DVT

- Continue warfarin therapy for 3 months
- TED Hose
- Monitor effectiveness of warfarin; no clinically significant interactions with propranolol or ranitidine
- Monitor INR and review possible symptoms of bleeding with TM such as ecchymosis, epistaxis, hemoptysis, and gingival bleeding; report melena and hematuria immediately.

Problem 4: Motion Sickness

- Discontinue scopolamine transdermal system
- Initiate nonpharmacologic therapy
- Advise to avoid food immediately before travel; restrict fluid intake for several hours before travel

ANSWERS

1. c. Heartburn
2. a. Allows retrograde flow of gastric contents into esophagus
3. b. Anticholinergic activity of scopolamine transdermal system
4. a. Motion sickness
5. a. Nonsurgical visualization of esophagus
6. The mechanisms of pharmacologic and nonpharmacologic interventions for TM's GERD are:
   1. Pharmacologic interventions:
      a. Combination antacid containing aluminum hydroxide, magnesium carbonate, alginic acid, and sodium bicarbonate; increases pH of gastric contents and increases LES pressure
      b. Ranitidine competitively blocks action of histamine on H_2 receptors of stomach parietal cells, reducing gastric acid secretion
   2. Nonpharmacologic/lifestyle modifications that increase LES pressure:
      a. Weight loss
      b. Smoking cessation
      c. Reduce ethanol consumption
      d. Elevate head of bed 6–8 inches to reduce reflux
7. d. CrCl <50 mL/min
8. d. Minimal reduction in warfarin clearance
9. Pharmacologic and nonpharmacologic treatment problem(s) in TM's treatment plan:
   1. Pharmacologic:
      a. Drug-induced GERD due to scopolamine therapy
      b. Continued aggressive antacid use without relief
      c. Decreased LES pressure with nicotine, ethanol, and verapamil
      d. Possible increase in GERD symptoms with verapamil, nicotine, and ethanol
   2. Nonpharmacologic:
      a. No mention of previous lifestyle modifications
      b. Adherence to recommended lifestyle modifications
10. c. Severe, erosive esophagitis occurs
11. Psychosocial factors that may affect TM's adherence to pharmacologic and nonpharmacologic therapy
    1. Issues the patient must address:
       a. Smoking cessation
       b. Reduce ethanol intake
       c. Change dietary habits
       d. Elevating the head of bed
       e. Weight reduction
       f. Use of new medications
    2. Other barriers:
       a. Family support
       b. Adequate finances to purchase medications
12. The health care provider's role relative to the psychosocial factors identified is to:
    a. Develop an individualized plan for the pharmacologic and nonpharmacologic therapy.
    b. Provide patient education and positive reinforcement.
    c. Refer to local support groups and additional health care providers as needed.
13. Pharmacoeconomic considerations relative to TM's plan of care may include:

1. Costs of GERD therapy
   a. Pharmacotherapy costs
2. Costs of lifestyle modifications
   a. Smoking cessation therapy
   b. Weight reduction program
3. Costs of severe GERD
   a. Health care providers fee
   b. Diagnostic tests
   c. Costly pharmacotherapy
14. Key points are:
    a. GERD is a syndrome associated with an ineffective or incompetent lower esophageal sphincter (LES), which allows reflux of gastric contents into the esophagus, producing an epigastric burning sensation known as "heartburn."
    b. Several different medications and lifestyle practices can decrease the LES and predispose one to GERD symptoms. Lifestyle modifications may effectively reduce the symptoms of mild GERD. First line therapy with antacids should be initiated when lifestyle changes are no longer effective. Over-the-counter H_2-antagonists can be used for mild GERD.
    c. Higher doses of H_2-antagonists, proton pump inhibitors, or prokinetic agents can be utilized in moderate to severe GERD. These may be used alone, or in combination to heal esophagitis. Long-term therapy may be warranted for recurrences.

CASE 35

PROBLEM LIST

1. Gastroesophageal Reflux Disease (GERD)
2. Constipation
3. Gout/Hyperuricemia

SOAP NOTE

S: "I am having occasional heartburn and a bitter taste in my mouth after eating. It started 1 month ago while camping. I ate very heavy meals of fatty and spicy foods usually prior to bedtime. I also would drink a few beers with meals on the weekend. Now I'm also experiencing constipation. I've had some heartburn relief with antacid use."

O: Heartburn, and mild epigastric discomfort; BP 105/80, HR 68, RR 18, T 37.5°C, Wt 80 kg, hard stool

A: **Problem 1:** Mild GERD secondary to high fat, spicy meals eaten late in the evenings

  Problem 2: Constipation secondary to aluminum hydroxide content of antacid; also low fiber in diet

Problem 3: Gout not currently active; evaluate colchicine for potential drug interactions

P: **Problem 1: GERD**

- Discontinue aluminum hydroxide antacid
- Initiate famotidine 10 mg PO BID, over-the-counter brand
- Optimize therapy with antacid to provide 40–80 mEq of acid neutralizing capacity (ANC)
- Initiate hydroxymagnesium aluminate antacid, 3 TSP as needed after constipation resolves
- Monitor adverse effects and potential drug interactions
- Initiate lifestyle modifications for GERD
- Eat smaller meals during the day
- Avoid meals prior to bedtime
- Eliminate spicy, high fat foods from diet
- Elevate head of bed 6–8 inches for straight plane incline to reduce reflux
- Reduce ethanol consumption
- Recommend weight reduction

Problem 2: Constipation

- Educate on need to discontinue aluminum hydroxide antacid
- Recommend a gradual increase in fiber intake, ensure adequate fluid intake; encourage regular exercise
- Monitor for recurrence of constipation

Problem 3: Gout

- No intervention needed at this time; colchicine previously prescribed for acute gout attacks
- Educate on cross-sensitivity of NSAIDs to aspirin; emphasize importance of avoiding OTC and prescription products; encourage consultation with a health care provider prior to purchasing OTC agents
- Discuss dietary modification (i.e., avoid high-purine–containing foods) and emphasize importance of reducing ethanol consumption

ANSWERS

1. a. High-fat, spicy meals eaten late at night
2. d. Heartburn
3. c. Ethanol use
4. a. Backward flow of gastric contents into esophagus
5. a. Serum Creatinine 3.5 mg/dL
6. The mechanism of pharmacologic and non-pharmacologic interventions for PR's GERD are:
   1. Pharmacologic interventions:
      a. Hydroxymagnesium aluminate antacid—increases pH of gastric contents and indirectly assists in preventing backward flow of gastric contents
      b. Famotidine—competitively blocks action of histamine on H_2 receptors of stomach parietal cells, reducing gastric acid secretion
   2. Nonpharmacologic interventions:
      a. Alter diet, eliminate offensive foods
      b. Reduce ethanol consumption
      c. Elevate head of bed with blocks; reduces backward flow of gastric contents
      d. Weight loss
7. b. Aluminum content of antacid
8. Pharmacologic and nonpharmacologic treatment problem(s) present in PR's treatment plan:
   1. Pharmacologic:
      a. Constipation secondary to aluminum hydroxide antacid
   2. Nonpharmacologic:
      a. Ethanol use
      b. Diet of high-fat, spicy foods
9. c. Omeprazole
10. a. Reduces gastric acid secretion
11. Psychosocial factors that may affect PR's adherence to both pharmacologic and nonpharmacologic therapy are:
    1. Issues that patient must address
       a. Change in eating habits
       b. Reduce ethanol consumption
       c. Elevate head of bed
       d. Weight reduction
       e. Cost of over-the-counter medications
       f. Adherence to new medications
    2. Common emotional disorders presenting in the patient
       a. Anxiety
       b. Low self-esteem
    3. Other barriers:
       a. Family support
       b. Appropriate finances to purchase medication
12. The health care provider's role relative to the proposed psychosocial factors identified is to:
    a. Develop an individualized plan for the pharmacologic and nonpharmacologic treatments
    b. Educate PR about various over-the-counter medications for GERD, potential drug interactions and adverse effects; provide positive reinforcement
    c. Referral
13. Pharmacoeconomic considerations relative to PR's plan of care may include:
    1. Costs of GERD therapy
       a. Pharmacotherapy costs
    2. Costs of severe GERD
       a. Health care providers fees
       b. Diagnostic tests
       c. Costly prescription pharmacotherapy
14. Key Points are:
    a. GERD is a syndrome associated with the backward flow or reflux of gastric contents into the esophagus, producing an epigastric burning sensation known as "heartburn." Such reflux of gastric contents occurs when the lower esophageal sphincter (LES) is ineffective or incompetent.
    b. Different lifestyle practices and a variety of medications can decrease the LES pressure and predispose one to

GERD. Initiation of lifestyle modifications is an important and effective way to reduce the symptoms of mild GERD. Therapy with antacids should be initiated when lifestyle changes are no longer effective. Mild GERD may also be treated with over-the-counter H_2 antagonists.

c. Higher doses of H_2-antagonists, proton pump inhibitors, or prokinetic agents can be used alone or in combination to heal esophagitis associated with moderate to severe GERD. Long-term therapy may be warranted for recurrences.

CASE 37

PROBLEM LIST

1. UC (Proctosigmoiditis)
2. Sulfa Intolerance
3. Nutritional Support

SOAP NOTE

S: "For the past month, I have been feeling extremely fatigued. Two weeks ago I began experiencing an increase in the frequency of my bowel movements, rectal bleeding, and abdominal cramping which is usually relieved by defecation. I have about 6–7 bloody bowel movements per day."

O: Ulcerative colitis (UC) confirmed with rectal bleeding, diarrhea (6–7 bloody bowel movements/day), abdominal pain, malaise, and low-grade fever (37.5°C); BUN 8.9 (25); Hgb 102 (10.2); Lkcs 1.2×10^9 (1.2×10^3); Alb 30 (3); confirmative sigmoidoscopy report; abdominal tenderness with hyperactive bowel sounds; bloody, watery diarrhea; IBW 50.1 kg, actual Wt 45.5 kg

A: **Problem 1:** Recurrent UC secondary to lack of maintenance therapy being prescribed (following sulfasalazine intolerance)

Problem 2: Sulfa intolerance due to development of a dose-dependent adverse drug reaction while on sulfasalazine

Problem 3: Nutritional support secondary to malnutrition and malabsorption

P: **Problem 1: Recurrent UC**

- Give hydrocortisone enema 100 mg/60 mL QHS for 2–3 weeks; an alternate-night schedule may be used for an additional 2 weeks upon remission
- Initiate oral mesalamine (5-ASA) for maintenance therapy at appropriate starting dose for selected agent
- Monitor for signs of resolving UC symptoms, intact or partially intact tablets in the stool, and

development of skin rash, nausea, diarrhea, fever, or alopecia
- Continue PRN loperamide for diarrhea
- Educate on proper use of hydrocortisone enema and mesalamine drug therapy concerns; counsel on dietary intake, alcohol avoidance, and other psychosocial issues

Problem 2: Sulfa Intolerance

- Avoid use of any sulfur-derived products such as sulfasalazine
- Advise to contact health care provider if such a reaction ever experienced again secondary to drug therapy

Problem 3: Nutritional Support

- Aggressive nutritional replacement with a 1370 kcal/day diet with a protein requirement of 45.5 g/day; monitor weight daily
- Give B-complex multivitamin, 1 PO QD
- Monitor (by laboratory data) for iron, folic acid, and B_{12} deficiencies and treat appropriately; monitor cholesterol and triglycerides; serum electrolytes, BUN, and Cr routinely
- Instruct to limit only those foods that constantly produce symptoms

ANSWERS

1. c. Stress
2. a. Absent bowel sounds
3. b. Moderate
4. The patient education plan includes the following:
   1. Lifestyle modifications:
      a. Limitation of alcohol consumption as it may further irritate the gastric lining; a reduction in alcohol use to improve overall health.
      b. Stress management, as stress is a strongly suspected pathogenic factor.
      c. Dietary assessment for further insight into possible dietary antigens that may further exacerbate IBD. Instruct to avoid only foods that may worsen condition. Encourage proper eating habits in order to decrease the risk of further malnutrition.
   2. Medication use:
      a. Instruct to avoid NSAIDs as they may trigger inflammation of the bowels.
      b. Reinforcement of medication compliance.
      c. Educate on the use of hydrocortisone enema to induce remission and oral mesalamine for maintaining remission. Continue loperamide to relieve diarrhea.
      d. Instruct on the use of hydrocortisone enema. Enema to be instilled at bedtime in the supine position then changing to left, right, and prone positions for at least 20 minutes each in order to facilitate maximal topical coverage. A retention of 8 hours is also necessary.
   3. Indications for surgery:
      a. Failure of medical therapy
      b. Toxic megacolon

c. Colonic perforation or hemorrhage
d. Anal complications
e. Risk of developing colon cancer
5. b. More prevalent in females than males
6. Possible psychosocial factors to be addressed in DD's therapy include:
   1. Patient education
      a. Medication compliance
      b. Limited alcohol consumption
      c. Dietary restrictions
      d. Surgery as an elective
   2. Stress management
      a. Addressing work-related problems with management (supervisors, work crew leader, etc.)
      b. Reduction in late night working hours or increase rest in preparation for late night hours
   3. Common emotional disorders presenting in patients with IBD
      a. Depression
      b. Anxiety
   4. Social/family support
      a. Referral to self-help group
      b. Psychological referral
7. Pharmacoeconomic considerations relative to DD's plan of care include:
   1. Medication cost
      a. Cost-effectiveness of topical glucocorticosteroid for UC
      b. Expense of the newer oral 5-ASA medications
   2. Cost of surgery (if indicated)
8. a. Mesalamine
9. c. Plts 270 × 10⁹ (270 × 10³)
10. d. Iron-deficiency anemia
11. b. Rectal 5-ASA suppositories are indicated for distal ulcerative proctitis.
12. Key points are:
    a. Patient education and improvement in health-related quality of life parameters contribute to improvement in IBD patient outcomes. Questionnaires may be used to facilitate gathering pertinent data.
    b. A colectomy is curative in UC and may rid the patient of systemic complications.
    c. Because the acquisition cost of the newer 5-ASA formulations exceed that of SASP, they should be reserved for SASP-intolerant UC patients and men concerned about fertility.
    d. Antidiarrheals are contraindicated in severe IBD because they may precipitate toxic megacolon.

CASE 39

PROBLEM LIST

1. Constipation
2. Iron Deficiency Anemia/Anemia of Chronic Disease
3. CRF
4. HTN
5. BPH
6. Parkinson's Disease

SOAP NOTE

S: "Over the past 3 weeks I have had to strain during bowel movements. My stools are hard to pass. I have only had two bowel movements per week, and taking laxatives does not help. I often feel very tired and weak. My doctor recently changed my blood pressure medicine."

O: Abdomen tender with decreased bowel sounds; GU: soft, enlarged asymmetrical prostate gland: RECT: guaiac negative; barium enema: no obstruction; dry mucous membranes; Hgb 83 (8.3); Hct 0.24 (24); MCV 75 (75); MCH 24 (24); MCHC 300 (30); Retic 0.0005 (0.5); Plts 180 × 10⁹ (180 × 10³); Fe 7 (40); TIBC 81 (450); ferritin 9.0 (9.0); folate 11 (5); cranial nerves II-XII WNL; strength 5/5 bilaterally upper extremities; 5/5 lower extremities; gait with small steps and reduced arm swing; (+) slow resting hand tremor; sensory intact; alert × 3; new antihypertensive: verapamil; phosphate binder (aluminum hydroxide) for complications of CRF; benztropine and levodopa/carbidopa sustained release for Parkinson's disease

A: **Problem 1:** Drug-induced constipation secondary to verapamil; benztropine, aluminum hydroxide suspension, and insufficient fluid intake are contributing factors; Parkinson's disease itself may cause chronic constipation

Problem 2: Iron deficiency anemia secondary to blood loss during dialysis and underlying renal failure contributing to anemia of chronic disease

Problem 3: CRF secondary to hereditary renal disease (mother has chronic renal failure) and history of HTN

Problem 4: HTN controlled on verapamil but is causing constipation

Problem 5: Currently not taking any medications for BPH

Problem 6: Parkinson's disease: currently managed with sustained-release levodopa/carbidopa; benztropine added for treatment of tremor

P: **Problem 1: Constipation**
- Discontinue offending agents: verapamil, aluminum hydroxide; slowly taper benztropine; explain reason for discontinuation
- For acute constipation, recommend glycerin suppository 1 per rectum; for chronic constipation,

recommend a bulk-forming laxative (i.e., psyllium, methycellulose) 1 rounded teaspoon in 8 oz. of liquid PO TID followed by an additional glass of fluid
- Discontinue PRN use of magnesium sulfate salt since ineffective and may cause magnesium accumulation in CRF
- Educate on importance of increased fluid intake and exercise
- Monitor frequency and consistency of stools until returning to "normal" pattern of defecation
- If hard stools continue, consider adding a stool softener, docusate sodium 1 to 2 capsules PO BID (no longer than 1 week)

Problem 2: Iron Deficiency Anemia/Anemia of Chronic Disease

- Oral iron inappropriate due to constipation; parenteral iron is necessary
- Assess total iron deficit:
  - Total iron (mg) = (0.66) (71 kg) [100 − (100) (8.3)/14.8] = 2058 mg
  - Volume of iron dextran injection: = 2058 mg × 1 mL/50 mg elemental iron = 41 mL iron dextran
- Initiate 25 mg IM test dose; monitor × 1 hour for anaphylactic reaction
- Give daily injections of <250 mg by Z- track method until total dose given
- Following iron supplementation, initiate recombinant erythropoetin therapy at 50–100 units/kg body weight IV 3 times per week as postdialysis dose
- Monitor Hct (target range 30–36%) twice weekly until stabilized and maintenance dose established
- Monitor CBCs, platelets, blood chemistry, BP, iron, TIBC, and ferritin, before and after treatment

Problem 3: Chronic Renal Failure

- Management aimed at minimizing worsening renal function
- Monitor renal function and electrolyte levels
- Use caution when initiating renally cleared medication; adjust for decreased renal function; avoid nephrotoxic agents
- Recommend alternative phosphate binder with fewer gastrointestinal effects such as calcium carbonate 650 mg 1 tablet PO TID
- Discontinue PRN use of magnesium sulfate salt due to possible magnesium accumulation in presence of renal dysfunction
- Educate regarding importance of dietary restriction of phosphate (i.e., minimize intake of dairy products, legumes, sodas, protein-rich foods)

Problem 4: HTN

- BP controlled on current regimen, but verapamil causing constipation
- Discontinue verapamil and initiate doxazosin 1 mg PO QD since DH has HTN and BPH
- Check BP and HR within 1–2 weeks; increase to 2 mg if BP not controlled
- Counsel to enroll in a smoking cessation program that includes a support group

Problem 5: BPH

- Recommend initiation of doxazosin 1 mg PO QD to reduce the tone of the bladder neck and urethra
- Initiate first dose at bedtime due to first-dose syncope and possible additive BP lowering effect
- Educate regarding other side effects of doxazosin (e.g., edema, palpitations, nausea, dry mouth)

Problem 6: Parkinson's Disease

- Continue sustained release levodopa/carbidopa since responded well to this formulation
- Slowly taper benztropine over 7–10 days, and discontinue since it is contributing to constipation; benztropine may also interfere with short-term memory and cause hallucinations
- Presently slow tremor at rest is not a disabling symptom; if symptom becomes disabling, a trial of diphenhydramine 25 mg 3–4 times daily may provide relief; careful monitoring of constipation and other anticholinergic side effects would be necessary

ANSWERS

1. b. Change in antihypertensive medication to verapamil
2. c. Parkinson's disease
3. d. Fecal impaction
4. c. Blood chemistry
5. Important patient information regarding nonpharmacologic treatment of constipation:
   a. Incorporate regular exercise into lifestyle
   b. Increase the amount of daily fluid intake especially as fiber is added to diet
   c. Increasing fiber in the diet may be useful in preventing symptoms
   d. Respond to the urge to defecate
6. b. Intestinal and esophageal obstruction
7. a. 15–30 minutes
8. d. Gender
9. Advice to patient on the use of bisacodyl for 2 weeks by DH:
   a. Bisacodyl is a stimulant laxative
   b. Chronic use of this agent beyond 1 week is not recommended
   c. Discontinue use of agent
10. d. Chronic renal failure
11. Mechanism of action of recombinant erythropoietin in anemia of chronic renal failure:

a. The primary cause of anemia of chronic renal failure is a decrease in erythropoietin production by the kidneys in response to hypoxia.

b. Erythropoietin stimulates bone marrow to produce erythroid cells

12. Psychosocial issues that may influence DH's adherence to nonpharmacologic and pharmacologic interventions for constipation:

a. Patient beliefs about bowel function:

b. Bowel habits—patient's perception of what is a normal frequency of bowel movements

c. "Autointoxication"—fecal matter is noxious and may promote aging; may lead to overuse of laxatives

d. Sedentary lifestyle may inhibit need for regular exercise to reduce symptoms of constipation

13. Pharmacoeconomic issues to be considered about DH's plan of care:

a. Cost of pharmacologic intervention—medications for constipation generally OTC; lack of insurance reimbursement

b. Laxative use associated with higher patient usage of health care system

c. Cost of increasing fiber in diet—high-fiber foods often more expensive (i.e., fresh fruit, vegetables)

14. Key points are:

a. Constipation is a common disorder of the gastrointestinal system that is often self-limiting; however, may require nonpharmacologic or pharmacologic intervention.

b. Definitions of constipation may vary, but most often incorporate straining, hard or firm stool, less frequent defecation, feeling of incomplete evacuation.

c. Nonpharmacologic management of constipation focuses on the prevention of symptoms and includes regular exercise and increased fluid intake. Increased fiber intake may play a role in prevention of symptoms.

d. Agents available for the treatment of constipation include: bulk-forming agents, stool softeners, lubricants, saline, and stimulant laxatives. In general, there are no differences in efficacy between laxatives, but there are differences in their uses.

e. Laxative use should not exceed 1 week of self-medication nor should they be used in the presence of abdominal pain/cramping, nausea, or vomiting.

SECTION 7 / HEPATIC AND PANCREATIC DISORDERS

CASE 41

PROBLEM LIST

1. Bleeding Esophageal Varices
2. Hepatic Encephalopathy
3. Coagulopathy
4. Cirrhosis
5. Ascites

SOAP NOTE

S: Altered mental status and is semi-conscious since early this morning; getting progressively worse after hematemesis; complaining of increasing nausea and abdominal pain for the past 2 weeks with 4 bloody stools during that time per report of husband.

O: Heme +, + tilt test, nystagmus, slightly increased girth, + hepatomegaly, + fluid wave, spider angiomas, possible fetor hepaticus, asterixis, muscle wasting in arms and legs, + nail clubbing, + palmar erythema, little to no hair on extremities, oriented to person only, altered mental status

Hct 0.27, Hgb 90, Plts 50 × 10⁹, Na 132, K 5.2, Mg 0.7, protein 54, albumin 24, INR 1.4, PT 18 , AST 3.2, ALT 0.55, T Bili 87, ammonia 88
Endoscopy shows actively bleeding esophageal varices

A: Problem 1: Bleeding esophageal varices per endoscopy, decreased Hct and Hgb, + tilt test

Problem 2: Hepatic encephalopathy—mental status changes, asterixis, nystagmus, possible fetor hepaticus, increased ammonia

Problem 3: Coagulopathy—increased prothrombin time and INR, decreased Hct and Hgb, bleeding esophageal varices and heme +

Problem 4: Cirrhosis most likely caused by long-term drinking history; also has a history of ascites and now has further complications of esophageal varices and coagulopathy

Problem 5: Ascites; increased abdominal girth and + fluid wave

P: Problem 1: Bleeding Esophageal Varices

• Give fresh frozen plasma (FFP) and 2 units of

packed red blood cells (PRBC) to restore volume and correct hypotension.
- Endoscopic band ligation is performed on the bleeding during endoscopy.
- Monitor for recurrent episodes of bleeding, volume and color of future vomitus, guaiac testing, and for further decreases in Hgb and Hct.
- Start famotidine 20 mg IV BID. Change to PO when able to take oral medications.
- Start somatostatin 100 μg IV bolus then 50 μg/hr by continuous infusion. Give for 3 days. Taper on the third day to 25 μg/hr.
- As an outpatient, start propranolol 20 mg PO BID. Titrate the dose to a resting heart rate of around 60. Monitor for bradycardia, weakness, lethargy, CNS side effects, and decreased blood pressure.

Problem 2: Hepatic Encephalopathy

- Place nasogastric tube and begin lactulose 30 mL every 1–2 hours to induce a bowel movement then adjust the dosage to produce 4–5 soft stools a day for the first 2 days, then titrate to 2–3 soft stools a day to bind ammonia. Monitor for diarrhea and clearing of sensorium. When more stable and fully conscious, the nasogastric tube may be removed and the lactulose and famotidine given orally.
- Keep NPO for 48 hours. When mental status has returned to normal, begin advancing a liquid diet.
- Monitor diarrhea, mental status, electrolytes, and renal and hepatic function.

Problem 3: Coagulopathy

- Administer blood transfusions as mentioned in problem 1 to keep Hct ≥0.3 (30).
- Give vitamin K, 10 mg subcutaneously daily for 3 days or until the prothrombin time is normalized.
- Monitor PT, INR, Hct, Hgb, BP, and HR.
- Advise to avoid all over-the-counter NSAIDs, acetaminophen, and aspirin-containing products.

Problem 4: Cirrhosis

- Treat symptoms supportively as discussed in problems 1–3.
- Recommend a diet that restricts daily protein intake to 40 g/day.
- Advise to abstain from alcohol consumption.
- Recommend a daily multivitamin.
- Check B_{12} and folate levels and evaluate the need for replacement.
- Monitor LFTs, albumin, PT, INR, T Bili, signs and symptoms of bleeding, bruising, and mental status changes.

Problem 5: Ascites

- Increase spironolactone to 100 mg PO QD;

monitor potassium and blood pressure, and look for signs and symptoms of gynecomastia
- Monitor weight, abdominal girth, fluid wave, renal function, and peripheral edema
- Educate about a salt-restricted diet and weighing self daily

ANSWERS

1. d. Vomiting
2. a. Bleeding into the GI tract
3. Dietary ingestion of food or bleeding into the gastrointestinal (GI) tract introduces a rich source of protein into the intestinal tract. Ammonia is produced in the lower GI tract when these proteins and urea are metabolized by bacterial enzymatic action. The ammonia is then absorbed into the blood stream and converted to ammonium ion. Normally, the liver converts ammonium into urea for excretion by the kidney, but when the liver is malfunctioning or blood is being shunted away from it, as in advanced cirrhosis, serum ammonium levels increase, and encephalopathy ensues.

   An alternative explanation concerns derangements in plasma and brain amino acid patterns. Characteristically, there is a relative elevation in methionine and aromatic amino acid (AAA) levels (e.g., phenylalanine, tyrosine, and tryptophan) and a corresponding relative deficiency in branched chain amino acid (BCAA) levels (e.g., valine, leucine, and isoleucine). These derangements lead to an imbalance of brain neurotransmitters, causing elevated levels of serotonin, octopamine, and phenylethanolamine and a decrease in dopamine and possibly norepinephrine, resulting in encephalopathy.
4. ST can be fed enterally. She has a functioning GI tract and already has a NG tube in place. Consider Hepatic-Aid, an enteral feeding formula with a modified protein component consisting of more BCAA than AAA. It is reasonable to estimate that ST would require around 30 kcal/kg/day in her current state. This would equal 1830 kcal/day. Hepatic-Aid has 1 kcal/mL; therefore, ST would need around 76 mL/hr. This would provide 1824 kcal/day. Monitoring should consist of residual checks every 6 hours. If residual >150 mL, hold feedings for 4 hours and recheck, continue to hold if >150 mL or restart when <150 mL. Perform Accuchecks every 6 hours and give regular insulin per a sliding scale as needed. Monitor input and output, electrolytes, mental status, CBC, renal, and hepatic status.
5. c. Chest pain
6. b. Gram-negative bacilli
7. a. Ciprofloxacin 750 mg PO every Monday
8. 1. Pharmacologic interventions
   a. Famotidine competitively inhibits histamine at the H_2 receptors of the gastric parietal cells, which inhibits gastric acid secretion.
   b. Somatostatin reduces portal pressure and blood flow to assist in controlling variceal bleeding.
   c. Propranolol, a beta blocker, decreases portal venous pressure, which may help prevent GI bleeding associated with portal hypertension.

d. Lactulose is a synthetic disaccharide that is neither absorbed nor hydrolyzed in the small bowel. It decreases the pH of colonic contents to an endpoint of approximately 5.5. As the colon becomes more acidic, the ratio of ammonium ion to ammonia increases and less absorption of ammonia occurs.

e. Vitamin K, or phytonadione, promotes liver synthesis of clotting factors (II, VII, IX, and X).

f. Spironolactone competes with aldosterone for receptor sites in the distal renal tubules, increasing sodium, chloride, and water excretion while conserving potassium and hydrogen ions.

g. Multivitamin as a dietary supplement.

2. Nonpharmacologic interventions

a. Endoscopic band ligation involves endoscopic placement of a small rubber band over a distal bleeding varix to stop variceal bleeding.

b. Fresh frozen plasma and packed red blood cells to volume resuscitate, correct orthostatic hypotension, and replace lost blood volume.

c. Protein restricted diet (40–60 g/day) may decrease hepatic encephalopathy exacerbations; however, this is still an area of debate.

d. Sodium restricted diet (2 g/day) will help prevent volume overload secondary to fluid retention.

9. Discontinuation of drinking. The goal should be total abstinence from alcohol.

a. Spontaneous bacterial peritonitis prophylaxis if needed

b. Diuretics

c. Encephalopathy prevention (lactulose, reduce protein in diet)

d. Vitamin supplementation (vitamin K to prevent bleeding)

e. Variceal bleeding prevention (propranolol)

f. Dietary modifications (1g/kg or protein with an intake of 2000–3000 calories/day is acceptable).

10. d. Should be dosed BID to TID

11. c. Tachycardia due to inhibition of the vagus nerve is the most commonly observed side effect

12. a. Diarrhea is uncommon with neomycin

13. Psychosocial issues for an alcoholic patient include:

a. Decreased productivity

b. Increase in vehicular accidents

c. Criminal behavior

d. Physical problems

e. Mental illness

f. Disruption of family and employment

14. Key points are:

a. Discontinuation of alcohol intake in patients with proven cirrhosis is of primary importance.

b. Therapy for cirrhosis is focused mainly on symptomatic management of the complications of this disorder. Specific complications of the disease are treated to reduce morbidity and the need for frequent hospitalizations.

c. Ascites, esophageal varices, hepatic encephalopathy, spontaneous bacterial peritonitis, and hypoprothrombinemia are all complications associated with cirrhosis.

d. Generally, adherence to a diet of 1 g/kg/day of protein and 2000–3000 kcal/day is an acceptable nutritional guideline for patients with cirrhosis. Fluid and electrolytes should be monitored regularly and replaced as needed.

e. Limited pharmacokinetic dosing research and guidance is available for the hepatically impaired patient. Empiric dosage reductions continue to be done since data quantifying the degree of adjustment necessary in liver impairment are generally unavailable. This is particularly important with medications that are primarily metabolized by the liver.

CASE 42

PROBLEM LIST

1. Hepatitis C Positive
2. Depression
3. Hypertension

SOAP NOTE

S: Right upper quadrant pain, fatigue, anorexia and N/V, and has been feeling progressively worse for about a year; has lost 9 kg (20 lb) over this year

O: + anti-HCV, bridging fibrosis and moderate degrees of inflammation and necrosis on liver biopsy, no evidence or history of decompensated liver disease (ascites, jaundice, bleeding varices, or encephalopathy), AST 1.63, ALT 1.87, HCV RNA 585,000 copies/mL, hepatitis C genotype 1

A: **Problem 1:** Hepatitis C positive

Problem 2: Depression—stable on sertraline

Problem 3: Hypertension—controlled on HCTZ

P: **Problem 1: Hepatitis C Positive**

• Begin interferon 3 million units SC three times a week and ribavirin 200 mg PO, 2 tablets in the morning and 3 tablets in the evening.

• Start the hepatitis A and B vaccination series.

• Advise not to become pregnant while on therapy or until 6 months after completion of therapy. Inform that ribavirin is pregnancy category X, and explain what that means. Discuss birth control options (birth control pills, condoms, spermicide, etc.).

• Counsel on safe contact with other members of household. (Don't share razors, toothbrushes, or anything that might have blood on it.) The rate of sexual transmission of hepatitis C is low, especially in a long-term monogamous relationship. Husband should be tested for hepatitis C; but there is probably no need to use barrier methods for protection.

• Educate on subcutaneous injection techniques.

• Monitor: ALT and CBC with differential week 1, 2,

and 4 of therapy. Then, monthly monitor: ALT, CBC with differential, Cr, and electrolytes as well as evaluation of side effects associated with ribavirin and interferon. Thyroid function test should be monitored every 3 months during treatment.

- Evaluate depression at every visit. Increase sertraline if needed. Tell to contact health care provider immediately if should feel suicidal.
- Evaluate other common side effects such as fatigue, myalgias, fever, anemia, leukopenia, neutropenia, and thrombocytopenia.
- At 6 months of therapy, check viral load. If there is a detectable viral load or elevated ALT, therapy with interferon and ribavirin should be discontinued. If viral load is undetectable and ALT has returned to normal, therapy should be continued for 1 year.
- If criteria for continuing therapy is met, viral load should be checked at the end of therapy to document response and at 6 months after therapy is completed to document if a sustained responder.

Problem 2: Depression

- Continue present therapy.
- Monitor for depression throughout course of therapy and adjust current medication, decrease interferon, or discontinue the combination regimen if necessary.
- Discontinue therapy if becomes suicidal and refer to specialist for further evaluation.

Problem 3: Hypertension

- Continue present therapy.
- Monitor BP at appropriate intervals.

ANSWERS

1. Flu-like symptoms
   Neutropenia
   Thrombocytopenia
   Depression
   Hypo- or hyperthyroidism
   Acute exacerbation of liver disease (could be indicative of autoimmune induction of liver injury and interferon should be stopped immediately)
2. a. Anemia (hemolysis)
3. The response to therapy should be assessed at 6 months by the HCV RNA level (viral load) and ALT. If the viral load is undetectable and the liver enzymes have returned to normal limits, the patient should continue the full 12-month treatment. If either of these parameters remains elevated at this 6-month evaluation, treatment with combination therapy should be discontinued as it is very unlikely there will be a response to therapy.
4. Thyroid disorders and depression that are controlled on medication are not contraindications to treatment with interferon. Since interferon can cause hypo- or hyperthyroidism as well as depression, it is important to monitor these parameters while the patient is on therapy. TSH and FT4 should be assessed every 3 months while the patient is on therapy, as well as should signs and symptoms of hypo- and hyperthyroidism and depression. Efforts should be made to correct any abnormalities with medications before adjusting the dose of interferon. If patients remain unresponsive to medication adjustment, then consider decreasing the dose or discontinuing combination therapy. If the patient becomes suicidal, combination therapy should be stopped immediately and appropriate care given.

5. c. High iron in liver
6. d. Restore lost hepatic function
7. b. The fecal/oral route
8. a. Anti-Hbe positive is the lab test that confirms the presence of hepatitis B
9. a. Chronic hepatitis is a slowly progressive disease and most patients live for many years after diagnosis.
   b. Must exercise caution not to transmit virus to others (do not share products which might become contaminated with blood (razors or toothbrushes).
   c. Treatments are available that provide clinical improvement or cure in some patients, and lifestyle changes like discontinuation of ethanol consumption and illegal drug use may be helpful in prolonging life.
   d. Treatment is difficult, lasting for a year and involving the injecting of drugs 3 times a week; support from family and friends is helpful.
   e. Side effects can be dose limiting or cause discontinuation of drug therapy.
   f. Patients may become depressed while being treated and may feel worse during treatment than before they started.
   g. For patients not responding to therapy, liver transplantation may be an option.
10. c. Interferon alfa-2B 5 million IU SC QD and 100 mg PO BID for 4 months
11. b. Decrease ribavirin to 300 mg PO BID, and decrease interferon to 1.5 million units SC three times a week. Tell patient to report any fevers or infection immediately. Check again at next month's appointment.
12. a. There is a vaccine available
13. Key points are:
    a. Treatment of chronic hepatitis B and C with interferon and/or antiviral therapy can help with clearance of the virus, improve liver function tests and liver histology, as well as prolong life.
    b. Maintaining compliance with therapy is essential to efficacy
    c. Many patients will have difficulty tolerating interferon therapy. Evening dosing and judicious use of acetaminophen (<2 grams per day) for fevers and headaches may improve tolerability.
    d. Ribavirin is a teratogenic substance, pregnancy category X. Patients should not become pregnant while on therapy or for 6 months upon discontinuation of the medication.
    e. Patients should stop consuming alcohol and using illicit drugs to preserve existing liver function and slow progression of the disease.

SECTION 8 / RHEUMATIC DISEASES

CASE 45

PROBLEM LIST

1. Rheumatoid Arthritis (RA), Active
2. Diarrhea of Recent Onset
3. Dehydration
4. Anemia
5. Recent DVT
6. GERD
7. Hypothyroidism
8. Postmenopausal Female
9. Obesity
10. Chronic Tobacco Use

SOAP NOTE

S: "I have been experiencing diarrhea for the past week and feeling fatigued. I am still having morning stiffness, and swelling of my hands, elbows, and knees. My mouth has also been really dry and I have heartburn every night after eating."

O: Swelling and tenderness in joints of hands and elbows, with tenderness in knees; major restriction in performing work or self-care activities, guaiac negative stool, BP 110/70 (supine), 90/60 (sitting), HR 84 (supine), 112 (sitting), Wt 80 kg, Ht 150 cm; platelet count 440 × 10^9, Fe 4.5 (25), ferritin 205, TIBC 43 (240), Na 141, BUN 8.9 (25), Cr 115 (1.3), BUN:Cr ratio (19:1), Hct 0.30 (30), Hgb 120 (12.0), MCV 84 (84), INR 2.3

A: **Problem 1:** Active RA despite several trials of NSAID therapy and 3 months of auranofin therapy

Problem 2: Diarrhea, likely due to increased auranofin dose

Problem 3: Mild dehydration due to recent onset diarrhea

Problem 4: Anemia of chronic disease (normochromic, normocytic) indicated by slightly decreased hemoglobin, hematocrit, and serum iron with decreased TIBC and slightly elevated serum ferritin level

Problem 5: Recent DVT on anticoagulation therapy

Problem 6: Gastroesophageal reflux disease (GERD), currently untreated

Problem 7: Hypothyroidism without recent TSH level

Problem 8: Postmenopausal, not on hormone replacement therapy (HRT)

Problem 9: Obesity

Problem 10: Chronic tobacco use

P: **Problem 1: RA, Active**

- Discontinue auranofin therapy
- Initiate methotrexate 5 mg PO 1 × weekly
- Obtain baseline laboratory assessment of AST, ALT, alk phos, albumin, T. bili, CBC with platelet count, and hepatitis B and C studies; monitor CBC with platelet count, AST, and albumin every 1–2 months during treatment with methotrexate
- Consider treatment with low-dose oral corticosteroid (prednisone 2.5 mg/daily) to decrease swelling and tenderness while waiting for response to methotrexate (2 to 3 weeks)
- Discontinue piroxicam therapy; begin celecoxib 200 mg BID; closely monitor INR (especially during first few days after celecoxib initiation) and for signs and symptoms of GI bleed, while patient remains on warfarin therapy
- Educate patient regarding adverse effects associated with medications used in treatment of RA
- Discuss need for proper balance of rest and exercise, as well as appropriate nutrition
- Refer to physical and occupational therapy
- Educate patient and family members about RA and refer to support groups if not done previously

Problem 2: Diarrhea of Recent Onset

- Discontinue auranofin as stated in Problem 1
- Discuss the implications of diarrhea caused by auranofin therapy

Problem 3: Dehydration

- While in clinic, begin oral rehydration therapy with commercially available solution containing glucose (<5%), sodium, potassium, chloride, and water to reverse dehydration; instruct patient to continue oral rehydration solution at home to ensure adequate fluid intake
- Monitor for correction of serum sodium, BUN:Cr ratio along with improvement of diarrhea after discontinuation of auranofin
- Monitor blood pressure and pulse rate; instruct to rise slowly when attempting to stand until adequately hydrated
- Discuss clinical signs of dehydration with patient and family member if possible (i.e., hypotension, muscle cramps, altered mental status, decreased urine output, weight loss, dry mucous membranes); encourage to report any further signs/symptoms

Problem 4: Anemia of Chronic Disease

- Inform anemia may improve with adequate treatment of RA
- Monitor anemia as plan outlined in Problem 1 is implemented
- Consider treatment with recombinant human erythropoietin if anemia worsens or persists after improvement of RA

Problem 5: Recent DVT on Anticoagulant Therapy

- Continue warfarin therapy at current dose; has been treated for 8 weeks (3 months is typical duration for patient with first-time DVT)
- Monitor INR closely while initiating celecoxib; if INR in therapeutic range during that time (INR 2–3), monitor monthly (monitor more frequently if making alterations to drug regimen that may affect bleeding risk)
- Educate about signs and symptoms of bleeding, DVT, and PE
- Discuss vitamin K intake and have limit foods rich in vitamin K
- Educate about importance of consulting health care provider before taking any OTC or natural/herbal products, and specifically discuss need to avoid taking extra doses of NSAIDs or aspirin
- Encourage mobility, as limited mobility likely contributed to recent DVT

Problem 6: GERD

- Discontinue PRN antacid therapy
- Initiate ranitidine 150 mg PO BID and continue for 6–12 weeks; if symptoms recur, consider maintenance therapy
- Inform to avoid triggering foods (spicy foods, tomato juice, coffee, peppermint, etc.), especially during the evening or at bedtime; also discuss eating smaller meals
- Encourage a weight reduction plan involving healthy diet and exercise as tolerated with RA
- Inform to elevate the head of the bed 6–8 inch high to achieve a straight incline from foot to head to improve symptoms
- Encourage patient to stop smoking
- Avoid alcohol, which may exacerbate heartburn
- Encourage patient to take plenty of liquids with esophageal mucosa irritating medications, such as NSAIDs

Problem 7: Hypothyroidism

- Check TSH, FT_4D, or FT_4I annually
- Discontinue aluminum hydroxide-containing antacid to avoid impairing the absorption of levothyroxine from the gastrointestinal tract
- Educate about signs and symptoms of hypothyroidism and hyperthyroidism

Problem 8: Postmenopausal Female

- Refer patient for annual breast and pelvic examinations, as well as mammography and lipid profile if not recently performed
- Discuss risks/benefits of hormone replacement with estrogen/progestin therapy
- For prevention of osteoporosis, encourage adequate calcium intake (1500 mg elemental calcium/day) in combination with vitamin D (400 IU/day), including supplementation if not obtained through diet

Problem 9: Obesity

- Counsel on appropriate diet
- Encourage involvement in appropriate exercise activities as tolerated

Problem 10: Long-Term Tobacco Use

- Discuss need for smoking cessation; explain possible benefits including improvement of GERD symptoms, osteoporosis prevention, as well as risks of cardiovascular and respiratory diseases, and cancer with continued smoking
- Educate about nicotine replacement therapies (e.g., nicotine patches, gum, or drug therapy to aid in smoking cessation)

ANSWERS

1. b. TNF-alpha
2. c. Ulnar deviation
3. a. Dry mouth
4. c. Class III
5. a. Elevated platelet count
6. c. Vitamin E supplementation provides a small amount of pain relief in RA that is additive to anti-inflammatory drug effects
7. d. Schizophrenia
8. d. Symptoms of constipation
9. Baseline laboratory assessments that should be performed if methotrexate therapy is initiated in CJ include:
   a. Liver enzymes (AST, ALT, alk phos)
   b. Albumin
   c. SCr
   d. Total bilirubin
   e. CBC with platelet count
   f. Hepatitis B and C studies
10. Factors that may increase the risk of pulmonary toxicity with methotrexate therapy in CJ include:
    a. Age
    b. Smoking history
11. Signs and symptoms that might indicate methotrexate-pulmonary toxicity include pneumonitis with symptoms of shortness of breath and/or fever and then progression to pulmonary fibrosis
12. Although concurrent therapy with aspirin and methotrexate is associated with increases in methotrexate hepatotoxicity, a recent study (Iqbal MP, Baig JA, Ali AA, et al. The effects of non-steroidal anti-inflammatory drugs on the disposition of

methotrexate in patients with rheumatoid arthritis. *Biopharm Drug Disp* 1998; 19: 163–167) found no clinically relevant effects of NSAIDs (aspirin, diclofenac, ibuprofen, indomethacin, and naproxen) on methotrexate pharmacokinetics. While high-dose methotrexate may be much more toxic when used with NSAIDs, the low doses of methotrexate used to treat RA are usually safely administered with most NSAIDs.

13. Pharmacoeconomic considerations relative to CJ's plan of care may include:
    1. Direct medical
       a. Treatment and complications
          • Drug costs—celecoxib, methotrexate, warfarin, famotidine, levothyroxine
          • Adverse events—treatment, prophylaxis, laboratory monitoring
       b. Increased use of health resources
          • Costs of physical, occupational therapy
    2. Direct nonmedical
       a. Travel, hotel, meals in the event of hospitalization
       b. Lost wages (family)
    3. Indirect personal
       a. Activities of daily living, productivity, disability
       b. Quality of life
    4. Intangible personal
       a. Pain, suffering, emotional stressors
14. Key points are:
    a. Rheumatoid arthritis (RA) is a chronic autoimmune disease of unknown etiology that affects joints and other tissues and organs; the variable course of RA may or may not be altered by the drug and nondrug therapies.
    b. Nonpharmacologic therapies are used to help the patient cope and maintain or correct the problems associated with RA.
    c. NSAIDs are used as one of the baseline measures to treat the acute inflammation associated with RA.
    d. Slow-acting antirheumatic drugs may diminish the progression of joint destruction and thus are indicated in patients with potentially reversible, progressive, and erosive disease.
    e. The current second-line drugs of choice appear to be methotrexate for moderate to severe disease and sulfasalazine for mild to moderate RA.
    f. Early intervention in patients with unresponsive inflammation, progressive disease, and/or high rheumatoid factor titers will hopefully diminish the relentless progression of the disease in 10–15% of those who will develop severe RA.

CASE 48

PROBLEM LIST

1. Acute Gout Attack/Hyperuricemia
2. HTN
3. Hypokalemia

SOAP NOTE

S: "I woke up early this morning with excruciating pain in my left big toe. Over the past few hours, it has become red, swollen, and hot. I have had some pain in my toe before, but never this intense."

O: Redness, heat, and swelling of left first metatarsophalangeal joint; medication for hypertension: hydrochlorothiazide; T 38.8°C; BP 150/99; K 3.2 (3.2); Lkcs 12.0 × 10^9 (12.0 × 10^3); Sed Rate 55 (55); uric acid 530 (8.9); synovial fluid aspirate (left metatarsophalangeal joint) is cloudy with protein and glucose WNL, Gram stain (−), leukocyte count 19.5 × 10^9/L (predominance of PMNs), and reveals needle-shaped crystals (approximately 5 μm in length); 24-hour uric acid clearance pending

A: **Problem 1:** Acute gout attack/hyperuricemia: hydrochlorothiazide most likely contributed to hyperuricemia

Problem 2: Poorly controlled BP

Problem 3: Hypokalemia (asymptomatic) secondary to hydrochlorothiazide and alcohol consumption

P: **Problem 1: Acute Gout Attack**
• Discontinue hydrochlorothiazide
• Avoid use of indomethacin and other NSAIDs since DW has hypersensitivity to aspirin.
• Initiate colchicine 0.5–1.2 mg PO × 1 dose, followed by 0.5–0.6 mg every hour until improvement of adverse GI effects (i.e., nausea, vomiting, or diarrhea) or maximum of 8–10 mg has been administered
• Assess need for maintenance treatment of hyperuricemia based on patient's clinical condition, results of 24-hour uric acid excretion, frequency of attacks, and evidence of joint destruction, tophi formation, and renal involvement
• Discuss dietary modifications (i.e., limit ethanol [ETOH] consumption) and weight reduction

Problem 2: Hypertension
• Discontinue hydrochlorothiazide as stated in problem 1
• Initiate treatment with beta-blocker (atenolol 25 mg PO QD) to reduce BP (target <40/90); educate regarding potential adverse effects
• Reinforce lifestyle modifications; emphasize importance of proper diet and exercise for weight reduction and of limiting ETOH consumption for the management of hypertension as well as hyperuricemia
• Schedule follow-up visit for BP check within 4 weeks

Problem 3: Hypokalemia

- Discontinue hydrochlorothiazide as stated in problem 1
- Recommend an increase in dietary potassium, preferably from food sources such as fresh fruits and vegetables
- DW currently asymptomatic; counsel on the symptoms suggestive of hypokalemia (i.e., muscle weakness)
- Check K^+ level during the follow-up visit for BP check; provide further recommendations, if necessary

ANSWERS

1. b. Hydrochlorothiazide therapy
2. The signs and symptoms of an acute gout attack present in DW are:
   a. Excruciating pain in left big toe which became red, swollen, and hot after a few hours
   b. Recall of past less intense episodes of pain in same toe
   c. WBC 12.0 (12,000)
   d. ESR 55 (55)
   e. Uric acid 530 (8.9)
   f. T 38.8°C
   g. Synovial fluid aspirate (left metatarsophalangeal joint): cloudy, protein WNL, glucose WNL, Gram stain (−), leukocyte count 19.5×10^9/L (predominance of PMNs), needle-shaped crystals (approximately 5 μm in length)
3. c. Monosodium urate
4. d. Tophus
5. b. Overproduction
6. a. Vitamin C intake
7. c. Colchicine possesses analgesic activity
8. Adverse effects associated with colchicine therapy are:
   a. GI effects (i.e., nausea, vomiting, or diarrhea)
   b. Rarely, bone marrow depression
   c. Rarely, loss of body and scalp hair, rashes, peripheral neuropathy, myopathy, vesicular dermatitis, anuria, renal damage, or hematuria with prolonged administration
   d. Increased serum alkaline phosphatase
9. Indomethacin would not be a good choice for treatment of acute gout in DW because:
   a. Possibility of cross-reactivity in aspirin allergic patient
   b. May increase sodium and water retention, adversely affecting hypertension
10. d. Allopurinol
11. a. Pruritic maculopapular rash
12. Pharmacoeconomic considerations relative to DW's plan of care may include:
    1. Direct medical
       a. Treatment and complications
          - Drug costs–colchicine, atenolol
          - Adverse events–treatment
       b. Use of health resources
          - Costs of medical care, laboratory monitoring
    2. Direct nonmedical

a. Lost wages during acute gout attack
3. Indirect personal
   a. Activities of daily living, productivity
   b. Quality of life
4. Intangible personal
   a. Pain, suffering, emotional stressors
13. Key points are:
    a. Gout is characterized by hyperuricemia that results from an overproduction or an underexcretion of uric acid, or both.
    b. Progression of gout is variable and patient-dependent, but risk of debilitating chronic disease is decreased today as a result of effective treatments.
    c. Treatment with hypouricemic agents for long-term control should be based on careful patient assessment, as treatment is lifelong when deemed necessary.
    d. Occasional gout or asymptomatic hyperuricemia may not require drug treatment; modifications in diet and lifestyle may be sufficient to keep some patients symptom-free.

CASE 49

PROBLEM LIST

1. SLE Exacerbation
2. Lupus Nephritis/Chronic Renal Failure
3. Depression
4. Dry mouth

SOAP NOTE

S: "I have had a fever for the past 2 days and am having increasing fatigue, joint tenderness and swelling, chest pain, and some shortness of breath. My mouth has also been dry. Since I found out I have lupus, I have been feeling sad and discouraged and don't spend much time with my family or friends. I usually don't sleep too well at night."

O: Mild SOB; low-grade fever (T 38.2°C); joint swelling and tenderness at ankles, knees, wrists (warm to touch); malar rash; 15 pound weight loss; BP 150/90; thrombocytopenia, Plts 145×10^9 (145×10^3), and leukopenia, Lkcs 3.0×10^9 (3.0×10^3); Sed Rate 50; low serum calcium 1.95 (7.8); elevated phosphate 1.78 (5.5); slightly elevated uric acid 446.1 (7.5); Cr 221 (2.5 mg/dL); BUN 14 (40); ANA + (titer 1:480, rim fluorescent pattern); LE cell test +, anti-DNA antibodies +; anti-Sm +; decreased serum complement; urinalysis: 3+ protein, granular casts

A: **Problem 1:** SLE exacerbation with clinical manifestations of joint involvement, malar rash, pleurisy with mild dyspnea, fatigue, weight loss, renal, hematologic, and CNS complications

Problem 2: Lupus nephritis/chronic renal failure secondary to progression of SLE

Problem 3: Depression with insomnia: a psychiatric manifestation of SLE; hydroxychloroquine may also contribute to insomnia

Problem 4: Dry mouth possibly due to treatment with amitriptyline

P: Problem 1: SLE Exacerbation

- Continue hydroxychloroquine with appropriate monitoring for ocular toxicity; continue to conduct ophthalmic examinations (funduscopy, visual acuity, color tests) every 6 months
- Discontinue sulindac since NSAIDs may contribute to decreased renal perfusion
- Initiate corticosteroid therapy for SLE flare involving major organs such as the kidney and lung; administer methylprednisolone 10–30 mg/kg/day intravenously for 3–6 days, followed by oral prednisone 0.5–1 mg/kg/day for several weeks until symptoms relieved and laboratory parameters and clinical manifestations improved
- Once clinical manifestations have been sustained for at least 2 weeks, slowly taper prednisone over 6 months to a year as dictated by disease fluctuations
- Instruct to minimize exposure to direct sunlight or fluorescent light and to apply a sunscreen (SPF 15) that blocks both UVA and UVB radiation liberally QID or as needed
- Educate about the manifestations of SLE; discuss SLE educational programs and support groups with PS and family/friends
- Discuss importance of proper exercise and rest habits
- Review adverse effects of all medications and educate not to abruptly discontinue corticosteroid therapy

Problem 2: Lupus Nephritis/Chronic Renal Failure

- Initiate methylprednisolone IV 10–30 mg/kg/day for 3–6 days followed by oral prednisone 0.5–1 mg/kg/day for several weeks
- If no improvement seen with corticosteroids, immunosuppressive therapy (e.g., cyclophosphamide or azathioprine) may be added (allowing for reduction of prednisone dose when used in combination)
- Continue to monitor electrolyte abnormalities especially potassium, calcium, phospate, bicarbonate; monitor hemoglobin, hematocrit, and platelets
- Continue to monitor urine output
- Add calcium supplementation with calcium bicarbonate, 500 mg PO TID
- Restrict dietary phosphorus through reduction of foods high in phosphorus (i.e., meat, milk, legumes, and colas); a low-protein diet will also reduce phosphorus intake
- Monitor uric acid, which is currently slightly elevated and educate patient regarding symptoms associated with gout attacks
- Continue to monitor blood pressure (target <140/90) to prevent further progression of renal failure secondary to hypertension
- Educate about the severity of renal impairment and renal prognosis

Problem 3: Depression

- Contact prescribing physician regarding dry mouth secondary to amitriptyline therapy; recommend discontinuation of amitriptyline therapy and initiation of a selective serotonin reuptake inhibitor (SSRI)
- Specialist should reassess depression, as not adequately managed; encourage patient to continue psychological therapy with specialist
- Determine if PS and her family have been involved with support groups and offer services if not previously received information
- Discuss neuropsychiatric effects related to SLE as well as those due to medications such as corticosteroids and hydroxychloroquine, which both can cause insomnia
- Discuss proper sleep hygiene to decrease insomnia

Problem 4: Dry Mouth

- Discuss anticholinergic effects of amitriptyline, including dry mouth, and assess severity of the problem
- Contact prescribing physician regarding dry mouth and recommend an SSRI, which would produce fewer anticholinergic and cardiovascular effects than tricyclic antidepressants
- If dry mouth persists after discontinuation of amitriptyline or is accompanied by dry eyes, refer to physician to assess possible Sjogren's syndrome

ANSWERS

1. a. Anti-Sm antibodies
2. a. Inflammation
3. c. Oral ulcers
4. a. Acute cutaneous lupus erythematosus (ACLE)
5. d. Abrupt onset of symptoms
6. a. First-degree relative with SLE
7. Clinical, laboratory, and pathological findings of lupus nephritis and chronic renal failure present in PS are:
   1. Clinical findings
      a. Hypertension
   2. Laboratory findings

    a. Urinalysis—3+ proteinuria, granular casts

    b. Decreased serum complement

    c. Electrolyte abnormalities: low serum calcium level of 1.95 (7.8), elevated phosphate level of 1.78 (5.5), slightly elevated uric acid level of 446.1 (7.5)

    d. Serum creatinine level of 221 (2.5 mg/dL)

    e. BUN of 14 (40)

    f. Calculated creatinine clearance = 26.4 mL/min

  3. Pathological findings

    a. Positive anti-DNA antibodies

8. c. Rash

9. Adverse effects that may occur with antimalarial medications are:

    a. Gastrointestinal (epigastric burning, abdominal bloating, nausea, vomiting)

    b. Cutaneous lesions, pigment changes

    c. Neurological effects (headache, insomnia, nervousness)

    d. Neuromuscular syndrome (lower extremity muscle weakness, abnormal creatine kinase levels, abnormal muscle biopsy results)

    e. Ocular toxicity

10. b. Cyclophosphamide

11. Treatment goals for PS's SLE include:

    a. Relieve symptoms of the disease

    b. Slow or prevent the inflammatory response and subsequent tissue destruction

    c. Improve the overall quality of life for the patient

    d. Prolong survival

    e. Closely monitor for disease manifestations

    f. Avoid precipitating factors

    g. Educate about the manifestations of the disease and the side effects of drug therapy

12. An appropriate prednisone taper schedule for PS would be as follows:

    a. 20 mg PO QD for 2 weeks

    b. 17.5 mg PO QD for 3 weeks

    c. 15 mg PO QD for 4 weeks

    d. 15 mg alternating with 12.5 mg PO QD for 2–4 weeks

    e. 15 mg alternating with 10 mg PO QD for 2–4 weeks

    f. 15 mg alternating with 7.5 mg PO QD for 2–4 weeks

    g. 15 mg alternating with 5 mg PO QD for 2–4 weeks

    h. 15 mg alternating with 2.5 mg PO QD for 2–4 weeks

    i. 20 mg alternating with 0 mg PO QD for 4 weeks

    j. 17.5 mg alternating with 0 mg PO QD for 4 weeks

    k. 15 mg alternating with 0 mg PO QD for 4 weeks, etc.

    l. Schedule may take longer if disease exacerbations occur

13. Issues that should be addressed with PS related to SLE and pregnancy are:

  1. Effect of pregnancy on lupus activity (flares)

    a. 50–60% of pregnant patients experience flare, usually during third trimester

    b. Toxemia can be a maternal complication

  2. Impact of SLE on fetal outcome and premature delivery

    a. SLE activity during pregnancy can cause 12–30% more fetal loss and 20–50% more premature deliveries than in patients without lupus

  3. Use of medications for SLE in pregnant patients

    a. Most patients will need to maintain SLE medications during pregnancy

    b. Corticosteroids are considered the drugs of choice due to efficacy and relatively few adverse effects

    c. Data on use of antimalarials during pregnancy sparse (Pregnancy category C); doses of antimalarials used for SLE have been associated with a few case reports of congenital abnormalities with chloroquine appearing more teratogenic than hydroxychloroquine

    d. Despite the possible risk associated with the use of antimalarials in pregnancy, a patient with uncontrolled (active) lupus may have a greater chance of experiencing spontaneous abortion or neonatal death than teratogenic risk; therefore, a patient taking an antimalarial when she becomes pregnant should remain on the medication throughout pregnancy

    e. NSAIDs and aspirin are relatively safe (Pregnancy category B) during first and second trimesters, but considered harmful during third trimester (Pregnancy category D); restrict use to first trimester only and the lowest possible dose

    f. Immunosuppressant medications (azathioprine, cyclophosphamide) should be avoided if possible due to association with teratogenicity

    g. Patient should be advised to consult physician or pharmacist before taking any new OTC or herbal products

14. Issues the patient must address include:

    a. Reduced activity due to symptoms (fatigue, joint pain, chest pain, and dyspnea)

    b. Chronic medications and associated adverse effects

    c. Development of proper exercise and rest habits

Common emotional disorders presenting with SLE:

    a. Depression

    b. Anxiety

    c. Mania

    d. Psychoses

    e. Organic brain syndrome

    f. Psychosomatic complaints (insomnia, fatigue)

Other barriers:

    a. Family dynamics (small child to care for)

    b. Other stressors in life

    c. Financial resources may be limited, affecting ability to purchase medications

15. The health care provider's role relative to PS's proposed plan of care is:

    a. Individualize a plan for patient: both pharmacologic and nonpharmacologic

    b. Provide patient education regarding both disease state and drug therapy

    c. Provide positive reinforcement

    d. Referral

16. Pharmacoeconomic considerations relative to PS's plan of care may include:

  1. Direct medical

    a. Treatment and complications

- Drug costs–hydroxychloroquine, prednisone, calcium supplements, SSRI
- Adverse events–treatment, prophylaxis, laboratory monitoring
  b. Use of health resources
  - Costs of medical and psychological therapy
2. Direct nonmedical
  a. Travel, hotel, meals during hospitalization
  b. Lost wages
  c. Child care expenses
3. Indirect personal
  a. Activities of daily living, productivity, disability
  b. Quality of life
4. Intangible personal
  a. Pain, suffering, depression, emotional stressors
17. Key points are:
  a. Systemic lupus erythematosus is a chronic inflammatory disease involving many organ systems; the disease occurs primarily in black or Hispanic women under 40 years of age.
  b. The symptoms and prognosis for each patient are determined by the organs affected, with early involvement (<30 years) of the renal and central nervous systems being poor prognosticators. Common symptoms include joint and muscle pain, fatigue, fevers, and weight loss.
  c. Anti-inflammatory medications (NSAIDs and low-dose corticosteroids) and hydroxychloroquine are used to treat mild disease flare ups such as joint and muscle pain, fatigue, and rashes.
  d. High-dose corticosteroids, azathioprine, and cyclophosphamide are used to treat severe exacerbations involving the renal, cardiac, and central nervous systems. If patients are unresponsive or cannot tolerate these medications, cyclosporine and methotrexate can be utilized to suppress the inflammation associated with SLE.
  e. Laboratory values are used to assess disease activity or monitor drug toxicity. Common lab values monitored include the antinuclear antibody (ANA) test (increased with disease activity), double-stranded DNA antibodies (increased with disease activity), serum complement (CH_{50}, decreased with disease activity), serum creatinine (increased with disease activity and drug toxicity), and the complete blood cell count (CBC: RBC, Hgb, Hct, decreased with disease activity and drug toxicity).

CASE 50

PROBLEM LIST

1. Osteoporosis
2. Peptic Ulcer Disease
3. Chronic Alcoholism
4. Rheumatoid Arthritis
5. Anemia

SOAP NOTE

S: "I have had pain in my back for 2 days and increasing joint pain. My stomach hurts pretty often and antacids don't help."

O: Palpable liver, hepatomegaly; guaiac-negative stool; muscle atrophy in dorsal musculature and joint swelling of both hands; decreased hemoglobin 100 (10); low hematocrit 0.25 (25); decreased albumin 25 (2.5); low serum folate 9.064 (4); low Lkcs 3.0×10^9 (3.0×10^3) and Plts 100×10^9 (100×10^3); increased MCV 105 (105); *H. pylori* (−)

A: **Problem 1:** Osteoporosis with several risk factors (postmenopausal, history of hip fracture, chronic alcoholism, long-term corticosteroid therapy, and smoking)

Problem 2: Peptic ulcer disease (NSAID induced), currently on maintenance therapy with ranitidine and antacids PRN; alcohol use and smoking are likely contributing to ulcer disease

Problem 3: Chronic alcoholism with malnutrition and anemia

Problem 4: Rheumatoid arthritis for ten years; currently with joint pain

Problem 5: Anemia, macrocytic, secondary to alcoholism; peptic ulcer disease may also be contributory

P: **Problem 1: Osteoporosis**

- Evaluate current dietary calcium intake and initiate calcium supplementation with calcium carbonate (1500 mg/day elemental calcium) and vitamin D (400–800 IU PO QD)
- Recommend hormone replacement therapy (HRT); discuss benefits and risks of HRT; initiate HRT with estrogen 0.625 mg plus medroxyprogesterone 2.5 mg PO QD
- Discuss lifestyle changes including discontinuation of alcohol consumption, smoking cessation, and limiting caffeine intake
- Discuss options for weight-bearing exercise and modest weight training; emphasize a balance of rest and exercise, which is important for concomitant management of RA

Problem 2: Peptic Ulcer Disease (PUD)

- Increase ranitidine dose to 150 mg PO BID for 6 to 8 weeks, then return to maintenance dose of 150 mg PO QHS
- Discuss importance of discontinuation of alcohol and smoking
- Discontinue current antacid therapy as calcium carbonate is initiated for osteoporosis and H_2-antagonist dose increased

Problem 3: Chronic Alcoholism

- Counsel on the benefits of discontinuing alcohol consumption; discuss alcohol rehabilitation and management of withdrawal symptoms and recommend support groups for TF and family
- Monitor nutritional status; start daily multivitamin with iron, folic acid 1 mg PO QD to improve status and anemia
- Initiate thiamine 100 mg PO QD to prevent Wernicke's encephalopathy
- Monitor folate, hemoglobin, hematocrit, albumin, and vitamin B_{12} levels
- Discuss the role of alcohol in insomnia; discuss proper sleep hygiene

Problem 4: Rheumatoid Arthritis (RA)

- Continue prednisone, 5 mg PO QD
- Assess need for additional agent to control RA; evaluate options of second-line anti-rheumatic agents with careful consideration of risks and potential benefits of each agent
- Initiate trial of capsaicin cream to relieve pain associated with joint inflammation
- Educate about proper nutrition and importance of rest and exercise
- Refer to physical and occupational therapy

Problem 5: Anemia

- Initiate treatment with folic acid 1 mg PO QD in addition to daily multivitamin with iron
- Discontinue alcohol consumption
- Continue to monitor folate, hemoglobin, hematocrit, and MCV; increase in hematocrit should be seen within 2 weeks and return to normal within 2 months
- Discuss signs/symptoms of PUD-related bleeding; encourage to report if these occur

ANSWERS

1. d. Ranitidine therapy
2. c. Back pain
3. c. 20–50%
4. The mechanism of action of the pharmacologic and nonpharmacologic interventions employed in the treatment of osteoporosis in this case are:
   1. Pharmacologic interventions:
      a. Calcium—adequate intake essential for attaining peak bone mass and may affect the rate of bone loss; vital for adequate response to other antiosteoporotic agents
      b. Vitamin D—enhances gastrointestinal absorption of calcium; combined with calcium has been shown to decrease incidence of nonvertebral fractures in elderly
      c. Estrogen with progestin—preserves bone mineral density; increasing evidence that estrogen is beneficial for women greater than 10 years postmenopausal for

attenuation of further bone loss; progestin for patient with intact uterus to prevent endometrial tissue hyperplasia
   2. Nonpharmacologic interventions:
      a. Cessation of tobacco use abates osteoporosis risk/contributory factor
      b. Reduction or elimination of alcohol consumption; abate osteoporosis risk/contributory factor
      c. Weight-bearing exercise; minimize risk; protective factor
5. d. 1500 mg/day
6. a. Calcium carbonate
7. b. Calcitonin
8. c. Prednisone
9. a. Thromboembolism
10. Benefits of estrogen therapy other than prevention of osteoporosis that should be discussed with TF are:
    a. Relief from conditions associated with menopause (vasomotor symptoms, urogenital atrophy)
    b. Favorable effect on lipid profile
    c. Possible reduction in risk of dementia and colorectal cancer
11. b. Hydrochlorothiazide
12. Appropriate patient counseling points to address with a patient receiving alendronate are:
    a. Alendronate should be taken upon arising in the morning; tablet should be taken with 6–8 ounces of water, at least 30 minutes prior to ingestion of other foods, beverages, or other medications
    b. Patients should not lie down for 30 minutes after ingestion of alendronate due to risk of esophagitis
    c. Adequate calcium and vitamin D intake is necessary to assure optimal increases in bone mineral density
    d. Side effects that may occur with therapy are abdominal pain or distention, nausea, dyspepsia, constipation, flatulence, and dysphagia
    e. Alendronate should be used cautiously in patients with history of preexisting gastrointestinal problems
13. Pharmacoeconomic considerations relative to TF's plan of care may include:
    1. Direct medical
       a. Treatment and complications
          - Drug costs—calcium carbonate, vitamin D, HRT, ranitidine, folic acid, multivitamin/iron, thiamine, prednisone, capsaicin cream
          - Adverse events—treatment, prophylaxis, laboratory monitoring
       b. Use of health resources
          - Costs of medical, physical, or occupational therapy and alcohol rehabilitation
    2. Direct nonmedical
       a. Travel, hotel, meals in event of hospitalization
       b. Lost wages (daughter/caregiver)
    3. Indirect personal
       a. Activities of daily living, productivity, disability
       b. Quality of life
    4. Intangible personal
       a. Pain, suffering, emotional stressors
14. Key points are:

a. Osteoporosis is a disease characterized by loss of bone mass and is clinically silent until a fracture occurs.

b. As the population ages, there will be a significant increase in the number of persons at risk for osteoporotic fractures.

c. Preventive measures such as exercise and risk avoidance are key to maximizing bone mass and reducing risk of fractures.

d. Adequate calcium, through diet or supplementation, should be recommended for all patients.

e. Identification of patients at risk, through risk assessment and bone mineral density measurements, can lead to early intervention and decreased risk of fractures.

f. Patients on medications that may cause bone loss, such as glucocorticoids, should institute preventive measures and be monitored closely for the development of osteoporosis.

g. Estrogen therapy, with or without progestin supplementation, prevents postmenopausal bone loss and also provides possible benefits to the cardiovascular system, but risk of cancer may be increased in some patients.

h. Alendronate, a bisphosphonate, decreases the risk of fractures in women with established osteoporosis and prevents bone loss in nonosteoporotic postmenopausal women.

i. Raloxifene, a selective estrogen receptor modulator, maintains bone and possibly the cardiovascular benefits of estrogen, while minimizing its adverse effects on uterine and breast tissue.

j. In addition to decreasing bone resorption, calcitonin provides significant analgesic benefit for patients who have back pain caused by vertebral compression fractures.

SECTION 9 / RESPIRATORY DISEASES

CASE 51

PROBLEM LIST

1. Acute Exacerbation of Steroid-Dependent Asthma
2. Theophylline Toxicity
3. Cushingoid Signs and Symptoms and Adrenal Insufficiency

SOAP NOTE

S: "Prednisone was making me sick, and I stopped taking it 2 days ago. Then I started using my inhalers more often because I was short of breath, but inhalers just aren't working anymore. I also have difficulty sleeping, and sometimes have nausea, vomiting, and tiredness. After I was started on cimetidine my stomach got better."

O: SOB; BP 100/60 (sitting); BP 90/50 (standing); RR 27; HR 130; SCr 2.4; BUN 30; Na 125; K 5.9; Cl 94; cushingoid appearance; inspiratory/expiratory wheezing; 15% increase in FEV_1/FVC with β_2-agonist dose; oriented $\times$ 2, alert, but confused; abrupt discontinuation of prednisone; ECG shows atrial fibrillation that was stable before admission; theophylline level of 25 mg/L

A: Problem 1: Acute exacerbation of steroid-dependent asthma secondary to abrupt discontinuation of prednisone

Problem 2: Theophylline toxicity secondary to drug interaction with cimetidine via enzyme inhibition

Problem 3: Cushingoid signs and symptoms and adrenal insufficiency secondary to long-term treatment and abrupt discontinuation of prednisone

Problem 4: GERD possibly induced by erythromycin

P: Problem 1: Acute Exacerbation of Steroid-Dependent Asthma

- Start nebulized albuterol, 5–10 mg in 0.3 mL normal saline, followed by 2–5 mg in 0.3 mL normal saline every 20 minutes until symptoms improve
- Monitor arterial blood gases, chest examination, respiration rate, and breathing patterns to assess efficacy of nebulizer treatment
- Start methylprednisolone, 125 mg IV q8h
- Change IV steroid therapy to PO when appropriate; start prednisone, 20 mg PO QID with a slow taper (start with a decrease of 5 mg every 3 days and titrate to symptoms)
- Instruct on proper use of inhalers
- When acute symptoms resolved: albuterol, 2 puffs QID PRN; beclomethasone, 4 puffs QID

- Discontinue cromolyn and monitor response as an outpatient

Problem 2: Theophylline Toxicity

- Hold next theophylline dose (based on calculated pharmacokinetic parameters, theophylline half-life is 16.5 hours)
- Reevaluate use of theophylline
- Evaluate necessity for GERD therapy as discussed below; if theophylline and cimetidine therapy continued, reduce theophylline dose by 50%; alternatively, switch GERD therapy to ranitidine to reduce potential of interaction
- Monitor theophylline level after 2–3 days
- Monitor ECG, heart rate
- Continue to monitor theophylline level at clinic visits every 2 months when stable

Problem 3: Cushingoid Signs and Symptoms and Adrenal Insufficiency

- Taper steroid therapy as discussed above
- Monitor electrolytes, BUN, and SCr
- Initiate 0.9% normal saline and titrate to blood pressure and urine output
- Educate about adherence and signs and symptoms of disease exacerbation and adrenal insufficiency

Problem 4: GERD Possibly Induced by Erythromycin

- Consider trial discontinuation of erythromycin and therapy for GERD; may cause GERD symptoms; expect serum theophylline levels to decrease between 4–8 mg/L within 1 week
- If GERD symptoms decrease with these changes, discontinue GERD therapy and consider alternative antibiotic for coverage of *Streptococcus pneumoniae*, *Haemophilus influenzae*, or *Moraxella catarrhalis*

ANSWERS

1. b. Cimetidine drug interaction
2. BJ has been treated with prednisone, 20 mg daily (approximately equivalent to 80 mg of hydrocortisone) for a prolonged period of time. Hydrocortisone production is regulated by several feedback systems, both positive and negative. When amount of exogenous steroids exceeds the baseline production of endogenous hydrocortisone (approximately 30 mg) over a long-term period, the pituitary-adrenal axis shuts down due to negative feedback, and the body stops producing endogenous hydrocortisone.
   In turn, the pituitary-adrenal axis requires time to recuperate from exogenous steroid intake, so steroids are normally tapered to prevent the symptoms of adrenal insufficiency.
3. c. Cough
4. d. To reduce risk of side effects
5. The proper technique for metered-dose inhaler use is:
   a. Remove cap
   b. Shake canister
   c. Exhale (to functional residual capacity or fully if slow exhalation)
   d. Hold MDI upright and place lips around mouthpiece, or place mouthpiece ~2 inches or 2 fingerwidths from mouth, or place lips around spacer mouthpiece (if using a spacer device)
   e. Start to inhale slowly
   f. Actuate MDI while continuing to inhale
   g. Inhale completely and hold breath for 10 seconds (or at least 4–5 seconds)
   h. Wait 1 minute
   i. Repeat treatment (steps b–h) if more than one inhalation prescribed
   j. For inhaled steroids, rinse mouth with water or mouthwash and expel contents
6. c. Adrenal insufficiency
7. a. Hyperthyroidism
8. Pharmacoeconomic considerations relative to BJ's asthma management include:
   1. Direct costs
      a. Inpatient hospitalization
      b. Outpatient services
      c. Physician services
      d. Emergency room services
      e. Medications
   2. Indirect costs
      a. Lost school days
      b. Loss of outside employment or housekeeping productivity because of restricted activity or days spent in bed
      c. Mortality costs
9. b. Salmeterol MDI, 2 puffs BID PRN
10. d. After inhalation of corticosteroids, rinse mouth with water or mouthwash and expel contents
11. Psychosocial factors that may affect BJ's adherence to both pharmacologic and nonpharmacologic therapy are:
    1. Issues the patient must address
       a. Reduced activity due to symptoms
       b. Chronic medications
       c. Dietary restrictions
    2. Other barriers
       a. Depression
       b. Family dynamics—limited support system
       c. Limited financial resources
12. b. Respiratory distress
13. Key points for steroid-dependent asthma are:
    a. Prevent chronic and troublesome symptoms (e.g., coughing and breathlessness in the night, early morning, or after exertion)
    b. Maintain "normal" pulmonary function
    c. Maintain normal activity levels (including exercise and other physical activity)
    d. Prevent recurrent exacerbation of asthma and minimize the need for emergency department visits or hospitalizations
    e. Provide optimal pharmacotherapy with least amount of adverse effects

f. Meet patients' and families' expectations of and satisfaction with asthma care

CASE 52

PROBLEM LIST

1. Theophylline Toxicity
2. COPD
3. Hypertension
4. Angina
5. Hyperuricemia and Gout

SOAP NOTE

S: Complains of nausea, agitation, tremors, relatively new-onset chest pain on exertion, and recent anginal pain accompanied by palpitations; suffered first gouty attack 1 week ago

O: FEV_1/FVC is 35%; FEV_1 increased 200 mL after bronchodilator; theophylline level is 21 mg/L; BP 155/95; mild AV nicking on examination; uric acid 9.8

A: **Problem 1:** Theophylline toxicity secondary to smoking cessation

Problem 2: COPD has been controlled on current regimen

Problem 3: Hypertension was previously well controlled on hydrochlorothiazide; current high blood pressure reading possibly related to theophylline toxicity, noncompliance to drug therapy, or worsening disease

Problem 4: Angina secondary to insufficient control with isosorbide dinitrate, noncompliance to drug therapy, or worsening disease

Problem 5: Hyperuricemia secondary to hydrochlorothiazide therapy

P: **Problem 1: Theophylline Toxicity**
• Hold theophylline
• Reevaluate use of theophylline
• If theophylline therapy continued, check theophylline level within 2–3 days, decrease theophylline dose by 30%
• Monitor HR, ECG

Problem 2: COPD
• Discontinue albuterol
• Start ipratropium inhaler, 2 puffs QID
• Administer pneumococcal and *Haemophilus influenzae* vaccine
• Encourage continued abstinence from cigarettes

Problem 3: Hypertension
• Discontinue hydrochlorothiazide
• Start diltiazem CD, 120 mg PO QD; may titrate up as needed and tolerated
• Monitor blood pressure closely; goal is SBP below 140 mm Hg and DBP below 90 mm Hg
• Monitor pulse

Problem 4: Angina
• Continue isosorbide dinitrate, 30 mg PO TID
• Start diltiazem as above in treatment of hypertension
• Consult cardiology team
• Continue PRN use of SL nitroglycerin; educate about proper use of SL nitroglycerin

Problem 5: Hyperuricemia and Gout
• Discontinue hydrochlorothiazide and alcohol intake
• Recheck uric acid level in 3 months

ANSWERS

1. d. Ipratropium
2. b. Is recommended every fall for COPD patients
3. c. History of smoking
4. The effects of theophylline on the respiratory and cardiac systems include:
   1. Respiratory system:
      a. Bronchodilation
      b. Improved respiratory muscle contractility and reserve
      c. Stimulation of central ventilatory drive
      d. Increased mucociliary clearance
   2. Cardiac system:
      a. Decreased mean pulmonary artery pressure and pulmonary vascular resistance
      b. Increased collateral ventilation
      c. Improved biventricular cardiac performance
5. Goals of therapy for SB's COPD:
   a. Alter environmental influences
   b. Correct airflow obstruction
   c. Improve patient's functional status
   d. Prevent acute disease exacerbations
   e. Optimize drug therapy regimens
   f. Maintain adequate nutrition
6. a. Isosorbide dinitrate
7. d. Once open, the tablets have an expiration date of 1 month
8. c. Pharmacologic therapy with an appropriate agent is indicated
9. a. Congestive heart failure (CHF)
10. Psychosocial factors that may affect SB's adherence to both pharmacologic and nonpharmacologic therapy are:
    1. Patient issues
       a. Chronic medications
       b. Reduced activity due to symptoms
       c. Dietary restrictions

2. Other barriers
    a. Depression
    b. Limited financial resources
    c. Family dynamics–limited support system
11. The costs associated with COPD include:
    1. Direct costs
        a. Medications
        b. Emergency room services
        c. Inpatient hospitalization
        d. Outpatient services
        e. Physician services
    2. Indirect costs
        a. Lost school days
        b. Loss of outside employment or housekeeping productivity because of restricted activity or days spent in bed
        c. Mortality costs
12. Key points are:
    a. COPD is a potentially preventable disease
    b. Cessation of smoking would dramatically decrease its incidence. Public education about the hazards of smoking should continue.
    c. Once COPD develops, those affected with moderate-to-severe disease are faced with a multitude of drug therapies with clearly debatable efficacy.
    d. The progressive nature of disease means the cost to the patient, both personally and financially, and the cost to society is high.

CASE 55

PROBLEM LIST

1. COPD Exacerbation
2. Atrial Fibrillation
3. Hypokalemia
4. Congestive Heart Failure (CHF)
5. Hypertension

SOAP NOTE

S: "I woke up short of breath, wheezing, and coughing for the last several days. I also have tightness in my chest and palpitations that kept me awake. This morning my wife took my temperature, she said it was 102°F."

O: Confused and pale elderly male in acute respiratory distress, complaining of chest pain and palpitations; BP 145/94, HR 140, RR 26, T 39.9°C; + JVD, inspiratory and expiratory wheezing, rales, and rhonchi; hepatojugular reflux, hepatomegaly, 2+ pedal edema, A&O × 1; Na 134 (134), K 3.1 (3.1), Cl 95 (95), HCO$_3$ 20 (20), BUN 12 (35), SCr 213 (2.8), WBC 8.9 × 10^9 (8.9 × 10^3), Mg 1.1 (2.2); theophylline: 4 μg/mL, digoxin: 0.7 ng/mL;

prebronchodilator FEV$_1$: 1.5 L; postbronchodilator FEV$_1$: 2 L; ECG: irregularly irregular; ABG: pH 7.4, PO$_2$ 52, PCO$_2$ 50

A: **Problem 1:** COPD exacerbation secondary to inadequate use of inhaler, recent addition of beta-blocker, and/or a subtherapeutic theophylline level

Problem 2: Atrial fibrillation possibly due to hypoxia, hypokalemia, nonadherence to therapy, insufficient control with monotherapy with digoxin, or worsening disease state

Problem 3: Hypokalemia possibly secondary to hydrochlorothiazide

Problem 4: Worsening of congestive heart failure possibly secondary to nonadherence to drug therapy, worsening of disease state, or inadequate dosage

Problem 5: Uncontrolled hypertension secondary to nonadherence to drug therapy, worsening of disease state, or inadequate dosage

P: **Problem 1: COPD Exacerbation**

- Start metaproterenol 0.2–0.3 mL in 2.5 mL of normal saline solution with nebulizer; after adequate response achieved, restart MDI with spacer
- Start ipratropium inhaler
- Reassess the need for theophylline; if indicated, reload with 375 mg aminophylline or 300 mg PO IR theophylline to achieve therapeutic level
- Increase maintenance theophylline dose to 300 mg BID and monitor theophylline level
- Instruct on proper use of inhalers; educate regarding importance of adherence to her therapy
- Stress importance of smoking cessation

Problem 2: Atrial Fibrillation

- Correct hypoxia and hypokalemia as stated in problems 1 and 2, respectively
- Discontinue digoxin and monitor heart rate
- Start warfarin, with INR goal of 2–3 to prepare for cardioversion, if necessary

Problem 3: Hypokalemia

- Give bolus KCl, 40 mEq IV over 4 hours
- Start daily potassium supplementation, 20–40 mEq/day; monitor for increases following changes in CHF therapy, below

Problem 4: Congestive Heart Failure

- Discontinue hydrochlorothiazide
- Start furosemide 20–40 mg PO daily
- Begin enalapril as addressed below; goal for reducing CHF mortality is 5–20 mg QD to BID
- Consider spironolactone and beta-blocker use

- Monitor weight and adjust furosemide dose for adequate diuresis
- Monitor electrolytes
- Discontinue effervescent aspirin tablet

Problem 5: Hypertension

- Start enalapril at 2.5 mg PO BID and titrate to response and as tolerated; goal: SBP below 140 and DBP below 90

ANSWERS

1. b. 5–15 μg/mL
2. c. Decreased liver function
3. d. Contains high sodium content, which should be avoided in patients with hypertension and congestive heart failure
4. The mechanisms of action of the pharmacologic and nonpharmacologic interventions in this case are:
   1. Pharmacologic interventions
      a. Hydrochlorothiazide inhibits sodium reabsorption in the distal tubules, causing increased excretion of sodium and water as well as potassium and hydrogen ions
      b. Nadolol competitively blocks response to β_1- and β_2-adrenergic stimulation
      c. Theophylline has a bronchodilator effect via inhibition of phosphodiesterase
      d. Albuterol relaxes bronchial smooth muscle by action on β_2-receptors
      e. Digoxin has indirect inotropic effect through inhibition in the transport enzyme Na^+-K^+ ATPase, leading to increased intracellular Ca^{+2}–ultimately enhancing myocardial contractility; parasympathomimetic; neurohormonal; decrease plasma renin activity
   2. Nonpharmacologic interventions
      a. Sodium-restricted diet
      b. Adherence to medications
5. b. Tachycardia
6. a. Hospital stay less than 48 hours
7. c. If patient remains hypokalemic, hypomagnesemia cannot be corrected
8. Pharmacologic and nonpharmacologic treatment problem(s) present in MM's treatment plan are:
   1. Pharmacologic

   a. Insufficient theophylline dosing or noncompliance by MM
   b. Hydrochlorothiazide-induced hypokalemia
   c. Alka-Seltzer-induced hypertension
   d. Insufficient dosing for blood pressure medication
   e. Nadolol-induced exacerbation of COPD and CHF
   2. Nonpharmacologic
      a. Lack of proper MDI and spacer device use
9. c. That he requires nursing home services
10. Psychosocial factors that may affect MM's adherence to both pharmacologic and nonpharmacologic therapy are:
    1. Patient issues
       a. Chronic medications
       b. Reduced activity due to symptoms
       c. Dietary restrictions
    2. Other barriers
       a. Depression
       b. Limited financial resources
       c. Family dynamics–limited support system
11. Costs associated with COPD include:
    1. Direct costs
       a. Medications
       b. Emergency room services
       c. Inpatient hospitalization
       d. Outpatient services
       e. Physician services
    2. Indirect costs
       a. Lost school days
       b. Loss of outside employment or housekeeping productivity because of restricted activity or days spent in bed
       c. Mortality cost
12. Key points are:
    a. COPD is a potentially preventable disease
    b. Cessation of smoking would dramatically decrease COPD incidence; public education about the hazards of smoking should continue
    c. Once COPD develops, those affected with moderate-to-severe disease are faced with a multitude of drug therapies with debatable efficacy
    d. The progressive nature of disease means the cost to the patient and to society is high, both humanistically and financially

SECTION 10 / CARDIOVASCULAR DISORDERS

CASE 56

PROBLEM LIST

1. Warfarin Toxicity
2. Atrial Fibrillation
3. Gastroesophageal Reflux Disorder/Heartburn

SOAP NOTE

S: Complains of palpitations and weakness; has had three nosebleeds in the last week; abdominal discomfort and lack of appetite; currently not complaining of any symptoms of heartburn

O: Irregularly irregular HR of 125 bpm, atrial

enlargement, and electrocardiographic evidence supporting the diagnosis of atrial fibrillation, with rapid ventricular rate. INR of 3.9 and bruising on the arms and knees; elevated respiratory rate (25/min); history of heartburn at night, symptoms currently controlled

A: Problem 1: Warfarin toxicity secondary to cimetidine *and/or* recent ethanol abuse. Use of an alternative H$_2$-antagonist such as ranitidine or famotidine with less potential for drug interactions is desirable.

Problem 2: Afib (not in NSR) with a rapid ventricular response; maintained in NSR for 3 years on procainamide therapy, rate effectively controlled with digoxin. Recent ethanol and pseudoephedrine use for the patient's cold may be the reason for the recent exacerbation. Noncompliance with procainamide due to recent heavy alcohol use could also be a contributing factor.

Problem 3: GERD symptoms appear to be well controlled. Use of an alternative H$_2$-antagonist such as ranitidine or famotidine with less potential for drug interactions is desirable.

P: Problem 1: Warfarin Toxicity

- Hold warfarin for 2–3 days, repeat INR, if INR <2.0, then restart at 6 mg PO QD; well controlled on this dose previously
- Reassess INR within the following 5–7 days
- Goals of therapy: INR between 2–3 (for atrial fibrillation) and prevention of any further episodes of bleeding
- Counsel to eat a steady diet of vitamin K-containing foods and avoid OTC medications without consulting with his health care provider
- Although warfarin is the antithrombotic drug of choice in patients greater than 65 years of age, aspirin is an alternative agent in individuals who are at risk for warfarin-induced bleeding
- If this patient continues to abuse alcohol, use aspirin rather than warfarin

Problem 2: Atrial Fibrillation

- Goals of therapy are to maintain ventricular response <100 bpm, maintain NSR, and provide effective anticoagulation (goal INR 2–3)
- See Problem 1 for warfarin management
- Discontinue OTC pseudoephedrine as cold resolved. Instruct to avoid OTC medications without first contacting his health care provider
- Reeducate the patient to avoid ethanol use and the need for a continuing support group
- If after 1 week the patient's rate is not controlled on digoxin, consider an alternative (beta-blocker, diltiazem or verapamil) instead of digoxin for rate control
- If digoxin is continued, monitor for toxicity since the serum concentration is at the upper portion of

the "therapeutic range" and thus at greater risk for toxicity
- Continue procainamide SR; maintained NSR for 3 years prior to recent exacerbation
- Monitor for signs/symptoms of procainamide toxicity such as drug-induced lupus erythematosus syndrome, GI side effects, and rash

Problem 3: GERD

- Discontinue cimetidine therapy and use alternative GERD regimen. Alternatives are OTC H$_2$-antagonist (except cimetidine) or antacid therapy
- Suggested alternative: famotidine 10 mg PRN

ANSWERS

1. d. Addition of pseudoephedrine therapy
2. c. Bruising on arms and legs
3. d. Elevated INR
4. b. Atenolol
5. c. Drug-induced lupus erythematosus syndrome
6. The target INR values for the following conditions in patients receiving anticoagulation therapy with warfarin is:
   a. Non-rheumatic atrial fibrillation: 2.0–3.0
   b. Mechanical prosthetic heart valves: 2.5–3.5
   c. Treatment of deep vein thrombosis: 2.0–3.0
7. d. ESR
8. c. Cholestyramine
9. a. Amiodarone
10. The pharmacologic and nonpharmacologic treatment problems present in this patient's treatment plan include:
    1. Pharmacologic
       a. OTC cimetidine/warfarin potential interaction
       b. Possible excessive warfarin use by the patient
       c. Pseudoephedrine-induced atrial fibrillation
    2. Nonpharmacologic (assuming alcohol is non-pharmacologic)
       a. Ethanol-induced atrial fibrillation
       b. Ethanol-induced INR elevation
       c. Maintenance of "steady" diet without any major changes
11. Alcoholism is the major psychosocial factor that affects the adherence to pharmacologic therapy in this patient. The underlying problems related to this patient's recent binge drinking (death of a close friend) must be addressed. If the patient's alcohol use continues, an alternative antithrombotic therapy must be considered.
12. Pharmacoeconomic considerations relative to this patient's atrial fibrillation plan of care may include:
    1. Costs of chronic atrial fibrillation treatment
       a. Direct medical
          - Drug costs
          - Health care provider costs
    2. Costs of atrial fibrillation (uncontrolled) to patients and families (i.e., hospitalizations)
       a. Direct medical
          - Hospital personnel and overhead
          - Treatment and complications
       b. Direct nonmedical
          - Travel, hotels, meals
          - Lost wages (family/patient)

   c. Indirect personal
     • Decreased productivity
     • Quality of life
   d. Intangible personal
     • Suffering
13. Key points:
   a. Atrial fibrillation is the most common sustained arrhythmia. It affects approximately 2–4% of patients over the age of 60.
   b. The goals of therapy for atrial fibrillation are to maintain ventricular response <100 bpm, convert to and maintain NSR (if possible) and provide effective anticoagulation (goal INR 2–3).
   c. Avoid drugs and/or conditions that may predispose to the development of an atrial fibrillation recurrence.
   d. Rate control is accomplished utilizing beta-blockers, calcium channel blockers (diltiazem and verapamil), and digoxin.
   e. After initial rate control (during an acute episode), pharmacologic or electrical methods may be used for conversion to normal sinus rhythm, in the appropriate patients.
   f. If conversion to normal sinus rhythm is successful, maintenance therapy of normal sinus rhythm is initiated. In patients with chronic atrial fibrillation effective anticoagulation (warfarin: goal INR 2–3) should be utilized. In certain situations (low-risk patients, patients at risk from warfarin therapy, etc.) aspirin therapy may be utilized.

CASE 58

PROBLEM LIST

1. Atrial Fibrillation (Afib)
2. Hypertension (HTN)
3. Hyperlipidemia

SOAP NOTE

S: Patient complains of dizziness, SOB, palpitations

O: BP 145/90, HR 146, pulse irregularly irregular, ECG: Afib, history of HTN for 20 years, mild AV nicking, mild LVH; total cholesterol 240 mg/dL, LDL-C 170 mg/dL, HDL-C 34 mg/dL, TG 180 mg/dL

A: Problem 1: Atrial fibrillation: Potential causes are history of childhood rheumatic heart disease and 20-year history of HTN; on echocardiogram, the atria are enlarged, and mild hypertrophy of the left ventricle is noted; symptoms of Afib for at least 2 days; no thrombi observed on the transthoracic echocardiogram.

Problem 2: Hypertension: Reasonably well controlled (current 145/90 mm Hg, previous clinic visit BP 145/85 mm Hg); control imperative, because end-organ damage present (AV nicking, LVH), and the risk for coronary artery disease must be decreased.

Problem 3: Hyperlipidemia: Two risk factors are present for development of coronary artery disease (HTN, age [male >45], HDL <34); claims adherence to step II diet for 2 years; based on NCEP ATP II treatment guidelines and randomized trials, drug therapy is needed with a goal LDL-C concentration of <130 mg/dL (percent reduction in LDL needed is ~24%). Gemfibrozil as primary prevention in a patient with normal TGs not recommended.

P: Problem 1: Atrial Fibrillation

• Digoxin is not a good choice for rate control due to palpitations during exercise
• Start either IV verapamil (5–10 mg IV over 2–3 min, repeated in 30 min if needed and 5 mg/hr infusion titrated to ventricular rate <100 beats/min and SBP >90 mm Hg) or diltiazem (0.25 mg/kg IV over 2 minutes followed by 0.35 mg/kg in 15 min if needed) to control ventricular rate
• Plan cardioversion (either direct current or chemical cardioversion) in 3 weeks
• Initiate anticoagulation with warfarin for 3 weeks before and 4 weeks after conversion to NSR; goal INR is 2–3
• Alternative to anticoagulation and conversion in 3 weeks in selected patients is transesophageal echocardiography to determine if an atrial thrombus is present with immediate cardioversion if no thrombus present
• Educate regarding warfarin use and adverse effects associated with the drug

Problem 2: Hypertension

• Continue lisinopril
• Start diltiazem or verapamil IV as above with conversion to oral dose that controls the ventricular rate and blood pressure
• Once oral daily dose is established, assess need for multiple drugs for hypertension
• Consider D/C of lisinopril if blood pressure can be controlled with calcium channel blocker (CCB) alone
• Since an additional drug, CCB, is being utilized to treat atrial fibrillation, D/C furosemide if additional HTN therapy needed in the future, consider hydrocholorothiazide

Problem 3: Hyperlipidemia

• Discontinue gemfibrozil
• Start pravastatin 20 mg daily in the evening, titrate upward to 40 mg daily
• Educate about the most common adverse effects of

pravastatin: GI related, such as diarrhea, nausea, vomiting, and flatulence
- Counsel patient to report muscle pain, tenderness, or weakness, especially if accompanied by fever or malaise
- Follow up in 4–6 weeks with lipoprotein analysis and liver function testing
- Continue step II diet

ANSWERS

1. b. History of rheumatic heart disease
2. a. Digoxin
3. b. AV nicking
4. b. <30% of total calories from fat, ≤7% of total calories from saturated fat and <200 mg cholesterol/day.
5. c. D/C gemfibrozil and initiate fluvastatin therapy
6. c. Three weeks
7. b. Continue lisinopril and D/C furosemide
8. Adverse effects associated with chronic verapamil therapy for rate control in atrial fibrillation include:
   a. Reduced myocardial contractility: heart failure
   b. AV/SA nodal conduction disturbances: bradycardia and atrioventricular block
   c. Hypotension, flushing, headache, dizziness, edema, constipation
9. d. Phytadione
10. The nonpharmacologic treatment problems present in this patient's treatment plan include:
    a. Maintenance of Step II diet to enhance drug efficacy
    b. Exercise-induced atrial fibrillation (this should be minimized with appropriate selection of drug therapy for rate control)
11. Psychosocial factors that may affect this patient's adherence to both pharmacologic and nonpharmacologic therapy include:
    a. Exercise-induced atrial fibrillation. If this patient continues to experience exercise-induced atrial fibrillation, he may choose to discontinue his exercise program.
    b. Discontinuing his exercise program may have an adverse effect on the management of this patient's hypertension and hyperlipidemia. Providing appropriate treatment will minimize these episodes of atrial fibrillation.
12. Pharmacoeconomic considerations relative to this patient's hypertension plan of care may include:
    1. Direct medical
       a. Drug costs
       b. Health Care Provider costs
13. Key points are:
    a. Hypertension is a very common condition affecting approximately 50 million Americans.
    b. Untreated or undertreated hypertension is a major risk factor for the development of coronary artery disease.
    c. Lifestyle modifications should be initiated in this patient to reduce the risk of the development of cardiovascular disease.

d. The goal of hypertension therapy in this patient is to reduce and maintain blood pressure less than 140/90 mm Hg with lifestyle modifications and drug therapy.
e. Since this patient has atrial fibrillation, drugs that manage both atrial fibrillation and hypertension are preferred. Avoid drugs and/or conditions that may predispose to the development of an atrial fibrillation occurrence.

CASE 59

PROBLEM LIST

1. Acute Ischemic Stroke
2. Atrial Fibrillation with Rapid Ventricular Response
3. Hypothyroidism (Overmedicated with Levothyroxine)
4. Osteoarthritis
5. Osteoporosis

SOAP NOTE

S: MB is unable to respond to questions and cannot give history because of stroke.

O: Lethargic, weak-appearing elderly female unable to speak, respond to questions, or walk; ECG: Afib, ventricular rate 115; HR 110 (irregular); finger and hand deformities, increased ESR, thin hair, patches of baldness; TT_4 150 (12), TSH 3 (3), RT_3U 0.3 (30), FT_4 index 3.6

A: Problem 1: Acute stroke: Probable cardioembolic cerebrovascular accident (CVA) secondary to Afib. Based on ACCP guidelines thrombolytic therapy is not recommended.

Problem 2: Atrial fibrillation with rapid ventricular response: Afib since 1990 with no anticoagulation; likely due to excessive thyroid hormone therapy and/or recent viral infection; large left-ventricular thrombus noted on echocardiogram.

Problem 3: Hypothyroidism: Overmedicated with levothyroxine; appropriate dosage approximately 1 to 2 μg/kg (average 1.7 μg/kg).

Problem 4: Osteoarthritis: Caution must be exercised with the concomitant use of NSAID therapy for osteoarthritis and anticoagulation therapy needed for atrial fibrillation and cardioembolic stroke; likely to benefit from analgesic therapy with acetaminophen.

Problem 5: Osteoporosis: Currently receiving estrogen replacement therapy and calcium carbonate therapy; bone-density and x-ray (DEXA) testing needed to assess the severity of bone loss associated with osteoporosis and effectiveness of current therapy.

P: **Problem 1: Acute Stroke**
- Diagnosis confirmed as an embolic stroke, anticoagulant therapy indicated
- Baseline CBC, platelet count, and aPTT (for control)
- Initiate heparin therapy with a bolus dose of 75–80 U/kg (4350–4640 U). Initiate a continuous infusion of heparin 15–20 U/kg/hr (870–1160 U/hr). The infusion should be started at the lower range due to the increased risk of bleeding.
- Goal aPTT 1.5–2.5 times control and should first be evaluated 6 hours after the bolus dose and infusion adjusted accordingly
- Monitor for bleeding and appropriate laboratory studies (e.g., CBC, platelets, stool guaiac, urinalysis) daily for the first few days and every other day thereafter
- Warfarin therapy should be started on the first day with a maintenance dose of 4–5 mg/day; goal INR 2.0–3.0
- Heparin and warfarin therapy should overlap for 4–5 days and a therapeutic INR obtained on 2 consecutive days before the heparin is discontinued
- Hyperthyroidism potentiates warfarin effects by accelerating the clearance of the vitamin K-dependent clotting factors without influencing the pharmacokinetics of warfarin. Warfarin dosing requirements may be reduced once patient thyroxine concentrations return to "normal."

Problem 2: Atrial Fibrillation with Rapid Ventricular Response
- D/C digoxin and start atenolol, 25 mg daily, titrating to keep heart rate <100 bpm
- Reassess the need for rate control when levothyroxine dose is optimized
- Chronic anticoagulation to reduce the risk of recurrent embolic events

Problem 3: Hypothyroidism (Excessive Levothyroxine for Treatment of Hypothyroidism)
- Hold levothyroxine for 1 week, restart at 0.1 mg/day PO
- Reevaluate thyroid function test results in 4–6 weeks.

Problem 4: Osteoarthritis
- D/C naproxen 375 BID
- Initiate acetaminophen 650 mg q4h PRN for osteoarthritis

Problem 5: Osteoporosis
- The risk and benefits of estrogen replacement therapy (ERT) must be evaluated in the setting of a CVA

- Assess the need to ERT based on appropriate bone density and x-ray studies
- Increase calcium carbonate dose to 1500 mg/day and add 600–800 units of vitamin D PO daily
- Separate administration of calcium and thyroid preparations

ANSWERS

1. d. Aphasia
2. b. Lethargic
3. a. Protein binding displacement of warfarin from albumin, resulting in transient increases in warfarin effect (i.e., increased INR)
4. c. D/C naproxen, start APAP 650 mg PO q6h
5. a. Hyperthyroidism
6. c. The time since the onset of her symptoms is uncertain
7. a. Warfarin 5 mg for 3 days, adjust based on INR goal of 2–3
8. b. Platelets, Hgb/Hct, aPTT
9. The nonpharmacologic treatment problems present in this patient's treatment plan include:
   1. Outpatient
      a. Post-CVA rehabilitation (physical, emotional barriers that arise)
      b. Dietary considerations for warfarin therapy
10. Psychosocial factors that may affect this patient's adherence to both pharmacologic and nonpharmacologic therapy:
    a. The most important factor in determining patient's ability to adhere to treatment plan is the extent of recovery from current stroke. Significant rehabilitation will likely be needed and recovery will affect ability to take medications properly. Recovery will determine the extent of chronic care required.
    b. Physical and emotional support systems that will be necessary depending on the degree of recovery from the CVA.
11. Key points are:
    a. Atrial fibrillation is the most common sustained arrhythmia which affects approximately 2–4% of patients over the age of 60.
    b. The goals of therapy for atrial fibrillation are to maintain ventricular response <100 bpm, convert to and maintain NSR (if possible) and provide effective anticoagulation (goal INR 2–3).
    c. Avoid drugs and/or conditions that may predispose to the development of an atrial fibrillation recurrence.
    d. Rate control is accomplished utilizing beta-blockers, calcium channel blockers (diltiazem and verapamil), and/or digoxin.
    e. After initial rate control (during an acute episode), pharmacologic or electrical methods may be used for conversion to normal sinus rhythm, in the appropriate patients.
    f. If conversion to normal sinus rhythm is successful, maintenance therapy with anti-arrhythmics of normal sinus rhythm is initiated

g. In patients with chronic atrial fibrillation effective anticoagulation (warfarin: goal INR 2–3) should be utilized. If certain situations (low-risk patients, patients at risk from warfarin therapy) aspirin therapy may be utilized.

12. Alendronate must be taken at least 30 minutes before the first food, beverage, or medication of the day, with plain water only. Other foods and beverages will likely decrease the bioavailability of the drug. To enhance delivery of the drug to the stomach patients should be advised not to lie down for at least 30 minutes after the dose.

13. Pharmacoeconomic considerations relative to this patient's atrial fibrillation plan of care may include:
   1. Costs of chronic atrial fibrillation treatment
      a. Direct medical
         • Drug costs
         • Health care provider costs
   2. Costs of atrial fibrillation (uncontrolled) to patients and families (i.e., hospitalizations)
      a. Direct medical
         • Hospital personnel and overhead
         • Treatment and complications
      b. Direct nonmedical
         • Travel, hotels, meals
         • Lost wages (family/patient)
      c. Indirect personal
         • Decreased productivity
         • Quality of life
      d. Intangible personal
         • Suffering

CASE 60

PROBLEM LIST

1. Hypertension
2. Anticoagulation for Mitral Valve Replacement
3. Hyperlipidemia
4. Type 1 DM

SOAP NOTE

S: Complains of increasing headaches over the last 2 weeks. States noncompliance with cholesterol-lowering and low-sodium diet. Has noted blood spots on tissue after bowel movements for the past 2 days. Describes rectal bleeding but denies any blood in urine or any other signs or symptoms of bleeding. Complaining of polyuria, polydipsia, and general weakness. Has not tested his blood glucose for 1 week and states that his regular insulin is cloudy.

O: BP 190/98, AV nicking; small external hemorrhoid; INR 4.9, Hgb 142 (14.2); last visit 141 (14.1), Hct 0.34 (34), TC 7.2 (280), TG 3.6 (280), LDL 186, HDL 30, fasting blood glucose 22.2 (400), HbA$_{1C}$ 13.5, urine glucose 2+

A: **Problem 1:** Hypertension: As described above, has multiple risk factors for development of coronary artery disease (hypertension, hyperlipidemia, diabetes mellitus, and smoking). Has Stage 3 hypertension and JNC VI recommendations suggest blood pressure lowering should be more aggressive in diabetic patients with a goal of <130/85.

Problem 2: Anticoagulation for mitral valve replacement: Has an excessive INR on current warfarin regimen (Goal INR 2.5–3.5) Anticoagulation for mechanical valve replacement required for life. Dark stools could be a result of melena and/or from the FeSO$_4$. Blood on tissue secondary to hemorrhoid and/or rectal bleeding.

Problem 3: Hyperlipidemia: Patient has multiple risk factors for the development of coronary artery disease, including: diabetes mellitus, smoking, low HDL, high LDL, and hypertension. LDL cholesterol and TG are elevated. Will likely improve somewhat with effective glycemic control. Based on NCEP guidelines, goals for LDL lowering and TG lowering are: <130 mg/dL and 200 mg/dL respectively. The ADA goals for LDL lowering are <100 mg/dL. Has failed dietary therapy for hyperlipidemia.

Problem 4: Type 1 DM: Uncontrolled diabetes, even though compliant with insulin injections. Mixes his insulin and since regular is now whitish (cloudy), regular insulin has become contaminated.

P: **Problem 1: Hypertension**
   • Continue lifestyle modifications and stress medication and dietary compliance
   • Educate on the importance of smoking cessation and recommend treatment approaches (nicotine replacement, counseling, etc.) if necessary
   • JNC VI guidelines recommend ACEI therapy in patients with diabetes to prevent or slow the progression of diabetic nephropathy
   • Start enalapril 5 mg PO daily. Titrate to response (ultimate goal <130/85 mm Hg) up to 40 mg/day in single or divided doses
   • Assess potassium concentrations, systolic and diastolic blood pressure, BUN, and serum creatinine at the next visit (within 1 week)
   • Encourage patient to report any persistent cough, rash, or signs of infection (e.g., fever, sore throat) and to not use salt substitutes or potassium supplements unless recommended by health care provider

Problem 2: Anticoagulation for Mitral Valve Replacement

- Hold warfarin dosing for 2–3 days, repeat INR and if <3.5, then restart warfarin 5 mg PO on Saturday and Sunday alternating with 7.5 mg PO Monday–Friday, to a target INR of 2.5–3.5.
- Recheck INR in 7 days and adjust dose accordingly based on the INR
- Provide education: examine all sites (urine, stool, mouth, etc.) regularly for bleeding, avoid aspirin or aspirin-containing medications, notify health care professionals when starting a new medication in order to avoid any drug interactions or bleeding, don't double up on warfarin if a dose is missed, do not abruptly change dietary habits.
- Monitor hemoglobin concentrations, hematocrit, and stool guaiac test results for blood loss.
- Due to the potential for gastric bleeding secondary to ASA or NSAID use, discontinue ibuprofen and instruct to take acetaminophen for headaches. Caution against excessive analgesic use.

Problem 3: Hypercholesterolemia

- Provide dietary advice and refer to dietician related to the importance of following a Step II diet/ADA diet
- LDL-C lowering required: 46%; TG lowering required: 38%
- Begin HMG CoA reductase inhibitor therapy. Choose an agent that will reduce LDL-C by the 46% required, however the effect on TG more variable. More effective diabetes control may help to lower TG concentrations.
- Begin simvastatin 20–40 mg PO daily at bedtime or atorvastatin 20 mg PO daily
- Educate on the most common adverse effects of simvastatin: GI related, such as diarrhea, nausea, vomiting, and flatulence.
- Counsel to report muscle pain, tenderness, or weakness, especially if accompanied by fever or malaise.
- Follow up in 4–6 weeks with lipoprotein analysis and liver function testing.

Problem 4: Type 1 DM

- Teach proper mixing technique to prevent contamination of regular insulin. Replace contaminated regular insulin.
- Continue with old regimen due to effective long-term control before this problem. Monitor blood glucose concentrations with goal of 4.4 and 7.02 (80 and 126) and HbA_{1C} <7.

- Treat hyperglycemia with insulin therapy acutely.
- Monitor for fatigue, signs and symptoms of hypoglycemia (irritability, difficulty concentrating, hunger, tremors, sweating, or tachycardia), or hyperglycemia (polyuria, dyspnea, or blurred vision).

ANSWERS

1. c. D/C enalapril and initiate diltiazem therapy
2. b. Renal disease
3. a. Atenolol
4. c. HbA_{1C}
5. d. NSAID-induced gastritis
6. d. Diltiazem
7. b. Hydralazine
8. c. <130/85 mm Hg
9. a. <100 mg/dL
10. The nonpharmacologic treatment for this patient's hypertension and dyslipidemia includes:
    a. Restriction of sodium to less than 100 mmol daily (6 g of sodium chloride or 2.4 g sodium)
    b. The JNC recommends that all overweight hypertensive patients (body mass index of 27 or greater) should lose weight
    c. Dietary therapy (Step I diet, DASH diet, ADA diet in this patient)
    d. Regular aerobic physical activity achieving a moderate level of physical fitness
    e. Smoking cessation
    f. Alcohol ingestion should be no greater than the equivalent of two beers/day
11. The risk factors for the patient developing cardiovascular disease
    a. Hypertension
    b. Hyperlipidemia
    c. Diabetes
    d. Smokes one pack of cigarettes per day
12. Key points are:
    a. Hypertension is a very common condition affecting approximately 50 million Americans.
    b. Untreated or undertreated hypertension is a major risk factor for the development of coronary artery disease.
    c. Lifestyle modifications should be initiated in this patient to reduce the risk of the development of cardiovascular disease.
    d. The goal of hypertension therapy in this patient is to reduce and maintain blood pressure less than <130/85 mm Hg with lifestyle modifications and drug therapy.
    e. Since this patient has DM, aggressive control of therapy is essential to avoid the development of cardiovascular disease.
13. List an antihypertensive that would be the preferred first-line therapy and one agent that would *not* be preferred as first-line therapy.
    a. Congestive heart failure
       ACE inhibitors (with or without diuretics and digoxin) reduce mortality

Diuretics alleviate congestive symptoms caused by sodium and water retention

Vasodilators: Hydralazine/ISDN have also been shown to be effective in CHF, but < ACEI losartan lacks mortality data in heart failure, but reduces symptoms

Beta-blockers reduce mortality

Avoid negative inotropes (i.e., beta-blockers, if patient is unstable, verapamil, and diltiazem) in those patients with extensive LV dysfunction

Avoid alpha1-antagonists alone

b. Diabetes mellitus

Close monitoring is needed with most drugs in this population

Beta-blockers: glucose intolerance, mask and prolong recovery of hyperglycemia

Diuretics: glucose intolerance

ACE inhibitors, CCBs, alpha1-blockers and central - agonists are acceptable agents

14. Pharmacoeconomic considerations relative to this patient's hypertension plan of care may include:

   1. Costs of chronic hypertension treatment
      a. Direct medical
         • Drug costs
         • Health care provider costs

CASE 62

PROBLEM LIST

1. Coronary Artery Disease (S/P Myocardial Infarction, Angina Pectoris)
2. Atrial Fibrillation (Afib)
3. Congestive Heart Failure
4. Hypercholesterolemia

SOAP NOTE

S: During a follow-up visit for management of angina pectoris, states that after last visit to the clinic, when medication adjustments were made, noticed an improvement in the number of anginal episodes experiencing during the first week following the visit. Since that time, has experienced an increase in the anginal episodes, back to the frequency before the last visit. Previous history of noncompliance with medications.

O: No fatigue, SOB, orthopnea, and PND; physical examination results are unchanged from the previous visit, with no JVD, HJR, or heart murmurs heard; does not have any peripheral edema. ECG: No ischemic changes in the absence of pain and atrial fibrillation with a ventricular rate of 65 beats /min; CV examination: heartbeat irregularly irregular; serum digoxin concentration: 1.8 nmol/L (1.4 ng/mL); INR 2.1; lipid panel: TC 5.2 mmol/L (200

mg/dL); LDL 3.00 mmol/L (115 mg/dL); VLDL 0.98 mmol/L, 38 mg/dL); HDL 1.2 mmol/L (47 mg/dL); TG 2.14 mmol/L (190 mg/dL)

A: **Problem 1:** Coronary artery disease (S/P myocardial infarction, angina pectoris): Worsening angina secondary to noncompliance with nitrate-free period resulting in nitrate tolerance. Given the need of warfarin therapy for atrial fibrillation, the addition of aspirin for CAD secondary prevention is unnecessary at this time, unless recurrent CAD events occur while on warfarin.

Problem 2: Atrial fibrillation: Chronic Afib; not a candidate for cardioversion.

Problem 3: Congestive heart failure: Baseline at present. Consider longer acting agent to improve compliance, since history of noncompliance. When ACE inhibitor maximized consider adding beta-blocker (carvedilol, etc.). This could eliminate the need for the nitrate to manage angina and potentially the digoxin to control ventricular rate.

Problem 4: Hypercholesterolemia: Currently receiving lovastatin therapy for secondary prevention of CAD. Goal LDL-C concentration: ≤100 mg/dL. Based on history it is unclear how long receiving lovastatin or what the initial LDL-C concentration was (necessary to determine if the dose should be increased or continued as is).

P: **Problem 1: Coronary Artery Disease**

• Continue nitroglycerin patch therapy
• Discuss the importance of removing the nitroglycerin patch at bedtime and applying the new patch each morning
• Instruct to call the clinic if continues to incur this much chest pain after using the NTG patch as directed
• Continue SL nitroglycerin therapy
• Remind to keep track of the number of anginal attacks and return for a follow-up appointment in 2–3 weeks

Problem 2: Chronic Afib

• Continue warfarin and digoxin therapy
• Reeducate regarding these two medications

Problem 3: CHF

• Continue digoxin and furosemide therapy
• Change captopril to lisinopril 10 mg PO daily (with goal of 20 mg PO daily) and evaluate at next appointment
• Remind to report any symptoms of dizziness, significant weight changes, or increased heart failure symptoms. Also review adverse effects associated with digoxin.

- When ACE inhibitor dose maximized, consider beta-blocker therapy

Problem 4: Hypercholesterolemia

- Obtain more information related to lovastatin therapy (i.e., duration of therapy, original dose, and LDL-cholesterol concentration)
- Remind to take lovastatin with the largest meal, preferably dinner
- No changes in medication warranted at this time
- Recommend an appointment with a dietician for reinforcement of dietary restrictions
- Obtain LFTs at next follow-up
- Review the adverse effects related to HMG CoA reductase inhibitors

ANSWERS

1. d. Provide a 10–12 hour nitrate-free period.
2. c. Lisinopril 20 mg daily
3. a. ECG findings
4. b. <100 mg/dL
5. d. Nitroglycerin
6. b. Serum concentrations obtained 1 hour after a digoxin dose are likely to be falsely elevated and not reflective of the true serum concentrations.
7. d. Acetaminophen
8. b. Weight gain of 2–3 pounds in 1 week.
9. The nonpharmacologic therapies for this patient's heart failure include:
   1. Patient/family education
      a. Discussions/pamphlets on signs and symptoms of heart failure and medications
      b. Emphasis on compliance with complete treatment agenda
      c. Instructions on when to contact health care providers (see Table 40.5 in textbook)
   2. Diet
      a. Daily weight chart
      b. Individualized diet according to needs/preferences/lifestyle
      c. Sodium restriction: mild (<3 g/day) or moderate (<2 g/day)
      d. Information regarding sodium and potassium content in foods
      e. Alcohol restriction
      f. Fluid restriction: ~2L/day
      g. Nutritional supplements (e.g., vitamins)
      h. Emphasize importance of compliance
   3. Pharmacologic treatment of hyperlipidemia, ischemic heart disease, atrial fibrillation, and hypertension
   4. Exercise program
   5. Intensive follow-up: telephone calls, home visits, outpatient clinic visits
10. Pharmacologic treatment problems present in this patient's treatment plan include:

a. Worsening angina secondary with noncompliance (patient noncompliance or misunderstanding of instructions) with nitrate-free period resulting in nitrate tolerance.
b. Inadequate ACE inhibitor dose for mortality reduction.
11. Psychosocial factors that may affect this patient's adherence to both pharmacologic and nonpharmacologic therapy include:
a. Emotional needs/presence of depression
b. Financial barriers
c. Complicated medical regimens
12. Key points are:
   1. Angina
      a. The goals of treatment for ischemic heart disease are to minimize the frequency and severity of angina and to reduce cardiovascular morbidity and mortality.
      b. Drug therapy with nitrates, beta-blockers, and calcium channel blockers, alone or in combination, are effective at reducing anginal episodes and reducing the frequency of anginal attacks.
      c. Given the underlying heart failure in this patient, prevention of ischemic episodes is essential to maintain left-ventricular function. Therapies for ischemic heart disease should complement heart failure therapies as much as possible. For example, we should attempt to treat two disorders with one drug whenever possible. Appropriate anti-anginal medications in this patient include: carvedilol (slowly titrated), nitrates, and amlodipine.
   2. Heart failure
      a. HF is a clinical syndrome that progresses to worsening symptoms and death largely as a consequence of maladaptive effects triggered by neurohormones and cytokines.
      b. HF can result from abnormalities in either systolic or diastolic dysfunction.
      c. Participation in cardiac rehabilitation programs can improve exercise tolerance and quality of life and may reduce mortality in HF patients.
      d. Patient education is extremely important especially with respect to facilitating compliance with dietary and medication treatment plans.
      e. Based on their ability to consistently improve both the clinical status of patients and their longevity, ACE inhibitors are considered first-line therapy in the management of HF patients. Initiation of ACE inhibitor therapy should begin with low doses that are slowly titrated to target doses.
      f. Alternative vasodilator therapy such as angiotensin receptor antagonists or the combination of nitrates plus hydralazine should be reserved for patients intolerant of ACE inhibitors.
      g. Beta-blockers are currently advocated in the management of stable NYHA Class II–III HF patients based on their ability to reduce mortality and hospitalization rates. The initiation of beta-blocking therapy begins with low doses that are slowly and carefully increased. Since this patient has angina, these agents are particularly useful in the prevention of

anginal episodes. Alternatives are nitrates (which this patient is receiving) and amlodipine.

   h. Diuretics are used in the management of HF in order to relieve symptoms.

   i. Digoxin can be used safely in most patients with HF due to systolic dysfunction with target serum digoxin concentrations between 0.7 and 1.2 ng/mL.

   j. Anticoagulant therapy is indicated in HF patients with coexisting atrial fibrillation or other conditions that predispose them to thromboembolic conditions.

13. Pharmacoeconomic considerations relative to this patient's coronary artery disease/angina plan of care may include:

   1. Costs of chronic coronary artery disease treatment
      a. Direct medical
         • Drug costs
         • Health care provider costs

   2. Costs of coronary artery disease (uncontrolled) to patients and families (i.e., hospitalizations)
      a. Direct medical
         • Hospital personnel and overhead
         • Treatment and complications
      b. Direct nonmedical
         • Travel, hotels, meals
         • Lost wages (family/patient)
      c. Indirect personal
         • Decreased productivity
         • Quality of life
      d. Intangible personal
         • Suffering

CASE 63

PROBLEM LIST

1. Pulmonary Embolism (PE)
2. Oral Contraception
3. MPV
4. PSVT
5. IBS
6. Iron (Fe) Deficiency Anemia

SOAP NOTE

S: JO complains of shortness of breath, chest pain, and hemoptysis; but no abdominal pain at present

O: Tachycardia, tachypnea, hypertension, abnormal findings on chest x-ray films, loud P2, V/Q mismatch, and pulmonary angiogram findings are all consistent with the diagnosis of PE; decreased Hct, Hgb, MCV; guaiac-negative stool; midsystolic click heard on auscultation

A: **Problem 1:** PE: Possibly due to oral contraceptive use, age, and smoking or due to an underlying disease process that has not been diagnosed as yet; requires immediate treatment; hemodynamically unstable so thrombolytic therapy controversial.

Problem 2: Oral contraception: Life-threatening condition potentially associated with oral contraceptive use; alternative methods of contraception should be recommended

Problem 3: MVP: Appears stable

Problem 4: PSVT: Presently in sinus tachycardia with no symptoms, likely secondary to PE

Problem 5: IBS: Stable symptoms

Problem 6: Fe deficiency anemia: Probable Fe deficiency anemia in young female with no evidence of active bleeding

P: **Problem 1: PE**

• Perform baseline CBC, platelet count, and aPTT (for control)
• Initiate heparin therapy with a bolus dose of 75–80 U/kg (4650–4960 U) and follow with continuous infusion of heparin 15–20 U/kg/hr (930–1240 U/hr).
• Goal aPTT is 1.5–2.5 times control and should first be evaluated 6 hours after the bolus dose and the infusion adjusted accordingly
• Monitor for bleeding and appropriate laboratory studies (e.g., CBC, platelets, stool guaiac, urinalysis) done daily for the first few days and every other day during the hospitalization thereafter
• Start warfarin therapy on the first day with a maintenance dose of 4–5 mg/day; goal INR: 2.0–3.0; once INR is "therapeutic" for 2 days discontinue the heparin
• Duration of therapy is 3 months

Problem 2: Oral Contraception

• Counsel about contraception and explore alternative birth control methods
• Discuss the available methods of contraception, their ease of use, their efficacy rates, and patient-specific factors, such as adverse effects or contraindications. Encourage patient to choose the method most acceptable to her
• Educate regarding the danger of becoming pregnant while being treated with warfarin

Problem 3: MVP

• Continue present treatment with atenolol
• Reeducate the patient regarding the need for antibiotic prophylaxis before dental procedures
• Alert dentist she is taking warfarin therapy

Problem 4: PSVT

• Continue atenolol treatment
• Tachycardia likely related to current PE; if it persists after control of PE, consider increasing atenolol dose or switching to alternative agent
• Monitor ECG, blood pressure, symptoms, and other atenolol adverse effects closely

Problem 5: IBS

- Continue psyllium
- Instruct to take psyllium in a large glass of water or fruit juice and to drink fluids throughout the day
- Encourage exercise and the avoidance of any foods that have proven to exacerbate the condition
- Use stool guaiac test results to identify possible bleeding
- Avoid use of other laxatives
- Instruct to avoid taking psyllium at the same time as other drugs (take 4 hours apart)

Problem 6: Iron Deficiency Anemia

- Check blood smear and iron, TIBC, and transferrin concentrations to assess the adequacy of treatment
- Increase the iron dosage to three times a day
- Monitor compliance and tolerance
- Encourage a proper diet, discuss avoidance of drug and food interactions with iron, proper storage of iron, and the need for 6 months of therapy
- Monitor CBCs and other laboratory tests (as outlined above) every 4–6 weeks, until a return to normal concentrations documented
- Continue therapy for at least 6 months depending on responsiveness to therapy and ability to tolerate oral iron therapy; consider alternatives if the patient can't tolerate oral iron
- Increase fiber in diet

ANSWERS

1. a. Midsystolic click heard best along the left lower sternal border
2. d. Constipation
3. a. Weight-based heparin dosing should be based on ideal body weight.
4. a. Oral contraceptive use
5. d. Amoxicillin 2 g PO × 1
6. a. Ventricular fibrillation
7. c. Oral contraceptives
8. c. At least 3 months
9. The nonpharmacologic treatment problems present in this patient's treatment plan include:
   a. Need for contraception, alternative to oral contraceptives
   b. Maintenance of a "steady" diet (no major fluctuations in vitamin K content) for warfarin therapy
   c. Maintenance of a diet high in fiber and fluid to help alleviate her constipation problem and manage her irritable bowel syndrome
10. Risks associated with warfarin use in pregnancy and alternatives for chronic treatment of venous thromboembolism include:
    a. Warfarin is a known teratogenic drug, and its use should be avoided during pregnancy because of the risk of congenital malformations, nasal bone deformities, and stippling of the bones.
    b. The actual incidence is not clearly established but is

around 1–2%. The first trimester of pregnancy is the most dangerous time, but abnormalities have been identified during the later stages of pregnancy.
    c. Women of childbearing age taking warfarin should be advised very strongly about the use of appropriate contraceptive methods.
    d. After the fetus has been delivered, warfarin may be taken safely because it does not cross into breast milk.
    e. LMWH is the recommended anticoagulant to be used chronically during pregnancy.
11. Psychosocial factors that may affect this patient's adherence to both pharmacologic and nonpharmacologic therapy include:
    a. The use of warfarin and associated risks, if the patient becomes pregnant, may make warfarin therapy difficult if the patient does not identify an acceptable form of contraception, aside from oral contraceptives
    b. Successful treatment of iron deficiency anemia with iron therapy will be difficult in this patient given her history of constipation. If the patient continues to experience constipation while on the iron therapy she may be unwilling to complete the required course of therapy
    c. Acceptance of alternative forms of contraceptives by sexual partners
    d. Fears associated with anticoagulant therapy
    e. Dietary and lifestyle changes required due to anticoagulant therapy
12. Pharmacoeconomic considerations relative to this patient's thromboembolic disorder plan of care may include:
    1. Costs of chronic thromboembolic disorder (3 months of warfarin therapy) treatment
       a. Direct medical
          - Drug costs
          - Health care provider costs
    2. Costs of thromboembolic disorder (uncontrolled) to patients and families (i.e., hospitalizations due to recurrence, noncompliance, etc.)
       a. Direct medical
          - Hospital personnel and overhead
          - Treatment and complications
       b. Direct nonmedical
          - Travel, hotels, meals
          - Lost wages (family/patient)
       c. Indirect personal
          - Decreased productivity
       d. Intangible personal
          - Suffering

CASE 65

PROBLEM LIST

1. Congestive Heart Failure (CHF)
2. Coronary Artery Disease (S/P MI and Angina)
3. Hypertension (HTN)
4. Crohn's Disease
5. Renal Insufficiency
6. Allergic Rhinitis

SOAP NOTE

S: Complains of leg edema, nocturia, and SOB

O: ECG shows sinus tachycardia with occasional premature ventricular contractions. Positive S3, positive S4 with gallop, positive JVD, hepatomegaly, bilateral rates, and 2+ ankle edema, elevated PT, BP 150/100, AV nicking and narrowing, retinal exudates; SCr 177 mmol/L (2.0 mg/dL), BUN 8.57 mmol/L (24 mg/dL)

A: **Problem 1:** CHF secondary to coronary artery disease (CAD) and HTN: Current increase in symptoms secondary to suboptimal diuretic therapy with HCTZ, steroid therapy, and potentially post-MI metoprolol therapy.

Problem 2: CAD (S/P MI and angina): 30 days S/P MI and did not receive revascularization therapy during recent hospitalization; currently receiving metoprolol for anginal symptoms (in addition to providing protection from sudden cardiac death post-MI). Lipids should be obtained to determine if therapy necessary for secondary prevention.

Problem 3: HTN: Long-standing, uncontrolled HTN. Goal BP 130/85–140/90 mm Hg.

Problem 4: Crohn's disease: Currently in remission

Problem 5: Renal insufficiency: Estimated CrCl of ~25 mL/min. Secondary to poorly controlled hypertension, renal insufficiency can affect the dosing of medication excreted unchanged by the kidneys.

Problem 6: Allergic rhinitis: Well controlled

P: **Problem 1: CHF**

- Discontinue the HCTZ, start furosemide 40 mg once daily in the morning
- Taper the prednisone as described below
- Start enalapril 2.5 mg BID (or captopril 12.5 mg TID or lisinopril 5 mg daily)
- Follow up in 1 week, measure BP, K, BUN, and Cr and adjust therapy accordingly. Goal dose: 10 mg PO BID and the dose should be titrated up over several weeks
- Discontinue the potassium supplement due to ACE inhibitor therapy in renal insufficiency; consider the need for chronic potassium therapy when the goal dose of patient is achieved

Problem 2: CAD–S/P Myocardial Infarction-Angina

- Educate about the risk factors of CAD and stress smoking cessation, weight control, and medication compliance
- Continue NTG SL PRN and ECASA therapy
- If exhibiting anginal symptoms on current beta-blocker therapy, consider adding long-acting nitrate (ISDN 10 mg TID, NTG patch daily, ISMN 20 mg BID, etc.)
- Remind to continue to keep track of the number of anginal attacks and the number of weekly NTG SL tablets used

Problem 3: HTN

- Goal BP more aggressive due to presence of heart failure and multiple other risk factors
- Control hypertension with heart failure and angina medications

Problem 4: Crohn's Disease

- Taper off the corticosteroid over the next 3–6 months
- Monitor closely for signs and symptoms of steroid withdrawal and flare of Crohn's disease and provide stress coverage as necessary
- Consider discontinuing the sulfasalazine

Problem 5: Renal Insufficiency

- Monitor and adjust dosing of all medications as necessary

Problem 6: Allergic Rhinitis

- Currently well-controlled

ANSWERS

1. d. +JVD
2. a. Bilateral rales
3. a. Coronary artery disease
4. c. Allergic rhinitis
5. c. Sulfasalazine
6. b. Methylprednisolone 6 mg daily
7. a. Hydrocortisone 100 mg IV q8h until the stress resolves
8. b. 0.125 mg daily
9. DA should be provided with the following information for using her nicotine gum correctly:
   a. The nicotine gum is used to help you stop smoking. It has a better efficacy rate if you enroll in a stop-smoking program.
   b. The gum should never be swallowed.
   c. Chew one piece of gum whenever you have the urge to smoke.
   d. Chew the gum very slowly until the taste of nicotine or a slight tingling in the mouth is perceived (about 15 chews). Then stop chewing the gum and put it to the side of your mouth.
   e. Once the tingling in the mouth is gone (usually about 1 minute), the chewing procedure should be repeated. This cycle should be repeated intermittently for about 30 minutes, then the gum should be thrown away.
   f. To get the best results from the gum, follow the instructions carefully. Do not chew as you would regular gum.
   g. Do not use more than 30 pieces of gum per day. (The average daily use is 10 to 12 pieces.)

10. Nonpharmacologic treatment options include:
    1. Patient/family education
        a. Discussions/pamphlets on signs and symptoms of heart failure and medications
        b. Emphasis on compliance with complete treatment agenda
        c. Instructions on when to contact health care providers (see Table 40.5 in textbook)
    2. Diet
        a. Daily weight chart
        b. Individualized diet according to needs/preferences/lifestyle
        c. Sodium restriction: mild (<3 g/day) or moderate (<2 g/day)
        d. Information regarding sodium and potassium content in foods
        e. Alcohol restriction
        f. Fluid restriction: ~ 2 L/day
        g. Nutritional supplements (e.g., vitamins)
        h. Emphasize importance of compliance
    3. Pharmacological treatment of hyperlipidemia and hypertension
    4. Exercise program
    5. Intensive follow-up: telephone calls, home visits, outpatient clinic visits
11. Pharmacoeconomic considerations relative to this patient's plan of care may include:
    1. Direct medical
        a. Drug costs
        b. Health care provider costs
    2. Costs of HF exacerbation (uncontrolled) to patients and families
        a. Direct medical
            • Hospital personnel and overhead
            • Treatment and complications
        b. Direct nonmedical
            • Travel, hotels, meals
            • Lost wages (family/patient)
        c. Indirect personal
            • Decreased productivity
            • Quality of life
        d. Intangible personal
            • SOB & suffering
12. Key points are:
    1. Heart failure
        a. HF is a clinical syndrome that progresses to worsening symptoms and death largely as a consequence of maladaptive effects triggered by neurohormones and cytokines.
        b. HF can result from abnormalities in either systolic or diastolic dysfunction.
        c. Participation in cardiac rehabilitation programs can improve exercise tolerance and quality of life and may reduce mortality in HF patients.
        d. Patient education is extremely important especially with respect to facilitating compliance with dietary and medication treatment plans.

    e. Based on their ability to consistently improve both the clinical status of patients and their longevity, ACE inhibitors are considered first-line therapy in the management of HF patients. Initiation of ACE inhibitor therapy should begin with low doses that are slowly titrated to target doses.
    f. Alternative vasodilator therapy such as angiotensin receptor antagonists or the combination of nitrates plus hydralazine should be reserved for patients intolerant of ACE inhibitors.
    g. Beta-blockers are currently advocated in the management of stable NYHA Class II–III HF patients based on their ability to reduce mortality and hospitalization rates. The initiation of beta-blocking therapy begins with low doses that are slowly and carefully increased. Since this patient has angina, these agents are particularly useful in the prevention of anginal episodes. Alternatives are nitrates (which this patient is receiving) and amlodipine.
    h. Diuretics are used in the management of HF in order to relieve symptoms.
    i. Digoxin can be used safely in most patients with HF due to systolic dysfunction with target serum digoxin concentrations between 0.7 and 1.2 ng/mL.
    j. Anticoagulant therapy is indicated in HF patients with coexisting atrial fibrillation or other conditions that predispose them to thromboembolic conditions.

    2. S/P myocardial infarction
        a. Myocardial infarction is one of the most common reasons for hospitalization in the western world. The actual mortality rate is about 15%; approximately 10% of patients will die during the first year after their AMI.
        b. Short-term and long-term survival depends on the extent and location of the coronary obstructive lesions and the prompt correction of post-MI complications.
        c. The presence or absence of mechanical, electrical, ischemic, and vascular abnormalities provides the necessary information to institute approximate medical and/or surgical treatment.
        d. Correction and treatment of all modifiable cardiovascular risk factors is essential in an effort to reduce the risk for future vascular events.
        e. Risk factor reduction should focus on hypertension management, smoking cessation, lipid-lowering therapy, antiplatelet therapy, and cardiac rehabilitation and exercise.
        f. Treatment of hypertension reduces cardiovascular morbidity and mortality.
        g. Smoking cessation is especially important in patients with ischemic heart disease. Smoking is associated with increased morbidity and mortality, silent ischemia, arrhythmias, and coronary vasospasm in patients with coronary artery disease. Pharmacologic and nonpharmacologic approaches are available for assisting patients with smoking cessation.

h. Lipid-lowering drug therapy in patients with angina and/or prior myocardial infarction with average and elevated serum cholesterol concentrations has been shown to reduce cardiovascular morbidity and mortality.

i. Exercise training reduces cardiovascular mortality, improves functional capacity, and attenuates myocardial ischemia and thus is an important lifestyle modification.

j. Other cardiovascular risk factor reductions should include weight loss if overweight, alcohol use only in moderation, and estrogen replacement therapy in postmenopausal women. Lastly, epidemiologic evidence suggests that the increased intake of vitamins (vitamin E, vitamin C, folic acid) are associated with reduced coronary artery disease risk; however, data from clinical trials are needed before these therapies gain widespread acceptance.

CASE 67

PROBLEM LIST

1. Deep Venous Thrombosis (DVT)
2. Alcohol Abuse
3. Abnormal LFTs
4. Anemia
5. WPW Syndrome
6. Obesity

SOAP NOTE

S: Swelling in his right calf and thigh accompanied by tenderness and redness

O: Enlarged, red painful right leg larger than left, 3+ pitting edema, decreased pulse, positive venogram: consistent with filling defect in right calf and thigh; increased concentrations on results of AST, ALT, LDH, T bili, PT, aPTT; slightly decreased concentrations of Na; icteric sclera, increased abdominal girth, peripheral edema, enlarged and palpable liver; increased MCV, borderline Hct and Hgb

A: **Problem 1:** DVT: Right-leg DVT without evidence of pulmonary embolism. Baseline coagulation studies are abnormal, which must be considered in initiating therapy. There is no evidence of bleeding, stool is guaiac-negative, and no ecchymoses are noted on physical examination.

Problem 2: Alcohol abuse: Alcohol use is affecting liver function and should be discontinued.

Problem 3: Abnormal LFTs; possible alcoholic liver disease; possible amiodarone-induced liver dysfunction.

Problem 4: Anemia: Megaloblastic anemia secondary to chronic alcohol abuse; asymptomatic

Problem 5: WPW syndrome: Currently stable on amiodarone

Problem 6: Obesity: Contributing to multiple medical problems

P: **Problem 1: DVT**

- Baseline aPTT: 30.2 s, goal aPTT: 45–76 s
- Initiate intravenous full-dose weight-based heparin therapy. Initiate with a bolus dose of 75–80 U/kg (9375–10,000 U) and infusion of 18 U/kg/hr (2250 U/hr).
- Recheck aPTT in 6 hours and adjust heparin infusion to maintain aPTT of 1.5–2.5 × control
- Begin warfarin on the first day of heparin therapy at 2.5 mg daily. Baseline INR already elevated, and on amiodarone, which will decrease warfarin requirements
- Stop heparin after 4–5 days of combined warfarin therapy when the INR >2.0 for 2 consecutive days
- Observe for bleeding, and monitor CBC, platelets, PT, aPTT, urinalysis, and stool guaiac daily for the first few days and periodically thereafter
- Continue warfarin for 3 months. If inadequate resolution or recurrence, therapy may be continued for a longer period of time
- To avoid future recurrences weight reduction mandatory
- Counsel on the need for frequent clinic attendance and absolute compliance
- Encourage patient to discontinue alcohol use and eat a well-balanced consistent diet
- Discontinue aspirin (contained in Alka-Seltzer). Refer to social worker and dietician for counseling

Problem 2: Alcohol Abuse

- Refer to inpatient detoxification unit and Alcoholics Anonymous
- Begin oxazepam, 10 mg PO q6h PRN for alcohol withdrawal
- Begin thiamine at 100 mg PO daily and folic acid 1 mg PO daily
- Monitor for alcohol withdrawal

Problem 3: Abnormal LFTs

- Discontinue alcohol use, provide dietary instruction, and obtain support through Alcoholics Anonymous
- Initiate spironolactone 50 mg and increase over 3–5 days, up to a maximum of 400 mg/day or an adequate response of 1 kg fluid loss per day
- Avoid more vigorous diuretics at this time because there are no pulmonary symptoms
- Serum and urinary electrolyte concentrations

should be monitored as well as daily weight and abdominal girth

Problem 4: Anemia

- Obtain a blood smear, folic acid concentration, vitamin B_{12} concentration, serum iron, and serum transferrin concentrations; calculate iron saturation
- Specific therapy should be directed by these findings

Problem 5: WPW Syndrome

- Continue amiodarone at 200 mg/day for present
- Obtain thyroid function tests
- Serious consideration of future alternatives, such as radiofrequency ablation therapy

Problem 6: Obesity

- Weight loss, dietary instruction, and a monitoring program essential to successful weight loss
- To avoid future recurrences of thromboembolic disease weight reduction mandatory

ANSWERS

1. a. Icteric sclera
2. c. Pulmonary fibrosis
3. a. Paroxysmal supraventricular tachycardia
4. d. Hypertension
5. c. Three months
6. b. Rebolus at 40 U/kg and increase the infusion rate by 2 U/kg
7. d. Reduced synthesis of vitamin K-dependent clotting factors by the liver
8. c. Plasma aldosterone concentrations
9. The effects of alcohol on warfarin therapy include:
   a. Acute alcohol consumption may result in an increased clearance of warfarin and a subsequent decrease in the INR.
   b. Chronic consumption may lead to a potentiation of effect, primarily because of a destructive effect on the liver. In a patient such as WM, the most likely effect is a potentiation of effect, because hepatic dysfunction is already evident. To further complicate the discussion, there is evidence that mild alcohol consumption (2 ounces per day) in patients who do not abuse or binge with alcohol may not influence warfarin at all.
10. Nonpharmacologic treatment problems present in this patient's treatment plan include:
    a. Maintenance of a "steady" diet (no major fluctuations in vitamin K content) for warfarin therapy
    b. Alcoholism
    c. Obesity
11. Psychosocial factors that may affect this patient's adherence to both pharmacologic and nonpharmacologic therapy include:
    a. Alcoholism will affect this patient's adherence to all therapies and potentially increase the risk associated with warfarin therapy.
12. Key points are:
    a. Acquired risk factors for the development of venous thromboembolism include (but are not limited to the following): immobility, surgery, trauma, obesity, malignancy, cardiovascular disease, and many others.
    b. The main goals of treating venous thromboembolic disorders are: prevention of embolic complications, reducing morbidity related to the acute event, and maximizing efficacy while reducing adverse effects and treatment cost.
    c. Weight-based unfractionated intravenous heparin therapy should be used during the acute treatment phase. Published dosing guidelines should be followed and patient-specific therapy adjusted based upon laboratory aPTT monitoring. An alternative to heparin therapy is low-molecular-weight therapy.
    d. Long-term anticoagulant therapy, usually with warfarin, should be instituted and continued for at least 3 months. Warfarin therapy should be monitored using INR.

SECTION 11 / SKIN DISEASES

CASE 69

PROBLEM LIST

1. Diffuse, Erythematous Maculopapular Rash
2. Pneumonia/Bronchitis
3. COPD
4. Seizure
5. Meningioma
6. Diarrhea

SOAP NOTE

S: "My breathing is better now, but my skin really itches."

O: Diffuse, erythematous, maculopapular rash; eosinophilia (0.08); serum theophylline concentration 38.85 (7); total serum phenytoin concentration 71.35 (18) with corresponding serum albumin value 32 (3.2); improved oxygenation, PO_2 10.7 kPa (80), and resolving hypercapnia, PCO_2 7.3 kPa (55) demonstrated by arterial blood gases; *Moraxella catarrhalis* isolated from sputum

A: **Problem 1:** Diffuse, erythematous maculopapular rash: drug-induced exanthem probably caused by ampicillin/sulbactam and/or amoxicillin/clavulanate; other potential causes include phenytoin or furosemide

Problem 2: Pneumonia/bronchitis: resolving acute exacerbation of chronic bronchitis (AECB) versus pneumonia caused by *M. catarrhalis*

Problem 3: COPD: resolving AECB with improved oxygenation and reduced hypercarbia

Problem 4: Seizure: possible etiologies: acute hypoxic episode; newly diagnosed meningioma; or new-onset seizure disorder; serum phenytoin concentration, adjusted for hypoalbuminemia, slightly elevated

Problem 5: Meningioma: newly diagnosed by CT following seizure activity

Problem 6: Diarrhea: probable antibiotic-associated diarrhea

P: **Problem 1: Diffuse, Erythematous Maculopapular Rash**

- Discontinue amoxicillin/clavulanate
- Begin ofloxacin, 400 mg PO BID
- Discontinue furosemide; if diuretic needed, use nonsulfonamide-related agent (e.g., ethacrynic acid)
- Administer diphenhydramine 50 mg IV or PO q6h PRN for pruritus

Problem 2: Pneumonia/Bronchitis

- Discontinue amoxicillin/clavulanate and continue ofloxacin for 14-day total duration of antimicrobial therapy

Problem 3: COPD

- Continue albuterol sulfate/ipratropium bromide MDI
- Assess MDI technique and incorporate spacer device if suboptimal
- Continue theophylline SR, 300 mg PO BID; repeat serum theophylline determination 1 week after discontinuing cimetidine to identify need to increase dosage
- Use peak flow meter to assess disease state

Problem 4: Seizure

- Continue phenytoin at reduced doses (230 mg per day); repeat serum phenytoin concentration 1 week after discontinuing cimetidine to determine if the serum phenytoin concentration has declined

Problem 5: Meningioma

- Relevance uncertain since most common benign brain tumor
- Refer to oncologist and/or neurosurgeon

Problem 6: Diarrhea

- Discontinue amoxicillin/clavulanate since diarrhea most common adverse drug reaction (especially with increased clavulanate doses)
- Assay stool sample for *Clostridium difficile* toxin; if positive, begin metronidazole 500 mg PO TID for 10 days
- Implement antidiarrheal such as loperamide if *C. difficile* result negative and patient complains of discomfort

ANSWERS

1. a. Topical application
2. c. Drug interaction
3. d. IgE production
4. d. 50
5. c. Erythematous pustules
6. a. Eosinophilia
7. a. With the first dose of therapy
8. c. Within 1–2 weeks
9. Cimetidine, an inhibitor of the cytochrome P450 enzyme system, may increase both the serum theophylline and phenytoin concentrations. Phenytoin, an inducer of the cytochrome P450 enzyme system, may decrease the serum theophylline concentration.
10. Unbound fraction of phenytoin is increased in patients with hypoalbuminemia:
    a. Free/unbound phenytoin concentration may be monitored to assess whether it is in the usual therapeutic range of 2–4 µmol/L (1–2 mg/L) or
    b. Total phenytoin concentration laboratory result must be adjusted; the formula below may be used to assess whether it is in the usual therapeutic range of 20–40 µmol/L (10–20 mg/L):

$$C_{adjusted} = \frac{C_{observed}}{0.2 \times Albumin\ (g/dL) + 0.1}$$

   c. For patient SA, the adjusted serum phenytoin concentration is above the usual therapeutic range and dosage reduction should be considered

$$C_{adjusted} = \frac{18\ mg/L}{0.2 \times (3.2) + 0.1} = 24.3\ mg/L$$

11. Active psychosocial issues that may affect SA's compliance with both pharmacologic and nonpharmacologic therapies include:
    1. COPD issues
       a. Reduced activity due to symptoms
       b. Chronic MDI use that may be technically difficult for SA to perform
       c. Disease progression, with need for temporary mechanical ventilation
       d. Possible depression and/or anxiety
    2. Emotional issues associated with new diagnoses
       a. Meningioma–possible need for surgery or chemotherapy
       b. Seizure disorder–anxiety and fear of future seizures, social stigma, and loss of driving privileges
12. The pharmacoeconomic considerations relative to SA's plan of care include:

1. Direct medical
   a. Medical personnel and overhead
   b. Treatment and complications
2. Direct nonmedical
   a. Lost wages
3. Indirect personal
   a. Decreased productivity
   b. Quality of life
4. Intangible personal
   a. SOB and suffering
13. Key points are:
   a. Allergic and drug-induced skin diseases encompass a varied spectrum of diseases.
   b. Although allergy is suspected in many cases, the specific allergen may be difficult to identify. Other mechanisms operate in some diseases, but the clinical presentation does not distinguish the etiology.
   c. Drug-induced conditions tend to be acute and resolve, particularly when the offending agent is removed.
   d. Topical corticosteroids, occasional short-term systemic corticosteroids in severe conditions, and antihistamines are the mainstay of drug therapy in addition to other nonspecific topical treatments.

CASE 70

PROBLEM LIST

1. Psoriasis
2. Smoking Cessation
3. Dysmenorrhea
4. Contraception

SOAP NOTE

S: "The skin on my elbows and knees has been red, scaly, and itchy for the past several weeks; I've been afraid to apply lotions to these areas: I'm also frustrated because I want to quit smoking but have failed three times."

O: Skin: erythematous, dry, scaling psoriatic plaques on elbows and knees bilaterally; BP: 120/70; medications: oral contraceptive for 10 years

A: **Problem 1:** Psoriasis—newly diagnosed; onset flare of relatively localized psoriasis

Problem 2: Smoking: motivated to stop smoking; attempted three times in the past on own without pharmacologic agent, but has failed due to symptoms typical of nicotine withdrawal

Problem 3: Dysmenorrhea; adequately treated with oral contraceptives for several years

Problem 4: Contraception: ten year history of heavy smoking while receiving oral contraceptives; current blood pressure–normal; no PMH of HTN or thromboembolic disease; LFTs: WNL

P: Problem 1: Psoriasis

- For initial management, use 6% salicylic acid in 60% propylene glycol with 20% ethyl alcohol to assist skin hydration and promote shedding of scaling epithelial cells; apply this preparation under occlusion at night; a combination preparation of tar and salicylic acid is an appropriate option
- Discuss potential side effects of salicylic acid such as tinnitus, nausea, and hyperventilation, but emphasize less likely to occur when only small-localized areas of skin treated
- Discuss potential side effects of tar, such as irritation and photosensitivity; tar may stain clothing and has an unpleasant smell
- Recommend a high-potency topical corticosteroid to reduce inflammation and irritation (e.g., clobetasol propionate) applied BID × 2 weeks; after 2 weeks, a mid-strength topical corticosteroid (e.g., triamcinolone acetonide 0.1% cream) can be applied BID × 2 weeks, followed by QD application thereafter
- Discuss potential local side effects of corticosteroid creams such as striae and skin atrophy
- Arrange follow-up appointment in 4 weeks to assess response to therapy and to make adjustments to therapy if necessary
- Educate about psoriasis and provide options for psychosocial support

Problem 2: Smoking Cessation

- Initiate high-dose nicotine patch for 4–12 weeks, depending upon the patch selected; if successful abstinence from smoking during initial period, continue therapy at reduced doses
- Discuss importance of completely stopping smoking while using nicotine patch, to avoid side effects of increased nicotine
- Apply patch to clean, dry, hairless area of skin on upper trunk or upper outer arm; rotate sites and avoid placing patch on damaged skin (avoid areas with psoriatic plaques)
- Monitor for symptoms of excess nicotine (increased heart rate and blood pressure, tremor, nausea, vomiting, and diarrhea) and adjust dose as necessary
- Discuss option of attending group sessions
- Offer problem solving and skills training (e.g., avoiding trigger times such as coffee break times; change routines; reward system with the money saved by not smoking)

Problem 3: Dysmenorrhea

- Continue current combination oral contraceptive (COC)
- Discuss the additional benefits of COC use,

including the significantly lower risk for developing endometrial or ovarian cancer

- Discuss the increased risk of cardiovascular disease in women in age group (>35) associated with smoking while taking COCs
- If BF continues to smoke, discontinue COC and institute alternative therapy such as an NSAID

Problem 4: Contraception

- Continue current COC regimen
- Monitor blood pressure
- If BF continues to smoke and is sexually active, other contraceptive options should be selected (e.g., diaphragm, IUD, cervical cap, sponge, or condoms) with appropriate counseling
- Reinforce the importance of monthly breast self-examinations and annual gynecological examinations

ANSWERS

1. a. Equal frequency in women and men
2. c. 30s
3. d. Melanoma
4. b. Axillae
5. b. An increase in epidermal cell proliferation is usually not observed
6. a. Hydrate the stratum corneum and prevent the increased transepidermal water loss observed in patients with psoriasis
7. a. Salicylic acid
8. d. HPA-axis suppression is generally irreversible after short-term use of potent topical corticosteroids
9. d. UVB
10. If a relapse has occurred:
    a. Ask for a recommitment to total abstinence
    b. Remind BF that a lapse can be used as a learning experience and review the circumstances that caused it; suggest alternative behaviors
    c. Identify problems encountered and anticipate challenges in the immediate future
    d. Praise efforts as she progresses through various phases of nicotine transdermal system therapy
    e. Continue the nicotine transdermal system
11. Should BF decide to use nicotine gum:
    a. Use 4 mg (rather than 2 mg) gum as BF is a highly dependent smoker (smokes greater than 25 cigarettes/day)
    b. Use one piece every 1–2 hours, use to respond to cravings
    c. Chew and "park" gum between cheek and gum every 1–5 minutes
    d. Repeat—use one piece no longer than 30 minutes
    e. Do not consume acidic food/beverages before or during use
    f. Patients often do not use enough gum to get maximum benefit
12. Active psychosocial issues that may affect BF's compliance with both pharmacologic and nonpharmacologic therapies include:
    1. Psoriasis issues
        a. Negative effects on appearance
        b. Anxiety and depression regarding incurable disease and disease progression
        c. Potential side effects of potent topical corticosteroids
    2. Smoking cessation issues
        a. Previous failures when attempting to quit smoking
        b. Nicotine withdrawal symptoms
        c. Anxiety and depression
13. The health care provider's role relative to BF's plan of care:
    a. Individualize a pharmacologic and nonpharmacologic plan for BF
    b. Provide patient education for both smoking cessation and psoriasis and positive reinforcement
14. The pharmacoeconomic considerations relative to BF's plan of care include:
    1. Direct medical
        a. Medical personnel
        b. Treatment and complications
    2. Indirect personal
        a. Decreased productivity
        b. Quality of life
    3. Intangible personal
        a. Suffering
15. Key points are:
    a. Psoriasis varies greatly in severity and treatment must be based on a risk-to-benefit ratio.
    b. The selection of therapy for psoriasis depends upon the location and clinical presentation.
    c. There is a wide range of therapies for psoriasis that must take into account the patient's quality of life.

CASE 72

PROBLEM LIST

1. Eczema Exacerbation
2. Asthma

SOAP NOTE

S: "I itch so much that I can't sleep at night."

O: Areas of erythematous, scaly rash; elevated IgE

A: **Problem 1:** Uncommon eczema exacerbation, primarily affecting the LUE, producing an itchy, erythematous, scaly rash; possible psychosocial component

Problem 2: Asthma currently well controlled with no wheezing on exam

P: **Problem 1: Eczema Exacerbation**

- Institute application of high-potency fluorinated corticosteroid cream, such as betamethasone dipropionate, applied BID × 2 weeks; after 2 weeks, a mid-strength topical corticosteroid, such as triamcinolone acetonide 0.1% cream, can be applied BID × 1 week
- Return to dermatology clinic in 3 weeks for follow-up

- Diphenhydramine syrup (1 mg/kg) PO at bedtime; caution patient and family regarding possible adverse effects such as drowsiness and potential for asthma worsening due to drying of respiratory secretions
- Recommend adding colloidal oatmeal to daily bath water to help relieve itching; adding an emollient to bath water is an alternative, but requires vigilant supervision of young children to prevent accidents, because tub surface slippery
- Assess for environmental "triggers," such as furry pets in the home (especially if one enters the patient's bedroom) or the placement of fabric toys on the bed, possibly contaminated with dust mites.
- Educate parents and provide contact information for self-help groups and other health care resources; (National Eczema Association for Science and Education (NEASE) = http://www.eczema-assn.org)
- Consult counselor or mental health professional for psychosocial issues

Problem 2: Asthma

- No changes recommended in current therapy

ANSWERS

1. d. Pruritus
2. d. Viral
3. b. Reduce the inflammation and itching
4. b. HPA suppression
5. a. Lichenoid plaques
6. c. Bathing in conjunction with lubricant application helps prevent dry skin
7. a. Pemphigus
8. b. Keeping the bedroom cool and using cotton bedding
9. Avoid sensitizing agents such as neomycin.
   1. Preferred agents include:
      a. Erythromycin
      b. Bacitracin
   2. Mupirocin is effective but more expensive
10. Psychosocial issues in children include:
    1. Itch-scratch cycle triggers
       a. Emotional stress
       b. Hostility from a parent
       c. Discord between parents
    2. Techniques used to stop scratching include:
       a. "Habit reversal"
       b. Behavioral and cognitive interventions
       c. Relaxation training
       d. Learning to express anger and to be assertive
11. Patients should benefit more from traditional H_1-blockers such as:
    a. Hydroxyzine 25 mg syrup (1–1.4 mg/kg) PO at bedtime
    b. Promethazine 25 mg syrup PO at bedtime

12. Key points are:
    a. Allergic and drug-induced skin disease encompass a varied spectrum of diseases.
    b. Atopic dermatitis, contact dermatitis, and idiopathic urticaria tend to be more chronic with exacerbations and remissions.
    c. Topical corticosteroids, occasional short-term systemic corticosteroids in severe conditions, and antihistamines are the mainstay of drug therapy in addition to other nonspecific topical treatments.

CASE 73

PROBLEM LIST

1. 60% TBSA burn
2. ABG Abnormalities
   a. Carbon Monoxide Poisoning (37%)
   b. Metabolic Acidosis
   c. Hypoxia
3. Hypovolemia
4. Hemochromogens in Urine
5. Hypophosphatemia
6. Stress-related Mucosal Damage (SRMD) Prophylaxis
7. Hyperkalemia
8. Absent Peripheral Pulses in Right Upper Extremity

SOAP NOTE

S: Critically injured patient in acute distress

O: 60% TBSA burn; coagulated blood vessels; pulseless RUE; laryngoscopic evidence of possible inhalation injury; oliguria; hemoglobinuria; hypoxia (PO_2 = 9.6 kPa); hyperkalemia (K = 5.2 mmol/L); hypophosphatemia (PO_4 = 0.30 mmol/L); hypocarbia (PCO_2 = 4.4 kPa); metabolic acidosis (HCO_3 = 14 mmol/L); carboxyhemoglobinemia (carboxyhemoglobin = 0.37)

A: **Problem 1:** 60% TBSA burn while trapped in a house fire, a critical and possibly life-threatening injury

Problem 2: ABG abnormalities from being trapped in an environment with a hostile atmosphere
a. Carbon monoxide poisoning (37%)
b. Metabolic acidosis
c. Hypoxia

Problem 3: Hypovolemia because of inadequate fluid resuscitation

Problem 4: Hemochromogens in urine; hemoglobin released from destroyed red blood cells and myoglobin from burned muscle tissue

Problem 5: Hypophosphatemia due to hypermetabolic state and anaerobic glycolysis

Problem 6: SRMD prophylaxis

Problem 7: Hyperkalemia secondary to intravascular hemolysis and release of intracellular potassium

Problem 8: Absent peripheral pulses in the right arm due to compartment syndrome produced by circumferential eschar

P: Problem 1: 60% TBSA Burn

- Excise full-thickness injuries and replace with skin grafts (autografts) on or after postburn day two; excise approximately 10–20% TBSA during each operation
- Apply an antimicrobial cream such as silver sulfadiazine to burns twice daily until grafted
- Biopsy eschar every other day and quantitatively analyze for microbes

Problem 2: ABG Abnormalities

a. Carbon monoxide poisoning (37%)

b. Metabolic acidosis

c. Hypoxia

- Increase the FIO_2 from 0.4 to 1.0
- Increase the rate of fluid administration (see problem 3)
- Withhold bicarbonate unless the arterial pH falls below 7.20
- Send a blood sample for cyanide concentration
- Perform chest escharotomies if inadequate respiratory excursion
- Administer phosphorus intravenously (see problem 5)
- Replace mafenide acetate cream with silver sulfadiazine or nitrofurazone cream

Problem 3: Hypovolemia

- Increase the rate of lactated Ringer's to 1100 mL per hour
- Attain and maintain a urine output of 0.5–1 mL/kg per hour
- Consider insertion of pulmonary artery (Swan-Ganz) catheter

Problem 4: Hemochromogens in Urine

- Increase urine flow to 75–100 mL per hour
- Administer mannitol if crystalloid alone does not achieve desired urine output
- Reduce rate of fluid administration when the pigments clear

Problem 5: Hypophosphatemia

- Administer phosphorus 0.2 mmol/kg intravenously over 2–3 hours; use sodium phosphates rather than potassium phosphates because of hyperkalemia

- Obtain follow-up serum phosphorus concentration in 6 hours
- Repeat dose until deficit corrected
- Continue parenteral or enteral phosphorus supplementation to meet daily needs

Problem 6: SRMD Prophylaxis

- Administer famotidine 20 mg IV q12h or an alternate H_2RA such as ranitidine or cimetidine

Problem 7: Hyperkalemia

- Monitor serum potassium concentrations
- Monitor ECG for evidence of uncorrected hyperkalemia
- Treatment not indicated at this time

Problem 8: Absent Peripheral Pulses in Right Upper Extremity

- Surgeon will incise the eschar laterally through its entire depth and extend the incision along the midlateral line of the arm until all circumferential eschar is cut and the constriction relieved
- Document that peripheral pulses established following the procedure
- Consider fasciotomy if pulses continue to be absent

ANSWERS

1. b. To maintain life
2. b. 10–20% TBSA
3. d. Full-thickness injury
4. a. Autograft
5. c. Mafenide acetate
6. d. 5 mg/kg/min
7. b. 8 hours
8. d. Radiotherapy
9. b. Carbonic anhydrase inhibition
10. Yes. The guidelines from the American College of Surgeons call for IM administration of 250 units tetanus immune globulin
11. a. Preferred parenteral benzodiazepine is lorazepam, which undergoes Phase II hepatic metabolism, since burn patients demonstrate impaired Phase I hepatic metabolism.

    b. Avoid use of succinylcholine administration in burn patients because severe and potentially fatal hyperkalemia is associated with its use.

    c. Decreased potency of nondepolarizing neuromuscular blocking agents such as pancuronium and atracurium is observed after the first postburn week and increased dosage is required; dosing can be guided by assessment of the degree of paralysis by a peripheral nerve stimulator
12. Enteral nutrition is preferable to parenteral nutrition and can be accomplished even in the absence of bowel sounds; because of gastric ileus, successful insertion of a nasoduodenal feeding tube may require use of an endoscope
13. Sulfonamide hypersensitivity is unlikely; a transient leukopenia is commonly observed following burn injury and is probably due to margination and movement of leukocytes from the systemic circulation

14. Active psychosocial factors that may influence JD's adherence to both pharmacologic and nonpharmacologic therapy include:
    1. Emotional disorders in patient and family members associated with life-threatening injury:
       a. Anxiety and depression about possible loss of life
       b. Altered body image
    2. Other barriers:
       a. Loss of wages; stress on financial reserves
15. The pharmacoeconomic considerations relative to JD's plan of care include:
    1. Direct medical
       a. Medical personnel and overhead
       b. Treatment and complications
    2. Direct nonmedical
       a. Lost wages
    3. Indirect personal
       a. Decreased productivity
       b. Quality of life
16. Key points are:

a. The complex clinical management and rehabilitation of a severely burned patient requires a multidisciplinary team including surgeons, nurses, pharmacists, dietitians, physical therapists, occupational therapists, respiratory therapists, and social workers.
b. A large TBSA full-thickness burn requires surgical excision and split-thickness skin grafting. Fluid requirements during the initial postburn period are surprisingly large, and guidelines for fluid resuscitation have been devised by experienced clinicians.
c. The pharmacist must be aware that the postburn hyperdynamic and hypermetabolic phase produces multiple pharmacokinetic and pharmacodynamic changes.
d. The nutritional requirements of burn patients can be substantial, with energy needs often approaching twice those of other hospitalized patients.
e. Prevention and treatment of infection in the burned patient is of paramount importance, since it is the most common cause of death in patients who survive initial resuscitation.

SECTION 12 / DISEASES OF THE EYE AND EAR

CASE 75

PROBLEM LIST

1. Acute Angle-Closure Glaucoma
2. Acute Anginal Attack; R/O MI
3. Gastritis; R/O Gastric Ulcer or Gastroesophageal Reflux Disease (GERD)
4. HTN
5. H/O Medication Noncompliance

SOAP NOTE

S: "What did you put in my eyes? It's killing me! This isn't helping my blurred vision."

O: Blurred vision; BP 150/95, HR 100, RR 20, T 37°C, Wt 80 kg, IOP 50 mm Hg; troponin I 1.1 (1.1); ECG readings negative for changes consistent with MI; UGI endoscopy: no visible gastric ulcerations; *Helicobacter pylori* culture: pending

A: **Problem 1:** Acute angle-closure glaucoma secondary to atropine eye drops

Problem 2: Acute anginal attack resolved; MI ruled out

Problem 3: Gastritis needing further workup to rule out GERD or duodenal ulcer

Problem 4: Poor control of HTN secondary to problem 5

Problem 5: Medication noncompliance as evident by missed propranolol; poor understanding of use of SL NTG

P: **Problem 1: Acute Angle-Closure Glaucoma**

- Pilocarpine 4%, 1 gtt q 5 min × 6; place finger on nasolacrimal duct to decrease systemic absorption; monitor for cholinergic side effects such as diarrhea and salivation
- Mannitol, 1 to 2 g/kg IV (80–160 g = 400–800 mL of 20% mannitol); monitor for headache, nausea, vomiting, dehydration, pulmonary edema, CHF, and hypersensitivity reactions
- Refer to ophthalmologist for consideration of laser iridotomy or peripheral trabeculoplasty

Problem 2: Acute Anginal Attack/Rule Out MI

- Restart propranolol at 20 mg PO BID; monitor HR,

BP, and potential CNS and sexual dysfunction side effects; instruct on the importance of medication compliance in relation to HTN and coronary artery disease (CAD)

- Give new prescription for NTG, 0.4 mg SL PRN for chest pain; explain that NTG should be kept in a dry area and replaced 6 months after opening; also, NTG should not be taken with alcohol, because it can cause severe hypotension; review other important patient education issues regarding SL NTG (see Chapter 42)
- Advise about the cardiovascular effects of smoking; offer smoking cessation therapy

Problem 3: Gastritis/Rule Out GERD or Duodenal Ulcer

- Await results of *H. pylori* culture; if positive, use eradicative therapy: 10-day, BID regimen of a proton pump inhibitor (omeprazole or lansoprazole) with two antibiotics (clarithromycin and either amoxicillin or metronidazole) to improve compliance
- Continue antacids as needed for severe pain
- Encourage lifestyle changes; discourage alcohol and smoking; raise head of bed 6–8 inches; encourage smaller meals rather than larger meals
- Avoid foods or medications that can decrease lower esophageal sphincter (LES) tone, such as calcium channel blockers, anticholinergic agents, theophylline, alcohol, coffee, cola, tea, peppermint, tomato juice, or onions
- If symptoms continue, consider propranolol as a rare cause of decreased LES tone

Problem 4: Hypertension

- Restart propranolol 20 mg PO BID
- Investigate psychosocial issues, such as lack of disease or medication education, insufficient funds or access to receive medications, which may be the cause of noncompliance
- Educate about the importance of propranolol therapy for both HTN and CAD; stress importance of not discontinuing therapy abruptly because of the risk of rebound HTN
- If adverse effects become bothersome or compliance not adequate, consider switching to an alpha-1 antagonist such as terazosin and discontinuing saw palmetto; dosage should begin at 1 mg PO QHS titrated to a goal of 10 mg PO QHS as tolerated; this therapy may also improve prostate symptoms, if present

Problem 5: History of Medication Noncompliance

- Examine psychosocial issues that may be the cause of noncompliance
- Determine whether compliance aids such as pill boxes, personalized calendars, or other methods would help MC better use his medications

ANSWERS

1. b. Miotic activity causes increase in aqueous humor outflow
2. b. Have the patient occlude the nasolacrimal duct for approximately 3–5 minutes following instillation of eye drops
3. Problems attributed to noncompliance include:
   a. Exacerbation of coronary artery disease secondary to poor understanding of how to use SL NTG and/or discontinuation of propranolol
   b. Uncontrolled HTN secondary to discontinuation of propranolol
4. Open-angle glaucoma is usually caused by a physical blockage within the trabecular meshwork, which leads to decreased outflow of aqueous humor. Patients who experience angle-closure glaucoma usually have a narrow anterior chamber or experience dilation of the pupil to the point that the iris comes into contact with the lens. There can be complete blockage of aqueous humor outflow, which is uncommon in open-angle glaucoma.
5. d. Scopolamine or atropine
6. The choice of *Helicobacter pylori* eradicative therapy for MC should be based on the following factors:
   a. Choice of a simplified regimen due to history of noncompliance
   b. Choice of a therapy with known successful eradication rates
   c. Choice of therapy that will minimize adverse effects and potential for drug-drug interactions and avoid any drug allergies
   d. Choice of therapy based upon any previous attempts to eradicate *H. pylori* to minimize failure due to possible resistance
7. b. He should allow for a nitrate-free interval of at least 4 hours a night
8. d. It may lead to blindness if not corrected
9. a. Troponin I
10. a. Laser iridotomy or peripheral trabeculoplasty
11. c. Serum troponin I levels
12. Patients experiencing acute angle-closure glaucoma typically experience pain. Because of this, the patient may experience anxiety and fear loss of vision. This is in contrast to symptoms of open-angle glaucoma, in which patients do not typically experience pain, and psychosocial factors, such as knowledge of the severity of disease, may be more important in the patient adhering to medical therapy.
13. Cost of medications necessary to treat acute angle closure glaucoma may be negligible compared to costs of untreated disease. If a patient is left untreated, blindness is essentially imminent, and indirect costs, such as lost productivity, may be tremendous. Additionally, the patient would certainly experience poorer quality of life following loss of vision.
14. Key points for acute angle-closure glaucoma include:
    a. Angle-closure glaucoma is an emergency that requires immediate medical attention.
    b. Medications that may precipitate open-angle and angle-

closure glaucoma differ due to differences in anatomical causes of disease.

c. A combination of topical agents and intravenous agents should be utilized until surgical therapy can be performed.

d. Surgical therapy, including laser iridotomy and peripheral trabeculoplasty are curative for patients who experience angle-closure glaucoma.

CASE 77

PROBLEM LIST

1. Acute Otitis Media (AOM)
2. Probable Upper Respiratory Tract Infection (URI)

SOAP NOTE

S: "Was grumpy" 5 days ago, often inconsolable, and pulling on left ear during this time period

O: Fever (maximum) 37.7°C (99.9°F); left tympanic membrane (TM) is erythematous, opaque, and slightly bulging; reduced mobility noted on pneumatic otoscopy; rhinorrhea is present (clear in color); Lkcs 12.4 × 10⁹ (12.4 × 10³), differential: Segs 0.76 (76), bands 0.12 (12), monos 0.6 (6), lymphs 0.6 (6)

A: Problem 1: Acute otitis media (AOM)

Problem 2: Probable upper respiratory infection/sinusitis

P: Problem 1: Acute Otitis Media (AOM)

- At risk for drug-resistant *Streptococcus pneumoniae* (DRSP), initial therapy should include amoxicillin 80 to 90 mg/kg (680 mg) given in three divided doses (225 mg) (Dowell SF, Butler JC, Giebink GS, et al. Acute otitis media: management and surveillance in an era of pneumococcal resistance—a report from the Drug-resistant *Streptococcus pneumoniae* Therapeutic Working Group. Pediatr Infect Dis J 1999 Jan;18(1):1–9)
- Monitor for resolution of symptoms (fever, pain, irritability) and for possible side effects (rash, diarrhea)
- Continue analgesic therapy with acetaminophen liquid 80 mg q6h for supportive therapy
- Follow-up in 3 days; if NK does not respond to therapy, an alternative agent such as amoxicillin-clavulanate should be selected; this combination therapy is effective against DRSP and beta-lactamase-producing pathogens
- A total of 10 days of therapy with an effective agent recommended
- Follow-up with physician within 3–6 weeks after infection resolved

Problem 2: Probable Upper Respiratory Infection (URI)/Sinusitis

- Selected plan for AOM (above) also recommended for URI; monitor for signs of improvement (decreased nasal congestion, rhinorrhea, and resolution of fever)

ANSWERS

1. c. *Streptococcus pneumoniae*
2. Common symptoms of acute otitis media which NK exhibits include:
   a. Fever
   b. Infant is inconsolable and increasingly irritable
   c. NK has been pulling on his left ear
3. a. Aspirin should be used to reduce fever and pain
4. d. Amoxicillin
5. An alternative to amoxicillin should be prescribed under the following conditions:
   a. Documented penicillin allergy
   b. Documented amoxicillin failure following 3 days therapy
   c. Previous failure of amoxicillin on at least 2 occasions
   d. Presence of resistant organism determined by culture
   e. Coexisting illness requiring a second-line medication
6. c. Previous exposure to amoxicillin
7. Anatomic changes in children that predispose them to otitis media include anatomical positioning (prone versus sitting/standing) and decreased Eustachian tube length and patency
8. b. Fussiness and inconsolability of the infant or child causes parents to ask physicians for "something" to alleviate the condition
9. c. These agents may be given less frequently and therefore have better compliance
10. a. Rebound congestion if used for periods of greater than 3 days
11. c. Antimicrobial resistance patterns of the medication(s) chosen
12. Pharmacoeconomic considerations for the treatment of acute otitis media include:
    a. First-line agents should be used when appropriate in an attempt to reduce costs of medications and development of antimicrobial resistance
    b. Topical antibiotics have not been shown to be effective and should not be used
    c. Repeat physician office visits and additional medical therapy should be considered in the overall cost of therapy
13. Key points of therapeutic, pathophysiologic, and disease management concepts for acute otitis media include:
    a. Treatment is aimed at preventing acute or chronic complications as a result of chronic or recurrent infections.
    b. Antimicrobial therapy should be reserved for acute episodes in children less than 2 years of age or in children with chronic or recurrent infections.
    c. Adjunctive therapies such as antihistamines and decongestants are of no value in the management of otitis media, but they are capable of causing side effects.
    d. Education of the parent or caregiver as well as judicious

selection and use of antimicrobial therapy will serve to improve the outcome of otitis media.

CASE 78

PROBLEM LIST

1. Acute Otitis Externa
2. Seasonal Allergies

SOAP NOTE

S: "I think I have an ear infection. It has been bothering me for the past couple of days. It's been really painful. Can I get some antibiotics? . . . I also need a refill of my antihistamine.

O: Left ear erythematous and tender; external auditory canal macerated; (+) serous drainage; T 37.0°C; TMs intact and normal appearance

A: **Problem 1:** Acute otitis externa secondary to prolonged exposure to water

   Problem 2: Seasonal allergies

P: **Problem 1: Otitis Externa**

   • Begin therapy with a corticosteroid/drying agent; an OTC combination product containing 1% hydrocortisone, 44% alcohol available
   • Instruct the placement of 4–6 drops of the solution into each ear canal four times daily. Alternatively, the drops may be placed onto a cotton or gauze wick which is placed in the ear canal
   • Advise avoidance of water contact while being treated; monitor for resolution of symptoms (decreased pain and swelling) which should generally occur within 5 days
   • Oral antibiotic therapy may be necessary if the infection spreads to the surrounding soft tissue (necrotizing otitis externa); choice of therapy should be guided by sensitivities of auditory canal fluid cultures
   • Advise that he may avoid future occurrences of otitis externa with careful aural hygiene and use of over-the-counter drying agents containing isopropyl alcohol or acetic acid

   Problem 2: Seasonal Allergies

   • Determine causative allergens; determine timing and severity of symptoms in relation to exposure to potential allergens
   • Reduction of symptoms may be possible by avoidance of known allergens, use of HEPA filters on indoor heating/ventilation systems and frequent cleaning, and use of a paper filter mask during outdoor activities

• Astemizole is not a viable alternative as it has been associated with numerous drug-drug interactions and is no longer marketed in the United States; begin therapy with loratadine 10 mg QD PRN; counsel to take this approximately 30–60 minutes prior to exposure to known allergens to improve efficacy

ANSWERS

1. b. Scuba diving
2. The most common pathogens are: *Pseudomonas aeruginosa, Staphylococcus aureus, Aspergillus,* or *Candida* species
3. d. Hypoalbuminemia
4. Key educational points regarding proper administration of ear drops include:
   a. Wash hands before administering
   b. Avoid touching the dropper to surface of the ear
   c. If drops are in suspension, gently shake for approximately 10 seconds
   d. Lie on side or tilt head to allow administration
   e. Medication may be applied to a gauze or cotton wick, which is then inserted in the ear canal and left in place
5. a. Cromolyn sodium
6. c. It is used as a drying agent
7. Psychosocial factors in this case which may contribute to treatment failure include:
   a. Failure to obtain OTC drying agent due to factors such as the perception that OTC product is not as "strong" as a prescription product
   b. LR's "love of the water" increases chances of noncompliance or concordance
   c. Belief that acute otitis externa is self-limiting may reduce chances that prophylactic aural hygiene is completed
8. d. For cases when the infection has spread to surrounding tissues of the ear
9. b. Benign prostatic hyperplasia symptoms
10. d. Tympanic membrane
11. c. Perforated tympanic membrane
12. Prophylactic use of OTC drying agents can potentially reduce overall cost of care as well as improve patient quality of life. Costs avoided with successful prophylaxis include:
    a. Medication costs
    b. Physician office visit costs
    c. Costs of adverse effects related to therapy
    d. Costs associated with lost productivity
13. Key points of therapeutic, pathophysiologic, and disease management concepts for otitis externa include:
    a. Treatment of otitis externa involves meticulous aural hygiene in addition to topical pharmacotherapy.
    b. Patient education on the administration of otic preparations is essential, especially if the patient is going to self-administer the medication.
    c. Topical administration of antibiotic preparations such as neomycin or chloramphenicol may lead to adverse events, and their administration is generally not recommended.
    d. Oral antibiotics are only indicated if the infection has spread to the surrounding soft tissue.

CASE 79

PROBLEM LIST

1. Acute Migraine Headache
2. GERD
3. Chronic Migraine Headache
4. Status Post Deep Venous Thrombosis
5. Smoking

SOAP NOTE

S: "My head hurts so bad on this left side; I can't stand the light and vomiting anymore; laying down and taking my medicine has not helped at all and now my chest has a burning pain."

O: Complaining of pain, photophobia, emesis, and erythematous oral mucosa

A: Problem 1: Acute migraine lasting 1.5 days; no relief with NSAIDs

Problem 2: Exacerbation of GERD secondary to self administration of NSAIDs for acute migraine attack

Problem 3: Chronic migraine headache; more than 2 migraine attacks per month that are predictable and debilitating

Problem 4: Distal deep venous thrombosis 9 months ago; no long-term anticoagulation required; hematologic abnormalities ruled out

Problem 5: Smoking 2 PPD

P: Problem 1: Acute Migraine

- Discontinue ibuprofen
- Begin sumatriptan injection 6 mg SC; if relief occurs but pain returns, one additional SC injection may be given within the 24-hour period
- If no relief give morphine sulfate, 3–5 mg IV q2h PRN for acute headache pain

Problem 2: GERD

- Initiate famotidine 40 mg PO QHS or alternative H_2-antagonist
- Recommend avoidance of NSAIDs as dyspepsia is common with NSAID administration
- Educate on nonpharmacologic treatments to alleviate GERD
- Eat smaller meals during the day
- Avoid meals prior to bedtime
- Eliminate spicy, offensive foods from diet
- Elevate head of bed 6–8 inches for straight plane incline to reduce reflux

Problem 3: Chronic Migraine

- An appropriate candidate for prophylactic therapy due to many predictable headaches

- Initiate propranolol, 20 mg PO BID; titrate propranolol to an average dose of 80–240 mg QD BID to TID; maximum doses should not exceed 320 mg/day
- Monitor closely for hypotension and bradycardia, as well as changes in cholesterol and blood glucose levels

Problem 4: Status Post Deep Venous Thrombosis

- Educate on nonpharmacologic measures to prevent further clotting, such as walking, weight reduction, and smoking cessation

Problem 5: Smoking

- Educate regarding the importance of smoking cessation; encourage to set a quit date and enroll in a smoking cessation program that will help achieve this goal; recommend a decrease in the quantity of cigarettes smoked each day
- Consider for nicotine replacement if cessation desired; the dosage form preferred should be selected as part of the smoking cessation program
- Dietary counseling and physical activity should be incorporated as part of the management of smoking cessation to assist with weight loss and adequate nutrition maintenance

ANSWERS

1. Use of NSAIDs in this patient likely worsened underlying GERD due to dyspepsia; stress is unrelated.
2. Five attacks lasting 4–72 hours and two of the following characteristics: unilateral location, moderate or severe intensity, or aggravation by routine physical activity. At least one of the following should occur during the attack: nausea/vomiting or photophobia and phonophobia
3. Economic impact of lost productivity in a disease state affecting the young/middle-aged adult population should always be considered. Lost work days likely cost more than the cost of therapy
4. b. Selected for patients dependent on factors such as attack frequency and impact on quality of life
5. a. Status post deep venous thrombosis
6. Monitored closely for hypotension and bradycardia; cholesterol and blood glucose levels checked regularly, especially with her obesity
7. a. 5HT1B/1D Agonist
8. b. Avoid large meals especially before bed
9. d. Longer half-life
10. Tricyclic antidepressants due to delayed gastric emptying (worsens GERD); valproate may cause weight gain, which may worsen her obesity and thus her GERD and is a poor choice in a young female due to teratogenicity; methysergide is used only as a last resort and would not be appropriate at this point
11. a. Two to three times per week

12. d. SC sumatriptan
13. c. Associated symptoms
14. Key points are:
   a. Proper headache classification is key in choosing the correct therapy and secondary causes of headache should be ruled out as inappropriate headache management results in significant costs and impairs quality of life.
   b. Reduction of frequency and severity of headache attacks is the cornerstone of treatment and often involves both pharmacologic and nonpharmacologic means.
   c. Preventive therapy may not eliminate all headache; acute treatment is thus necessary for breakthrough attacks but should not exceed two to three times weekly to avoid rebound headache.

CASE 81

PROBLEM LIST

1. Idiopathic Generalized Epilepsy with Tonic-Clonic Seizures
2. Phenytoin Toxicity
3. Alcoholism for 15 Years
4. PUD & Gastritis
5. HTN
6. Hypokalemia

SOAP NOTE

S: "I've had an increase in number of seizures up to four monthly, and I am sick at my stomach. Since I've been on that new stomach medicine I've been sleepy and unsteady."

O: Alb 32 (3.2), Phenytoin 130 (32.5), HEENT: Gingival hyperplasia, (+) bilateral nystagmus on lateral gaze (at 45 degrees); ataxia, (+) Romberg sign, guaiac positive, BP 160/90, K (3.1)

A: **Problem 1:** Worsening of baseline seizure control with an increase in number of seizures

Problem 2: Phenytoin acute toxicity due to drug interaction with cimetidine; chronic gingival hyperplasia

Problem 3: Alcoholism: increase in ethanol consumption contributing to worsening seizure control

Problem 4: PUD diagnosed recently and gastritis: aggravated by smoking and heavy ethanol consumption; cimetidine therapy prescribed for management of PUD; currently remains guaiac positive with low hematocrit

Problem 5: HTN poorly controlled on current hydrochlorothiazide regimen taken intermittently

Problem 6: Hypokalemia (asymptomatic) secondary to hydrochlorothiazide therapy

P: **Problem 1: Seizure Disorder**

- Modification of seizure triggers (e.g., heavy alcohol intake, lack of sleep, stress) is necessary
- Discontinue cimetidine due to interaction with phenytoin
- If seizures persist after triggers modified, an alternative anti-epileptic drug may be added to the phenytoin until the new agent's serum concentration is therapeutic; then a plan to slowly taper phenytoin could be instituted

Problem 2: Phenytoin Toxicity

- Discontinue cimetidine and substitute ranitidine, 150 mg PO BID; follow up in clinic to assess drug therapy within 2 weeks

Problem 3: Alcoholism

- Strongly encourage participation in alcohol rehabilitation; emphasize how alcohol intake adversely affects seizure disorder
- Assess nutritional status, consider thiamine and folate if oral intake poor

Problem 4: PUD and Gastritis

- Admits to stopping cimetidine after 4 days since experiencing ataxia; reports still experiencing blood in stool and hematocrit still low; emphasize that adherence to ranitidine therapy essential; avoidance of irritating foods, ethanol, and NSAIDs also critical to ulcer healing
- May benefit from iron administration as he recovers from gastrointestinal (GI) blood loss; recommend iron sulfate, 325 mg PO TID; counsel to take this in between meals and that stools may become dark from the iron
- Should follow up with the gastroenterologist within 6–8 weeks to assess recovery

Problem 5: HTN

- Evaluate compliance with therapy and emphasize hydrochlorothiazide must be taken every day; recheck blood pressure in 7 days, if not under control at that time (<140/90 mm Hg) consider increasing dose to 25 mg of hydrochlorothiazide

Problem 6: Hypokalemia

- Consider potassium supplementation chronically (20 mEq daily) and recheck; may need 2 days of higher doses initially; an alternative would be a combination product, such as hydrochlorothiazide/triamterene to reduce the number of tabs per day
- Encourage an intake of dietary potassium, preferably from fresh fruits and vegetables high in potassium

ANSWERS

1. Concentration normal = (concentration observed)
   (4.4 g/dL/albumin of patient)
   (Alternative formulas may be acceptable)

$$44.7 = (32.5) \ (4.4 \ g/dL/3.2 \ g/dL)$$

2. Cimetidine is an enzyme inhibitor, which inhibits the metabolism of phenytoin, thus decreasing clearance and increasing the level of phenytoin
3. a. Ataxia
4. Alcoholism destroys compliance, worsens seizure control, affects phenytoin metabolism, predisposes patients to gastritis.
5. No, HK already has difficulty due to alcoholism in adhering to once daily phenytoin; if a new agent is initiated, there must be an overlap with phenytoin until the new agent is within the therapeutic range; then phenytoin would have to be slowly tapered; monotherapy is the most appropriate with an emphasis on compliance
6. HK needs to be educated on epilepsy and its triggers such as infection, sleep deprivation, stress, and ethanol intake; emphasize that taking medication regularly is key in preventing seizure recurrence
7. c. Alcoholism
8. d. Full-dose H$_2$-antagonist
9. b. Guaiac positive, low hematocrit
10. a. Discontinue smoking
11. d. Gingival hyperplasia
12. a. Gynecomastia
13. c. Seizure diary
14. Key points are:
    a. Patient-specific seizure precipitants should be identified and eliminated.
    b. Minimize the use of polydrug therapy and sedating AEDs whenever possible.
    c. Periodic monitoring of AED blood levels may be useful for guiding subsequent dosage adjustments (for phenytoin in particular), and for monitoring medication compliance, adverse effects, and the effects of drugs or conditions that alter AED clearance.

CASE 82

PROBLEM LIST

1. Status Epilepticus
2. Partial Epilepsy with Secondarily Generalized Tonic-Clonic Seizures
3. SLE
4. Chronic Pancreatitis

SOAP NOTE

S: Sister reports three seizures at home characterized by loss of consciousness, tongue biting, urinary incontinence, and muscle rigidity followed by jerking movements of all extremities; additional complaints of 3-week history of arthralgias, fatigue, and mild fever

O: Recurrent seizures witnessed by paramedics and emergency room staff without recovery of consciousness between attacks; bite wound on tongue, unresponsive to deep pain, increased BP, HR, Temp, and glucose level; carbamazepine level: 13 (3); erythematous malar (cheek) rash; moderate joint swelling of hands and feet; BUN 13.6 (38); CR 212 (2.4); Platelets 45 × 10^9 (45 × 10^3); (+) ANA (titer: 1:480); ESR 50; Amylase 3.67 (220)

A: **Problem 1:** Status epilepticus likely triggered by poor carbamazepine compliance; other potential causes such as metabolic abnormalities, and other primary central nervous system (CNS) disorders should be investigated

Problem 2: Partial and secondarily generalized tonic-clonic seizures with poor compliance likely due to every 8 hours dosing required for carbamazepine

Problem 3: Clinical and laboratory data suggest mild exacerbation of SLE; NSAIDs are effective for analgesic, anti-inflammatory, and antipyretic effects; naproxen may be contributing to poor renal function

Problem 4: Chronic pancreatitis of unknown cause: no clinical signs or symptoms of acute pancreatic inflammation or evidence of pancreatic insufficiency (e.g., malabsorption or inability to maintain normal blood sugar levels)

P: **Problem 1: Status Epilepticus**
- Give diazepam, 10 mg IV (or lorazepam, 4 mg IV) immediately and monitor respiratory status and seizure recurrence; diazepam already administered by paramedics and terminated seizures temporarily, recurrent seizure in the ER likely related to the short duration of diazepam's anticonvulsant effect; another dose of diazepam may be administered for immediate prevention of seizures, but additional anticonvulsant therapy (e.g., phenytoin) necessary to maintain seizure control; lorazepam also effective for aborting repetitive seizures, has a longer-lasting anticonvulsant effect (length of CNS activity rather than biological half-life) than diazepam, and may therefore be preferred
- Initiate phenytoin, 20 mg/kg (1200 mg) IV at a rate of approximately 50 mg/min; BP, HR, and ECG should be monitored during IV phenytoin infusion
- Complete neurologic evaluation necessary to assess other possible causes of seizures

Problem 2: Partial and Secondarily Generalized Tonic-Clonic Seizures

- Initiate a new BID sustained release form of carbamazepine and increase every 3–7 days as necessary to achieve therapeutic levels and seizure control; stop dose escalation when seizures are controlled or dose-limiting adverse effects occur
- Counsel regarding the importance of compliance with prescribed anti-epileptic drug regimen; encourage discussion of any adverse effects with health care providers

Problem 3: SLE

- Change NSAID therapy from naproxen to sulindac, 150 mg PO BID
- Monitor BUN and CR levels, urinalysis results, and BP for possible adverse effects of sulindac therapy
- Monitor signs and symptoms of SLE to assess improvement or worsening of this condition
- Counsel to avoid direct sunlight, as it may cause the rash to worsen
- Hydroxychloroquine (200–400 mg daily) is also effective for treating the skin lesions of SLE and should be considered if the rash does not resolve

Problem 4: Pancreatitis

- No specific treatment recommended for pancreatitis
- Monitor for signs and symptoms of acute pancreatitis (e.g., abdominal pain, alterations in fluid balance, malnutrition) or the complications of chronic pancreatic insufficiency
- Recommend a low-fat diet

ANSWERS

1. a. IV phenytoin 100 mg q8h
2. a. Baseline CBC and if pretreatments are normal then periodically
3. NSAIDs can adversely affect the kidney through immunologically mediated toxicity but this is rare; more commonly, NSAIDs decrease renal prostaglandin synthesis, thus causing a decrease in the beneficial vasodilatation induced by the renal prostaglandins.
4. a. Diplopia, nausea, ataxia
5. JZ will require ophthalmological monitoring every 6 months for ocular toxicity
6. The pharmacist's role in strengthening patient compliance includes:
    a. Counsel on benefits of the medication
    b. Counsel on management of side effects
    c. Provide written reinforcement
    d. Provision of a seizure diary to document seizure activity
    e. Provision of a pill box to act/trigger adherence to therapy
7. d. Carbamazepine 100 mg BID × 3 days, then 200 mg BID × 1 week, and then 200 mg of extended release product twice daily with titration to therapeutic levels
8. c. Autoinduction
9. a. Valproate
10. a. Gabapentin
11. a. Prednisone
12. Naproxen inhibits prostaglandin, which suppresses pain, inflammation, serositis, and the constitutional symptoms of SLE
13. Key points are:
    a. Monitor for clinical and laboratory evidence of adverse effects of drug therapy.
    b. The clinical status of the patient should be the ultimate guide regarding the necessity for dosage adjustments.
    c. In patients who have persistent seizures despite titration of therapy to the maximum tolerated dose, another AED should be gradually substituted for the original medication.
    d. Patients and their families require education and support regarding epilepsy, its treatment, and its effect on daily activities.

CASE 84

PROBLEM LIST

1. Chronic Parkinson's Disease with On/Off Syndrome
2. HTN
3. Osteoporosis
4. Hallucinations

SOAP NOTE

S: "My medicine is wearing off on me. I am getting some odd movements about 30 minutes after a dose of my medication for Parkinson's disease, and I am seeing things that I know are not there."

O: Gait with small steps and reduced arm swing, (+) cog-wheeled rigidity upper and lower extremities, (+) pill-rolling tremor upper extremities, (+) bradykinesia; BP 166/90

A: **Problem 1:** Chronic Parkinson's disease with poor control and on/off syndrome; a clear "peak" dose dyskinesia pattern and a wearing off of medication (carbidopa/levodopa) effect before the next dose

Problem 2: HTN not adequately controlled

Problem 3: Osteoporosis; patient is on estrogen replacement and calcium

Problem 4: Hallucinations; most likely etiology is drug-induced effect of carbidopa/levodopa, as AJ is insightful ("things I know are not there"), and are always visual, not auditory; thus true psychosis is unlikely

P: **Problem 1: Chronic Parkinson's Disease with On/Off Syndrome**

- Carbidopa/levodopa is well known to lose efficacy in Parkinson's disease

- Add bromocriptine, 1 mg PO QD; monitor for gastrointestinal (GI) distress, orthostasis, hallucinations, and other central nervous system (CNS) side effects; advise to monitor for additive side effects with carbidopa/levodopa
- Addition of bromocriptine will likely improve wearing off time; chronic disease treatment additive side effects of bromocriptine and carbidopa/levodopa can be troublesome; reduce carbidopa/levodopa to 25/100 mg and instruct to take one tablet QID to minimize peak levels and provide the suggested total daily dose reduction that is often necessary when beginning a dopamine agonist
- Continue to titrate up bromocriptine
- Encourage to continue a program of regular physical exercise, emphasizing activities that involve balance, range of motion, and fine motor movements
- Provide education to family and friends regarding Parkinson's disease

Problem 2: HTN

- Continue atenolol at current dosage since patient is tolerating well
- Add hydrochlorothiazide 12.5 mg and check a chemistry panel (including glucose, sodium, and potassium) and blood pressure in 1 week; monitor for hyponatremia, hypokalemia, and increased glucose
- Recommend adequate intake of potassium (approximately 90 mmol/day) preferably from food sources such as fresh fruits and vegetables; monitor K^+ on follow-up visits; in the future if the patient has hypokalemia the addition of other forms of K^+ supplementation may be warranted
- Reassess HTN monthly until target BP (<140/90 mm Hg) is achieved; thereafter follow up periodically
- Reinforce lifestyle modifications including physical activity and weight reduction

Problem 3: Osteoporosis

- AJ is already on estrogen replacement; ensure that yearly evaluations of bone density are being performed
- Recommend addition of vitamin D, 400–800 IU PO QD, along with current calcium supplementation regimen
- Emphasize that lifestyle modifications including exercise will be beneficial for osteoporosis, HTN, and Parkinson's disease; counsel to limit caffeine intake

Problem 4: Hallucinations

- Reduce daily carbidopa/levodopa intake to prevent AJ's hallucinations
- Assess for hallucination reoccurrence/worsening as bromocriptine's dosage is titrated upward
- Consider an atypical antipsychotic that is free of

extrapyramidal side effects if hallucination episodes are affecting quality of life

ANSWERS

1. a. Involuntary resting tremor
2. c. Nausea, abnormal movements
3. d. Idiopathic
4. c. Cisapride
5. Serum creatinine because amantidine must be dose adjusted in renal failure.
6. b. MAO-B inhibitor
7. Selegiline is metabolized to amphetamine and meth-amphetamine and may result in stimulation, affecting the patient's sleep patterns.
8. Hydrochlorothiazide increases renal reabsorption of calcium needed for bone maintenance.
9. d. Olanzapine
10. a. Dopamine agonist
11. As neuronal degeneration continues, the presynaptic neurons also degrade; dopamine agonists stimulate the postsynaptic receptor; thus, these agents may work longer than drugs that depend on an intact presynaptic receptor.
12. a. Bioavailability
13. Reassure AJ that the hallucinations are drug induced and that her cognitive function is intact; explain that dementia/cognitive impairment does not occur in the majority of Parkinson's disease patients.
14. Key points are:
    a. The causes of PD remain obscure. However, age-related changes, toxin exposure, and genetic predisposition are believed to play a role in promoting oxidant stress with subsequent neurodegeneration and depletion of nigrostriatal dopamine.
    b. Appropriate treatment can delay the onset of functional impairment, provide significant symptomatic relief, and improve quality of life. Toward improving quality of life, successful management depends on proper diagnosis, familiarity with pharmacologic and nonpharmacologic modalities, and individualized treatment.
    c. Levodopa with PDI remains the most efficacious form of pharmacotherapy, but the development of late-stage motor and neuropsychiatric complications remains problematic.
    d. Current recommendations favor the selective use of anticholinergic agents for young patients with tremor-predominant disease, direct dopamine agonists for young patients with akinetic-rigid disease, and levodopa and PDI for older adults. Additionally, early initiation of selegiline should be considered as a means of delaying the onset of functional impairment.

CASE 86

PROBLEM LIST

1. Seizures
2. Acute Postsurgical Pain Control
3. Postoperative Antithrombotic Therapy

SOAP NOTE

S: "My hip is hurting from the surgery and I am having headaches. Before today, I have not had a seizure for about 1 year."

O: Well-developed, obese female in severe distress; BP 160/104, HR 110, RR 22, T 37.0°C, Wt 72 kg, Ht 168 cm; HEENT: WNL; Normal S1, S2, positive S3; Chest: Clear, no rales or rhonchi; ABD: Soft, nontender, positive bowel sounds; Foley catheter in place; A and O × 3, but exhibits slowed speech and memory impairment; Pertinent laboratory tests: Na 145 (145), Hct 0.36 (36), LDH 2.0 (120), TSH 3, K 3.8 (3.8), Hgb 115 (11.5), Alk Phos 1.0 (60) T4 64 (5), Cl 108 (108), Lkcs 10 × 10^9 (10 × 10^3), Alb 38 (3.8), Phenytoin 48 (12), HCO$_3$ 22 (22), Plts 250 × 10^9 (250 × 10^3), Glu 11.1 (200), BUN 11.3 (30), MCV 86 (86), Ca 2.25 (9.0), Cr 115 (1.3), AST 0.83 (50), Mg 1.07 (2.6); urinalysis: WNL; chest x-ray: mild left ventricular hypertrophy

A: **Problem 1:** Current seizure precipitated by accumulation of normeperidine (metabolite of meperidine); renal impairment, secondary to NSAID use, caused accumulation of normeperidine; 800 mg phenytoin in last 48 hours; therapeutic phenytoin level; 4-year history of generalized seizures

Problem 2: Acute postsurgical pain: poor pain control at current dose of meperidine; needs more potent analgesic with less seizure risk

Problem 3: Postoperative antithrombotic therapy: postsurgical patient at risk for DVT and PE formation; received enoxaparin 30 mg SC BID × 3 days

P: **Problem 1: Seizures**

- Discontinue meperidine to prevent further accumulation of normeperidine
- Assess KM's adherence to current phenytoin regimen
- Recommend phenytoin level again in 5 days
- Monitor KM for seizure control
- Assess neurologically for toxicity (ataxia, nystagmus, dizziness, drowsiness)

Problems 2: Acute Postsurgical Pain

- Discontinue meperidine
- Discontinue ibuprofen and monitor renal function
- Start morphine sulfate elixir, 30 mg PO q4–6h
- Start senna, 187 mg PO PRN at bedtime to promote bowel movements
- Use promethazine, 25 mg PO q4h PRN for nausea
- Monitor respiratory rate, heart rate, and blood pressure
- Monitor for sedation, nausea, and bowel sounds

Problem 3: Postoperative Antithrombotic Therapy

- Continue enoxaparin at present dose until ambulatory
- Encourage continued ambulation and recommend elastic stockings to prevent venous stasis and thrombus formation

ANSWERS

1. b. Normeperidine
2. The oral:parenteral ratio is about 5:1 because of first pass metabolism. Thus, 10 mg/hr IV = 240 mg/day; 240 mg IV/5 = 48 mg PO morphine QD. Reduce the 48 mg by 25% = 16 mg. Morphine SR tablets are available as 15, 30, 60, 100, and 200 mg tablets. Round the 16 mg oral dose to the nearest available tablet and administer every 12 hours. The patient may need breakthrough pain coverage; immediate release morphine can be used. Narcotic therapy should include therapy for constipation such as a stool softener or laxative. Note: Morphine SR loses its extended release kinetics if it is broken in half or crushed.
3. Prophylactic therapy with enoxaparin should begin 12–24 hours after surgery to allow stabilization of hemodynamics and to reduce bleeding at surgical site.
4. b. Monitoring anticoagulation tests not required
5. c. Morphine
6. a. Hydromorphone
7. Cockcroft & Gault equation:

$$\text{CrCl} = \frac{(140 - \text{age})\,\text{IBW}}{72 \times \text{SCr}}\,(0.85 \text{ for females})$$

(IBW = 45 kg + 2.3 kg for each inch over 5 feet tall)
IBW = 58.8 kg (59 kg); CrCl ≈ 42 mL/min

8. It is not recommended to dose adjust because, while decreasing normeperidine accumulation and the seizure risk, the patient's pain control may be compromised if higher doses are required. Therefore, choosing an alternative pain medication, such as morphine, is more appropriate for a patient with renal insufficiency. Factors that predispose KM to further normeperidine-induced seizures include doses greater than 400–600 mg/day, previous seizures, and her poor renal function.
9. d. Salsalate
10. c. Phenytoin metabolism
11. a. Acetaminophen
12. Psychosocial factors include
    1. Barriers to therapy
       a. Afraid of "pain-pills" and "addiction"
       b. Misuse/overuse, resulting in abuse or side effects
    2. Physical symptoms
       a. Pain exacerbation with under-treatment
       b. Poor sleep patterns
       c. Increased heart rate (autonomic responses)
       d. Increased blood pressure
       e. Sweating
    3. Emotional symptoms
       a. Irritability

b. Anxiety
c. Depression from chronic pain
d. Debilitation
e. Isolation
f. Fear
4. Social pain
a. Relationship problems
b. Financial difficulties
13. c. Naloxone
14. It is not economically beneficial to obtain another phenytoin level at this time. The current level was obtained shortly after the seizure and was therapeutic. Therefore, the economic expenditure to obtain the level is not justified. The pharmacokinetics of phenytoin extended release

capsules requires at least 48–96 hours to reach steady state. Thus, medically a duplicate level has no benefit.
15. Key points are:
a. Knowledge of equianalgesic dosing is important for converting routes of administration or to other various opioid analgesics.
b. Clinical understanding of medication pharmacodynamics can reduce adverse effects while optimizing efficacy.
c. Normeperidine is a renally eliminated metabolite that can exacerbate pre-existent seizure conditions.
d. NSAID therapy can compromise renal function and alter platelet aggregation.
e. Opioids often cause constipation, nausea, and vomiting that may require adjunctive therapy.

SECTION 14 / PSYCHIATRIC DISORDERS

CASE 87

PROBLEM LIST

1. Generalized Anxiety Disorder (GAD)
2. Iron Deficiency Anemia
3. GI Blood Loss
4. Atopic Eczema

SOAP NOTE

S: "I am anxious and on edge. The hydroxyzine doesn't do much for my nerves. My stomach has been giving me more trouble lately. The hydrocortisone cream does not help much with my rashes. Is there anything that can be done for my menstrual cramps?"

O: Appears mildly anxious, hypervigilant, diaphoretic; pale conjunctiva; several mild eczematous lesions on R and L anticubital fossae and face; pale nail beds; decreased RBC, ferritin, Hct, and Hgb; peripheral smear shows microcytic RBCs; guaiac-positive stools

A: Problem 1: Generalized anxiety disorder not responding to hydroxyzine

Problem 2: Iron deficiency anemia resulting from excessive use of NSAIDs to treat dysmenorrhea symptoms

Problem 3 GI blood loss related to OTC NSAID use

Problem 4: Atopic eczema not responding to OTC hydrocortisone

P: Problem 1: GAD

- Recommend cognitive-behavioral psychotherapy to help patient cope with the symptoms of anxiety
- Discontinuation of hydroxyzine as ineffective and compliance poor
- Start diazepam 2 mg PO TID
- Titrate the dose as needed to improve anxiety symptoms
- Educate that may experience relief in the first week of treatment
- Inform that may experience drowsiness and decreased coordination initially, so should use caution if driving or operating machinery
- Inform that diazepam has been associated with birth defects, so contraception recommended if sexually active
- Inform that physical dependence may occur during prolonged therapy

Problem 2: Iron Deficiency Anemia

- Ferrous sulfate 325 mg PO TID, and continue treatment for 3–6 months after normalization of CBC
- Educate about potential adverse effects of iron such as nausea, epigastric pain, cramps, and constipation
- Advise to keep iron out of reach of children, because it is toxic in overdose
- Inform that stools may turn a darker color with iron use

Problem 3: GI Blood Loss

- Discontinue use of OTC oral NSAIDs
- Educate about NSAID-induced GI blood loss
- Recommend referral to work up GI bleeding

- Begin omeprazole 20 mg QD

Problem 4: Atopic Eczema

- Discontinue hydrocortisone cream since ineffective
- Begin betamethasone 0.1% cream and apply TID to rash for itching
- Reevaluate lesions after 2 weeks

ANSWERS

1. b. Excessive noradrenergic activity
2. a. Hypervigilance
3. b. Diazepam has a rapid onset of action
4. a. Diaphoresis
5. The MOA of diazepam is related to potentiation of the neurotransmitter, GABA. This results in enhanced inhibitory effects on the central nervous system.
6. d. Memory impairment
7. a. Alcohol use
8. Pharmacologic and nonpharmacologic treatment problems present in TB's treatment plan include:
   1. Pharmacologic
      a. Use of OTC NSAIDs for dysmenorrhea
      b. Use of OTC hydrocortisone for eczema
      c. Use of hydroxyzine for generalized anxiety disorder
   2. Nonpharmacologic
      a. Lack of stress reduction, exercise, or counseling for GAD
9. c. Lorazepam
10. a. Counseling
11. Psychosocial factors that may improve or worsen TB's anxiety include:
    a. Her father's health
    b. Her relationships with the opposite sex
    c. Stress level at work
    d. The complexity of her medical regimen
    e. Financial considerations
12. Pharmacoeconomic considerations relative to TB's plan of care include:
    a. Cost of diazepam
    b. Cost of counseling
    c. Time involved devoted to transportation to see counselor
    d. Indirect costs of illness related to personal suffering
    e. Loss of time at work due to illness
13. Key points are:
    a. The treatment of generalized anxiety disorder should include cognitive-behavioral psychotherapy.
    b. The symptoms of generalized anxiety disorder include anxiety over several life situations lasting at least 6 months. Associated symptoms include restlessness, easily fatigued, difficulty concentrating, irritability, muscle tension, and disturbed sleep.
    c. Benzodiazepines are the mainstay of pharmacotherapy. They work by potentiating the inhibitory neurotransmitter, GABA.
    d. Patients who are prescribed benzodiazepines for generalized anxiety disorder should be informed about adverse effects such as drowsiness, impaired coordination, memory impairment, and the risk of dependence.

CASE 89

PROBLEM LIST

1. Suicidal Ideation Secondary to Depression
2. Mild Intermittent Asthma

SOAP NOTE

S: Depressed following layoff from his job; drinking heavily, wife left him; complains of mild nausea

O: Lethargic; acetaminophen 2 hours postingestion 330 (5); other labs: WNL

A: Problem 1: Suicidal ideation secondary to depression

Problem 2: Mild intermittent asthma

P: Problem 1: Suicidal Ideation Secondary to Depression

- Initiate supportive psychotherapy and counseling
- Begin antidepressant therapy with a drug unlikely to be lethal in overdose, such as fluoxetine
- Monitor for clinical improvement over several weeks
- Monitor for potential adverse effects such as anxiety, headache, insomnia, sweating, nausea, and anorexia

Problem 2: Mild Intermittent Asthma

- Continue metaproterenol inhaler PRN shortness of breath
- Advise to report any increase in the frequency of use of metered dose inhaler

ANSWERS

1. d. Combination of personal losses and genetic predisposition
2. b. Heavy drinking
3. d. Fluoxetine will inhibit the metabolism of tricyclic antidepressants
4. a. Weight loss
5. The epidemiology of depression as it pertains to suicide: The lifetime prevalence of depression is 17%. The incidence is more common in women than men. Women are more likely to attempt suicide, but men are more likely to succeed than women. The risk of completed suicide in patients with major depression is 15%, which is 30 times higher than the general population.
6. c. Insomnia
7. d. Doxepin
8. Pharmacologic and nonpharmacologic problems in MK's treatment plan include:
   1. Pharmacologic
      a. Lethality of some potential pharmacotherapies
      b. Risk of drug interaction with alcohol
      c. Depression, currently untreated
   2. Nonpharmacologic
      a. Lack of social support
      b. Recent history of suicide attempt
9. a. Supportive psychotherapy
10. Psychosocial factors that may decrease or increase MK's risk of suicide include:

1. Decreasing factors
    a. Gainful employment
    b. Marriage
    c. Abstinence from drug and alcohol use
2. Increasing factors
    a. Psychosocial factors that may increase MK's risk for suicide are the opposite of those factors that reduce the risk.
11. Pharmacoeconomic considerations relative to MK's plan of care include:
    a. Cost of fluoxetine
    b. Unemployment and financial problems
    c. Further treatment for depression required (6–9 months)
    d. Counseling required
    e. Time and travel expense to and from counseling sessions
12. Key points are:
    a. Depression is a major risk factor for suicide attempts.
    b. Suicide attempts are more common in women, but men are more likely to be successful at suicide.
    c. Depressed patients are 30 times more likely to commit suicide than the general population.
    d. Risk factors for suicide include financial difficulty, unmarried status, and alcohol/drug abuse
    e. Tricyclic antidepressants should be avoided when there is a risk of suicide. SSRIs are safer, since they are non-lethal in overdose.

CASE 92

PROBLEM LIST

1. Insomnia
2. Angina
3. COPD
4. Hypertension
5. Hypercholesterolemia
6. Gout

SOAP NOTE

S: "I really need something to help me sleep. I just can't get to sleep unless I am in my own bed."

O: He reports frequent symptoms of insomnia when he is in a new environment. Bilateral rales and rhonchi; uric acid 7 g/dL; 24-hour uric acid excretion 900 mg; total cholesterol 320 mg/dL; triglycerides 120; BP 160/90; has nicotine-stained fingers

A: **Problem 1:** Insomnia

Problem 2: Angina

Problem 3: COPD

Problem 4: Hypertension

Problem 5: Hypercholesterolemia

Problem 6: Gout

P: **Problem 1: Insomnia**

- Begin triazolam 0.25 mg orally QHS. Benzodiazepines are the drugs of choice for transient insomnia
- Monitor for complaints of insomnia and for improvement in sleep quality
- Educate the patient about the possibility for rebound insomnia if he takes the drug nightly for more than a few nights

Problem 2: Angina

- Continue the nitroglycerin and verapamil. Increase the isosorbide dinitrate dose to 20 mg BID, at breakfast and in the afternoon. This should provide enough of a nitrate-free interval to reduce risk of tolerance
- Monitor the patient for headache, dizziness, postural hypotension
- Counsel SF to take sublingual nitroglycerin before exercise to prevent angina

Problem 3: COPD

- Encourage SF to quit smoking and refer him to a comprehensive smoking cessation program. Smoking cessation will have a greater impact on SF's pulmonary function than any other intervention
- Continue use of ipratropium, consider switching to a combined ipratropium/albuterol inhaler at 4 puffs QID to simplify his metered dose inhaler regimen and increase the likelihood of adherence to his therapy. Assess SF's MDI technique
- Monitor for tachycardia since SF takes theophylline. Tachycardia will increase his oxygen demand and worsen his angina

Problem 4: Hypertension

- SF is receiving a diuretic, which can increase his uric acid. His other antihypertensive is verapamil, which improves his angina symptoms. Continue the verapamil but discontinue hydrochlorothiazide since it may be exacerbating his gout.
- SF may need additional treatment for hypertension. An agent should be selected that will not exacerbate any of his disease states. A beta-blocker would help his angina but may exacerbate his COPD. A cautious trial of a low dose of a cardioselective beta-blocker, such as atenolol 25 mg PO QD, may be initiated in the hospital. Monitor closely for exacerbation of his COPD symptoms
- Encourage caloric restriction, exercise, and weight loss, and a no-added-salt diet

Problem 5: Hypercholesterolemia

- Order fasting lipid profile to determine LDL and HDL; target LDL in this patient is 100 mg/dL
- Begin simvastatin 20 mg QD

- Monitor for signs and symptoms of myositis and hepatitis as well as LFTs
- Encourage a low-fat diet, exercise, and weight loss

Problem 6: Gout

- Discontinue hydrochlorothiazide and potassium chloride.
- Discontinue allopurinol since hydrochlorothiazide may have been causing the hyperuricemia.
- Monitor uric acid, and monitor for signs and symptoms of gout.

ANSWERS

1. b. Change in environment
2. a. Transient
3. a. Effects should not persist into the next day
4. a. Theophylline level of 20 μg/mL
5. The mechanism of action of benzodiazepines with regard to sleep induction involves potentiation of GABA, an inhibitory neurotransmitter. Benzodiazepines bind to the benzodiazepine receptor subunit, which increases GABA binding and increases chloride influx into the neuron. This hyperpolarizes the neuron, leading to decreased nervous conduction and central nervous system depression.
6. b. COPD
7. d. Erythromycin
8. Pharmacologic and nonpharmacologic treatment problems include:
   1. Pharmacologic
      a. Use of high dose of hydrochlorothiazide in patient with gout
      b. Failure to combine albuterol and ipratropium in a single metered dose inhaler
      c. Lack of treatment for hypercholesterolemia
      d. Inadequate nitrate therapy and subtherapeutic antihypertensive treatment
   2. Nonpharmacologic
      a. Lack of exercise; dietary fat and sodium restriction
      b. Continued use of tobacco
9. c. Eliminate daytime nap
10. Psychosocial factors that may improve or worsen SF's insomnia:
    1. Improve insomnia
       a. Good prognosis for his conditions
       b. Reassurance from healthcare providers
       c. Encouragement from support group
       d. Elimination of noise/distractions/stress in the evening
    2. Worsen insomnia
       a. Lack of good prognosis
       b. Lack of reassurance from healthcare providers
       c. Lack of adequate support group
       d. Increased noise levels in evening
11. Pharmacoeconomic considerations relative to SF's plan of care include:
    a. Cost of nicotine replacement versus cost of cigarettes
    b. Cost of one inhaler of combined albuterol and ipratropium versus one of each

c. Cost of atenolol versus cost of hydrochlorothiazide, potassium chloride, and allopurinol
d. Cost of statin drugs plus lab tests versus cost of exercise and dietary restriction
e. Cost of poorly treated or undertreated disease likely to be much higher than optimizing therapy

12. Key points are:
    a. Insomnia is classified as transient, short term, and long term.
    b. Transient insomnia is usually associated with a change in environment, such as hospitalization, and usually lasts just a few days.
    c. Treatment of transient insomnia generally involves a short course of benzodiazepines.
    d. The preferred benzodiazepines are those that have a rapid onset and a fairly short duration of action.
    e. Benzodiazepines with longer half-lives may cause residual sedation and daytime psychomotor impairments.

CASE 93

PROBLEM LIST

1. Heroin Overdose
2. RLL Pneumonia
3. Asthma
4. Risk for Opiate Withdrawal

SOAP NOTE

S: Semi-comatose, wife reports increased use of heroin by LB over past few days

O: Groggy, responsive only to pain, A & O × 0; in respiratory distress; pinpoint pupils; BP 80/50, HR 49, RR 8, T 37.8°C; decreased bowel sounds; skin cool to touch, needle-track marks noted on both arms; Tox screen: (+) morphine; chest x-ray: RLL infiltrate; sputum with gram-positive cocci in pairs and chains

A: **Problem 1:** Heroin Overdose

Problem 2: RLL Pneumonia

Problem 3: Asthma

Problem 4: Risk of Opiate Withdrawal

P: **Problem 1: Heroin Overdose**

- Administer naloxone 0.4 mg IV and repeat 4–5 times within 30–45 minutes as necessary to improve mental status and respirations
- Consider administering naloxone as a continuous infusion or on a scheduled basis since the methadone may be contributing to the overdose, and methadone is long acting
- Monitor the patient for improved cognition, increased respirations, and narcotic withdrawal

Problem 2: RLL Pneumonia

- Begin intravenous antibiotics to cover for pneumococcus. Since allergic to penicillin, begin levofloxacin 500 mg IV QD
- Continue IV levofloxacin until no longer hypotensive and has recovered from the opiate overdose. Switch to the oral route when WBC count decreases and symptoms improve. DC levofloxacin when LB clinically stable and afebrile at least 48 hours.
- Perform sputum culture and sensitivity testing, as well as blood cultures to determine presence of bacteremia.

Problem 3: Asthma

- Classify asthma when LB is able to speak, so that proper treatment can be initiated according to national (NHLB) recommendations
- When mental status is improved, perform pulmonary function testing to determine responsiveness to bronchodilation
- Educate about asthma and its treatment, and teach proper metered dose inhaler technique

Problem 4: Risk of Opiate Withdrawal

- Since LB will receive naloxone, an opiate antagonist, LB may experience non–life-threatening opiate withdrawal
- Once stable and no longer experiencing signs and symptoms of overdose, discontinue naloxone and monitor for signs of withdrawal
- Arrange for follow up in the methadone detoxification program, because LB may benefit from methadone maintenance therapy

ANSWERS

1. a. Heart rate 49
2. c. Increased use of other routes of administration
3. b. Naloxone is likely to wear off before methadone, leading to re-sedation
4. c. Needle-track marks
5. Naloxone is a potent opiate-receptor antagonist with a short half-life and duration of action. In the presence of opioid substances, naloxone serves as a competitive antagonist at the opioid receptor, preventing the opioid from producing its pharmacologic effects.
6. b. Opiate withdrawal
7. d. Nalbuphine
8. Pharmacologic and nonpharmacologic problems in LB's treatment plan include:
   1. Pharmacologic
      a. Lack of appropriate treatment for asthma
      b. Use of oral theophylline and beta-agonists for asthma
      c. Continued abuse of heroin
   2. Nonpharmacologic
      a. Poor adherence to detoxification program
      b. Lack of education about asthma treatment
      c. Lack of education about opiate dependence
      d. Poor insight into severity of dependence
9. a. Methadone maintenance
10. Psychosocial factors that may increase or decrease LB's risk for relapse include:
    1. Increase risk
       a. Poor insight into problem of dependence
       b. Lack of employer involvement in maintaining abstinence
       c. Lack of family support of need for abstinence
       d. Use of substances by wife
       e. Lack of access to a methadone maintenance program
       f. Social stigma associated with heroin dependence
    2. Decrease risk
       a. Employer involvement in program
       b. Enrollment in methadone maintenance
       c. Treatment of wife for codependence
11. Pharmacoeconomic considerations relative to LB's treatment plan include:
    a. Employer support of methadone maintenance
    b. Use of funds for appropriate treatment rather than heroin
    c. Ability to pay for medication treatment of substance dependence and asthma
    d. Cost of substance treatment program
12. Key Points are:
    a. Heroin use is increasing and the purity is higher than in the past.
    b. Non-IV use of heroin is becoming more common due to increased purity.
    c. Narcotic overdose may be life-threatening, and results in CNS and respiratory depression.
    d. Naloxone is the treatment of choice for narcotic overdose.
    e. Naloxone may have a shorter duration of action than the opiate itself.
    f. Naloxone may precipitate opiate withdrawal symptoms.
    g. Methadone maintenance is appropriate in patients who fail detoxification programs.

CASE 94

PROBLEM LIST

1. Chronic Bronchitis Exacerbation
2. Isolated Systolic Hypertension
3. Status Post MI
4. Nicotine Dependence

SOAP NOTE

S: "I'm short of breath all the time, and I have been coughing up green junk all week. I think I'm ready to quit smoking now, can you help?" "I just can't get around the way I used to."

O: Chronically ill appearing, barrel-chested; using accessory muscles to aid breathing; AV nicking noted; BP 170/80, HR 85, RR 18, T 39.5°C; WBCs 18.5; epinephrine MDI 2 puffs q4h PRN SOB; triamterene 37.5 mg/hydrochlorothiazide 25 mg QD for hypertension.

A: **Problem 1:** Chronic bronchitis exacerbation

Problem 2: Isolated systolic hypertension

Problem 3: Nicotine dependent

Problem 4: S/P Acute MI 6 months ago

P: **Problem 1: Exacerbation of Chronic Bronchitis**

- Begin treatment with combined ipratropium/ albuterol inhaler using spacer 4 puffs q2–4h PRN for shortness of breath
- Initiate antibiotic treatment with trimethoprim/sulfamethoxazole DS PO BID since febrile and has leukocytosis
- Monitor for improved symptoms, decreased temperature, decreased WBCs, decreased shortness of breath, decreased coughing, and decreased sputum production
- Instruct on proper use of MDI

Problem 2: Isolated Systolic Hypertension

- Continue thiazide diuretic therapy, since this is appropriate pharmacotherapy for ISH
- Encourage patient to maintain a low sodium diet
- Since BP is poorly controlled, add a low dose of a cardioselective selective beta-blocker, such as atenolol 25 mg PO QD, and monitor closely for worsening of respiratory symptoms

Problem 3: Nicotine Dependence

- Select a "quit date" and let friends and family know of plans to quit
- Discuss the health benefits of smoking cessation, such as reducing his decline in respiratory function and decreasing risk of another AMI
- Encourage participation in smoking cessation support group
- Initiate nicotine patch 21 mg and wear daily for 6–8 weeks
- Apply patch to a hairless area on the body between the neck and waist every morning after waking
- Dispose of used patches properly to reduce risk to children and pets

Problem 4: S/P Acute MI 6 Months Ago

- Restart aspirin every day to reduce his risk of another MI
- If tolerated, atenolol may reduce risk of MI

ANSWERS

1. b. 25% of adults
2. a. Cerebrovascular disease
3. b. Nicotine spray has most rapid absorption
4. a. Appetite
5. Nicotine affects both the sympathetic and parasympathetic nervous system. It increases CNS release of norepinephrine and dopamine, which are associated with pleasure, appetite suppression, and reward. Release of acetylcholine may enhance cognition and improve task performance. Smokers report simultaneous arousal and relaxation, improved attention, enhanced problem solving skills, and reduced stress.
6. b. Skin irritation
7. c. Theophylline
8. Pharmacologic and nonpharmacologic problems in TT's treatment plan include
   1. Pharmacologic
      a. Use of epinephrine for shortness of breath
      b. Lack of ipratropium for COPD
      c. Inadequate pharmacotherapy for ISH
      d. Lack of ASA for s/p MI
      e. Lack of beta-blocker s/p MI
      f. Continued nicotine use
   2. Nonpharmacologic
      a. Poorly educated about treatment of hypertension, COPD, and MI
      b. Poor follow-up after MI
9. a. behavioral modification
10. a. bupropion
11. Psychosocial factors that may increase or decrease TT's risk for relapse include:
    1. Increase risk
       a. Lack of support from friends and wife
       b. Lack of monitoring and support from health care professional
       c. Environmental exposure to smokers and cigarettes
       d. Lack of access to appropriate treatment
    2. Decrease risk
       a. Support from family and friends
       b. Access to health care facilities
       c. Removal from environments where tobacco products are used
12. Pharmacoeconomic considerations include:
    a. Insurance rarely covers smoking cessation products
    b. Patients perceive the cost of smoking cessation products as too high
    c. TT may not be able to afford a month's supply of medication at a time, whereas he may be able to buy one pack per day
    d. TT will need several new prescriptions, all of which will decrease the amount of money left for smoking cessation products
13. Key points are:
    a. Nicotine is a complex drug with sympathetic, parasympathetic, and CNS effects. The CNS effects are reinforcing, and lead to dependence
    b. Nicotine withdrawal symptoms perpetuate the smoking cycle

c. Smoking has numerous adverse health effects, including COPD and heart disease

d. Health care professionals may assist patients with smoking cessation by recommending specific nicotine replacement therapies, all of which have been demonstrated to increase the likelihood of smoking cessation

e. Smoking cessation has immediate health benefits to smokers

CASE 96

PROBLEM LIST

1. Attention-Deficit/Hyperactivity Disorder (ADHD) Suspected
2. Asthma
3. Eczema

SOAP NOTE

S: No recent complaints; has used OTC epinephrine MDI on 3 occasions in the past 4 months for SOB; has had some scaling and itching. Teacher has indicated that KR is not progressing at the educational rate of his peers. He is disruptive in class and his social interaction and self-esteem are both suffering as a result.

O: Pulmonary function test results consistent with diagnosis of bronchial asthma, but no wheezing is present; indicated that he has not used moisturizing lotion consistently and has been out of hydrocortisone for at least 6 months; has increased motor activity, short attention span, excessive impulsivity, and reading comprehension limitations in the presence of normal IQ results.

A: Problem 1: Attention-deficit/hyperactivity disorder (ADHD); impulsivity and short attention span; key target symptoms.

Problem 2: Mild asthma requiring more appropriate treatment.

Problem 3: Exacerbation of eczema secondary to regimen noncompliance.

P: Problem 1: ADHD

- Begin methylphenidate 5 mg PO BID at 8 AM and 12 noon with food.
- Counsel patient and family on potential adverse effects such as insomnia, GI upset, tremulousness, loss of appetite. Stress daily compliance as well as expected outcome of therapy. Stimulants should enable student to learn coping mechanisms and to minimize distractions (impulsivity) while in the classroom.
- Advise parents to consider placement of KR in special education classes for reading remediation with participation in regular second-grade classroom activities for all other subjects and activities.
- Urge education and/or counseling of teachers about his disorder and the pharmacologic treatment.
- Encourage participation in family therapy for all members of the family, not just isolated counseling for KR.
- Return to clinic in 4 weeks to monitor for efficacy and presence of adverse effects. Consider possible dose titration if efficacy not apparent.

Problem 2: Mild Asthma

- Change OTC epinephrine MDI to albuterol MDI PRN.
- Attempt to identify environmental triggers (pollen, ragweed) that may be contributing to periodic shortness of breath.
- Continue to monitor for exacerbation of respiratory symptoms.

Problem 3: Eczema

- Recommend consistent use of moisturizing lotion as previously used and 0.5% hydrocortisone to reduce rash.

ANSWERS

1. b. Decrease phenytoin metabolism
2. d. Utilization of drug holidays
3. a. Low abuse potential
4. d. Abnormal thyroid function
5. Methylphenidate can cause insomnia; therefore, do not take doses after 1 PM. Methylphenidate should be taken with food to minimize anorectant and GI irritation effects. CNS stimulation (internal tremulousness, piloerection, shaky hands, tachycardia, sweatiness) is usually mild and transient, if it occurs at all. Do not crush medication and try to take at same time of day. If behavior is not a problem on weekends or school breaks, consider use of drug holidays.
6. a. Initiate another stimulant
7. c. Dextroamphetamine
8. a. Mood disorders
9. c. Reduce resentment toward child with ADHD
10. Parents, as well as the ADHD child, must come to accept this disorder as having a biological basis just like any other disease. Familial involvement is recommended and can be rigorous: family counseling is suggested, noon-time doses often require cooperation between school nurses and parents, and methylphenidate's status as a C-II agent requires monthly, written prescriptions that must be physically picked up at the doctor's office. Low acceptance

of disease usually correlates to poor compliance. Treatment expectations must also be realistic and can be conveyed through appropriate clinician-directed education.

11. Pemoline is an effective stimulant in the treatment of ADHD. However, several cases of liver toxicity, some resulting in liver transplantation, have been correlated with pemoline usage. The FDA currently recommends informed consent and twice monthly LFT evaluation.

12. Key points are:

a. Stimulants are the most effective treatment option for ADHD. If therapeutic failure occurs with one stimulant, another stimulant should be preferentially utilized before resorting to other agents such as tricyclic antidepressants, clonidine, or bupropion. Family counseling is essential as it decreases familial resentment and educates the whole family. Daily compliance is necessary to enjoy full therapeutic benefit. Adverse effects with stimulants are usually mild and transient.

b. The optimal management of ADHD is contingent on a reliable and accurate diagnosis using DSM-IV criteria.

c. Treatment goals should be established jointly with the patient and family.

d. Treatment of ADHD must address multiple aspects of the child's disorder and should not be reduced to the use of medication alone.

e. The majority of patients will respond to one of the available stimulants. Although few differences have been found among the stimulants, methylphenidate is the most studied and most used stimulant.

f. Most randomized clinical trials have assessed short-term use of stimulants. There are no long-term studies evaluating stimulants or psychosocial therapy use over several years. Likewise, there are no long-term outcome studies assessing the effect of medication-treated ADHD on educational and occupational achievements, involvement with the judicial system, or other areas of social dysfunction.

g. Treatment with stimulants does not normalize behavior problems. Although there is improvement in core symptoms, there is little evidence of improvement in long-term academic performance or social skills.

h. The tricyclic antidepressants are the drugs of choice for the 30% of patients who fail to respond to stimulant medications or who cannot tolerate the side effects associated with stimulants. There is some evidence that patients who display greater anxiety, depression, or mood disturbances in conjunction with their ADHD may respond better to TCAs than stimulants. Likewise, some believe that patients who exhibit aggression may deteriorate on TCAs.

i. Decreased appetite, insomnia, and irritability are common with the stimulants. High doses of stimulants may cause CNS damage, hypertension, and possibly motor disorders.

j. Medically unexplained sudden death has been reported in children receiving normal doses of desipramine. The American Academy of Child and Adolescent Psychiatry recommends a baseline ECG, one within days of a dosage increase, and another once steady-state at maximal doses is achieved.

13. d. CNS hyperstimulation

CASE 97

PROBLEM LIST

1. Benzodiazepine Overdose
2. Alcohol Dependence
3. Cocaine Abuse
4. Seizure Disorder
5. Guaiac Positive

SOAP NOTE

S: History of taking oral diazepam 5–30 mg PO QD for stress relief; has had frequent blackouts. RS's friend states that RS was shooting an "eight ball of snow" before coming to ED. History of a single seizure 15 years ago and history of noncompliance with phenytoin.

O: Decreased BP 80/50, HR 55, RR 6, O × 0, responsive only to painful stimuli; RS is a binge drinker (two bottles of wine before this ED visit); Alb 25 (2.5), ALT 7.8 (470), AST 1.75 (105), Alk Phos 2.5 (150), PT 13.5, INR 1.3; guaiac positive and distended, nontender abdomen (wt increased by 2 kg); urinalysis is positive for cocaine and ecgonine (cocaine metabolite); CXR shows mild cardiomegaly. PHT 0 (0).

A: Problem 1: Benzodiazepine overdose exacerbated by decreased clearance due to hepatic dysfunction

Problem 2: Alcohol dependence and abuse with medical sequelae (increased LFTs, guaiac positive, blackouts); currently at risk for alcohol withdrawal

Problem 3: Cocaine overdose secondary to IV cocaine use, mild cardiomegaly as per ECG; not in acute distress due to primary CNS depression with alcohol and benzodiazepines (see above)

Problem 4: Seizure disorder (by history) questionable

Problem 5: Guaiac positive secondary to esophageal varices or direct irritant effects of alcohol on gut

P: Problem 1: Benzodiazepine Overdose

- Administer flumazenil 0.2 mg IV over 15 seconds. After the initial dosage, if the desired level of consciousness not obtained, give a second dose.
- Continue monitoring for at least 4 hours after the last dose of flumazenil to ensure that competitive inhibition at the benzodiazepine receptor sites occurred.
- Expect flumazenil onset of action in 1–2 minutes and peak effect within 6–10 minutes.

Problem 2: Alcohol Dependence/Withdrawal

- Monitor electrolyte, vital signs (BP, RR, HR, T), and for signs and symptoms of alcohol withdrawal (nausea, vomiting, sweating, agitation, tremors, and possibly seizures).
- Begin thiamine 100 mg IV QD to prevent Wernicke-Korsakoff psychosis induced from chronic alcohol use/dependence.
- Rehydrate with D5W and monitor blood glucose, since at risk for hypoglycemia after alcohol consumption and possibly decreased nutritional intake.
- Monitor for possible seizure activity, especially 48–72 hours post last alcohol consumption.

Problem 3: Cocaine Overdose

- Counsel and provide information about the physical dangers of cocaine use.
- Counsel on the risks of HIV infection from intravenous drug abuse and shared needles.

Problem 4: Grand Mal Seizure (by History)

- Discontinue phenytoin.
- Monitor for seizures.

Problem 5: Guaiac Positive

- Give stress ulcer treatment with ranitidine 50 mg IV q8h, and when oral medication ingestion possible, change to ranitidine 300 mg PO QHS.
- Monitor Hct and Hgb levels, stool guaiac test results, PT, INR, and vital signs.
- R/o varices, active PUD.
- Educate about peptic ulcer disease, risk factors, and the need to discontinue alcohol consumption.
- Encourage patient to join Alcoholics Anonymous or a similar alcohol-abstinence therapy group.

ANSWERS

1. a. CAGE
2. a. Thiamine
3. a. Diazepam
4. a. Paranoid schizophrenia
5. a. Lactation
6. a. Nicotine
7. d. Positive quality of life
8. b. Females
9. b. Total abstinence
10. c. Intravenous
11. Substance abuse affects not only the person misusing substances, but also immediate family members, employers, and society itself through decreased productivity and disproportionate utilization of healthcare resources. Crime and violence are increased, as are rates of mortality. Family members are encouraged to participate in organizations such as Al-Anon and Al-Teen. Family therapy seeks to teach acceptance of the person without endorsing the substance abuse.
12. The first phase of rehabilitation is medical stabilization through detoxification from abused substance. The second phase of treatment focuses on education, patient acceptance of illness, and aftercare. Moderate or periodic (social) use of drugs or alcohol after treatment is unrealistic. Total abstinence is indicative of treatment success.
13. c. Crack
14. d. Gingival hyperplasia
15. d. LSD
16. c. Disproportionate healthcare utilization
17. Key points are:
    a. Substance abuse and dependence is a prevalent medical illness that requires professional assistance to treat.
    b. Substance abuse and dependence results in increased mortality, absorbs a disproportionate share of total healthcare costs, and is associated with increased disease comorbidity, especially other psychiatric disorders.
    c. Substance dependence is characterized by a maladaptive pattern of substance use that leads to adverse cognitive, behavioral, and psychological symptoms. Repeated self-administration occurs despite adverse effects. Tolerance, withdrawal, and compulsive substance use are characteristic of dependence.
    d. Etiological theories are inconclusive but probably entail a combination of behavioral, genetic, and biological components.
    e. Heroin supplies in the United States are currently at a higher level of purity than in the past two decades, which has allowed ingestion via smoking or snorting, as opposed to the traditional intravenous method of administration.
    f. Opioid withdrawal is usually medically benign. Agents such as methadone, LAAM, and buprenorphine are effective treatment options during narcotic detoxification.
    g. Sedatives and anxiolytic drugs are some of the most commonly used medications, with almost 15% of the U.S. population having had a benzodiazepine prescribed by a physician. Anxiolytic/sedative withdrawal is accomplished through gradual tapering of a cross-tolerant medication and provision of supportive care and emergent symptomatic treatment.
    h. Cocaine abuse, especially in the smokable form of crack, is epidemic in certain segments of the U.S. Crack is cheap, readily available, produces an immediate and profound high, and is very addictive.
    i. Current levels of amphetamine abuse in the U.S. are being fueled by the relatively easy synthesis and production of synthetic supplies in small "meth labs."
    j. Plant source hallucinogen use dates to 500 B.C. in some cultures. Synthetic hallucinogens became available in the 1940's with the synthesis of lysergic acid diethylamide (LSD). Addiction to hallucinogens is rare and users seldom report for medical assistance, except in the case of "bad trips" or severe paranoia.
    k. Marijuana is the most commonly used illicit drug in the U.S. Patients requesting detox or medical assistance for marijuana abuse alone is rare. Samples of marijuana in the U.S. have gradually increased in percentage of THC, the psychoactive compound found in marijuana, over the past three decades.
    l. Inhalant abuse is associated with younger patients. Techniques such as "huffing" or "bagging" are associated with increased mortality.

CASE 98

PROBLEM LIST

1. Significant Weight Loss (Anorexia Nervosa)
2. Dehydration
3. Electrolyte Disturbances (Hypokalemia, Metabolic Alkalosis)
4. Dental Caries
5. Amenorrhea
6. Acne

SOAP NOTE

S: Pronounced emaciation; intense exercising and restrictive diet; self-image of being overweight despite weight loss; progressive weakness and fatigue; reduced intake of fluids in conjunction with diet and use of diuretics and laxatives to lose weight.

O: Significant weight loss of 10 kg (56 kg down to 46 kg) over past month; elevated BUN consistent with muscle/protein wasting. Poor skin turgor and dry mucous membranes; reduced blood pressure (BP 85/60); electrolyte abnormalities consistent with dehydration; reduced body weight; K 2.7, Cl 70, pH 7.58; PCO_2 40; PO_2 90; HCO_3 36; BE +11; absence of menses for over 4 months

A: Problem 1: Anorexia nervosa with 35% weight loss

Problem 2: Dehydration secondary to anorexia nervosa, complicated by periodic use of diuretics, laxatives, and vomiting

Problem 3: Hypokalemia and hypochloremia with associated metabolic acidosis

Problem 4: Dental caries secondary to enamel erosion via vomitus (stomach acid)

Problem 5: Amenorrhea

Problem 6: Acne vulgaris, R/O age related vs stress induced

P: Problem 1: Anorexia Nervosa (AN)

- Begin correction of nutritional abnormalities with gradual weight increase (0.1–0.3 kg/day)
- Encourage to take food orally, use tube feedings if refuses
- Supervision of daily meals initially, with daily record of weight gain progress
- Positive incentives or rewards if weight gain goals attained
- Supportive and behavioral therapy as soon as TD medically stable
- Education on dangers of self-starvation and abuse of laxatives and diuretics
- Consider serotonergic antidepressant (fluoxetine, others) if significant depression develops
- Schedule regular follow-up appointments to monitor progress

Problem 2: Dehydration

- Initiate standard maintenance IV solution of D5W with NS supplemented with KCl 20 mEq/L at a rate of 50–100 mL/hr
- Continue IV rehydration until blood pressure within normal, electrolyte imbalances stabilized, and marked improvement in skin turgor and dried mucous membranes present
- Encourage use of oral route of fluid administration if possible
- Monitor electrolytes and blood pressure

Problem 3: Electrolyte Disturbance

- Use of IV solution in problem 2 should reverse both metabolic acidosis and electrolyte imbalance
- Close monitoring of electrolytes, especially during first 24–48 hours, to avoid overcompensation
- Increased dietary intake of potassium, either through supplements or food-based (oranges, bananas) after initial electrolyte stabilization

Problem 4: Dental Caries

- Caries are likely to be secondary to exposure to stomach acids (periodic vomiting to control weight)
- Refer to dental clinic for work-up
- Educate about sequelae to vomiting

Problem 5: Amenorrhea

- As body weight returns to normal, menses will return to normal cyclical pattern
- Instruct to note when menses returns to normal and contact clinician with any subsequent changes

Problem 6: Acne

- Daily facial cleansing with mild soap
- Topical application of 5% benzyl peroxide BID
- Refer to dermatologist if acne persists

ANSWERS

1. c. Purging
2. b. Avoidance of exercise
3. a. Major depressive disorder
4. d. Females age 13–18 years old
5. c. Incidence of anorexia decreases with increased economic status
6. b. Amenorrhea
7. c. Cardiac complications
8. c. Papillomacular rash
9. d. Abrasions or calluses on the dorsum of the dominant hand
10. a. Fluoxetine
11. b. Higher than those recommended for depression
12. c. Side effect profile and drug interactions
13. The goals of psychotherapy should include individual and

family therapy sessions. Aid should be given in overcoming patient denial and improving self-confidence. Psychotherapy should also help build self-identity.

14. Common side effects of the SSRIs include GI disturbance, insomnia, and sexual dysfunction.

15. Normal-weight bulimia is difficult to detect due to lack of obvious weight loss and patient tendency to hide binge-purge activity.

16. Counseling should include medication indication, strength, schedule, possible side effects, and compliance. Patients should be advised to avoid operation of heavy machinery until aware of how the medication will affect them. Education should include avoidance of doubling up on doses and what to do in case of missed dose. As with all medications, safe storage should also be discussed.

17. a. Loss of self-esteem

18. Key points are:
   a. The incidence of obesity is increasing, not only in the adult population, but also in children and adolescents, and has become the second leading cause of preventable death.
   b. Obesity occurs from a complex interplay of physiological, hereditary, psychological, and metabolic influences.
   c. Skinfold thickness measurements coupled with body mass index (BMI) gives a convenient measurement and accurate evaluation of the degree of obesity.
   d. Waist circumference should be measured and used with BMI to assist in determining the degree of obesity, associated risks, and morbidity.
   e. Many serious disorders (hypertension, diabetes, cardiovascular disease, and gastrointestinal disorders) are associated with obesity and detrimental to the longevity of the individual.
   f. Treatment of obesity should involve dietary therapy, exercise, behavior therapy, and if necessary pharmacotherapy and surgery.
   g. Pharmacotherapy provides a temporary means of weight loss, and must be used in combination with other treatment modalities to gain lasting results.
   h. The two classic eating disorders (EDs) are anorexia nervosa (AN) and bulimia nervosa. AN is a syndrome characterized by self-starvation, extreme weight loss, excessive exercise, body image disturbance, and an intense fear of becoming obese, despite being grossly underweight. Bulimia nervosa is characterized by binge eating usually followed by some form of purging, such as self-induced vomiting, medication-induced vomiting (ipecac), laxative abuse, or associated behaviors such as diuretic use, diet pill use, or compulsive exercising.
   i. The most common type of ED is normal-weight bulimia, which involves patients who are within 10% of ideal weight despite purging.
   j. EDs are classified as psychiatric illnesses. Diagnosis is based on criteria from the fourth edition of the American Psychiatric Association's *Diagnostic and Statistical Manual* (*DSM-IV*).
   k. Complications associated with AN can affect virtually every physiological organ system.
   l. A particularly dangerous practice is the repeated induction of vomiting with syrup of ipecac.
   m. Chronic absorption of ipecac can lead to a potentially fatal cardiac, gastrointestinal, and neuromuscular toxicity.
   n. The treatments of AN and bulimia require a multidisciplinary approach, often incorporating psychotherapy and pharmacotherapy. Psychotherapy is the mainstay of treatment for EDs and should not be replaced, overlooked, or downplayed when medication therapy is decided upon. In general, bulimia nervosa responds more favorably to medication therapy than does AN.
   o. Antidepressants, specifically SSRIs and TCAs, have shown success in the treatment of EDs and appear to provide symptomatic relief in patients who are clinically depressed. Other pharmacotherapeutic modalities such as cyproheptadine, anticonvulsants, and opiate antagonists have also been studied.

CASE 99

PROBLEM LIST

1. Schizophrenia × 30 Years
2. History of Generalized Tonic-Clonic Seizures Secondary to Head Injury 5 Years Ago (1–2 Seizures per Year)
3. Anticholinergic Side Effects (Sedation, Constipation)
4. Tardive Dyskinesia (TD)

SOAP NOTE

S: Depressed and reports hearing voices again for the past 2 weeks

O: Speech is slurred, with her tongue protruding from her mouth. MJ has choreiform and athetoid movements (involuntary moving of arms and legs); MJ is lethargic, thirsty, and constipated

A: Problem 1: Poor control of schizophrenic symptoms

Problem 2: Seizures generally controlled (1–2 per year), phenytoin level within normal

Problem 3: MJ is experiencing mild anticholinergic symptoms secondary to antipsychotic use

Problem 4: Mild to moderate tardive dyskinesia secondary to 20 year history of haloperidol

P: Problem 1: Schizophrenic Symptoms
- Increase haloperidol to 10 mg BID
- Monitor MJ for decreased auditory hallucinations and clinical improvement
- Follow for changes in TD, EPS, and anticholinergic effects per problems discussed below
- If unresponsive, or if adverse effects remain

problematic, consider switch to atypical antipsychotic such as risperidone or quetiapine

Problem 2: Generalized Tonic-Clonic Seizures

- Continue with phenytoin
- Monitor for seizures and the possibility of drug interactions, especially combination of phenytoin and estrogen and/or ibuprofen
- Educate MJ on the potential side effects of phenytoin (e.g., nystagmus, ataxia, slurred speech, confusion, gingival hyperplasia)

Problem 3: Anticholinergic Side Effects

- For thirst, recommend increased fluid intake and sucking on sugarless gum or candy
- For constipation, increase docusate 100 mg PO BID with a high-fiber diet
- Review carefully the other clinical symptoms of anticholinergic effects, such as blurry vision and urinary hesitancy
- Monitor anticholinergic side effects; if improvement is not noted in 2–4 weeks, MJ should return to clinic for assessment and possible switch to atypical antipsychotic

Problem 4: Tardive Dyskinesia

- Start amantadine 100 mg PO BID
- Monitor for improvements in the symptoms of TD, which should be seen in about a week if amantadine is effective
- Assess for continued signs of TD utilizing Abnormal Involuntary Movement Scale (AIMS) quarterly
- The best treatment for TD is prevention; attempt to utilize lowest possible effective dose of antipsychotic

ANSWERS

1. a. Mesoridazine
2. d. Males tend to develop schizophrenia earlier than females
3. a. Female gender
4. d. Paranoia
5. b. Auditory
6. b. Auditory hallucinations
7. d. Depot preparations are indicated in the chronically noncompliant.
8. Total daily PO dose is multiplied by 10. 20mg/daily (PO) $\times$ 10 = 200mg. 200mg would then be given IM every 4 weeks.
9. b. Dystonic reaction, diphenhydramine 50 mg IM q 30 minutes until resolution
10. b. 37.5 mg IM every 2 weeks
11. c. WBC <3,500 and neutrophil count <1,500
12. MJ is a good candidate for clozapine. She has exhibited

treatment resistance, has a long history of illness, and does not appear to have any blood dyscrasias. MJ would also be a candidate for decanoate therapy.

13. Psychosocial factors that limit medication compliance include:
    a. Lack of insight
    b. Lack of education
    c. Lack of funds
    d. Peer pressure to abandon antipsychotic therapy
    e. High percentage of drug abuse in the schizophrenic population
    f. Confusing/inconsistent insurance coverage
14. c. Clozapine
15. c. Cost of frequent monitoring of complete blood count
16. Key points are:
    a. Schizophrenia is a chronic condition that necessitates daily compliance with antipsychotics.
    b. When compliance is compromised or questionable, the use of a decanoate injection or a newer atypical antipsychotic is suggested, noting that newer medications can be cost prohibitive.
    c. Continuous efforts at basic education/medication counseling are recommended.
    d. The primary goal of antipsychotic therapy is to reduce psychotic symptoms while minimizing adverse effects so that the schizophrenic may attempt to lead as normal a life as possible.

CASE 100

PROBLEM LIST

1. Type 1 Diabetes
2. Depression
3. Angina
4. Hypothyroidism
5. Hypertriglyceridemia
6. Hypertension
7. Chronic Renal Insufficiency

SOAP NOTE

S: Complaints of "being depressed," numbness/tingling in her left foot, and blurred vision

O: Nervous-appearing, depressed; BP 100/60, HR 70, Wt 60 kg, Glu 5.6 (100), HbA$_{1C}$ 10, TSH 5.2 (5.2), free T$_4$ index 1.2, Chol 3.9 (150), HDL chol 0.52 (20), TG 40 (350), BUN 7.14 (20), Cr 310 (3.5); urinalysis: pH 1.020, glucose ($-$), protein ($3+$), casts ($+$)

A: **Problem 1:** Uncontrolled diabetes, type 1, due to noncompliance

Problem 2: Treatment of depression required

Problem 3: No angina problem in 6 years

Problem 4: Hypothyroidism not responding to levothyroxine dose

Problem 5: Current therapy not appropriate for hypertriglyceridemia

Problem 6: Hypotension

Problem 7: Chronic renal insufficiency secondary to longstanding type 1 diabetes

P: Problem 1: Type 1 Diabetes
- Stress importance of compliance with insulin usage and glucose monitoring
- Discuss long-term complications of uncontrolled diabetes, including current symptoms indicating peripheral neuropathy and pigmentary retinopathy
- Suggest daily diary of glucose checks
- Evaluate ability to self-administer insulin; consider pen-type devices as administration aids
- Reevaluate at next visit

Problem 2: Depression
- Start sertraline 50 mg PO q AM
- Counsel patient that full benefits of sertraline probably will not be seen for 4 weeks
- Counsel patient on expected ADRs during first few weeks of therapy, including nervousness, insomnia, and GI complaints

Problem 3: Angina
- Consider discontinuation of NTG due to no chest pain in 6 years

Problem 4: Hypothyroidism
- Increase levothyroxine to 0.125 mg PO QD
- Obtain free T$_4$ index and TSH after 8 weeks on new dose
- Provide patient education about possible side effects of levothyroxine
- Review signs and symptoms of hypo/hyperthyroidism

Problem 5: Hypertriglyceridemia
- Discontinue cholestyramine
- Start gemfibrozil 600 mg PO BID
- Monitor lipid levels and LFTs every 6 months
- Discuss possible side effects of medication, including gastrointestinal symptoms and abdominal pain

Problem 6: Hypertension
- Discontinue clonidine due to potential depressive effects
- Discontinue hydrochlorothiazide due to impaired renal function and current hypotension

- Monitor blood pressure and reevaluate for hypertension treatment if necessary
- Consider angiotensin-converting enzyme inhibitor for antihypertensive and renal-protective effect in diabetes; begin fosinopril 10 mg PO QD

Problem 7: Chronic Renal Insufficiency
- Consider ACE inhibitor as above
- Monitor daily weights, serum electrolytes and BUN, creatinine; instruct to contact office if she experiences edema in extremities
- Renally adjust medications; instruct to check with health care provider before taking any OTC or herbal remedies

ANSWERS

1. d. Physical ailments
2. d. Previous response to antidepressants
3. Psychosocial factors include:
   a. Financial stressors due to increased absenteeism from work or decreased ability to hold down a job
   b. Decreased social contact due to self-alienation and alienation by peer group
   c. Decreased self-esteem and disturbances in family relationships
4. c. Anhedonia
5. d. When did you last take fluoxetine?
6. b. Nefazodone and astemizole
7. a. Nausea
8. a. Every other day dosing
9. c. Peripheral edema
10. d. Female gender
11. c. May cause weight gain, so weigh self regularly
12. a. Bupropion
13. b. Most persons who attempt suicide communicate their intention
14. a. Clomipramine
15. a. Fluoxetine
16. b. DSM-IV criteria
17. Possible side effects include nausea, insomnia, headache, diarrhea, agitation, and sexual dysfunction. Response usually requires 3–4 weeks of treatment. Duration of treatment varies among patients. Most receive medication for at least 6 months, while some require longer treatment courses due to relapses.
18. Key points are:
    a. DSM-IV criteria should be used to diagnose depression
    b. Treatment forms available include psychotherapy, medications, and electroconvulsive therapy
    c. Treatment plans should be individualized to fit the patient
    d. Failure to treat at the very least affects quality of life and can lead to suicide

CASE 101

PROBLEM LIST

1. Requires Scheduled Immunizations
2. Parents Require Poison Prevention Counseling

SOAP NOTE

S: Mother reports patient experienced a "bad reaction" after the last vaccination; mother anxious about immunizations; mother states BG had fever of 40°C after his last DTwP and "he was crying and fussy for hours"; BG's sister found playing with an open bottle of BG's vitamins

O: Normal physical exam; normal laboratory values; BG completed HBV and HiB series; received one dose of MMR, three doses of OPV, and four doses of DTwP; had chickenpox at 15 months of age and has not received the varicella vaccine

A: Problem 1: Requires scheduled immunizations: BG has received all necessary immunizations to date; does not require vaccination for varicella as he has already had chickenpox; at this visit BG should receive IPV or OPV, as well as a DTP shot; experienced fever, irritability, and crying after the DTwP; acellular vaccine has since become available and would be the preferred vaccine in this patient; either IPV or OPV would be appropriate at this visit; mother will require counseling to alleviate concerns regarding prior reactions to the DTwP

Problem 2: Parents require poison prevention counseling: BG and his sister are in an age group at risk for accidental ingestions; BG's parents should be counseled about poison prevention as well as the steps to take if a drug, plant, or other potentially harmful substance is ingested

P: Problem 1: Requires Scheduled Immunizations

- Counsel mother on the advantages and disadvantages of IPV or OPV
- Administer OPV or IPV
- Counsel mother on the availability of the DTaP vaccine, the differences between the DTaP and DTwP, and the risk of pertussis if BG does not receive the vaccine or receives only the DT vaccine; also counsel mother on the potential adverse effects of the DTaP
- Administer DTaP

- Pretreat BG with 240 mg of acetaminophen (10–15 mg/kg) and instruct mother to administer a second dose within 4–8 hours; repeat doses q4–6h PRN (not to exceed 5 doses per 24 hours)

Problem 2: Parents Require Poison Prevention Counseling

- Instruct parents to "child-proof" their home and store all medicines in child-resistant bottles; keep all medicines and cleaning agents in their original containers and store them out-of-reach of children. Safety latches should be installed on cabinets containing harmful substances
- Instruct parents to keep the number of the poison control center near the phone
- Encourage parents to keep a bottle of ipecac in the house and to call the poison control center before administering this agent

ANSWERS

1. Toxoids are modified nontoxic products of microorganisms or exotoxins. Vaccines are products derived directly from microorganisms; they may be killed, inactivated, live attenuated, polysaccharide, or composed of components of a microorganism that are antigenic.
2. c. *Haemophilus influenzae* type B
3. a. IM
4. b. *Corynebacterium diphtheriae, Bordetella pertussis, Clostridium tetani*
5. a. MMR
6. c. VAERS
7. b. Polysaccharide vaccines
8. Meningococcal vaccine, pneumococcal vaccine, and influenza vaccine
9. d. OPV
10. b. Varicella vaccine
11. b. The IPV has not been associated with VAPP
12. Psychosocial factors include:
    a. Some parents may feel that immunizations are unnecessary since the incidence of the disease prevented is low
    b. Some parents may be anxious about the adverse effects associated with certain vaccines
    c. Some religious groups object to the use of products that are from a human source
    d. Some parents refuse or defer vaccination due to the pain associated with the injections
13. Key points are:
    a. The benefits of the administration of the DTaP immunization outweigh the risks associated with the adverse effects. Adverse effects associated with an acellular vaccine should be less than those associated with a whole cell vaccine.

b. The immune status of the patient, as well as household contacts, must be taken into consideration when administering immunizations. Live vaccines, such as the OPV, should not be given to patients who are immunocompromised or who may come into contact with immunocompromised individuals.

c. Certain disease states, such as sickle cell anemia, may affect a patient's risk of contracting certain infections. Additional immunizations may be indicated in these patients.

d. The psychosocial concerns of parents regarding vaccines should be addressed. Parent's concerns should be acknowledged and they should be counseled on the benefits of the vaccine, as well as the adverse effects that may occur.

CASE 103

PROBLEM LIST

1. Acute Otitis Media
2. Viral Upper Respiratory Tract Infection
3. Diaper Rash

SOAP NOTE

S: Mom states her child has a "cold with runny nose and cough"; lethargy and irritability; mild, nonproductive cough; clear, watery rhinorrhea; sore throat; tugging on right earlobe; warm to touch; poor appetite

O: T 39°C; pale skin; right tympanic membrane red and bulging; erythematous throat; erythema, tenderness, and inflammation over entire diaper area with vesicular satellite lesions on periphery of redness

A: **Problem 1:** Acute otitis media of bacterial or viral origin

Problem 2: Upper respiratory infection likely of viral origin since LW has clear, watery rhinorrhea and both parents are recovering from the "flu"

Problem 3: Diaper rash dermatitis consistent with *Candida albicans*

P: **Problem 1: Acute Otitis Media**

• Initiate amoxicillin/clavulanate oral suspension 300 mg PO BID (40 mg/kg/day) × 10 days
• Monitor for amoxicillin/clavulanate adverse events (mainly hypersensitivity reactions and diarrhea)
• Monitor symptoms for clinical improvement including number of times LW tugs on right ear, appetite, and improved energy
• Monitor temperature
• Return to clinic if LW is not improving after 3 days or she has persistent fever

Problem 2: Viral Upper Respiratory Infection

• Acetaminophen 150 mg PO q4h PRN fever and pain
• Recommend Cardec-DM pediatric drops 1 mL PO QID PRN cough and congestion

Problem 3: Diaper Rash

• Remove diaper and gently wash and rinse diaper area with plain water
• Clotrimazole cream applied to affected area QID until rash is resolved

ANSWERS

1. Pathophysiology of otitis media in children includes:
   a. Eustachian tube is short and connects to the middle ear at a 10° angle
   b. Obstruction of eustachian tube leads to fluid accumulation (typically observed in the setting of a viral upper respiratory infection)
   c. Congested eustachian tube is an excellent medium for bacterial proliferation
2. b. 6 months to 1 year
3. a. Day-care settings
4. c. Winter
5. Possible etiologic pathogens of otitis media in LW include:
   a. Viral: influenza, rhinovirus, respiratory syncytial virus, and parainfluenza
   b. Bacterial: *Streptococcus pneumoniae*, *Haemophilus influenzae*, and *Moraxella catarrhalis*
6. c. 10 days
7. Rationale for amoxicillin/clavulanate: Otitis media could be a relapse bacterial infection. LW should have received a 10-day course of amoxicillin instead of 5 days since short-course therapy is not recommended for children under 2 years of age. Otitis media could be due to a penicillin-nonsusceptible *Streptococcus pneumoniae* which would not have responded to the original therapy of amoxicillin 50 mg/kg/day.
8. b. Diarrhea
9. Therapeutic advantages of amoxicillin/clavulanate include:
   a. Clavulanate is a beta-lactamase inhibitor
   b. Increased spectrum of activity against beta-lactamase-producing microorganisms that cause otitis media, such as *Haemophilus influenzae* and *Moraxella catarrhalis*
   c. Activity against *S. pneumoniae*-intermediate susceptibility to penicillin
10. d. No follow-up is required as long as LW remains asymptomatic
11. a. Association of aspirin use and Reye's syndrome in children with influenza
12. c. Antipyretic
13. Care of diaper rash
    a. Change the diaper as soon as it is wet or at least every 2–4 hr including a change at night until the rash is resolved
    b. Apply cornstarch as a drying agent
    c. Avoid overnight use of plastic pants
    d. Expose the diaper area to air as frequently as possible

e. Apply antifungal creams (e.g., clotrimoxazole applied to affected area QID)

f. Apply 0.5–1% hydrocortisone ointment BID for up to 1 week when severe inflammation is present

14. Key points are:

a. Acute otitis media is an infection often observed in children with viral upper respiratory infections.

b. Amoxicillin is the consensus drug of choice. There is no evidence that extended spectrum beta-lactam oral antibiotics are more efficacious than amoxicillin.

c. Higher doses of amoxicillin are recommended in children living in areas where penicillin-nonsusceptible *Streptococcus pneumoniae* is prevalent.

d. Duration of therapy is 3–5 days except in children <2 years old where therapy should be for 10 days.

CASE 105

PROBLEM LIST

1. Pneumococcal Pneumonia
2. COPD
3. Steroid-Induced Gastritis
4. Alcohol Abuse
5. Seizure Disorder
6. Degenerative Joint Disease

SOAP NOTE

S: Fever; chest pain; chills; purulent rust-colored sputum production; shortness of breath; malaise; lethargy; dyspnea; gastric pain

O: Chest x-ray shows consolidation; hypoxic; elevated WBC with left shift; T 39.5°C; tachycardia; tachypnia; sputum Gram stain reveals gram-positive in pairs (many); guaiac-positive stools; BUN 59 (21); Cr 106.1 (1.2)

A: **Problem 1:** Pneumococcal pneumonia requiring empiric therapy

Problem 2: COPD exacerbation secondary to acute respiratory infection with immediate goal to correct air flow obstruction and to improve his pulmonary function

Problem 3: Steroid-induced gastritis (with guaiac-positive stools) in a noncompliant patient in which systemic steroids are not indicated; ulceration is minimal since hematocrit and hemoglobin are stable.

Problem 4: Alcohol abuse: sober for approximately 1 year; enrolled in Alcoholics Anonymous

Problem 5: Seizure disorder: secondary to alcohol withdrawal during period of alcohol abuse; no seizures during current period of alcohol abstinence

Problem 6: Degenerative joint disease but currently asymptomatic on acetaminophen (and presumably from prednisone)

P: **Problem 1: Pneumococcal Pneumonia**

- Initiate ceftriaxone 1 g IV QD
- Monitor temperature, leukocyte count with differential, chest x-ray
- Determine final sputum and blood culture report and confirm if pneumococcus is sensitive to penicillin
- Evaluate JS clinically after 48–72 hr and adjust antibiotic therapy as indicated (i.e., switch from IV to PO)

Problem 2: COPD

- Begin methylprednisolone 60 mg IV q6h with a rapid taper down to oral prednisone 30 mg PO QD within 3 days
- Taper prednisone until discontinuation over next 14 days
- Monitor for signs of steroid withdrawal
- Implement COPD treatment strategy with inhaled steroids
- Instruct JS on the proper use of inhalers
- Begin nebulized metaproterenol 0.3 mL of a 5% solution diluted in 2.5 mL of normal saline q4h
- Consider scheduled metaproterenol inhalations plus PRN rather than just PRN
- Continue ipratroprium inhalations 2 puffs QID
- Monitor ABGs, chest examination, heart rate, respiration rate
- Begin maintenance fluids to ensure adequate hydration

Problem 3: Steroid-Induced Gastritis

- Begin taper of systemic steroids after acute COPD exacerbation resolves, with goal of discontinuing prednisone
- Monitor for steroid withdrawal symptoms
- Maalox 30 mL PO QID PRN gastritis

Problems 4: Alcohol Abuse

- Provide support and encouragement to JS to continue attending Alcoholics Anonymous meetings and participate in their support groups
- Commend JS for his ability to remain sober for 1 year

Problem 5: Seizure Disorder

- Discontinue phenytoin since JS has abstained from alcohol for about 1 year

Problem 6: Degenerative Joint Disease

- Maintain current therapy with acetaminophen
- Monitor for onset of symptoms of DJD (currently JS is asymptomatic, which may change after steroid withdrawal)

- Monitor acetaminophen ingestion
- Reevaluate if acetaminophen requirements increase (>3–4 g/day)
- Monitor liver function tests

ANSWERS

1. b. Cost
2. d. Vitamin C deficiency
3. d. Diabetes mellitus
4. c. Seizures
5. b. Guaiac-positive stools
6. *Streptococcus pneumoniae*

In Vitro Susceptibility of *S. Pneumoniae*	Preferred Antibiotic
Penicillin susceptible (MIC < 0.1 mg/L)	Penicillin G or Penicillin V
Penicillin intermediate (MIC 0.1–1.0 mg/L)	High-dose penicillin G (IV), ceftriaxone, or cefotaxime
Highly penicillin resistant (MIC > 2.0 mg/L)	Vancomycin

7. Ceftriaxone versus aqueous penicillin
   - Due to the increased level of penicillin resistance in the United States, penicillin can no longer be safely recommended as empiric therapy for community-acquired pneumonia
   - Empiric therapy with a 3rd generation cephalosporin or a fluoroquinolone is recommended pending culture and sensitivity report
8. c. De-efervescence
9. Disease management plan for pneumococcal pneumonia in JS
   a. Switch to penicillin V-K 500 mg PO QID for the duration of 10-day therapy, since JS has improved after 72 hr and the organism is sensitive to penicillin
   b. Observe for hypersensitivity reaction with history of ampicillin rash years ago
   c. The ampicillin rash occurred years ago and it was associated with no complications; perhaps the rash was concurrent with a mono-like viral illness
   d. Monitor temperature, chest examination, sputum production, and chest x-ray
   e. Follow-up in clinic with administrations of pneumococcal vaccination and yearly influenza vaccination
10. d. Ofloxacin has unreliable pneumococcal sensitivities and should not be used
11. Steroid withdrawal symptoms versus relapse infection
    a. Flu-like syndrome, diaphoresis, and acute exacerbation of COPD symptoms suggest steroid withdrawal
    b. JS is receiving adequate dose of oral penicillin V-K and presumably has good absorption since he has not had nausea or vomiting
    c. JS remains afebrile and has no increase sputum production, making relapse infection unlikely
12. b. CHF patient
13. Patient instructions for use of inhalers
    a. Shake the canister thoroughly
    b. Place the mouthpiece between the lips, making sure the teeth and tongue are out of the way
    c. Hold the breath at full inspiration for 10 sec
    d. Pause at least 1 min, preferably 5 min, before the next inhalation from the canister
14. a. Erectile dysfunction
15. Key points are:
    a. Appropriate empiric therapy for suspected pneumococcal pneumonia should take into account the geographic pattern of penicillin resistance, especially in children or others who have been exposed to many antibiotics.
    b. In general practice, it may be reasonable to select an antibiotic that is likely to cover intermediate or highly resistant penicillin pneumococci until the sputum culture proves otherwise.
    c. Patients with an appropriate clinical response within 48–72 hr can be switched from parenteral to oral antibiotic therapy for the remainder of the total 10-day course of treatment.
    d. Active immunization with the pneumococcal vaccine is recommended in patients at high risk (e.g., >50 years of age, immunosuppressed patients, alcoholics, smokers, nursing home residents, COPD patients).

CASE 107

PROBLEM LIST

1. Active Tuberculosis
2. HIV Infection with AIDS
3. Mild Macrocytic Anemia
4. PCP–Secondary Prophylaxis
5. Depression
6. Prevention of Exposure to Pathogens

SOAP NOTE

S: "Since I started the HIV medications I was feeling better; but, these past few weeks, I've been so tired and have lost ten pounds; I've had fevers, chills, night sweats, and cough too."

O: PPD tuberculin skin test positive; chest radiograph reveals apical fibrocavitary infiltrates; generalized lymphadenopathy; eleven pound weight loss since last clinic visit; AFB smear positive for mycobacteria; culture and sensitivity pending; RBC 3.6×10^{12} (3.6×10^6), Hct 0.30 (30), Hgb 100 (10), MCV 115 (115)

A: **Problem 1:** Active tuberculosis secondary to tuberculosis exposure that progressed from infection to disease

Problem 2: HIV infection with AIDS; currently

receiving antiretroviral therapy; previous clinic visit reveals viral load undetectable and CD4 count increased

Problem 3: Mild macrocytic anemia secondary to zidovudine (in Combivir); other possible additive causes include HIV disease, use of trimethoprim/sulfamethoxazole, and tuberculosis

Problem 4: PCP–secondary prophylaxis; currently receiving therapy

Problem 5: Depression; currently receiving sertraline and responding well

Problem 6: Prevention of exposure to pathogens

P: Problem 1: Active Tuberculosis with HIV Infection

- Place in an AFB isolation room
- Conduct close contact investigation and screen contact(s) for tuberculosis infection and disease
- Avoid rifampin since receiving nelfinavir, a protease inhibitor; substitute rifabutin for rifampin (rifabutin; a less potent inducer of cytochrome P450; initiate rifabutin at one-half the usual dose since nelfinavir, an inhibitor of cytochrome P450, increases levels of rifabutin
- Initiate antituberculous therapy: isoniazid, 300 mg PO QD, along with pyridoxine, 50 mg PO QD; rifabutin, 150 mg PO QD; pyrazinamide, 750 mg PO QD; ethambutol, 750 mg PO QD; administer isoniazid (plus pyridoxine), rifabutin, pyrazinamide, and ethambutol for 8 weeks followed by 16 weeks of isoniazid (plus pyridoxine) and rifabutin; minimum total duration of antituberculous therapy is 6 months, but 9 months or longer may be necessary
- Monitor aspartate aminotransferase (AST, SGOT), renal function (BUN, serum creatinine), and uric acid
- Obtain baseline eye examination, followed by monthly exams to assess visual acuity while receiving ethambutol; also check for other eye abnormalities (e.g., uveitis while on rifabutin)
- Recommend alternative form(s) of contraception during therapy; document counseling
- Counsel to report any of the prodromal symptoms of hepatitis, any changes in visual acuity, or other adverse effects to physician; take isoniazid on an empty stomach and avoid foods with high histamine or tyramine content; rifabutin may impart an orange discoloration to the urine, stool, sputum, saliva, tears, and sweat; soft contact lenses may be permanently discolored
- Implement DOT therapy and explain the importance of adherence to the antituberculous regimen for the complete duration of therapy
- Repeat sputum examinations following initiation of

antituberculous therapy; perform at least at monthly intervals until sputum conversion documented; if sputum converts to negative following 2 months of therapy, perform at least one further sputum smear and culture at the completion of therapy
- Notify when no longer infectious and can return to daily activities

Problem 2: HIV Infection with AIDS

- Continue with current antiretroviral regimen at the same dosages
- Nelfinavir: monitor for diarrhea; also monitor glucose, lipid profile, blood pressure, bilirubin, liver function tests, and physical features associated with lipodystrophy syndrome
- Combivir: monitor for anemia, neutropenia, and thrombocytopenia
- Obtain viral load and CD4 count after current illness has been adequately treated

Problem 3: Mild Macrocytic Anemia

- Macrocytosis expected with zidovudine and currently no therapy warranted
- Avoid other medications that can cause bone marrow suppression if possible
- Significant anemia can be managed by transfusion support or with recombinant erythropoietin

Problem 4: PCP–Secondary Prophylaxis

- Continue trimethoprim/sulfamethoxazole at current dose; also provides protection against conventional bacterial infections
- Monitor for common adverse effects such as rash, fever, and leukopenia; also monitor liver function tests and renal function
- Previous CD4 cell count was 205 cells/mm^3; until more data available, continue prophylaxis even if CD4 cell count rises in response to antiretroviral therapy
- Reinforce importance of adherence to therapy

Problem 5: Depression

- Continue with current sertraline dosage and notify RC's psychiatrist of her recent admission
- Responding well to therapy; however, psychiatrist can identify if depression, anxiety, fear, or feelings of isolation have been precipitated by current illness
- Psychosocial aspects of tuberculosis should be addressed; educate about the disease and assure that having tuberculosis should not be viewed as shameful

Problem 6: Prevention of Exposure to Pathogens

- Advise on the following measures to prevent exposure to pathogens:

- Wash hands after bathroom use or contact with animals or soil
- Do not eat undercooked meats, poultry, eggs, or seafood; wash produce before eating
- Avoid drinking water from untreated source
- Safer sex
- Check that routine vaccinations recommended in persons with HIV disease are up-to-date; prior to travel, discuss other necessary vaccines, chemoprophylaxis, and immunoprophylaxis

ANSWERS

1. a. Inhaling airborne particles of Mycobacterium tuberculosis from an individual with active tuberculosis
2. Signs and symptoms noted upon RC's presentation: weight loss, fatigue, productive cough; history of fevers, chills, and night sweats; abnormal chest radiograph, positive PPD, positive AFB smear, and generalized lymphadenopathy. Other findings in patients co-infected with HIV disease include chest pain and hemoptysis; if TB disease is disseminated, hypotension and acute respiratory distress may be present; localized signs and symptoms depend on the organs involved and coexisting HIV-related complications
3. HIV disease, which is the most potent risk factor for the development of active tuberculosis among individuals previously infected with mycobacterial infection
4. Abnormal chest radiograph, weight loss, positive PPD tuberculin skin test, positive AFB sputum smears; positive culture for the organism, which confirms the diagnosis.
5. a. RC should be counseled to use alternative forms of birth control while receiving this agent
6. c. RC should receive supplementation with pyridoxine while receiving isoniazid to reduce the occurrence of isoniazid-induced side effects in the central and peripheral nervous system
7. b. Hepatotoxicity
8. b. The most toxic effect of this agent is optic neuritis; thus, RC should receive baseline examination of visual acuity prior to initiation of therapy, followed by monthly eye examinations
9. c. Monitor BUN and serum creatinine; baseline and periodic audiometric testing is also recommended
10. c. Antituberculosis therapy should not be initiated in a patient suspected of tuberculosis until the diagnosis is confirmed by positive culture results
11. c. Isoniazid, rifampin, pyrazinamide, and ethambutol; pyridoxine should also be added
12. Pharmacologic and nonpharmacologic problems that can occur include:
    1. Pharmacologic
       a. Mild macrocytic anemia secondary to use of zidovudine (in Combivir)
    2. Nonpharmacologic
       a. Close contact investigation and screening; advice on prevention of potential exposure to pathogens

13. Psychosocial factors that may affect RC's adherence to both pharmacologic and nonpharmacologic therapy are:
    a. Issues the patient must address
    b. Inability to work during the infectious period
    c. Reduced activity due to symptoms of tuberculosis
    d. Chronic medications adherence to complex regimen for tuberculosis, along with antiretroviral therapy and other medications
    e. Undesirable adverse effects of antituberculous drugs
14. Common emotional disorders presenting in the patient diagnosed with tuberculosis include:
    a. Anxiety
    b. Fear
    c. Depression
    d. Feelings of isolation and/or shame
    e. Family dynamics–limited support system
    f. Significant psychological problems may interfere with medication compliance
    g. Managing tuberculosis along with other chronic diseases (e.g., HIV infection)
15. The health care provider's role relative to the proposed psychosocial factors identified includes:
    a. Individualized plan for patient: both pharmacologic and nonpharmacologic
    b. Provide compassionate care
    c. Offer support services to patient and caregivers
    d. Identify if depression, anxiety, fear, or feelings of isolation are present; refer to RC's psychiatrist, who has been treating her for depression
16. Pharmacoeconomic considerations relative to RC's plan of care may include:
    1. Cost of treating drug-sensitive tuberculosis versus multi-drug-resistant tuberculosis
       a. Cost of treating tuberculosis
    2. Direct medical
       a. Hospital personnel and overhead
       b. Treatment, including implementation of DOT and complications
    3. Direct nonmedical
       a. Lost wages (family/patient)
       b. Travel, hotels, meals
    4. Indirect personal
       a. Inability to work during infectious period
       b. Quality of life
    5. Intangible personal
       a. Suffering related to the disease, including emotional suffering
17. Key points are:
    a. Tuberculosis is spread to a susceptible person via aerosolized droplet nuclei produced by coughing or sneezing in patients with pulmonary or laryngeal tuberculosis.
    b. Identification of close contacts of an individual with active tuberculosis is an important component of tuberculosis prevention and control.
    c. Goals of tuberculosis therapy are to cure the sick and impede transmission in the community; utilize combination regimen of antituberculous agents that provides optimal efficacy, minimal toxicity, and enables the shortest duration of therapy possible.

d. Use of DOT is encouraged in all settings and is highly recommended in patients co-infected with HIV infection.

CASE 109

PROBLEM LIST

1. Complicated Cystitis, Recurrent UTIs
2. Pelvic Inflammatory Disease (PID)
3. History of Sexually Transmitted Diseases (STDs)

SOAP NOTE

S: Complains of frequency, pain, and burning upon urination; complains of abdominal pain; brown foul-smelling vaginal discharge

O: Urine positive for bacteria and WBCs; gram-negative rods on urine Gram stain; cervical motion tenderness; adnexal tenderness; foul-smelling vaginal drainage; *Chlamydia trachomatis* and gram-negative diplococci in vaginal discharge; past history of gonorrhea and *Chlamydia*

A: **Problem 1:** Complicated cystitis; recurrent UTIs

Problem 2: PID

Problem 3: History of STDs

P: **Problem 1: Complicated Cystitis, Recurrent UTIs**

- Goal: treat current UTI; evaluate need for future prophylaxis
- Allergic to TMP-SMX (probably the SMX component), start norfloxacin 400 mg PO BID for 7 days; provides coverage for the most likely bacterial urinary pathogens such as *E. coli, Proteus* spp., and *Staphylococcus saprophyticus*
- Candidate for prophylaxis because of having more than 3 UTIs in a year
- TMP alone; effective prophylactic alternative in patients with TMP-SMX allergy
- Trimethoprim 100 mg PO QHS for 6 months, then reevaluate
- Monitor for response to therapy, relief of symptoms
- Monitor for recurrence of UTI, allergies, and adverse effects related to antibiotics such as rash, N/V, diarrhea, or yeast infection
- Repeat urinalysis after treatment course is complete
- Counseling on protected sex and sex with multiple partners

Problem 2: PID

- Goal: eliminate the clinical symptoms of infection (abdominal pain, cervical motion tenderness, adnexal tenderness, and vaginal discharge)

- Outpatient treatment is appropriate since minimal fever and no leukocytosis
- Single dose of ceftriaxone 125 mg intramuscularly to treat the gonorrhea
- Administer azithromycin 1 g PO as a single dose to treat the *Chlamydia*
- Return to clinic in 3 days for follow-up evaluation
- If symptoms still present after 3 days of therapy, inpatient admission warranted

Problem 3: History of STDs

- Evaluate AM's current and recent sexual contacts for STDs and treat if needed
- Strongly recommend HIV testing to AM and her sexual contacts
- Counseling on HIV infection and risk factors
- Counseling on the use of latex condoms to prevent STDs and HIV

ANSWERS

1. d. Vaginal discharge
2. c. Past history of tubal ligation
3. d. *E. coli*
4. b. The number of UTIs AM has had this year
5. a. Norfloxacin
6. The mechanism of action of the pharmacologic and nonpharmacologic interventions in this case are:
   1. Pharmacologic interventions
      a. Norfloxacin inhibits DNA gyrase required for DNA replication and transcription, DNA repair, recombination, and transposition
      b. Trimethoprin inhibits folic acid reduction to tetrahydrofolate and thereby inhibits microbial growth
      c. Ceftriaxone inhibits bacterial cell wall synthesis by binding to one or more of the penicillin-binding proteins which inhibits the final transpeptidation step of peptidoglycan synthesis in bacterial cell walls
      d. Azithromycin inhibits RNA-dependent protein synthesis at the chain elongation step; binds to the 50S ribosomal subunit resulting in blockage of transpeptidation
   2. Nonpharmacologic interventions
      a. Education
      b. Counseling on STD prevention
      c. HIV counseling
7. a. Azithromycin 1 g PO × 1
8. c. 7 days
9. b. Avoid unnecessary or prolonged sun exposure
10. The health care provider's role relative to the proposed psychosocial factors identified is:
    a. Individualizing a plan: both pharmacologic and nonpharmacologic
    b. Initiate treatment of sexual contacts
    c. Provide patient education and counseling to AM and sexual contacts

d. Provide positive reinforcement when the treatment plans are adhered to by AM and her sexual contacts

e. Referral to financial and social support services for AM and her sexual contacts if necessary

11. Psychosocial factors that may affect AM's adherence to both pharmacologic and nonpharmacologic therapy:
    1. Issues the patient must address
       a. Consequences of continuing high-risk sexual behavior
       b. Chronic treatment of recurrent UTIs with prophylactic antibiotics
       c. Cost of therapy and risk of adverse effects
    2. Other barriers
       a. Lifestyle and willingness to change
       b. Possible life stressors
       c. Financial resources, medications, condoms, etc.

12. Key points are:
    a. UTIs can involve the bladder (cystitis), the kidney (pyelonephritis), or other urinary structures.
    b. The highest prevalence of UTIs is in young to middle-aged women.
    c. Uncomplicated UTIs occur in otherwise healthy persons.
    d. Uropathogens originate primarily from the bowel, with *E. coli* as the most prevalent pathogen.
    e. The most common symptoms associated with cystitis are dysuria, frequency, and urgency.
    f. Recurrent uncomplicated UTIs can be managed with prophylactic or self-initiated therapy.

CASE 110

PROBLEM LIST

1. Primary Peritonitis or Spontaneous Bacterial Peritonitis (SBP)
2. Chronic Active Hepatitis with Cirrhosis
3. Coagulopathy
4. Ascites
5. Posttraumatic Seizure Disorder

SOAP NOTE

S: "I have fevers, chills, and abdominal pain. I'm always tired and haven't been eating much for the past 2 days."

O: T 39°C; anicteric; increased girth; + hepatosplenomegaly; + fluid wave; + abdominal pain; + diffuse tenderness; hypoactive bowel sounds; 2+ edema; no asterixis; Na 129 (129); Lkc 12.1×10^9 (12.1×10^3); Lkc differential: Neutrophils 0.80 (80%), bands 0.09 (9%); Plts 84×10^9 (84×10^3); AST 3.72 (223); ALT 2.87 (172); Alb 35 (3.5); T Bili 36 (2.1); PT 13.7 (13.7); INR 1.4; phenytoin serum concentration 49.5 μmol/L (12.5 mg/dL); anti-HCV positive; HCV-PCR quantitative: 1.2 million copies/mL; urinalysis: WNL; paracentesis: cloudy ascitic fluid, pH 7.18,

PMN 540 cells/m³; Gram stain (ascitic fluid): gram-negative rods; chest x-ray: WNL; EEG: WNL; liver biopsy: 20% bridging necrosis

A: Problem 1: Primary peritonitis, no evident source of infection; ascites is a risk factor; common pathogens: aerobic gram-negative bacilli (e.g., *E. coli, Klebsiella*)

Problem 2: Chronic active hepatitis with cirrhosis secondary to HCV

Problem 3: Coagulopathy; thrombocytopenia most likely the result of hypersplenism secondary to portal hypertension a complication of cirrhosis; increased prothrombin time secondary to cirrhosis

Problem 4: Ascites secondary to cirrhosis

Problem 5: Posttraumatic seizure disorder secondary to head trauma from an automobile accident; phenytoin serum concentration 49.5 μmol/L (12.5 mg/dL); phenytoin concentration adjusted for low Alb: 61.8 μmol/L (15.6 mg/dL)

P: Problem 1: Primary Peritonitis

- Start empiric antibiotic therapy: cefotaxime, 2 g IV q8h
- Monitor Cr, BUN, signs of clinical improvement (temperature, Lkc count, neutrophils, bands, ascites fluid, cultures, abdominal pain, tenderness), and adverse effects (e.g., rash, hypersensitivity reactions, nausea, diarrhea)
- Once cultures and antibiotic sensitivities are reported, adjust antibiotic therapy as needed
- Treat for at least 7 days
- Start selective gut decontamination, norfloxacin, 400 mg PO QD (upon discharge) for prophylaxis of primary peritonitis
- Discuss the benefits of primary peritonitis prophylaxis and recommend lifestyle modifications to assist with adherence
- Monitor nausea, vomiting, rash, hypersensitivity reactions, LFTs

Problem 2: Chronic Active Hepatitis with Cirrhosis

- Start interferon alpha-2b, 3 million units SC 3 times weekly and ribavirin, 400 mg PO q AM and 600 mg PO q PM
- Monitor liver function tests (LFTs), complete blood count (CBC) and Lkc differential [pretreatment, 2 and 4 weeks], TSH, severe psychiatric adverse events (depression and suicidal behavior), dyspnea, pulmonary infiltrates
- Counsel that "flu-like" symptoms (headache, fatigue, myalgia, and fever) are common and may be minimized with HS administration of interferon alpha-2b
- Begin hepatitis A and B vaccine series if Plts > 50 $\times 10^9$ (50×10^3); although vaccines administered

via IM route the benefits of hepatitis prophylaxis outweigh risks of developing a hematoma
- Monitor for side effects: injection site (soreness, induration, redness, swelling), headache, malaise, fatigue, fever, gastrointestinal (GI) upset
- Start multivitamin, 1 PO QD; thiamine, 50–100 mg PO QD; folic acid, 1 mg PO QD; and vitamin C, 500 mg PO QD for nutritional deficiency; hold if malabsorption or gastrointestinal (GI) tract dysfunction occurs (i.e., absent bowel sounds, no flatulence or bowel movements)
- Counsel on avoidance of alcohol, hepatotoxic drugs (e.g., acetaminophen) and certain alternative remedies (e.g., certain herbal teas)
- Warn: not to share personal items (e.g., razors), to cover open wounds, not to donate blood, to disclose HCV positive status to dentist

Problem 3: Coagulopathy

- Transfuse if Plts $< 25 \times 10^9$ (25×10^3) or signs of bleeding
- Monitor for bleeding (gum bleeding, epistaxis, bruising), Plts, Hgb, Hct, PT, PTT, INR
- Avoid, if possible, IM and SC injections, rectal examinations, suppositories, and enemas (risks vs. benefits)
- Avoid aspirin and NSAIDs
- Administer vitamin K, 10 mg slow IVP (do not exceed 1 mg/min) if PT/INR continues to rise
- Monitor for anaphylaxis (convulsive movements, cardiac irregularities, chest pain, bronchospasm, dyspnea, rapid weak pulse, etc.)

Problem 4: Ascites

- Reinforce low sodium diet
- Administer furosemide, 40 mg IV to reduce ascites fluid and peripheral edema; double q 3 days until desired response obtained; do not exceed a fluid loss of $>$1–2 L/day
- Increase spironolactone, 200 mg PO QD; double every 3 days until desired response obtained; do not exceed a fluid loss of $>$1–2 L/day; hold if malabsorption or gastrointestinal (GI) tract dysfunction occurs (i.e., absent bowel sounds, no flatulence or bowel movements)
- Restart furosemide, PO therapy upon discharge (conversion: IV dose 50% of PO dose)
- Monitor for dehydration (skin turgor, hypotension, dry mucous membranes), Cl, HCO_3, K, Na, BUN, Cr, urine output, daily weights, total intake and output
- Discuss the importance of controlling ascites (i.e., if ascites decreased less likely to develop primary peritonitis) and lifestyle modification to assist with adherence

Problem 5: Posttraumatic Seizure Disorder

- Goal: phenytoin total serum concentration, 40–80 mmol/L (10–20 mg/L); phenytoin free serum concentration, 4–8 mmol/L (1–2 mg/L)
- Continue phenytoin, 300 mg PO QHS; convert to IV if malabsorption or gastrointestinal (GI) tract dysfunction occurs (i.e., absent bowel sounds, no flatulence or bowel movements, a subtherapeutic phenytoin serum concentration not attributable to a drug interaction)
- Monitor phenytoin serum concentration in 5 days or earlier if seizures or signs of toxicity (nystagmus, slurred speech, ataxia, drowsiness, diplopia, behavioral changes, cognitive impairment) and adverse effects (rash, complete blood count, LFTs)
- Monitor Alb, BUN, CR, urine output; hypoalbuminemia and renal failure (CR $<$ 25 mL/min) may affect free phenytoin concentration

ANSWERS

1. b. Ascites
2. Signs and symptoms of primary peritonitis in MS: fever, chills, abdominal pain, nausea, chronic fatigue, and loss of appetite
3. T 39°C, hypoactive bowel sounds, increased girth, Lkcs 12.1 $\times 10^9$ (12.1 $\times 10^3$), + fluid wave, Lkc differential: neutrophils 0.80 (80%), bands 0.09 (9%), + abdominal pain, paracentesis: cloudy ascitic fluid, PMN 540 cells/m³, + diffuse tenderness, Gram stain (ascitic fluid): gram-negative rods
4. b. Pathogens most likely to cause primary peritonitis include *Escherichia coli*, *Klebsiella* spp., and other gram-negative bacilli
5. Pharmacologic and nonpharmacologic treatment problem(s) present in MS's treatment plan include:
   1. Pharmacologic
      a. Omission of norfloxacin or trimethoprim/sulfamethoxazole for primary peritonitis prophylaxis
      b. Omission of interferon alpha-2b and ribavirin for treatment of chronic HCV
   2. Nonpharmacologic
      a. Mental health referral
      b. Adherence with complex medical issues/regimen
      c. Diet to help control ascites and maintain adequate nutrition
      d. Maintain close follow-up with medical providers to monitor progress/adverse effects
6. b. Surgical debridement combined with appropriate antibiotic coverage is the standard of care
7. d. Clindamycin
8. d. MS should be assured that HCV is not communicable
9. a. Aminoglycosides are effective in the treatment of abscesses because of the low oxygen tension environment
10. c. Spironolactone inhibits aldosterone-mediated retention of Na and water, making it an effective agent in ascites

11. a. Phenytoin is 90% protein bound and should be adjusted in patients who are hypoalbuminemic and/or with severe renal failure

12. Psychosocial factors that may affect MS's adherence to both pharmacologic and nonpharmacologic therapy are:
    1. Issues the patient must address
       a. Dietary—decreased desire and/or inability to maintain an adequate nutritional intake
       b. Chronic medications—adherence to painful injections and long-term regimens
       c. Disease transmission—inconvenience and social stigma of being a carrier of a communicable disease
    2. Common emotional disorders presenting in MS
       a. Depression
       b. Anxiety
       c. Anger
    3. Other barriers
       a. Family dynamics; limited support system
       b. Other stressors in life
       c. Limited financial resources; unable to purchase medications

13. Pharmacoeconomic considerations relative to MS's plan of care may include:
    1. Costs of chronic active hepatitis with cirrhosis and the related complications at home
       a. Pharmacotherapy
    2. Costs of acute exacerbations from the complications of cirrhosis to patients and families
       a. Direct medical
          • Hospital personnel and overhead
          • Treatment
       b. Direct nonmedical
          • Travel, hotels, meals
          • Lost wages (family/patient)
       c. Indirect personal
          • Decreased productivity
          • Quality of life
       d. Intangible personal
          • Suffering

14. Key points are:
    a. Most cases of primary peritonitis are monomicrobial aerobic gram-negative bacilli.
    b. Empiric therapy for intra-abdominal infections should target the suspected organisms in each individual infection. Subsequently, therapy should be modified according to results of culture and sensitivity testing.
    c. In the treatment of primary peritonitis, ampicillin plus an aminoglycoside is commonly used. However, other agents such as a second- or third-generation cephalosporin are also appropriate treatment regimens.

CASE 112

PROBLEM LIST

1. Viral Gastroenteritis
2. Dehydration

SOAP NOTE

S: JP's mom states that he has "runny diarrhea and doesn't want to play with his two sisters"; vomiting; fever; no appetite; thirsty; lethargic; restless and irritable; decreased alertness; minimal interaction with siblings

O: 8–10 loose watery stools in 24 hr; pale appearance; tachycardia (HR 125); hypotension (BP 90/70 supine); 1.2 kg wt loss; sunken eyes; absent tearing; decreased skin turgor; Na^+ 131 (131), K^+ 3.0 (3.0), HCO_3 20 (20), BUN 8.9 (25); urinalysis: pH 7.4, SG 1.005, clear but dark yellow, no organisms seen

A: **Problem 1:** Viral gastroenteritis acquired from children infected at day care

   Problem 2: Dehydration secondary to viral gastroenteritis

P: **Problem 1: Viral Gastroenteritis**
   • Oral rehydration solution with Pedialyte
   • Monitor frequency of stools
   • Monitor weight
   • Monitor Na^+, K^+, HCO_3, and glucose
   • Start feedings initially with easily digested foods such as bananas, applesauce, and cereal, and advance as tolerated
   • Subsequent foods can include complex carbohydrates (potatoes, bread), lean meats, yogurt, vegetables, and fresh fruits
   • Avoid free water, caffeine, carbonated soft drinks, hyperosmolar fruit juices (i.e., specifically apple juice since this is what JP has been consuming), and foods high in simple sugars and fats

   Problem 2: Dehydration
   • Supportive care as outlined above
   • Counsel parents on how to monitor for JP's condition (i.e., keep records of stool counts, oral intake, and JP's mental alertness)
   • Recommend that parents bring JP back to clinic if he continues to produce frequent large-volume, watery stools

ANSWERS

1. b. Norwalk virus
2. c. Adults are immune to rotavirus gastroenteritis
3. c. Adenovirus
4. a. Fecal-oral contamination
5. a. 2 days; 3–8 days
6. a. Rotavirus
7. b. Moderate (5–10%)
8. d. Comparable rate of rehydration in patients with severe dehydration (>10% fluid deficit)
9. Since JP is moderately dehydrated, the following schedule is recommended:

a. Rehydration phase with ORS: Pedialyte 1450 mL (100 mL/kg based on wt before diarrhea) within 4–6 hr

b. Maintenance phase with ORS: Pedialyte 145 mL (10 mL/kg) for each diarrheal stool (not to exceed 150 mL/kg/day)

c. Start feeding and advance as tolerated as described in the SOAP report

10. Instructions to JP's mom:

a. Attempt to give the recommended volume of ORS to JP without forcing him to drink the solution to avoid aspiration

b. Do not give JP any antidiarrheal agent

c. Avoid apple juice until diarrhea abates

d. Return to clinic if JP continues to produce frequent large-volume, watery stools

e. Touch his lips to see if they are no longer dry and rough

11. Psychosocial factors to consider relative to JP's outcome include:

a. Assure JP's mom that her child will respond well if he can consume adequate oral fluid intake with Pedialyte as described previously

b. Ascertain if mom, dad, or a caretaker familiar with JP can care for him during this bout of viral gastroenteritis because JP will not be able to attend day care

c. Make sure parents are knowledgeable about how to monitor JP's conditions by keeping records of stool counts, oral intake, child's mental alertness

d. Reassure mom that she should not hesitate to call you or the clinic if she has any questions

12. Key points are:

a. Viral gastroenteritis is usually a self-limiting infection that may require supportive care, especially in infants, young children, and the elderly.

b. The primary goals for treatment of viral gastroenteritis involve providing supportive care, appropriate oral fluid and electrolyte therapy, and nutritional management.

c. Oral rehydration therapy is the preferred method of rehydration. Numerous commercially available solutions are marketed and can be purchased in pharmacies.

d. Free water, soft drinks, fruit juices, or sports drinks are not recommended for oral rehydration therapy because they provide inadequate electrolyte replacement and contain excess sugars.

e. Feeding should be advanced as tolerated commensurate with oral rehydration therapy.

f. Antidiarrheal agents should not be used as adjunct therapy for viral gastroenteritis.

CASE 113

PROBLEM LIST

1. Prosthetic Valve Bacterial Endocarditis
2. Increased Anticoagulation Effect
3. Anemia

4. Benzodiazepine Addiction

SOAP NOTE

S: Fever, chills, night sweats, weakness, headaches, and a decreased appetite; pale appearance

O: T 39°C; Roth spots; heart murmur; 3.5 kg weight loss; embolic lesions; ecchymosis; guaiac (+) stools; (+) vegetation; low Hct; elevated INR; prolonged PT; Cr 106 (1.2); Hct 0.30

A: **Problem 1:** Prosthetic valve bacterial endocarditis postdental procedure

Problem 2: Elevated INR with evidence of bleeding complications secondary to warfarin toxicity; possible causes include change in diet, change in regimen; drug interaction with OTC products

Problem 3: Anemia secondary to blood loss

Problem 4: Benzodiazepine dependence since mitral valve replacement 2 years ago for anxiety disorders and is now dependent on these agents

P: **Problem 1: Prosthetic Valve Bacterial Endocarditis**

• Start vancomycin 1 g IV QD

• Monitor vancomycin concentrations (target peak 30–45 mg/L, trough 10 mg/L)

• Start gentamicin 60 mg IV BID × 5 days

• Monitor gentamicin concentrations (target peak 3–5 mg/L, trough < 0.5 mg/L)

• Monitor Cr

• Start rifampin 300 mg PO q8h

• Review medication chart for potential drug interactions with rifampin and adjust or monitor drug therapy as indicated

• Inform SF that rifampin causes body fluids (e.g., tears, urine) to turn orange and that this discoloration does not cause any problems and does not indicate that any damage is occurring to your body; SF wears eyeglasses and has no intention to purchase contact lenses so discoloration of contact lenses is not an issue

• Monitor temperature (every shift)

• Daily white blood cell count (with differential) and blood cultures

Problem 2: Increased Anticoagulation Effect

• Ask SF what dose of warfarin she was taking at home and if she has been taking any OTC products

• Ask SF if there has been any changes in her diet while she was at home

• Hold warfarin dose until INR of 2.5–3.5

• Vitamin K 1 mg SC × 1 dose

• Repeat vitamin K dose if INR at 24 hr is high

- Restart warfarin at a lower dose and titrate to INR 2.5–3.5

Problem 3: Anemia

- Multivitamin with iron 1 tablet PO QD
- Monitor Hct

Problem 4: Benzodiazepine Dependence

- Discontinue diazepam and alprazolam
- Chlordiazepoxide 50 mg PO TID × 5 days, then taper over an additional 5 days
- Monitor symptoms of benzodiazepine withdrawal (e.g., anxiety, insomnia, irritability, sensitivity to light and sound, and muscle spasms)

ANSWERS

1. b. Duration of therapy is 10–14 days
2. d. Tricuspid valve
3. d. Angina
4. Transient bacteremia occurred from one or both scenarios:
   - Dental procedure despite prophylaxis
   - Dental flossing resulted in gingival bleeding since BF has increased anticoagulant effect (elevated INR)
5. b. *Staphylococcus aureus*
6. Gentamicin is advocated only during the first 3–5 days of therapy for *S. aureus* endocarditis. Potentially achieve more rapid clearance of bacteremia and reduce the time patients are febrile. Gentamicin peak concentration of 3–5 mg/L is synergistic with a cell wall-active antibiotic (e.g., nafcillin, vancomycin) against *S. aureus.*
7. d. At least 6 weeks
8. a. Switch vancomycin to oxacillin
9. Clear bacteremia; sterilize prosthetic valve; afebrile; prevent relapse; reduce further embolic events; minimize adverse events
10. b. Rifampin will induce the metabolism of warfarin
11. a. Continue current antibiotics and ask the microbiology lab to test the strain for tolerance.
12. Dental care instructions in SF should include:
    a. Understand the importance of reducing gingival bleeding while flossing
    b. Do not floss until the INR is within desired therapeutic target
    c. Use soft bristle toothbrush and brush gently
    d. Consult your dentist about brushing technique
    e. May need to reduce personal flossing and visit your dentist more often for teeth cleaning (requires prophylactic antibiotics)
13. a. SF is likely to be concerned about the need for surgical replacement of the prosthetic mitral valve
14. a. Oxacillin
15. Key points are:
    a. Infective endocarditis is a potentially life-threatening infection that requires aggressive and prolonged therapy with bactericidal antibiotics.
    b. High-dose antimicrobial therapy is needed for

endocarditis because of an absence of host defenses and poor antibiotic penetration within the infected vegetation.
    c. Combination therapy is required for treatment of endocarditis due to enterococcal species, *Pseudomonas aeruginosa,* tolerant organisms, or staphylococcal infections of prosthetic heart valves.
    d. Prosthetic valve endocarditis of bacterial origin requires at least 6 weeks of antibiotic therapy due to the difficulty of eradicating the infection and sterilizing the prosthetic valve.
    e. Prevention of infection is best achieved by recognition of patients at risk, identification of clinical situations likely to produce transient bacteremia, and use of the recommended prophylactic regimen.

CASE 115

PROBLEM LIST

1. Osteomyelitis with Overlying Decubitus Ulcer
2. Diarrhea
3. Parasitic Infection
4. Depression
5. Alcohol/Tobacco Abuse

SOAP NOTE

S: "I feel hot and my body aches; there is fluid coming out of the wound on my buttock; I also have more diarrhea that is hard to control; I drank a bit more lately because I am so upset that I have to live this kind of life."

O: Hypotension (BP 100/57), tachycardia (HR 107), elevated temperature (39.4°C); dehydration (dry mucous membranes); mental confusion; extensive and deep wound with drainage on right buttock with apparent bone erosion; abdominal rash; Foley catheter in place; head lice; increased leukocytes (Lkcs 14.7) with left shift (8 bands); increased ESR (75); borderline electrolytes (K 3.4, Na 134); low hematocrit (0.34) and hemoglobin (114); wound Gram stain results abnormal (indicating infection); x-ray results indicate osteomyelitis

A: Problem 1: Osteomyelitis; likely due to longstanding and extensive decubitus ulcer; paraplegia responsible for vascular insufficiency, pressure sores, decreased sensation, and pain; preliminary microbiologic results indicate polymicrobial bone infection; consider Enterobacteriaceae (presence of diarrhea and history of UTIs)

Problem 2: Diarrhea; possible cause: antibiotic-associated pseudomembranous colitis (due to

Clostridium difficile) as result of recent clindamycin use, or gastrointestinal infection; self-treatment with high doses of loperamide; rash may be adverse effect of loperamide

Problem 3: Parasitic infection; head lice; possibly associated with homeless status and improper hygienic conditions

Problem 4: Depression; probably related to difficult life circumstances; currently treated with trazodone; CNS, cardiac, and GI problems may be related to adverse drug effects, or potential abuse

Problem 5: Alcohol/tobacco abuse; possibly means for 'coping' with personal problems; CNS and GI problems may be associated with acute alcohol intoxication and/or withdrawal symptoms

P: Problem 1: Osteomyelitis

- Treat osteomyelitis empirically with broad-spectrum antibiotic therapy including coverage for gram-positive (staphylococci, streptococci), gram-negative, and initially anaerobic organisms; choose parenteral agents with good bone penetration
- Avoid using clindamycin until final stool culture report
- Potential empiric regimen:
  - Gentamicin IV 5 mg/kg/QD* (or ciprofloxacin 400 mg IV q12h)
  - + nafcillin/oxacillin 2 g IV q6h
  - + metronidazole 500 mg IV q6–8h
  - *(Dose/schedule based on pharmacokinetic monitoring)
- Evaluate extent of osteomyelitis by CT scan
- Need surgical debridement of avascular tissue and necrotic bone, and drainage of abscesses and sinus tracts if necessary
- Treat decubitus ulcer with local wound care; provide warm and clean environment; may apply absorbent dextranomer or polyurethane films
- Avoid pressure, shearing forces, and friction to skin and bone; reduce urinary contamination by optimal catheter care
- Provide high-protein diet; may consider oral ascorbic acid supplement (500 mg BID) to promote wound healing
- Evaluate empiric regimen as soon as final wound/bone culture and sensitivity reports available; tailor antibiotic therapy to infecting organism(s) and sensitivity profile(s)
- Monitor response based on amelioration of signs and symptoms, normalizing WBC, ESR, and improvement in radiographic findings
- Treat at least for 4–6 weeks
- Consider oral antibiotic therapy if good response to

parenteral therapy. Potential drugs include penicillins (i.e., dicloxacillin, augmentin), cephalosporins (i.e. cephalexin, cefepim), fluoroquinolones (i.e., ciprofloxacin, levofloxacin)

- Monitor antibiotic therapy for adverse effects, e.g., hypersensitivity reactions (i.e., penicillins, cephalosporins, quinolones), renal toxicity and ototoxicity (aminoglycosides), CNS and gastrointestinal reactions (metronidazole, quinolones)
- Assure adherence to drug regimen; may have visiting nurse or other institution monitor as outpatient
- Goal: treat acute osteomyelitis; prevent chronic complication; provide optimal local wound environment and nutritional status for enhanced wound healing

Problem 2: Diarrhea

- Investigate recent contacts and exposure to contaminated water or food
- Evaluate use of clindamycin and/or other drugs associated with causing diarrhea, especially antibiotic-associated pseudomembranous colitis (AAPC)
- Rehydrate with fluid and electrolyte therapy including adequate amounts of water, sodium, potassium, bicarbonate, and glucose; may use World Health Organization Oral Rehydration Solution (WHO-ORS)
- Stop loperamide therapy; inform of inappropriate dose (max. 16 mg/day) and adverse effects (i.e., drowsiness, rash)
- Await stool examination results; if *Clostridium difficile* infection suspected (AAPC), start metronidazole 250 mg PO TID–QID for 10–14 days. (Increase dose to 500 mg if drug is also continued for oral treatment of osteomyelitis)
- Inform of metronidazole's potential adverse effects (metallic taste, GI and CNS effects) and interactions with alcohol (disulfiram reaction)
- Goal: Find cause of diarrhea; correct dehydration and electrolytes; treat potential pathogen, if diarrhea not self-limiting

Problem 3: Parasitic Infection

- Inspect clothes and body parts with tight contact to clothing for potential lice infection
- Evaluate especially skin areas with itching, excoriation, and infection from scratching (i.e., rash on abdomen)
- Clean and wash the affected areas well; sterilize clothing
- Apply sufficient amount of permethrin 1% topical liquid to saturate hair and scalp and leave on hair for 10 minutes

- Rinse areas carefully with water and comb out nits and dead lice with fine-tooth comb
- Goal: Resolution of parasitic infection; increase patient's knowledge and understanding of the disease

Problem 4: Depression

- Evaluate efficacy of trazodone regimen and adherence
- Rule out potential abuse and adverse reactions, especially CNS (i.e., confusion, dizziness), gastrointestinal (i.e., diarrhea), cardiac (i.e., hypotension, tachycardia) effects
- Counsel regarding appropriate use, potential adverse effects, and interactions, especially with alcohol
- May increase trazodone dose (by 50 mg PO QD every 3–7 days; maximum dose of 600 mg/day in 3 divided doses); or switch to another antidepressant
- Refer to psychosocial service for further evaluation
- Goal: Minimize depressive episodes; psychological support

Problem 5: Alcohol/Tobacco Use

- Check alcohol level to rule out acute intoxication
- Investigate usual drinking habits and nutritional status, and check LFTs to rule out liver disease
- Check albumin and magnesium level for potential deficiencies
- Give thiamine 100 mg PO QD to prevent or treat Wernicke's syndrome often observed in alcoholics
- Check iron and folic acid level; if low give $FeSO_4$ 300 mg PO TID for 3 months, and folic acid 1 mg PO QD until both cessation of alcohol use and adequate nutrition can be assured
- Counsel regarding complications of alcohol and tobacco use; offer options for smoking cessation (i.e., bupropion); inform about support groups
- Refer to social worker
- Goal: Treatment/cure of alcohol-associated deficiencies; reduction/discontinuation of alcohol and tobacco use

ANSWERS

1. c. Contiguous osteomyelitis
2. c. In elderly patients osteomyelitis may involve the vertebral bodies infected from foci in the gastrointestinal and urinary tract
3. d. Achieving antibiotic bone concentrations considerably above the MIC of the infecting organisms
4. AM presents with a large and deep decubitus ulcer exposing bone; there is yellowish-green drainage and redness; pain is attenuated probably due to underlying paralysis; fever, chills and myalgias may be due to bacteremia (usually more common in hematogenous osteomyelitis); there is an elevated WBC with shift to the left, ESR, and positive wound culture; other signs and symptoms may include swelling and tenderness; in chronic cases one can find vascular thrombosis and/or sequestra, as well as necrotic bone.
5. a. *Staphylococcus aureus*
6. Preliminary wound culture shows polymicrobial infection; important to find out if correlation with microbial flora inside the bone; need to get culture of bone biopsy specimen. Wound contamination with infected urine or fecal flora (diarrhea) needs to be considered. Patient had frequent UTIs in the past; helpful to know pathogen(s), treatment, and sensitivities. Need to select empiric broad-spectrum antibiotic regimen including coverage for gram-positive, gram-negative, and anaerobic organisms. Choose optimal, cost-effective parenteral, and eventually oral therapy given the patient's homeless status, likely lacking health insurance and missing support system. Question patient about other potential drug allergies.
7. c. Peak serum sample should target a SBT $\leq$ 1:8
8. Pharmacologic and nonpharmacologic treatment problems include:
   1. Pharmacologic
      a. Stage IV decubitus ulcer with erosion into bone tissue
      b. Polymicrobial spectrum with pathogens possibly originating from fecal or urinary source
      c. Consider resistant organisms; investigate rationale for clindamycin use in the past
      d. Differentiate acute from chronic osteomyelitis because diminished pain sensation
      e. Treat AAPC if diagnosed
      f. Dosing adjustment necessary for potential aminoglycoside and vancomycin treatment
   2. Nonpharmacologic problems
      a. Paraplegia, pressure sore(s), poor nutritional status, and smoking significant risk factors for osteomyelitis
      b. Diarrhea and Foley catheter contributing factors
      c. Alcohol abuse risk for drug interactions and compliance
      d. Homeless status, depression, and lack of support influence choice of antibiotic regimen, adherence, and therapeutic outcome
9. a. Ciprofloxacin
10. c. In contrast to clindamycin metronidazole does not interact with alcohol.
11. d. Minimizing development of resistance, especially *Staphylococcus aureus*
12. Psychosocial factors that may affect AM's adherence to both pharmacologic and nonpharmacologic therapy are:
    1. Issues patient must address:

a. Prolonged antibiotic course with parenteral and oral agents; adherence to drug regimen

b. Undesirable adverse effects of antibiotic and antidepressant

c. Optimal wound and skin care; reduction of pressure and friction on affected area

d. Optimal body hygiene (head, mouth, and genital area), catheter care and prophylactic measures; prevention of infection

e. Smoking cessation, alcohol abstinence, optimal diet–lifestyle modification

2. Emotional disorders presenting in the patient

   a. Depression

   b. Frustration

   c. Anxiety

3. Other barriers

   a. Psychological problems may interfere with compliance

   b. Homeless status, limited access to optimal sanitary, food, and housing conditions, as well as missing family/friend support system may interfere with lifestyle modification efforts

   c. Limited financial and health care resources may prevent initiation and continuation of medications or appropriate foods

13. The health care provider's role relative to the proposed psychosocial factors identified is:

   a. Individualize a plan for patient: both pharmacologic and nonpharmacologic

   b. Provide patient education regarding drug therapy, adherence, lifestyle modification

   c. Investigate medication access programs for needy people

   d. Referral to social worker, dietitian, psychiatrist

   e. Show empathy and a caring attitude

14. The pharmacoeconomic considerations relative to AM's plan of care may include:

   a. Reduction of inpatient costs by rapid initiation of individualized, cost-effective therapy; referral to other institutions or to ambulatory centers for outpatient parenteral or oral follow-up antibiotic therapy; decreased hospital stay; reduction of overall health care costs; reducing morbidity; prevention

15. Key points are:

   a. The diagnosis of osteomyelitis needs to be made early in the course of the disease because rapid and adequate treatment influences prognosis.

   b. In contiguous osteomyelitis superficial wound cultures may not represent the microbial spectrum inside the bone.

   c. Although *Staphylococcus aureus* is the most common pathogen causing osteomyelitis, other microorganisms can often be found depending on the age of the patient, concomitant diseases, and risk factors.

   d. There is no specific laboratory test for osteomyelitis. Monitoring parameters include signs and symptoms, culture results, trends of the WBC count with differential, ESR, and results of radiologic imaging studies.

   e. Optimal osteomyelitis treatment includes adequate debridement procedures, identification of the organism, correct antibiotic selection, and delivery of adequate quantities to the bone for a prolonged time period.

f. The best cure rates for acute osteomyelitis are obtained when parenteral therapy is administered for a minimum of 4–6 weeks.

g. Following several weeks of parenteral therapy, oral antibiotic regimens may be instituted as long as they reach serum concentrations high enough to kill the pathogen(s).

CASE 116

PROBLEM LIST

1. Syphilis–Secondary Stage
2. Trichomoniasis
3. HIV Infection with AIDS
4. *Pneumocystis carinii* Pneumonia (PCP)–Primary Prophylaxis
5. Prevention of Exposure to Pathogens

SOAP NOTE

S: "I have a rash spread over various areas of my body that includes the palms of my hands and soles of my feet, as well as oral lesions." Over the past few days I've also noted a yellow-green vaginal discharge and vaginal irritation."

O: Maculopapular rash, oral lesions, generalized lymphadenopathy, elevated VDRL, positive FTA-abs; elevated ESR; wet mount reveals numerous trichomonads, malodorous vaginal discharge (yellow-green)

A: **Problem 1:** Syphilis–secondary stage; requires treatment and follow-up

Problem 2: Trichomoniasis; requires treatment

Problem 3: HIV infection; currently receiving antiretroviral therapy; viral load undetectable at previous clinic visit; CD4 count increasing

Problem 4: PCP–primary prophylaxis; currently receiving therapy

Problem 5: Prevention of exposure to pathogens

P: **Problem 1: Syphilis–Secondary Stage**

- Initiate treatment with benzathine penicillin 2.4 million units IM once
- Partner should be contacted, evaluated, and receive treatment
- Report syphilis case to the U.S. Public Health Service (syphilis is a reportable disease with a health department tracking mechanism)
- Inform patient regarding the Jarisch-Herxheimer reaction that may occur hours after the penicillin is administered; reaction subsides spontaneously in

12–24 hours; treat symptomatically with antipyretics if necessary
- Follow up to evaluate therapeutic outcome; HIV-infected persons should be evaluated clinically and serologically at 3, 6, 9, 12, and 24 months after therapy; VDRL titer should fall and become nonreactive within 2 years after effective treatment of secondary syphilis; if a fourfold reduction in titer over a 3-month period not demonstrated, retreatment necessary; patients with a fourfold increase in titer between tests also require retreatment

Problem 2: Trichomoniasis

- Initiate treatment with metronidazole 2 g PO once with food
- Partner should also be evaluated and receive the same treatment simultaneously
- Counsel that this agent may cause darkening of the urine; a metallic taste may also be noted upon administration
- Counsel to avoid alcoholic beverages and alcohol-containing products/food during metronidazole treatment and at least 1 day after completion of therapy
- Counsel CS and her partner to avoid sexual intercourse until cured (upon completion of therapy and asymptomatic)
- Follow-up unnecessary for both if asymptomatic after treatment or if initially asymptomatic (partner may be asymptomatic)

Problem 3: HIV Infection with AIDS

- Continue current antiretroviral regimen at the same dosages
- Combivir: Continue to monitor for anemia; currently mild macrocytic anemia; no treatment necessary; also monitor for neutropenia and thrombocytopenia
- Indinavir: monitor for nephrolithiasis and reinforce importance of adequate hydration and proper administration; also monitor glucose, lipid profile, blood pressure, bilirubin, liver function tests, and physical features associated with lipodystrophy syndrome
- Obtain viral load and CD4 count after current illnesses adequately treated

Problem 4: PCP–Primary Prophylaxis

- Continue trimethoprim/sulfamethoxazole at current dose; also provides protection against conventional bacterial infections
- Monitor for common adverse effects such as rash, fever, and leukopenia; also monitor liver function tests and renal function

- Previous CD4 cell count was 240 cells/mm³; until more data available, continue prophylaxis even if CD4 cell count rises in response to antiretroviral therapy; future data may support discontinuation of primary prophylaxis
- Reinforce importance of adherence to therapy

Problem 5: Prevention of Exposure to Pathogens

- Notify when syphilis treatment successful and VDRL titer decreases and becomes nonreactive
- Advise on the following measures to prevent exposure to pathogens:
  - Wash hands after bathroom use or contact with animals or soil
  - Do not eat undercooked meats, poultry, eggs, or seafood; wash produce before eating
  - Avoid drinking water from untreated source
  - Safer sex
- Check that routine vaccinations recommended in persons with HIV disease are up-to-date; prior to travel, discuss other necessary vaccines, chemoprophylaxis, and immunoprophylaxis

ANSWERS

1. b. Inhaling airborne particles of the organism
2. b. Rash on the palms of the hands and soles of the feet
3. Risk factors present in CS that increase the risk for syphilis:
   a. HIV infection
   b. Co-infection and previous infection with other sexually transmitted diseases
4. a. Dermatologic manifestations: hallmark of secondary syphilis; skin rash may be macular, papular, maculopapular, papulosquamous, or pustular; localized or generalized, with classic localization on the palms of the hands and soles of the feet
   b. Mucous patches that are highly infectious may occur in one of several places such as the oral cavity (as in CS), the lips, pharynx, and genitalia
   c. Nontreponemal test: VDRL positive (titer 1:32); treponemal test: FTA-abs positive
5. b. Wet mount examination of vaginal discharge that reveals numerous trichomonads
6. d. Benzathine penicillin, 2.4 million units IM once
7. d. Desensitize CS and treat with benzathine penicillin
8. c. Benzathine penicillin, 2.4 million units IM once
9. d. This is an allergic reaction to the therapeutic agent used
10. c. Metronidazole, 2 g PO once
11. Syphilis and trichomoniasis monitoring include:
    a. Syphilis: Follow-up recommended to evaluate therapeutic outcome; since HIV infected, evaluate clinically and serologically at 3, 6, 9, 12, and 24 months after therapy; VDRL titer should fall and become nonreactive within 2 years after effective treatment of secondary syphilis; if a fourfold reduction in titer over a 3-month period is not demonstrated, retreat; if a fourfold increase in titer between tests occurs, also retreat

b. Trichomoniasis: Follow-up unnecessary for CS and her partner if they become asymptomatic after treatment or for those who are initially asymptomatic (partner(s) may be asymptomatic)

12. Psychosocial factors that may affect CS's adherence to both pharmacologic and nonpharmacologic therapy are:
  1. Issues the patient must address
    a. Reduced activity due to symptoms
    b. Transmission of syphilis or trichomoniasis to partners during the infectious period
    c. Identify partner(s) that should be evaluated and treated for syphilis and trichomoniasis
    d. Chronic medications adherence to antiretroviral therapy during treatment for other STDs
    e. Avoidance of alcohol during metronidazole therapy
  2. Common emotional disorders presenting in a patient with STDs
    a. Depression
    b. Anxiety
    c. Feelings of isolation and/or shame
    d. Fear
  3. Other barriers
    a. Family dynamics–limited support system
    b. Significant psychological problems may interfere with medication compliance
    c. Managing syphilis and trichomoniasis along with other chronic diseases (e.g., HIV infection)

13. The health care provider's role relative to the proposed psychosocial factors identified:
  a. Individualize a plan for patient; both pharmacologic and nonpharmacologic
  b. Provide compassionate care
  c. Offer support services to patient, partner(s), and caregivers
  d. Identify if depression, anxiety, fear, or feelings of isolation and/or shame are present; refer to a specialist if necessary

14. Pharmacoeconomic considerations relative to CS's plan of care may include:
  1. Direct medical
    a. Hospital personnel and overhead
    b. Treatment and complications for CS and her partner(s)
  2. Direct nonmedical
    a. Lost wages (patient and partner)
  3. Indirect personal
    a. Decreased productivity
    b. Quality of life

15. Key points are:
  a. Patients with STDs, such as syphilis and trichomoniasis, and their sexual partners must be identified, appropriately treated, and counseled about the nature of their disease as well as prevention methods.
  b. Safe, efficacious, easy to administer, and relatively inexpensive treatment regimens are available for the management of syphilis and trichomoniasis.
  c. Adherence has improved for several STDs with the development of regimens that require only a single dose of medication.

CASE 118

PROBLEM LIST

1. Lipodystrophy (Abnormal Central Fat Redistribution and Peripheral Wasting)
2. PCP–Secondary Prophylaxis
3. Cryptococcal Meningitis Maintenance Therapy
4. Prevention of Potential Exposure to Pathogens

SOAP NOTE

S: "Overall I feel fine; however, I've noticed my arms, legs, buttocks, and face thinning and my abdomen becoming larger over the past several months."

O: Increase in abdominal girth; weight 74 kg (previous weight 3 months ago 74.5 kg); total cholesterol slightly elevated; viral load undetectable and CD4 cell count 250 cells/mm^3

A: **Problem 1:** Lipodystrophy syndrome probably due to indinavir; borderline high blood cholesterol but at low risk for CHD

Problem 2: PCP–secondary prophylaxis; currently receiving prophylaxis

Problem 3: Cryptococcal meningitis maintenance therapy; currently receiving suppressive therapy

Problem 4: Prevention of potential exposure to pathogens

P: **Problem 1: Lipodystrophy Syndrome**
  • Currently, optimal management of lipodystrophy unknown
  • Continue current antiretroviral regimen since viral load undetectable and CD4 cell count increasing; obtain viral load and CD4 cell count in 3 months; follow-up visit should also include physical exam to assess progression of peripheral wasting, central obesity, and potential development of fat pads and other abnormalities
  • Discuss importance of dietary intervention, physical activity, and risk factor reduction to control lipid abnormalities while continuing current antiretroviral therapy; pharmacotherapy not warranted at this time; obtain lipoprotein analysis in 3 months to assess measurement of fasting levels of total cholesterol [target goal < 5.2 mmol/L (200 mg/dL)], total triglyceride [target goal < 2.3 mmol/L (200 mg/dL)], LDL [target goal < 4.1 mmol/L (160 mg/dL), and HDL [target ≥ 0.9 mmol/L (35 mg/dL)]
  • If lipodystrophy syndrome worsens pharmacologic therapy should be initiated in addition to current nonpharmacologic interventions for

hypercholesterolemia, hypertriglyceridemia (if present), and insulin resistance (if present); if lipodystrophy progressively worsens with the addition of pharmacologic therapy, future options include discontinuation of protease inhibitor and changing to an antiretroviral from another class, growth hormone therapy, and surgery

Problem 2: PCP–Secondary Prophylaxis

- Continue trimethoprim/sulfamethoxazole at current dose; also provides protection against conventional bacterial infections
- Monitor for common adverse effects such as rash, fever, and leukopenia; also monitor liver function tests, and renal function
- CD4 cell count currently 250 cells/mm^3; until more data are available, continue prophylaxis even if CD4 cell count rises in response to combination antiretroviral therapy
- Reinforce importance of adherence to therapy

Problem 3: Cryptococcal Meningitis Maintenance Therapy

- Continue fluconazole therapy at current dose for suppressive therapy; monitor liver function tests
- Consider potential drug interactions with fluconazole, a less potent inhibitor of cytochrome P450 oxidase system than ketoconazole, if other medications are added in the future
- Reinforce importance of adherence to therapy

Problem 4: Prevention of Potential Exposure to Pathogens

- Advise on the following measures to prevent exposure to pathogens:
  - Wash hands after bathroom use or contact with animals or soil
  - Do not eat undercooked meats, poultry, eggs, or seafood; wash produce before eating
  - Use care in handling of cat; precautions when changing litter box
  - Avoid drinking water from untreated source
  - Safer sex
- Check that routine vaccinations recommended in persons with HIV disease are up-to-date; prior to travel, discuss other necessary vaccines, chemoprophylaxis, and immunoprophylaxis

ANSWERS

1. a. Indinavir
2. Presents with peripheral wasting of the buttocks, face, and extremities, central obesity, and borderline hypercholesterolemia; other findings in patients include insulin resistance, hypertriglyceridemia, vascular disease,

augmented breast size in women, "buffalo hump" and fat pads in other areas

3. Mechanism of action of antiretroviral agents:
   a. Indinavir, a protease inhibitor, inhibits HIV protease, an enzyme essential for normal viral replication; by inhibiting this enzyme immature noninfectious virions are generated
   b. Stavudine and lamivudine are nucleoside reverse transcriptase inhibitors, which competitively inhibit reverse transcriptase and act as chain terminators of viral DNA synthesis
4. b. Didanosine, zalcitabine, and nelfinavir
5. Factors that should be considered when selecting an appropriate antiretroviral regimen:
   a. Potency of antiretroviral regimen–combination therapy is now considered the standard of care
   b. Complexity of the dosing schedule (i.e., dosing frequency and food compatibility) and patient's predicted adherence
   c. Underlying conditions that may be exacerbated by specific antiretroviral agents
   d. Potentially significant drug-drug, drug-food, drug-disease state interactions
   e. Acquisition of drug-resistant HIV-1
   f. Cost and access to drugs
6. a. Continuation of the current antiretroviral regimen
7. c. 12 weeks
8. c. Peripheral neuropathy
9. a. Indinavir
10. a. Indinavir
11. b. Nephrolithiasis
12. Pharmacologic and nonpharmacologic treatment problem(s) present in JR's treatment plan are:
    1. Pharmacologic
       a. Lipodystrophy syndrome; etiology is unknown but thought to be related to the use of protease inhibitors
    2. Nonpharmacologic
       a. Advice on prevention of potential exposure to pathogens
13. Psychosocial factors that may affect JR's adherence to both pharmacologic and nonpharmacologic therapy are:
    1. Issues the patient must address
       a. Complex antiretroviral regimen–patient adherence to a large pill burden and complexity of the dosing schedule
       b. Undesirable adverse effects of antiretroviral agents
    2. Common emotional disorders presenting in the patient with HIV include
       a. Depression
       b. Anxiety
       c. Denial
    3. Other barriers
       a. Significant psychological problems may interfere with adherence to medications
       b. Limited financial resources
14. The health care provider's role relative to the proposed psychosocial factors identified is:
    a. Individualize a plan: both pharmacologic and nonpharmacologic

   b. Provide patient education and support services

   c. Referral

15. Pharmacoeconomic considerations relative to JR's plan of care may include:

   a. Use of antiretroviral regimens that include a protease inhibitor increase drug costs but reduce nondrug costs

   b. Mortality rates and hospitalization days have decreased with such regimens, lowering inpatient costs

16. Key points are:

   a. Highly active antiretroviral therapy (HAART) has prolonged survival, delayed disease progression, and improved the overall health and well-being of patients with HIV infection/AIDS.

   b. The goals of therapy are to improve survival by attaining maximal viral suppression, prevent the emergence of resistance, and prevent treatment failure.

   c. The standard of care in managing HIV infection is the initiation of HAART with a minimum of two nucleoside analogues and one to two protease inhibitors (PI) or a non-nucleoside reverse transcriptase inhibitor (NNRTI).

   d. Disturbing side effects of the protease inhibitors include lipodystrophy syndrome, which may include glucose and lipid abnormalities, and vascular disease.

   e. Patient adherence to HAART is essential to minimize the emergence of drug resistance and treatment failure.

CASE 120

PROBLEM LIST

1. PCP
2. Hyperkalemia
3. Macular Rash
4. Elevated Serum Transaminases
5. Central Nervous System (CNS) Reactions
6. Newly Diagnosed HIV Infection with AIDS
7. Substance Abuse

SOAP NOTE

S: On admission, RT complained "I am tired, can't catch my breath, and I become winded when climbing stairs." Other complaints include fatigue and nonproductive cough. Additionally, on day 4 of hospitalization, RT told the clinician that her hands were shaking and she felt very "agitated" and has a "headache."

O: Tachycardia; tachypnea; rales; hypoxia; bilateral infiltrates on chest x-ray films; positive bronchoalveolar lavage for *Pneumocystis carinii;* macular rash; hyperkalemia; elevated serum transaminases; fine peripheral motor tremors; (+) HIV RNA 238,910 copies/mL; low CD4 cell count of 123/μL

A: **Problem 1:** *P. carinii* pneumonia resulting from immunosuppression caused by HIV infection. RT currently receiving TMP-SMX (day 5 of therapy) and prednisone; now complaining of agitation, headache, tremors, and has a rash, which are most likely caused by TMP-SMX

Problem 2: Hyperkalemia secondary to TMP-SMX

Problem 3: Macular rash secondary to TMP-SMX

Problem 4: Elevated serum transaminases secondary to TMP-SMX

Problem 5: Central nervous system reactions (fine tremors, agitation, headache) most likely due to TMP-SMX; other contributing causes include steroid-induced CNS effects or other concurrent diseases or infections that need to be ruled out

Problem 6: Newly diagnosed HIV infection with AIDS-defining illness (PCP); HIV-RNA viral load measurement and CD4 count reflect significance of HIV infection

Problem 7: Substance abuse—intravenous drug use (heroin) and crack cocaine; management of drug withdrawal and psychosocial issues need to be addressed

P: **Problem 1: PCP**

- Discontinue TMP-SMX
- Start pentamidine (4 mg/kg) 265 mg IV q24h
- Continue prednisone 40 mg PO BID × 5 days, then 40 mg PO QD × 5 days, then 20 mg PO QD × 5 days, then 10 mg PO QD × 5 days, then D/C
- Monitor Cr, liver function tests, and blood glucose daily for pentamidine toxicity
- Monitor arterial blood gas daily for clinical improvement
- Following successful response to 21 days of acute therapy, switch RT to secondary PCP prophylaxis
- Explain the importance of adherence to prophylaxis. Provide as much educational and emotional support as needed to assure adherence.

Problem 2: Hyperkalemia

- Discontinue TMP-SMX as this is the most likely culprit of hyperkalemia in RT
- Monitor K⁺ levels daily
- This adverse event should resolve without any intervention after TMP-SMX has been stopped

Problem 3: Macular Rash

- Monitor resolution of rash since TMP-SMX was discontinued
- No supportive interventions are necessary as long as rash is nonpruritic or not worsening
- Closely observe mucous membranes for tissue

sloughing or development of vesicular lesions that preempt severe types of dermatologic reactions such as exfoliative dermatitis or Stevens-Johnson syndrome

Problem 4: Elevated Serum Liver Transaminases

- Discontinue TMP-SMX
- Monitor ALT, AST, and alkaline phosphate daily
- Caution is advised since pentamidine is also hepatotoxic

Problem 5: Central Nervous System Reactions

- No interventions are necessary since TMP-SMX was discontinued
- Monitor resolution of CNS reactions
- Other contributing issues that should be considered if symptoms do not resolve after stopping TMP-SMX include steroid-induced CNS changes and increased anxiety secondary to RT knowing about her HIV status

Problem 6: Newly Diagnosed HIV Infection

- Following successful therapy for acute PCP, RT will need to begin highly active antiretroviral therapy
- Emotional response to diagnosis must be addressed by a specialist
- Risk reduction counseling should be reinforced; counsel RT about prevention of potential exposure to pathogens
- Educate RT about the advantages (improved outcome) and disadvantages (complexity and toxicity of medications) of antiretroviral therapy
- Once the acute infection is controlled, obtain baseline CD4 cell counts and viral load measurements before initiating therapy (determine baseline viral load by averaging two viral loads taken within a few weeks apart; use the same assay for viral load measurement)
- If RT is amenable to treatment, combination antiretroviral therapy should be initiated; recommend 2 nucleoside reverse transcriptase inhibitors and a protease inhibitor
- Schedule follow-up visit to clinic monthly for the first 3 months, then every 3–4 months thereafter or more frequently if needed
- Routine monitoring of viral load every 8–12 weeks after initiation of therapy
- Maximal reduction in viral load may not occur until 4–6 months after starting therapy

Problem 7: Substance Abuse

- Initiate clonidine 0.1 mg PO TID
- Titrate clonidine dose upward PRN relief of opiate withdrawal symptoms
- Monitor BP supine and standing positions q-shift
- Promethazine 25–50 mg PO PRN N/V

- Acetaminophen 650 mg PO PRN, T > 38.0°C
- Kaolin-pectin suspension 30–60 mL PRN after each loose stool
- RT needs to receive counseling on a daily basis from persons experienced in the treatment of substance abuse; enroll in a substance abuse program

ANSWERS

1. c. Headache
2. b. PaO$_2$ and LDH
3. Adjunctive glucocorticoids (prednisone or equivalent) is indicated within 72 hours of starting antipneumocystis therapy in HIV-infected patients with severe PCP defined as a PaO$_2$ on room air of < 75 mm Hg. Glucocorticoids relieve the acute inflammatory reaction that occurs due to lysis of *P. carinii* cysts following exposure to TMP-SMX.
4. a. Concentration-dependent toxicity due to excessive TMP-SMX dose
5. d. Arrhythmias
6. Trimethoprim is akin to a potassium-sparing diuretic. Thus, high doses of TMP can result in hyperkalemia. This adverse reaction is concentration-dependent.
7. b. Serum creatinine
8. d. Stat Accu-check to determine blood glucose
9. Pentamidine exerts a lytic effect on pancreatic β-cells, causing a sudden influx of insulin into the systemic circulation with resultant hypoglycemia.
10. a. TMP-SMX 1 double-strength tablet PO every Monday, Wednesday, Friday
11. a. Continue PCP prophylaxis until the long-term outcome of withdrawing prophylaxis is established from clinical trials.
12. RT learned on this admission that the reason for her PCP was due to her immune system being ravaged by the destructive nature of HIV infection. RT could become depressed, perhaps even suicidal. Severe emotional response to diagnosis of her HIV infection must be addressed by a specialist. She needs education about HIV infection in terms of how it is caused, transmitted, and the various treatment options available. She should be encouraged to enroll in a chemical dependency program. Supportive care is one of the most fundamental keys to assuring RT that she can have a good quality of life. Supportive care interventions include housing and food assistance, access to treatment, and continuity of care.
13. Key points are:
    a. TMP-SMX is the drug of choice for acute therapy and prophylaxis of PCP.
    b. Macular rash is a common adverse effect of sulfonamides in patients with AIDS, but does not preclude further use of this drug.
    c. Adjunctive glucocorticoids should be administered within 72 hours of starting antipneumocystis therapy for severe PCP defined as a PaO$_2$ less than 75 mm Hg.
    d. Patients need secondary PCP prophylaxis indefinitely.

CASE 121

PROBLEM LIST

1. *Aspergillus* Pneumonia
2. Renal Failure
3. HTN
4. Type 1 DM
5. CRT
6. Hyperlipidemia/Hypertriglyceridemia
7. Deep Venous Thrombosis (DVT) prophylaxis

SOAP NOTE

S: "I feel short of breath. My cough has worsened and I have chest pain and fevers."

O: Decreased breath sounds; rales; BP 150/92; RR 26; T 39.2°C, HCO_3 21 (21); BUN 24.6 (69); Cr 221 (2.5); Total Chol 5.69 (220); Trig 3.16 (280); Lkcs 9.1 × 10^9 (9.1 × 10^3); Lkc differential: neutrophils 0.70 (70.0%), bands 0.07 (7.0%), monos 0.10 (10.0%); Alb 31 (3.1); Glu 18.9 (342); cyclosporine whole blood concentration (monoclonal RIA): 300 µg/L; SaO_2 0.9 (90%) on room air; bronchoscopy culture: *Aspergillus fumigatus;* urinalysis: mild proteinuria, few WBC; chest x-ray: RLL infiltrate; VQ scan: low probability for PE; renal biopsy: no cellular infiltrate, scarring consistent with other chronic form of renal failure; receiving immunosuppressant agents: azathioprine, cyclosporine, and prednisone; Type 1 DM; transplant rejection 1 month PTA treated with pulse high-dose steroids

A: **Problem 1:** *Aspergillus* pneumonia secondary to immunosuppression (e.g., receiving azathioprine, cyclosporine, and corticosteroids); DM also a risk factor

Problem 2: Renal failure (post transplant) most likely secondary to cyclosporine therapy (dose related)

Problem 3: HTN secondary to immunosuppressive medications (prednisone and cyclosporine) and impaired graft function

Problem 4: Type 1 DM; prednisone and cyclosporine can contribute to glucose intolerance

Problem 5: CRT secondary to ESRD

Problem 6: Hyperlipidemia/hypertriglyceridemia secondary to prednisone and cyclosporine (dose related); lipids and triglyceride levels–borderline high; two risk factors for coronary artery disease (CAD) (i.e., DM and HTN)

Problem 7: DVT prophylaxis secondary to immobility

P: **Problem 1:** *Aspergillus* **Pneumonia**
- Administer induction therapy with IV lipid-formulated amphotericin B for 2–4 weeks, according to guidelines in product information
- Monitor HCO_3, Cr, BUN, Mg, K, microbiologic cultures, CXR, and clinical signs of fungal infection
- Discharge maintenance therapy with itraconazole, 200 mg PO TID × 3 days followed by 200 mg PO BID; treat for 12 weeks
- Monitor liver function tests (LFTs) and skin for rash

Problem 2: Renal Failure
- Adjust renally cleared medications accordingly for estimated creatinine clearance of 30 mL/min; adjust insulin according to desired blood glucose levels
- Monitor K, PO_4, Mg, Ca, Cr, BUN, Wt, urine output, and total input and output
- Renal function may improve after reduction in cyclosporine dose or worsen if amphotericin B nephrotoxicity occurs; dose medications accordingly

Problem 3: HTN
- Titrate to BP ≤ 130/85
- Increase isradipine to 10 mg PO BID
- Place on a restricted sodium diet
- Monitor for gingival hyperplasia since on isradipine and cyclosporine

Problem 4: Type 1 DM
- Goal plasma glucose: 8.3–11.1 mmol/L (150–200 mg/dL) in acutely ill to relieve signs and symptoms of diabetes, prevent hyperglycemia, and avoid hypoglycemia
- Discontinue insulin 20 units NPH SC q AM and 10 units regular SC q AM/q PM
- Place on sliding scale insulin while acutely ill, an example is the following:

Blood Glucose		
SI (mmol/L)	Traditional (mg/dL)	Recommended Treatment
<3.3	<60	Give ampule of $D_{50}W$ and contact physician
<11.1	<200	No insulin required
11.1–13.8	201–250	Give 2 units regular insulin SC
13.9–16.6	251–300	Give 4 units regular insulin SC
16.7–19.4	301–350	Give 6 units regular insulin SC
19.5–22.2	351–400	Give 8 units regular insulin SC
>22.2	>400	Give 10 units regular insulin SC and contact physician

- Monitor blood glucose (fingersticks) q4–6h
- Change treatment for diabetic gastroparesis to metoclopramide, 5 mg PO QID 30 min before

each meal and HS; cisapride contraindicated in patients taking itraconazole due to potential occurrence of life-threatening arrhythmias

- Monitor for adverse effects: drowsiness, restlessness, fatigue, and less frequently occurring acute dystonic reactions, parkinsonian symptoms, and tardive dyskinesia

Problem 5: CRT

- Adjust immunosuppressive agents during treatment of *Aspergillus* pneumonia as follows: discontinue azathioprine, reduce dose of prednisone, 10 mg PO QD and cyclosporine (normal maintenance dose: cyclosporine, 150–450 mg PO BID)
- Check trough cyclosporine level; target concentration below therapeutic range (i.e., monoclonal RIA whole blood concentration 100 μg/L)

Laboratory Test	Therapeutic Serum Concentration (μg/L)	Therapeutic Whole Blood Concentration (μg/L)
Polyclonal radio-immunoassay (RIA)	100–250	200–800
Monoclonal RIA	50–125	150–400
High-performance liquid chroma-tography (HPLC)	50–125	150–400

- Discontinue immunosuppressive agents if patient's clinical status decompensates severely from *Aspergillus* infection; subsequently, graft rejection will occur, requiring surgical removal and placement on hemodialysis
- Monitor cyclosporine levels closely and adjust dose accordingly; itraconazole and prednisone frequently increase cyclosporine levels; metoclopramide may increase absorption of cyclosporine; trimethoprim/sulfamethoxazole may decrease cyclosporine levels
- Monitor LFTs, complete blood count (CBC), Plts, electrolytes, Trig, BUN, CR, urine output, BP, and glucose
- Monitor for signs and symptoms of graft rejection or graft versus host disease (GVHD) (fever, malaise, edema, flank tenderness, hypotension) and neurotoxicity (tremor, headache, paresthesias, and seizures)
- Administer cytomegalovirus (CMV) prophylaxis for 3 months post transplant: discontinue acyclovir and start ganciclovir 500 mg PO BID; take with food
- Administer *Pneumocystis carinii* pneumonia (PCP) prophylaxis for 6–12 months post transplant: start trimethoprim/sulfamethoxazole, 80/400 mg PO QD; take with 8 fl. oz. glass of water

- Administer thrush prophylaxis for 3 months post transplant: start nystatin, 5 mL swish and swallow QID

Problem 6: Hyperlipidemia/ Hypertriglyceridemia

- Evaluate risks versus benefits of lipid lowering therapy since lipid lowering may arrest or prevent complications of atherosclerosis and may also promote renal graft survival
- Reinforce diet modification and physical activity when well
- Discuss the importance of maintaining IBW
- After completion of treatment for *Aspergillus* pneumonia, consider starting pravastatin, 10 mg PO HS; do not exceed 20 mg PO QD while on cyclosporine
- Obtain baseline and follow-up CPK levels (every 6 months); cyclosporine reduces the clearance of pravastatin and may increase the risk of drug-induced rhabdomyolysis
- Discuss the signs of rhabdomyolysis (i.e., myalgias)
- Monitor LFTs
- Reassess lipoprotein analysis in 3 months

Lipids	Goal Serum Concentration	
	SI (mmol/L)	Traditional (mg/dL)
Fasting total cholesterol	<5.2	<200
Total triglycerides	<2.3	<200
Low-density lipoproteins	<3.4	<130
High-density lipoproteins	≥0.9	≥35

Problem 7: DVT Prophylaxis

- Administer heparin 5,000 U SC q12h until ambulatory

ANSWERS

1. c. Prednisone
2. Signs and symptoms of acute invasive pulmonary aspergillosis in RT include:
   a. Dry cough
   b. Fever
   c. Chest pain
   d. Dyspnea
   e. Hypoxia
   f. Abnormal chest radiograph
3. Findings that support diagnosis of *Aspergillus* pneumonia include: T 39°C, SaO$_2$ 0.9 (90%) on room air, RR 26, Lkcs 9.1 × 10^9 (9.1 × 10^3), decreased breath sounds; bronchoscopy culture: *Aspergillus fumigatus* normal; rales; chest x-ray: RLL infiltrate; Lkcs differential: neutrophils 0.70 (70.0%), bands 0.07 (7%), monos 0.10 (10.0%)
4. a. Lipid-formulated amphotericin B does not cause nephrotoxicity
5. d. RT should be advised to take itraconazole with an H2-

antagonist because the drug requires an alkalotic environment for adequate absorption

6. d. A standardized method for in vitro testing of molds is commonly performed to evaluate response to therapy

7. b. ACE inhibitors in combination with cyclosporine increase glomerular filtration and are considered an effective treatment for RT's HTN

8. Pharmacologic and nonpharmacologic treatment problem(s) present in RT's treatment plan are:
   1. Pharmacologic
      a. Opportunistic infection secondary to immunosuppression
      b. Cyclosporine-induced renal failure, HTN, and possibly hyperlipidemia
      c. Cyclosporine and prednisone contributing to glucose intolerance
      d. Acyclovir dose not adjusted for decreased renal function
      e. Omission of trimethoprim/sulfamethoxazole for PCP prophylaxis
      f. Omission of nystatin or clotrimazole for thrush prophylaxis
   2. Nonpharmacologic
      a. Adherence to complex medical issues/regimen
      b. Diet to maintain diabetes, blood pressure, and lipid control
      c. Maintain close follow-up with medical providers to monitor progress
      d. Education on signs and symptoms of graft rejection
      e. Mental health referral

9. b. Diabetes mellitus

10. c. Rhabdomyolysis

11. a. Itraconazole and cisapride are contraindicated because of the potential of causing life-threatening arrhythmias

12. Psychosocial factors that may affect RT's adherence to both pharmacologic and nonpharmacologic therapy are:
    1. Issues the patient must address
       a. Chronic medications–adherence to complex regimens at varying times
       b. Dietary regimens which are often unpalatable and inconvenient
       c. Laboratory test–commitment to life-long monitoring
    2. Common emotional disorders presenting in the renal transplant patient
       a. Anxiety
       b. Depression
    3. Other barriers
       a. Family dynamics–limited support system
       b. Other stressors in life
       c. Limited financial support–unable to purchase medications or appropriate foods

13. Key points are:
    a. Fungi causing systemic infections can be classified as endemic or opportunistic. *Coccidioides immitis, Histoplasma capsulatum,* and *Blastomyces dermatitidis* are major endemic pathogens. Opportunistic pathogens, such as, *Candida* spp., *Aspergillus* spp. and *Cryptococcus* spp. can cause invasive disease in patients who are immunocompromised.

b. In practice, empiric therapy for invasive aspergillosis is initiated based on clinical, radiological, and/or microbiological features prior to establishing a definitive diagnosis. Because the associated mortality with aspergillosis is extremely high in the immunocompromised host, aggressive therapy is warranted.

c. Lipid-based amphotericin B products are more expensive than conventional amphotericin B; however, they are associated with a lower incidence of nephrotoxicity and are indicated for refractory infections.

CASE 123

PROBLEM LIST

1. Head and neck surgical procedure
2. HTN
3. COPD/Smoking
4. Alcohol abuse
5. Psoriasis

SOAP NOTE

S: "Wet cough"; questionable alcohol abuse reported by wife

O: BP 135/85; pulse 78; pharynx–left tonsillar fossa, there is a white ulcerated lesion extending to the base of the tongue; chronic wet cough; however, lungs are clear; fifty pack years of smoking

A: **Problem 1:** Head and neck surgical procedure; excision of left tonsillar carcinoma, left radical neck resection, and tracheostomy

Problem 2: Hypertension; controlled

Problem 3: COPD/smoking; moderate-to-severe; risk of nicotine withdrawal

Problem 4: Alcohol abuse: questionable abuse reported by wife; risk of alcohol withdrawal

Problem 5: Psoriasis; mild; not active

P: **Problem 1: Head and Neck Surgical Procedure**
- NPO at least 12 hours prior to the procedure
- Surgery classified as a clean-contaminated procedure
- Most common pathogens for this procedure are oral aerobes and anaerobes, *S. aureus,* and streptococci
- Should receive cefazolin 1 g IV and clindamycin 600 mg IV preinduction
- Depending on the degree of risk, may also receive cefazolin 1 g IV q8h and clindamycin 600 mg IV q8h for 3 additional doses

- Monitor for possible adverse effects and allergic reactions to the antibiotics
- Postoperative medications should include ascorbic acid 500 mg PO TID, zinc sulfate 220 mg PO BID, bacitracin applied to neck wound, morphine sulfate 1–4 mg IV q4h PRN pain, and IV fluids
- Monitor pain control via a pain scale
- Monitor for major adverse effects of morphine, such as respiratory and circulatory depression and constipation, along with dose-related signs of intoxication, including miosis, drowsiness, decreased rate and depth of respiration, bradycardia, and hypotension
- Institute enteral feedings via nasogastric feeding tube as tolerated
- Monitor for any signs or symptoms of infection, pain control, and nutritional status including electrolyte and fluid status
- Postoperative speech and occupational therapy

Problem 2: HTN

- Monitor BP and HR during and after surgery
- Continue HCTZ 50 mg PO QD
- BP goal less than 140/90

Problem 3: COPD/Smoking

- Monitor respiratory status during and after surgery
- Continue albuterol and ipratropium bromide as prescribed but convert to nebulized formulations administered through tracheostomy
- Monitor for signs and symptoms of nicotine withdrawal postoperatively since in a smoke-free hospital setting
- Start nicotine patch 21 mg/24 hr postoperatively; apply 1 patch daily to a nonhairy area of the body; rotate site of application daily
- Encourage smoking cessation at discharge
- Inform that you are available to support him when ready to stop

Problem 4: Alcohol Abuse

- Start folic acid 1 mg PO QD, MVI 1 tab PO QD, and thiamine 100 mg PO QD, which should be continued until you can be reasonably sure he has stopped drinking and resumed an adequate dietary intake
- Monitor for signs and symptoms of alcohol withdrawal postoperatively
- If experiences alcohol withdrawal, treat appropriately with benzodiazepines such as lorazepam

Problem 5: Psoriasis

- Monitor for possible exacerbation of his psoriasis since physiological stress may be trigger

ANSWERS

1. b. Decrease the incidence of postoperative bleeding
2. c. Increase the overall percentage of nosocomial infections
3. a. Age
4. c. Clean-contaminated
5. b. *Staphylococcus aureus*
6. b. Cefazolin 1 g IV and clindamycin 600 mg IV
7. c. Vancomycin 1 g IV and clindamycin 600 mg IV
8. a. Preinduction
9. Psychosocial factors that may affect CT's adherence to both pharmacologic and nonpharmacologic therapy are:
   1. Issues the patient must address
      a. Reduced physical activity
      b. Chronic medication adherence to complex regimens at varying times
      c. Dietary regimens and feeding difficulties
      d. Speech impairment
      e. Social acceptance of physical appearance
   2. Common emotional disorders
      a. Anxiety
      b. Panic disorders
      c. Depression
   3. Other barriers
      a. Family dynamics
      b. Other stressors in life
      c. Limited financial resources
10. The health care provider's role relative to the proposed psychosocial factors identified is:
    a. Individualize a plan for patient: both pharmacologic and nonpharmacologic
    b. Provide patient education and positive reinforcement
    c. Referral (i.e. social services, psychologist, etc.)
11. Pharmacoeconomic considerations relative to CT's plan of care may include:
    1. Direct medical
       a. Hospital personnel and overhead
       b. Treatment and complications
    2. Direct nonmedical
       a. Travel, hotels, meals
       b. Lost wages
    3. Indirect personal
       a. Decreased productivity
       b. Quality of life
    4. Intangible personal
       a. Pain
       b. Suffering
12. Key points are:
    a. Identification of patients at risk for postoperative infection should be based on surgical wound classification and patient-specific risk factors.
    b. Antibiotics should be tailored to provide adequate coverage of the expected micorflora exposure.
    c. Antibiotics should provide adequate tissue concentrations at the surgical site.
    d. Antibiotic dosing should be timed in order to maintain adequate tissue concentrations for the anticipated duration of the surgical procedure.

e. Antimicrobials should be administered for the shortest effective period postoperatively.

CASE 124

PROBLEM LIST

1. Fever with Neutropenia
2. ALL
3. Thrombocytopenia
4. Oral Candidiasis
5. Nausea/Vomiting
6. Rheumatoid Arthritis
7. *Pneumocystis carinii* Pneumonia Prophylaxis

SOAP NOTE

S: Fever; nosebleeds; painful oral lesions; N/V; central line site is tender

O: T 39.8°C; ANC 0; Plts 13×10^9 (13×10^3); ecchymosis and petechiae on the extremities; white oral plaques (+ *C. albicans*); Hickman catheter site is erythematous; red lumen of Hickman catheter is (+) *S. aureus*

A: **Problem 1:** Central catheter line infection in a febrile neutropenic cancer patient with ANC 0 due to chemotherapy-induced bone marrow suppression

Problem 2: ALL being treated with induction chemotherapy

Problem 3: Thrombocytopenia secondary to cytotoxic ALL induction chemotherapy; BF is also receiving naproxen, which can inhibit platelet aggregation

Problem 4: Oral candidiasis secondary to immunosuppression caused by chemotherapy, which requires treatment because he is symptomatic and at risk for disseminated fungemia

Problem 5: Nausea/vomiting caused by the emetogenicity of chemotherapy

Problem 6: Rheumatoid arthritis; currently asymptomatic

Problem 7: PCP prophylaxis; currently receiving primary prophylaxis

P: **Problem 1: Fever with Neutropenia**
- Continue ceftazidime because BF is susceptible to infections caused by gram-negative bacilli
- Start vancomycin 1 g IV q12h; infuse over 1 hour for *S. aureus* central line (red lumen) infection
- Consider removal of central line if BF does not respond to 7–10 days of antibiotics

- Monitor BUN and CR for vancomycin-induced nephrotoxicity
- Monitor vancomycin concentrations since BF is at risk for nephrotoxicity because of concurrent nephrotoxic agents (methotrexate) and previous extensive use of NSAIDs for RA
- Consider G-CSF therapy if BF appears septic or systemic mycotic infection is suspected or documented

Problem 2: ALL
- Continue induction therapy per ALL protocol
- Repeat bone marrow biopsy to assess response to therapy per ALL protocol
- Provide supportive care for complications associated with induction chemotherapy as outlined with therapeutic plans for other problems discussed

Problem 3: Thrombocytopenia
- Give platelet transfusions to maintain platelet count $>20 \times 10^9$ (20×10^3)
- Discontinue naproxen

Problem 4: Oral Candidiasis
- Fluconazole 200 mg PO now, then 100 mg PO QD × 10 days
- Monitor serum liver enzymes and gastrointestinal effects (mainly nausea and vomiting) for fluconazole tolerance
- Monitor resolution of white plaques on oral mucosa

Problem 5: Nausea/Vomiting
- Continue prochlorperazine PRN
- Start ondansetron 0.15 mg/kg IV q4h × 3 doses
- Start acetaminophen 650 mg PO q4–6h PRN headache associated with ondansetron

Problem 6: Rheumatoid Arthritis
- Discontinue naproxen
- Monitor rheumatoid arthritis but do not anticipate BF to have any symptoms since he is receiving prednisone and methotrexate as part of ALL therapy

Problem 7: PCP Prophylaxis
- Assess tolerance to TMP-SMX by monitoring serum aminotransferase, neutrophil count, and rash
- Assess adherence with thrice-weekly TMP-SMX to determine if this is the most convenient dosing strategy for BF

ANSWERS

1. d. T >38.3°C; ANC <500
2. a. Bacteria

3. Indications for empiric therapy with vancomycin in a febrile neutropenic cancer patient:
   a. Catheter line infection
   b. Prophylaxis with fluoroquinolones
   c. Mucositis
   d. Colonization with resistant pneumococci or *S. aureus*
   f. Sepsis
   g. Meningitis (including CNS shunt infection)
   h. Soft tissue infection
4. *Staphylococcus aureus* may be resistant to the antistaphylococcal penicillins. Vancomycin can be changed to nafcillin or oxacillin if the organism is sensitive.
5. b. *Pneumocystis carinii* pneumonia prophylaxis
6. b. Gastrointestinal intolerance
7. a. BF did not appear septic and had no focus initially for gram-positive infection
8. b. Febrile after 5–7 days of broad-spectrum antibiotics
9. d. 10–14 days for line infection and afebrile with ANC >500
10. Patient compliance with topical therapy often is suboptimal because nystatin suspension has a bitter taste and clotrimazole troches require contact time for dissolution, which can be painful in patients with mucosal ulceration secondary to stomatitis. Overuse of fluconazole is leading to resistance of *Candida* non-albicans species.
11. b. Fluconazole 200 mg IV QD
12. G-CSF would be indicated in BF if his neutropenia was prolonged or he had a systemic mycotic infection. G-CSF is not likely to enhance resolution of *S. aureus* line infection. G-CSF is not indicated as adjunct therapy for oral thrush.
13. This is the first febrile neutropenic episode for BF, who was recently diagnosed with leukemia. Therefore, he and his family should be educated about the antibiotic management, which should include discussion on type and duration of antibiotics and indications for antifungals. GBF needs to be informed on monitoring ANC and length of time until ANC nadir.
14. Key points are:
    a. Use of vancomycin should be restricted to minimize emergence of resistance.
    b. Indications for vancomycin in febrile neutropenic patients include catheter-related or soft tissue infection; mucositis; prophylaxis with quinolones; colonized with resistant pneumococci or methicillin-resistant *Staphylococcus aureus;* sepsis; meningitis (including CNS shunt infection).
    c. An aminoglycoside (gentamicin or tobramycin) should be included in empiric therapy if any of the following conditions are present: catheter-related infection, sepsis, colonization with *Pseudomonas aeruginosa,* or parenteral administration of a cephalosporin within the previous 7 days.
    d. Monotherapy with ceftazidime is acceptable in patients without underlying conditions for use of vancomycin and aminoglycoside.
    e. Amphotericin B is indicated in febrile neutropenic cancer patients after 5–7 days of continued fever while receiving broad-spectrum antibiotics.

CASE 125

PROBLEM LIST

1. Gram-Negative Bacteremia
2. Mental Status Changes
3. Second- and Third-Degree Burns on Both Hands and Forearms

SOAP NOTE

S: "My burns are getting better but I feel weak; I need to get back to work by Saturday since I'm broadcasting a football game."

O: Intermittently oriented to person, place, and time; lethargic; hands and forearms bandaged and burns healing appropriately; currently receiving topical antibiotic cream; no current systemic antibiotic therapy; Lkcs 13.3×10^9 (13.3×10^3), Lkc differential: neutrophils 88%, bands 12%; blood: Gram stain shows gram-negative rods and cultures pending; urine and wound: no organisms on Gram stain and cultures pending; BUN 5.4 (15); Cr 100 (0.9)

A: **Problem 1:** Gram-negative bacteremia which requires antibiotic therapy; burn most likely source of infection

Problem 2: Mental status changes likely due to systemic infection; morphine may also contribute to mental status changes as receiving higher doses recently; CNS changes unlikely due to cimetidine since renal function normal; ICU psychosis also unlikely in this situation

Problem 3: Second- and third-degree burns on both hands and forearms: currently being treated with topical antibiotic and healing appropriately

P: **Problem 1: Gram-Negative Bacteremia**

- Initiate vancomycin 1.25 g IV q12h; provide coverage for methicillin-resistant *Staphylococcus aureus* (MRSA)
- Provide double coverage for *Pseudomonas aeruginosa*—several combinations for coverage may be appropriate; one example: ceftazidime 1 g IV q8h and tobramycin: initiate loading dose (220 mg); followed by maintenance dose (180 mg IV q8h); monitor renal function (BUN, Cr)
- Continue empiric regimen until culture and sensitivity results available; narrow therapy if possible based on results
- Repeat Lkcs with differential; monitor temperature and clinical response
- Continue antibiotics for approximately 10–14 days including 4–7 days afebrile and resolution of mental status changes

Problem 2: Mental Status Changes

- Monitor mental status changes during antibiotic therapy; reassess NEURO exam
- Assess total daily doses of PRN morphine; monitor use to ensure that pain is adequately treated but amount not excessive and contributing to mental status changes
- Provide adequate hydration

Problem 3: Burns

- Continue treatment with topical antibiotic
- Continue to monitor healing of burns

ANSWERS

1. c. Severe sepsis
2. d. Vancomycin, ceftazidime, tobramycin
3. a. Development of bacterial resistance
4. b. *Klebsiella pneumoniae*
5. c. Ciprofloxacin
6. d. Temporary deterioration is thought to be due to the release of bacterial endotoxins as a result of the bactericidal effects of antibiotic therapy
7. b. 8–12
8. Beta-lactam antibiotics exhibit concentration-independent killing above 4–5 times the MIC of an organism. The efficacy is related to the duration of time the drug concentration is above the MIC; thus, a continuous infusion would keep drug concentrations above the MIC 100% of the time and may be more effective than intermittent dosing that may allow a significant period of time when drug concentrations drop below the MIC. Due to a lack of controlled studies to date, it is unknown if continuous infusions offer a clinical advantage over traditional therapy.
9. 10–14 days including 4–7 days being afebrile and resolution of mental status changes; follow-up blood cultures should be negative if performed
10. No; none of these three therapies have been shown to improve mortality in patients with sepsis; corticosteroids may increase mortality due to secondary infections
11. c. Corticosteroids
12. d. 200%
13. Psychosocial issues related to SF's continuing care include:
    a. Ensure caregiver/home health care is available when discharged if patient is not able to perform daily functions with burned hands.
    b. Needs to be taught to properly care for burns at home.
    c. Needs occupational therapy rehabilitation.
    d. Needs workers' compensation benefits if eligible.
    e. Understands need to be compliant with antibiotics if taken at home.
14. Key points are:
    a. The successful management of sepsis relies on early clinical suspicion, rapid diagnosis, and appropriate antimicrobial therapy in addition to fluid and ventilatory support if required.
    b. The endotoxin-induced acute-phase response may cause rapid progression of the syndrome, which may result in

life-threatening conditions such as acute respiratory distress syndrome.
    c. Immunomodulatory adjunctive therapies such as monoclonal antibodies, corticosteroids, and other anti-inflammatory agents have not yet proved useful in decreasing mortality due to sepsis.

CASE 126

PROBLEM LIST

1. Severe Sepsis from Bacteremia, Possible Pneumonia
2. Hemodynamically Unstable
3. Respiratory Failure
4. Impending Malnutrition

SOAP NOTE

S: Currently sedated with morphine to facilitate mechanical ventilation; in MICU × 1 day following increasing shortness of breath, sputum production (thick, white), weakness, lethargy, fever × 2–3 days

O: Fever, requires mechanical ventilation, BP 90/65, HR 110, urine output < 10 mL/hr, CI 2.8, PAOP 6; leukocytosis with "left shift," blood cultures with gram-positive cocci, urine culture with gram-negative rods; respiratory acidosis (pH 7.26/pCO$_2$ 45), CXR with infiltrates

A: Problem 1: Severe sepsis from bacteremia and possible pneumonia

    Problem 2: Hemodynamic instability due to sepsis; signs of hypovolemia (decreased urine output, low PAOP)

    Problem 3: Respiratory failure due to sepsis, possible pneumonia, and underlying COPD; receiving mechanical ventilation

    Problem 4: Impending malnutrition

P: Problem 1: Severe Sepsis from Bacteremia, Possible Pneumonia

- Conduct microbiologic testing to rule out pneumonia
- Begin appropriate empiric antibiotic therapy for severe community-acquired pneumonia
- Risk factors that will influence choice of antibiotics include age, preexisting lung disease, and severity of disease (patient requires stay in ICU with mechanical ventilation)
- Narrow therapy, if possible, once organisms identified

Problem 2: Hemodynamic Instability

- Fluid therapy

- Monitor hemodynamic parameters and urine output closely
- Goal PAOP: 15–18 without signs of pulmonary edema
- Goal CI: 2.8–4.0 if possible considering preexisting disease

Problem 3: Respiratory Failure

- Continue albuterol because of preexisting lung disease

Problem 4: Impending Malnutrition

- Place nasogastric feeding tube
- Begin enteral feedings at 25 mL/hr with a high protein formula (1 kcal/mL, 62 g protein/L) to provide 30–35 kcal/kg/day and 1.5–2.0 g protein/kg/day
- Goal rate: 75 mL/hr
- Monitor and manage therapy

ANSWERS

1. *Streptococcus pneumoniae* with diminished penicillin sensitivity–most common cause of pneumonia (covered by cefepime)

   Pseudomonas aeruginosa–MA has structural lung disease (covered by cefepime and ciprofloxacin)

   Mycoplasma pneumoniae–possible, but not probable cause in MA (covered by ciprofloxacin)
2. b. Normal saline infusion
3. d. Bronchoscopy with BAL or PSB
4. a. Dobutamine
5. c. Low-dose dopamine
6. b. Penicillin G
7. d. 163
8. No. She has 2 of 3 criteria: $PaO_2:FiO_2$ ratio <200 and PAOP <18, patient does not have a chest x-ray characteristic of ARDS (diffuse, bilateral infiltrates)
9. c. Ipratroprium
10. a. Chest x-ray abnormalities
11. No. This is an unfortunate "disconnect" between laboratory standards and the clinical setting. Aminoglycosides exhibit concentration-dependent killing with best clinical results occurring when peak concentrations are at least 8–12 times the MIC of the organism. Normal serum peaks and troughs are 8–10 and <2 respectively. Aminoglycosides have poor penetration (<50%) into the lungs. It would be impossible to generate gentamicin concentrations in the lung at 8–12 times the MIC of this organism without massively overdosing the patient. Tobramycin or amikacin should be used if their MICs are better for this organism.
12. c. 7–9
13. Common psychosocial factors that can increase the risk of developing pneumonia include:
    a. Smoking diminishes mucociliary transport, results in increased gram-negative bacterial colonization
    b. Alcohol ingestion is associated with diminished macrophage activity
    c. Malnutrition is associated with diminished macrophage activity, results in increased gram-negative bacterial colonization
    d. Advanced age diminishes mucociliary transport and macrophage activity, results in increased gram-negative bacterial colonization
14. Key points are:
    a. The successful management of sepsis relies on rapid diagnosis, appropriate choice of empiric antimicrobial therapy based on clinical presentation and suspected infectious source, as well as various underlying patient factors.
    b. Hemodynamic and ventilatory support are fundamental to the clinical management of sepsis.
    c. An understanding of the pharmacokinetics and pharmacodynamics of antimicrobials as well as appropriate translation of culture and sensitivity data to the clinical setting are keys to developing an optimal antimicrobial regimen.

CASE 127

PROBLEM LIST

1. Cellulitis with ulceration
2. Morbid Obesity
3. HTN
4. Localized Fungal Infection (Athlete's Foot)
5. Smoking

SOAP NOTE

S: "I have pain in my left leg and there is an open spot; I also had a fever and chills the past few days. I am upset that I have to be here again. I cannot stand all these drugs."

O: BP 140/80; increased HR (96); slightly elevated temperature (37.9°C); inflammation and edema on left lower leg; painful to touch; about 5 cm × 5 cm ulceration; inflammation between toes and in skin folds on breast; overweight (150 kg); increased glucose (8.44); slightly decreased hematocrit (43%); increased leukocytes (16.1 × 10⁹) with 85% neutrophils; positive wound Gram stain results (gram-positive and gram-negative organisms found); skin culture results (toes, breast): *Candida* spp.

A: **Problem 1:** Cellulitis and ulceration; either not completely cured with recent regimen or new onset in the setting of obesity, dry skin, and leg edema.

Problem 2: Morbid obesity; AA's actual weight > 25% ideal body weight; major risk factor for HTN and also contributing factor for skin and soft tissue infection.

Problem 3: HTN; currently taking combination therapy of diuretic and calcium-channel blocker

Problem 4: Localized fungal infection; self-medication of feet

Problem 5: Smoking; ½ PPD × 15 years

P: Problem 1: Cellulitis–Skin Ulceration

- Include broad coverage for gram-positive and gram-negative organisms in empiric therapy
- Consider resistant organisms (i.e., MRSA), given previous hospitalizations and treatment
- Avoid beta-lactase given AA's drug allergy history
- Suitable empiric therapy: vancomycin 1.5 g IV BID and ciprofloxacin 750 mg PO BID; may add clindamycin (600 mg PO q8h) initially, if anaerobes are suspected
- The drug doses take AA's renal function (for vanco and cipro) and overweight (all drugs are dosed on higher side) into account (see also question 9)
- Alternatives: IV vancomycin + IV gentamicin (± clindamycin)
- Await final culture results and adjust antibiotic drug selection
- Switch to an all-oral regimen when AA is clinically improving. Possible regimen: levofloxacin (500 mg QD), either alone, or with clindamycin/metronidazole (if anaerobic coverage)
- Total treatment course should be 10–14 days
- Monitor signs and symptoms of cellulitis, ulcer size and drainage, temperature, leukocytes, renal function
- Obtain peak and trough level of vancomycin if drug is continued based on results of sensitivity
- Monitor for adverse drug reactions of vancomycin (i.e., "Red Man's syndrome," hypersensitivity reaction, nephrotoxicity, ototoxicity, thrombocytopenia, eosinophilia) and ciprofloxacin/levofloxacin (i.e., CNS reactions like headaches, dizziness; gastrointestinal problems; and dermatologic reactions such as rash), and potential drug interactions with quinolones (i.e., antacids, minerals, vitamins)
- Consider analgesic for pain (i.e., acetaminophen 650 mg q4–6h PRN; or acetaminophen and codeine if pain not controlled), cleansing of ulcer with normal saline or lactated Ringer's, and nonpharmacologic therapy with bedrest, elevation of legs, application of moist heat

Problem 2: Morbid Obesity

- Order dietary consult to design an individualized weight reduction program
- Include restriction of caloric intake through a suitable diet, instructions for physical exercise, and behavioral modification

- Recommend self-help programs (e.g., Weight Watchers, Nutrisystems, or Overeaters Anonymous) to provide psychological support and to increase motivation
- May initiate appetite suppressants at later time (if inappropriate response to diet, or after reaching a plateau with successful dieting)
- Rule out underlying hyperlipidemia or thyroid disease by checking lipid profile and thyroid function
- Rule out diabetes by rechecking blood glucose (oral glucose tolerance test or fasting plasma glucose)

Problem 3: HTN

- Continue current drug regimen
- Increase furosemide dose temporarily to 40 mg PO BID to reduce leg edema
- Monitor BP, HR, electrolytes, and renal function
- Analyze dietary intake of sodium and use of potassium-containing salt substitutes; encourage low-salt diet (2 g Na/day)
- Assess AA's knowledge about disease state and drug therapy, including potential side effects and drug interactions
- Emphasize adherence to medications

Problem 4: Localized *Candida* Infection

- Investigate usage pattern and success with tolnaftate
- Apply nystatin powder BID to moist lesions in skin fold areas, and use clotrimazole cream BID for lesions between feet; treatment duration may be few weeks
- Apply moisturizing cream to noninfected dry skin on legs
- Monitor for reduction in inflammation and itching, overall skin improvement, and adverse reactions of the drugs (i.e., skin irritation)
- Educate about risk factors for skin infections and measures to prevent them: employing good body hygiene; avoiding dry, cracked, and itchy skin; limit warm moist conditions on feet (e.g., due to wearing sneakers)

Problem 5: Smoking

- Educate about risks of tobacco use and benefits of quitting
- Encourage stopping smoking, especially in light of other medical problems and positive family history
- Inform about nonpharmacologic and pharmacologic options and support groups or programs
- Discuss various therapeutic options (nicotine gum, nicotine patches, bupropion) and their advantages and disadvantages

ANSWERS

1. b. Obesity
2. AA presents with pain, swelling, tenderness, erythema, and warmth on his leg as well as ulceration; he also had a low-grade fever, elevated white blood cell count, and a prodrome including chills. Other less frequent symptoms are lymphangitis and lymph node enlargement or tenderness.
3. a. Streptococci and staphylococci
4. AA had several previous episodes of cellulitis and was recently hospitalized for this. It would be important to know previous pathogens, sensitivities, drug regimen(s), duration, and efficacy. Did he complete a total course of antibiotics, and was he compliant with probable outpatient therapy? Unusual, nosocomial, and/or resistant organisms may be present, esp. MRSA. His preliminary wound culture shows polymicrobial spectrum; therefore, he empirically needs broad-spectrum therapy to cover for gram-positive and gram-negative organisms, and possibly anaerobes. When the culture results are back, his regimen should be adjusted accordingly, and if MRSA is excluded, vancomycin should be discontinued immediately. Also, conversion to an oral treatment regimen should be considered as soon as possible. His drug allergy information should be further investigated to not unnecessarily preclude beta-lactam antibiotics if they were indicated. Nonpharmacologic therapy for cellulitis includes leg elevation and rest, as well as application of moist heat to minimize edema around infected site.
5. c. "Red Man's syndrome"
6. d. Antacids
7. b. Concentration-dependent activity
8. Pharmacologic and nonpharmacologic problems include:
   1. Pharmacologic
      a. Recurrent cellulitis with polymicrobial spectrum and potential resistant organisms
      b. Drug allergies limiting antibiotic choice
      c. Dosing adjustment necessary
      d. Final pathogen(s) and final antibiotic regimen not yet identified
   2. Nonpharmacologic
      a. Obesity as significant risk factor for skin and soft tissue infection, hypertension, and potential diabetes (work-up needed)
      b. Smoking as risk factor for hypertension
      c. Diet and lifestyle
      d. Compliance
9. Actual body weight: 150 kg; height: 173 cm (69.2 in)
   To determine *vancomycin* dose the actual body weight should be used. To calculate creatinine clearance use ideal body weight.

$$\text{Ideal Body Weight (IBW) male} = 50 \text{ kg} + (2.3 \text{ kg} \times \text{each in} > 60 \text{ in})$$

IBW: $50 \text{ kg} + (2.3 \text{ kg} \times 9.2) = 71$. 16 kg (use 71 kg)

$$\text{Est. CrCl (male)} = \frac{(140 - \text{age})(\text{IBW})}{(72)(\text{SCr})}$$

$$\text{Est. CrCl} = \frac{(140 - 48) \times 71}{72 \times 1.1} = 82.5 \text{ mL/min}$$

The usual dose of vancomycin is 1 g or 10–15 mg/kg every 12 h. Based on AA's actual body weight he should receive 1.5 g vancomycin administered q12h. Dosing adjustment is necessary if CrCl < 60 mL/min. If vancomycin is continued drug levels need to be monitored because AA is obese. The usual dose for ciprofloxacin is 500–750 mg BID. Given his large weight, AA should receive a dose of 750 mg BID. Adjustments for renal function need to be made if CrCl < 30 mL/min.

10. c. Wait until final culture and sensitivities are identified (given his good renal function, one may only need to check peak level for efficacy).
11. c. Clindamycin
12. d. Aztreonam
13. Psychosocial factors that may affect AA's adherence to both pharmacologic and nonpharmacologic therapy are:
    1. Issues patient must address
       a. Prolonged antibiotic course and chronic antihypertensive therapy; adherence to drug regimen
       b. Undesirable adverse effects of antibiotic and antihypertensive agents
       c. Weight reduction and smoking cessation–acceptance of strict diet plan and lifestyle modification
       d. Appropriate skin care-preventive measures
    2. Emotional disorders presenting in the patient
       a. Depression
       b. Anxiety
       c. Frustration
    3. Other barriers
       a. Psychological problems may interfere with compliance
       b. Other stressors in life (i.e., competitive profession) may interfere with lifestyle modification efforts
       c. Limited financial resources may prevent purchasing of medications or appropriate foods
14. The health care provider's role relative to the proposed psychosocial factors identified is:
    a. Individualize a pharmacologic and nonpharmacologic plan for patient
    b. Provide patient education regarding drug therapy, compliance, lifestyle modification
    c. Referral
15. Pharmacoeconomic considerations relative to AA's plan of care may include:
    1. Reduction of inpatient costs
       a. Most cost-effective, individualized drug regimen
       b. Preferable oral therapy
       c. Decreased hospital stay
    2. Reduction of overall health care costs
       a. Reducing morbidity
       b. Prevention
16. Key points are:
    a. Skin and soft tissue infections usually result from a direct damage to the skin, but are often also associated with underlying diseases such as obesity, peripheral vascular disease, preexisting edema, and diabetes mellitus.
    b. The most common organisms associated with cellulitis are staphylococci and streptococci; however, polymicrobial infections can be seen in certain patients at risk.
    c. Signs and symptoms of cellulitis usually include pain,

erythema, warmth, swelling, and tenderness at the infection site; prodromal symptoms such as fever, chills, malaise, nausea, and vomiting can occur.

d. Uncomplicated cellulitis is empirically treated with agents effective against streptococci and staphylococci such as beta-lactamase-stable penicillins or first-generation cephalosporins. In patients with risk factors for gram-negative or anaerobic organisms, empiric regimens should be broadened and may include aminoglycosides, fluoroquinolones, metronidazole, clindamycin, or extended-spectrum penicillins.

e. Nonpharmacologic interventions include bed rest, elevation of affected area, application of moist heat, and analgesics.

SECTION 16 / NEOPLASTIC DISORDERS

CASE 128

PROBLEM LIST

1. Deep Vein Thrombosis (DVT)
2. Chronic Myelogenous Leukemia
3. Hypertension
4. GERD

SOAP NOTE

S: Pain, swelling in right calf; fatigue, 10 lb (4.5 kg) weight loss over 1 month, anorexia and abdominal fullness

O: BP 186/90, edema, erythematous right lower leg with positive Homans' sign; Lkcs 22×10^9 (22×10^3), Hct 0.22 (22%), Hgb 70 (7), Plts 150×10^9 (150×10^3), LAP 40 U/I; presence of Philadelphia chromosome; Doppler examination indicates extensive thrombosis in right popliteal vein

A: **Problem 1:** Deep vein thrombosis evidenced by: pain, edema, positive Homans' sign, and erythema; + Doppler examination

Problem 2: Chronic myelogenous leukemia (CML)

Problem 3: Hypertension—poorly controlled on his current regimen of hydrochlorothiazide 25 mg PO QD

Problem 4: Gastroesophageal reflux disease (GERD); currently controlled with famotidine

P: **Problem 1: Deep Vein Thrombosis**

- Obtain a baseline CBC with differential, platelet count, PT, INR, aPTT
- Begin enoxaparin 90 mg subcutaneous injection q12h
- Start warfarin on day 1 after beginning enoxaparin
- Monitor Hct, platelets, PT, and INR
- Discontinue enoxaparin when INR therapeutic × 48–72 hours
- Check PT/INR daily until therapeutic, 1–2/wk until INR is stable, then every 2 weeks until receiving stable warfarin dose
- Recheck INR if changes in therapy occur with interacting medications or dietary changes
- Goals: INR 2–3; resolution of DVT; requires therapy for at least 1.5–3 months

Problem 2: Chronic Myelogenous Leukemia

- Monitor CBC until stable, then twice weekly; aim for WBC between $2–4 \times 10^9$ and platelet count > 50×10^9
- Monitor cytogenetic response on bone marrow every 3 months during first year, then every 4–6 months
- Continue interferon alpha-2b 10×10^6 units (5×10^6 units/m^2) subcutaneous injection daily with plenty of fluids
- Premedicate with acetaminophen to lessen fever/chills
- Monitor liver function tests, electrolytes, T$_4$ and TSH; also monitor for depression and psychosis

Problem 3: Hypertension

- Continue hydrochlorothiazide 25 mg PO QD
- Add atenolol 50 mg PO QD; avoid calcium channel blocking agents and alpha-adrenergic agents because they may exacerbate GERD
- Monitor BP, HR, SCr, electrolytes, liver function tests, and lipid profile
- Counsel regarding potential for postural hypotension, to use caution when performing tasks which require alertness, and to avoid abrupt

discontinuation of atenolol to prevent rebound hypertension

Problem 4: GERD

- Currently controlled with famotidine 20 mg PO BID
- Monitor symptoms; goals of therapy are to decrease reflux, neutralize reflux, enhance esophageal clearance, and to protect esophageal mucosa
- Counsel on nonpharmacologic management of GERD, including: tilting head of bed, avoiding large meals and snacks prior to bedtime; minimizing intake of dietary fats, chocolate, peppermint, citrus juices, coffee, or alcohol, and avoiding smoking

ANSWERS

1. c. Allogenic bone marrow transplant
2. d. Exposure to large amounts of radiation
3. b. Chronic phase
4. b. Interferon alpha is capable of producing a complete cytogenetic response
5. Patients with CML are often minimally symptomatic at diagnosis. They are told that, without bone marrow transplant, they have an incurable disease. Because the chance of success with BMT is greatest if performed during the chronic phase and within the first year of diagnosis, patients are faced with the decision to face a life-threatening medical procedure when they are feeling otherwise healthy. If the patient decides to wait until his disease progresses, then the chance of a successful transplant is diminished. Family members may feel guilty if they are not eligible to be bone marrow donors. Additionally, the patient may face a great financial burden if he undergoes a bone marrow transplant. If the patient is not eligible for a bone marrow transplant, then he will be faced with the knowledge that his disease is incurable.
6. It is not valid; enoxaparin has only a minimal effect on activated partial thromboplastin time, but strongly inhibits factor Xa. Enoxaparin's dose may be adjusted based on anti-factor Xa levels. However, as anti-factor Xa levels are not yet widely available, they are not routinely monitored. Monitoring of enoxaparin therapy should include platelets, Hct, and anti-factor Xa levels (if available).
7. b. Prevent warfarin-induced skin necrosis
8. d. Inhibition of DNA synthesis
9. c. Myelosuppression
10. Counseling a patient receiving warfarin should include discussion on:
    a. Signs of bleeding
    b. Need for monitoring
    c. Duration of therapy
    d. Drug interactions
    e. Dietary considerations
    f. Need for altering health care providers of usage
11. a. Cimetidine
12. Key points are:

a. The earlier an allogeneic transplant is performed in the course of CML, the better the chance for long-term survival
b. Patients older than age 50, those without a donor, or those who are in poor health are not typically candidates for BMT
c. Alternatives to BMT include combination therapy with interferon alpha and hydroxyurea and/or cytarabine
d. The goal of using interferon in CML is to induce a cytogenetic and clinical remission to maintain normal blood counts. Cure is not likely with interferon therapy in CML.

CASE 129

PROBLEM LIST

1. Neutropenic Fever
2. Disseminated Intravascular Coagulation (DIC)
3. Intractable Nausea and Vomiting
4. Mucositis
5. Acute Myelogenous Leukemia (AML)

SOAP NOTE

S: Diaphoretic, weak-appearing, progressive fatigue, decreased energy, sore throat, nasal congestion, sweating, rigors, intractable nausea and vomiting, severe mouth pain 1 week after chemotherapy initiated

O: BP 110/56, HR 100, RR 20, T 39.5°C; + prominent gingival hyperplasia, erythematous buccal cavity; Lkc 0.3×10^9 (0.3×10^3), Plts 134×10^9 (134×10^3), Na 138 (138), K 3.1 (3.1), BUN 3.2 (9), Cr 88.4 (1.0), PT 24, INR 1.8, PTT 46.2, FiB 1.06 (106); bone marrow biopsy: hypocellular marrow; peripheral smear: no blasts; blood cultures negative to date; chest x-ray: WNL

A: Problem 1: Neutropenic fever associated with chemotherapy; probable infection

Problem 2: Disseminated intravascular coagulation (DIC) secondary to infection

Problem 3: Intractable nausea and vomiting following daunorubicin and ARA-C; delayed

Problem 4: Mucositis associated with daunorubicin and ARA-C

Problem 5: Acute myelogenous leukemia (AML) S/P induction therapy; unknown at this time whether induction successful

P: Problem 1: Neutropenic Fever

- Obtain blood cultures × 3 (include fungal stain); urine clean catch and culture

- Empiric ceftazidime 2 g IV q8h
- Monitor blood cultures, fever, vital signs
- If continues to spike fevers, add vancomycin
- Add amphotericin B if fevers continue 3 days after beginning ceftazidime

Problem 2: DIC

- Discontinue conjugated estrogens and medroxyprogesterone temporarily due to prothrombic tendency
- Monitor signs of vaginal bleeding and hot flashes
- Administer cryoprecipitate
- Monitor blood counts
- Transfuse PRBCs and platelets
- Begin heparin 5000 units SC q8h

Problem 3: Nausea and Vomiting

- Start chlorpromazine 10 mg IVP q4–6h PRN
- Lorazepam 0.5–1 mg IVP q6h PRN may be added
- For extrapyramidal symptoms, give diphenhydramine 25 mg IVP

Problem 4: Chemotherapy-Induced Mucositis

- Nystatin 5 mL swish and swallow QID
- Chlorhexidine 0.12% solution (swish and spit out) QID
- Salt-soda swishes QID
- Evaluate pain
- Morphine sulfate infusion 1 mg/hr; 2 mg IV q2h PRN breakthrough pain
- Consult dietitian to evaluate nutritional needs; obtain calorie count
- Begin parenteral nutritional support, if indicated

Problem 5: AML

- Repeat bone marrow biopsy 10–14 days post-completion of induction therapy; hold during acute illness
- If normal marrow elements are present and bone marrow < 5% blasts, initiate consolidation therapy as follows:
  - Cytarabine 3 g/m^2 IV q12h on days 1, 3, and 5; repeat × 2–4 cycles
  - Add steroid drops to prevent conjunctivitis
- Monitor CNS, cerebellar dysfunction, dysarthria, slurred speech, ataxia

ANSWERS

1. b. ANLL, M3
2. a. Liver failure
3. c. M1 FAB with Auer Rods
4. d. Hyperuricemia
5. Colony-stimulating factors should be initiated 24–48 hours after the completion of therapy in order to minimize duration of neutropenia. The use of colony-stimulating factors (CSF) in AML patients is controversial. G-CSF has a greater effect on cell differentiation and may stimulate maturation of the abnormal clone, while GM-CSF has a greater effect on cell proliferation and may increase the number of abnormal clones. It is therefore possible that some primary tumors would proliferate and that other abnormal cells would undergo leukemic transformation in response to CSFs. Despite the controversy surrounding their use, GM-CSF was approved by the US FDA for use in older patients with AML following high-dose induction chemotherapy. However, because of time lapse (3 weeks), EH is not likely to benefit from initiation of CSF
6. a. 15:17 translocation
7. c. DIC
8. d. Tumor-enhanced expression of interleukin-6
9. Recombinant erythropoietin (rh EPO), in general, is not cost effective compared to transfusions. However, quality of life and transfusion-related complications must be considered. Baseline erythropoietin levels may aid in predicting responsiveness to rh EPO. Iron deficiency must be corrected during rh EPO therapy for the maximum benefit.
10. a. Hypoxia
11. d. Dexamethasone
12. If EH needs an allogenic bone marrow transplant, her siblings will need to be HLA-typed to assess their compatibility to provide marrow. Family distress can be substantial if there are no suitable donors. Only approximately 25% of patients will have a compatible matched related donor. Family members may experience fear for themselves or the patient relative or guilt if they do not match.
13. Key points are:
    a. AML is typically a disease of adults while ALL is a disease of childhood.
    b. AML is generally more resistant to treatment than ALL.
    c. Initial presenting symptoms result from bone marrow failure and include fatigue, weight loss, fever, pallor, purpura, and pain.
    d. A diagnosis of acute leukemia is made by performing a bone marrow aspirate, which contains a minimum of 25% blast cells.
    e. Bone marrow transplant plays an important role in the treatment of AML.
    f. The treatment phases for AML include remission induction and postremission therapy with either chemotherapy or BMT.
    g. The 7 + 3 regimen (cytarabine + daunorubicin) is the standard of care in AML for induction of remission.
    h. Disseminated intravascular coagulation is a life-threatening complication primarily associated with M3 AML (promyelocytic leukemia).

CASE 131

PROBLEM LIST

1. Recurrence of Breast CA (Stage IV)
2. Increasing Shortness of Breath
3. Bone Pain

4. Hypertension (HTN)

5. Type 2 Diabetes Mellitus (DM)

SOAP NOTE

S: Complains of increasing shortness of breath over the past 2 weeks, accompanied by mild cough; mild/moderate bone pain in her left side

O: BP 120/88; RR 20; Wt 92 kg; well-healed scar left breast area; dullness of percussion over left lung bases, decreased breath sounds; Glu 7.7 (138), BUN 3.9 (11), Cr 106 (1.2); CXR: malignant left pleural effusion with cytology positive for breast adenocarcinoma; thoracentesis: glucose 5.3 mmol/L (95 mg/dL), LDH 234 (234), pH 7.5, specific gravity 1.025, protein 50 (5.0); Lkcs 2.6×10^9, RBC 110×10^{12} (110×10^6); cytology: adenocarcinoma breast; bone scan positive for multiple metastatic lesions to left lower ribs

A: **Problem 1:** Recurrent breast carcinoma with metastatic bone lesions and positive left pleural effusion requiring palliative care

Problem 2: Increasing shortness of breath secondary to malignant pleural effusion

Problem 3: Mild-moderate pain in left side due to bone metastases; confirmed by bone scan

Problem 4: HTN currently controlled

Problem 5: Type 2 DM currently controlled on present medications; carefully monitor sugar while on dexamethasone

P: **Problem 1: Recurrent Breast Carcinoma**

- Begin trastuzumab and docetaxel therapy; load with 4 mg/kg IV bolus dose of trastuzumab over 60 minutes for week 1
- Subsequent doses: 2 mg/kg of trastuzumab IV over 30–60 minutes administered every week; premedicate with acetaminophen 650 mg PO and diphenhydramine 25 mg PO 30 minutes prior
- Give docetaxel 100 mg/m² IV over 1 hour every 3 weeks; cycles should continue until MF has disease progression
- Give dexamethasone 4–8 mg PO BID × 3 days, beginning on day docetaxel administered
- Obtain baseline MUGA scan; liver function tests and CBC with differential should be obtained prior to initiating therapy
- Counsel about the possibility of edema, alterations in liver function tests, alopecia, suppressed bone marrow, and increased risk of infection, fever, chills, and myalgias

Problem 2: Increasing Shortness of Breath

- Remove pleural effusion fluid via thoracentesis

- Begin systemic therapy with trastuzumab and docetaxel

Problem 3: Bone Pain

- Obtain pain scale rating (0–10, 0 representing no pain)
- If pain rated 1–4: cautiously begin ibuprofen 800 mg PO TID with food
- Monitor renal function, platelets, hematocrit, signs/symptoms of bleeding; stool guaiac may be misleading with active hemorrhoids
- If pain rated 5–6: add combination opioid agent such as acetaminophen with oxycodone
- If pain rated ≥7: use opioid such as morphine sulfate in combination with NSAID
- Monitor for decreased pain; explain that pain may not completely resolve, but should be blunted and allow daily activities to resume
- Begin pamidronate 90 mg IVPB over 3 hours every 28 days
- Monitor calcium, phosphate, magnesium, potassium, CBC, differential, and hematocrit/hemoglobin

Problem 4: Hypertension

- Maintain current medications
- Monitor blood pressure as docetaxel and ibuprofen may cause fluid retention

Problem 5: Type 2 DM

- Continue current treatment regimen
- Monitor blood glucose; expect rise in glucose while taking dexamethasone
- Increase glyburide to 15–20 mg PO BID if necessary; may also consider adding sliding scale insulin as necessary
- Also consider changing daily dose of glyburide to QD regimen to improve compliance

ANSWERS

1. d. Smoking
2. a. Beginning at age 30, women should perform monthly breast self-exams
3. d. Improved QOL while receiving chemotherapy
4. c. Early stage (Stage I) breast cancer is easily controlled with surgery alone, or surgery and radiation
5. Trastuzumab in combination with taxanes have been reported to cause cardiotoxicity, including congestive heart failure, in 11% of patients. The exact mechanism of cardiotoxicity is not known. Congestive heart failure induced by trastuzumab is usually associated with left ventricular dysfunction. Trastuzumab and docetaxel therapy should be continued as long as her breast cancer continues to respond. Begin therapy with an angiotensin converting enzyme (ACE) inhibitor.

6. b. Enhanced microtubulin formation
7. c. Prevent edema
8. a. 10%
9. NSAIDs are excreted primarily by the kidneys and have been reported to cause acute renal failure, elevated BUN, decreased creatinine clearance, and glomerular and interstitial nephritis. MF's past medical history of hypertension combined with DM could contribute to renal dysfunction induced by ibuprofen. Acute renal failure associated with NSAID therapy is usually reversible upon drug discontinuation, so ibuprofen should be used cautiously.
10. Third spacing into pleural effusions and ascitic fluid can result in prolonged exposure to chemotherapy. This is well documented in patients receiving methotrexate. Extra fluid should be removed via thoracentesis and paracentesis.
11. c. Dexamethasone
12. Early detection of breast cancer may improve overall pharmacoeconomic outcomes by
    a. Being essentially without costs when referring to self-examination
    b. Increasing likelihood of arresting disease
    c. Decreasing need for radical surgeries and associated costs
    d. Decreasing costs associated with medical treatment
    e. Decreasing indirect costs associated with severe disease such as lost productivity
13. Key points are:
    a. Noninvasive breast cancer is generally easily controlled with surgery alone or surgery plus radiation.
    b. Locally advanced breast cancer is most effectively managed with combined-modality therapy. When all three modalities are combined, more than 90% of patients are disease free after treatment and may remain disease free for up to 3–5 years.
    c. The goals of treatment for metastatic breast cancer are to prolong survival and palliate symptoms. The choice of therapy depends on the site of disease involvement and patient-specific characteristics.

CASE 133

PROBLEM LIST

1. Pain
2. Nausea/Vomiting/Gastritis
3. Dehydration
4. Pancreatic Cancer

SOAP NOTE

S: Epigastric and right-sided abdominal pain not relieved by current oral medications, partially relieved by sitting forward; nausea, anorexia, and fatigue; admits to poor oral intake secondary to the nausea and vomiting

O: BP supine: 120/80 [HR 82], standing: 96/60 [HR 105], dry mucous membranes, slight oral erythema, poor skin turgor, tenderness in epigastrium and right upper abdomen, stool occult: guaiac positive; Na 148 (148), K 4.8 (4.8), Cl 106 (106), HCO_3 25 (25), BUN 13.6 (38), Cr 150 (1.7), Alk Phos 2.0 (122), Alb 30 (3.0), T Bili 18.8 (1.1), Ca 1.97 (7.9), PO_4 0.8 (2.4), Mg 1.2 (2.4); CT scan: mass in pancreas, liver metastases; CXR: WNL; KUB: no evidence of intestinal obstruction; upper endoscopy: diffuse erythema, small erosions, no definite ulcers

A: Problem 1: Pain secondary to pancreatic cancer; unable to tolerate oral medications; assess severity of pain.

Problem 2: Nausea, vomiting, gastritis; potentially caused by pancreatic cancer, chemotherapy, oral pain medications, or dehydration

Problem 3: Dehydration secondary to poor oral intake, nausea, vomiting, and diuretic use

Problem 4: Pancreatic cancer; s/p two cycles of chemotherapy; does not appear to be responding to current chemotherapy as evidenced by tumor progression and increased pain

P: Problem 1: Pain

- Assess pain using pain scale 0–10 (0 = no pain, 10 = worst pain imaginable)
- Discontinue acetaminophen with codeine
- Start hydromorphone 2 mg IV every 3 hr scheduled for pain control; patient may refuse
- Assess pain medication requirements and adjust
- Schedule pain medication (not PRN) and allow additional medication for breakthrough pain; may also consider patient-controlled analgesia (PCA) device using hydromorphone with a basal rate of 0.5–1.0 mg/hr and 0.5 mg every 30 min on demand. Assess patient needs; switch to oral hydromorphone by taking the total 24-hr PCA use and dividing into 4-hr increments
- May also switch to sustained-release product such as oxycodone SR; take 24-hr PCA total and give equianalgesic amounts q12h
- Start bisacodyl 5–10 mg QD
- Monitor: pain control, sedation, respiration rate, bowel function (constipation), mental status, rash or itching

Problem 2: Nausea and Vomiting

- Discontinue ibuprofen
- Start ranitidine 50 mg IV QD; switch to ranitidine 150 mg PO QD when able to tolerate oral medications
- Prochlorperazine 10 mg IV q6h PRN nausea; continue prochlorperazine 10 mg PO q6h PRN nausea when oral intake adequate

- Monitor: Nausea, vomiting, oral intake, stool guaiac, renal function, and side effects from prochlorperazine (sedation, dizziness, extrapyramidal symptoms)

Problem 3: Dehydration

- Obtain urine electrolytes and plasma osmolality to help evaluate dehydration
- Discontinue hydrochlorothiazide/triamterene 50/75 mg
- Replace fluid deficit over 48 hr; start normal saline at 250 mL/hr IV × 2 L, then D5 ¼ or D5 ½ normal saline at 150 mL/hr IV for next 36 hr
- Replace electrolytes in IV fluids as needed; monitor Na, K, BP, HR, urine output, skin turgor, and mucous membranes

Problem 4: Pancreatic Cancer

- Consider 5-fluorouracil infusion at 400–500 mg/m^2/day × 5 days, repeated monthly
- Monitor CBC with differential, platelets, mucositis, bowel movements
- If prognosis is < 6 months, enroll in hospice care

ANSWERS

1. c. Diabetes
2. a. Myelosuppression
3. b. After methotrexate
4. Advanced pancreatic cancer is considered incurable. Chemotherapy is palliative; therefore, the primary goal of treatment in a patient with advanced pancreatic cancer is to increase quality of life by diminishing symptoms, such as pain. Chemotherapy has been shown to decrease pain and improve quality of life. Increasing survival time is a secondary goal.
5. Gemcitabine improves disease-related symptoms and survival time compared to 5-FU.
6. b. Metamucil
7. d. Very low
8. c. 3:1
9. c. Meperidine
10. b. Who is unarousable
11. ML has a terminal illness. Issues with death and dying must be dealt with for him and his family. Focus must be on improving the remaining quality of his life.
12. a. Typically use less medication than those with scheduled pain medication administration
13. Key points are:
   a. Pancreatic cancer is one of the most lethal malignancies, resulting in death of over 95% of patients within 5 years of diagnosis.
   b. Most patients with pancreatic disease have advanced disease at diagnosis, leading to poor outcomes.
   c. Palliative care is important for patients suffering from pancreatic cancer; the goal of therapy is to improve quality of remaining life years.

CASE 135

PROBLEM LIST

1. Syndrome of Inappropriate Antidiuretic Hormone (SIADH)
2. Small Cell Lung Cancer (SCLC)
3. Drug-Drug Interaction

SOAP NOTE

S: 3 weeks prior: frequent hemoptysis, coughing, SOB, poor appetite, undesired 12-lb weight loss; family reports that GC has been confused and difficult to awaken

O: BP 140/82, HR 82, RR 17, T 38.3°C, Wt 53 kg, Ht 152 cm, BSA: 1.48 m^2; mild mucositis (Stage I), RRR; normal S1 and S2, no edema in extremities, clinically euvolemic, oriented to person only; Na 130 (130), Glu 5.55 (100), Lkcs 1.5 × 10^9 (1.5 × 10^3), ANC 253, Plts 70 (70); small cell lung cancer by histology

A: **Problem 1:** Syndrome of inappropriate antidiuretic hormone (SIADH); possibly tumor-induced

Problem 2: Small cell lung cancer (SCLC); to receive cisplatin/etoposide

Problem 3: Drug-drug interaction with erythromycin and cisapride; potentially life-threatening

P: **Problem 1: SIADH**

- Treat underlying cause (SCLC) as described below
- Add 3% NS to raise serum sodium
- Because of CNS symptoms, fluid restrict to 500 mL free water per day
- Monitor fluid status, edema, blood pressure, CNS symptoms, and serum sodium
- Add demeclocycline 300 mg PO BID after sodium corrected with 3% NS and mental status returns to baseline

Problem 2: SCLC

- Begin EP regimen (cisplatin 75 mg/m^2 per day IV D1 plus etoposide 100 mg/m^2 per day IV D1)
- Cycle: 3 weeks, continue for 4–6 cycles
- Monitor: potassium, magnesium, CBC, peripheral neuropathy, or hearing loss
- Anticipate myelosuppression with nadir occurring between 7–14 days; monitor closely for signs/symptoms of infection
- Continue nicotine gum as part of a comprehensive smoking cessation program, if able to swallow

Problem 3: Drug-Drug Interaction

- Discontinue cisapride and erythromycin
- No clear diagnosis for use of either agent; clarify

with primary care provider and discuss danger of this combination (cardiac arrhythmia and possible death) with primary care provider, patient, and patient's family

ANSWERS

1. c. 80%
2. d. Adenocarcinoma
3. a. Superior vena cava
4. c. Limited disease
5. Bupropion and nicotine patches may also be useful for smoking cessation. In combination, success rates as high as 35% have been achieved. Patients with history of seizures should not take bupropion. Patients must not smoke while using nicotine patches.
6. b. 7%
7. Chemotherapy has been shown to improve quality of life and reduce symptoms.
8. c. It produces less neurologic toxicity
9. For patients with extensive SCLC, the majority respond to chemotherapy, but less than 5% are alive at 5 years
10. Like many patients when first diagnosed with cancer, the diagnosis of lung cancer produces feelings of anger, shock, fear, and sadness. Patients with lung cancer may also feel guilt for having the disease secondary to life style factors, such as tobacco smoking.
11. Cisplatin is much more likely to produce renal toxicity compared with carboplatin. However, carboplatin produces much more bone marrow suppression than cisplatin.
12. According to the American Society of Clinical Oncology Guidelines for use of Hematopoietic Growth Factors, filgrastim would not be indicated for GC. Recommendations are for prophylactic use in patients receiving regimens likely to produce neutropenia in >40% of patients or in patients who experienced a neutropenic episode during prior cycles.
13. Key points are:
    a. Lung cancer continues to be the leading cause of death worldwide.
    b. Chemotherapy plus radiotherapy is the standard of care for patients with limited disease SCLC.
    c. Etoposide and cisplatin or cyclophosphamide, doxorubicin, and vincristine are the regimens most often administered to patients with limited disease SCLC.
    d. Prognosis is poor in patients with extensive disease SCLC, with less than 5% of patients alive at 5 years.
    e. Chemotherapy is the treatment of choice in patients with extensive disease SCLC.

CASE 137

PROBLEM LIST

1. Relapsed Ovarian Cancer
2. Anemia

SOAP NOTE

S: Abdominal discomfort and bloating

O: BP 110/60, HR 88, RR 18; ABD: distended, mild ascites, 15-cm mass extending to midline; GU: vagina smooth, narrow cervix small, smooth; uterus anteverted 5–6 cm with decreased mobility with tumor extension to midline; Hct 0.33 (33), Hgb 108 (10.8)

A: **Problem 1:** Relapsed ovarian cancer

    Problem 2: Anemia secondary to prior chemotherapy or anemia of chronic disease

P: **Problem 1: Relapsed Ovarian Cancer**

- Possible debulking of tumor for symptom relief; follow with paclitaxel 175 mg/m^2 IV over 3 hours on day 1; repeat cycle q 21 days
- Dexamethasone 20 mg PO 12 hr and 6 hr prior to start of paclitaxel
- Premedicate paclitaxel with diphenhydramine 50 mg IVP × 1, cimetidine 300 mg IV over 30 minutes × 1, and promethazine 25 mg IV q4h PRN nausea and vomiting
- Monitor CBC with differential and platelets
- Instruct to return immediately to hospital if experiences any sign of infection, such as fever, cough, or difficulty swallowing
- Monitor for hypersensitivity reactions, myalgias/arthralgias, and peripheral neuropathies

Problem 2: Anemia

- Obtain RBC indices, including reticulocyte count, MCV, MCHC, serum iron, TIBC, RDW, erythropoietin, and ferritin
- Guide pharmacotherapy, including parenteral or oral iron replacement, erythropoietin therapy, folic acid or vitamin B$_{12}$ administration based upon laboratory findings and positive identification of etiology of anemia

ANSWERS

1. c. Nulliparity
2. d. 1.5%
3. a. Epithelial
4. a. Lung
5. Although 80% of patients with ovarian cancer have elevations in CA-125, CA-125 may also be elevated in non-malignant conditions, leading to potential false-positive results.
6. d. 20%
7. c. Mucinous
8. Cytoreductive surgery allows better delivery of the chemotherapy to the tumor. In addition, more of the remaining tumor cells enter growth cycle, which makes chemotherapy more effective.
9. d. 6

10. In order to reduce the possibility of a hypersensitivity reaction, LL should be premedicated with dexamethasone, an H_2 antagonist and an H_1 antagonist antihistamine
11. d. 40–70%
12. a. From a purely economic standpoint, transfusions are not expensive. Recombinant erythropoietin is expensive, and over half the patients treated with erythropoietin may not benefit. Iron deficiency must be corrected to obtain optimal benefit.
    b. However, from the psychosocial aspect, erythropoietin improves quality of life and decreases the negative impact of the patient being transfusion-dependent.
13. Key points are:
    a. Ovarian cancer is less common than either endometrial or cervical cancers, yet is the leading cause of gynecologic cancer deaths.
    b. Ovarian cancer is usually not detected until disease is advanced.
    c. Screening may be helpful; however, screening methods are not yet ideal and may lead to either false positives or false negatives, depending upon the method used.
    d. Cytoreductive surgery should be used in combination with pharmacotherapy.

CASE 138

PROBLEM LIST

1. Capillary Leak Syndrome
2. Acute Renal Failure
3. Recurrent Malignant Melanoma
4. Fever
5. Tobacco Use

SOAP NOTE

S: Shortness of breath, lower extremity swelling, severe chills, lethargic

O: 2-cm mass in right inguinal node (removed); BP 104/64 (lying), HR 88, RR 16, T 39°C, Wt 78.5 kg (admission 68 kg), Tmax 39°C, rales, labored breathing; 2+ bilateral lower extremity edema; disoriented; Na 140 (140), K 3.6 (3.6), Cl 114 (114), HCO_3 17 (17), BUN 14.9 (42), SCr 265 (3.0); CT scan: consistent with metastatic disease

A: **Problem 1:** Capillary leak syndrome

Problem 2: Acute renal failure

Problem 3: Metastatic melanoma being treated with first cycle of biotherapy

Problem 4: Fever possibly induced by either interleukin-2 or interferon; must rule out infection by staphylococcal species (patient is at risk while receiving interleukin-2)

Problem 5: Tobacco use; requesting assistance with smoking cessation

P: **Problem 1: Capillary Leak Syndrome**
- Fluid bolus NS 250 mL; increase IV rate to 150 mL/hr
- Adjust ranitidine to 50 mg QD
- Start low-dose dopamine 2–5 μg/min/kg constant infusion, and discontinue diltiazem
- Discontinue naproxen to avoid renal toxicity
- Discontinue meperidine; normeperidine metabolite may accumulate in renal insufficiency
- Obtain blood cultures; consider adding anti-staphylococcal antibiotics
- Monitor I/O, blood pressure, chest x-ray, temperature, and electrolytes

Problem 2: Acute Renal Failure
- Estimated creatinine clearance 28.9 mL/min based on admission weight
- Renal function should improve as capillary leak syndrome resolves
- Discontinue aldesleukin, naproxen, meperidine as above
- Renally adjust all medications

Problem 3: Melanoma
- Monitor for side effects of aldesleukin: capillary leak syndrome, rash, neurotoxicity, infection
- Monitor for side effects of interferon alpha-2b: chills, fever, fatigue, leukopenia, increased hepatic enzymes
- Discontinue aldesleukin as Scr increased

Problem 4: Fever
- Obtain blood cultures as above
- Consider adding anti-staphylococcal antibiotics; vancomycin 15 mg/kg IV × 1
- Check random serum vancomycin level 20 hours post dose; if <15 μg/mL, continue vancomycin 15 mg/kg IV QD; if >15 μg/mL, re-dose based upon random level

Problem 5: Tobacco Use
- Encourage patient's willingness to quit tobacco use
- Nicotine replacement products (gum, patches, or inhalers) may be tried as part of an overall program; refer to support group such as American Lung Association
- If this approach fails, may be candidate for bupropion; antidepressant activity may be a desirable additional effect

ANSWERS

1. a. 20%
2. Adjuvant high-dose interferon alpha-2b has reduced relapse

rate and time to relapse in patients with malignant melanoma at high risk for relapse. High-risk patients are those with invasion of >4 mm or with lymph node involvement.

3. a. Theophylline
4. b. Liver transaminases
5. c. 15
6. a. Node involvement
7. d. Female gender
8. c. Stimulation of cytotoxic cells
9. Usually, fever and chills associated with interferon diminish with time. However, many patients do not tolerate fatigue. Length of treatment is also a factor as adjuvant interferon for melanoma lasts 1 year. Many third-party payers require the patient to receive injections in a physician's office.
10. Several steps can be suggested to allow improved tolerance to interferon therapy. Start with a lower dose and gradually increase to the total dose. Administer the interferon at night, usually following dinner. Prophylactic NSAIDs, acetaminophen, and diphenhydramine can help diminish symptoms. Assure the patient that most patients experience fewer symptoms with time.
11. d. Dexamethasone
12. Treatment for metastatic melanoma lasts for 1 year. Need to assess home situation for reliable transportation to medical appointments and availability of caregiver in the home. Due to age, unlikely to be able to tolerate toxicity of

biochemotherapy. If unable to tolerate treatment, consider enrollment into hospice program for supportive care. Insurance coverage may be important if outpatient prescription medications are not included in insurance benefits. Pharmacists can help by referring to available patient assistance programs.

13. Key points are:
   a. Treatment planning should consist of consideration of the type of skin cancer, anatomic location, size, general health and age of the patient, and whether the lesion is primary, recurrent, or metastatic.
   b. Surgical excision is the mainstay of therapy for all stages of melanoma; early detection is extremely important in overall outcome of disease.
   c. Adjuvant therapy with interferon alpha is indicated for patients with clinically positive lymph nodes after complete surgical resection of the primary lesion and any involved lymph nodes.
   d. The approved dose of interferon alpha for adjuvant therapy of melanoma consists of a prolonged regimen with high doses that are associated with significant toxicity.
   e. Many different regimens exist for biochemotherapy of melanoma; they are extremely toxic and often require hospitalization for administration or treatment of adverse effects.

SECTION 17 / PEDIATRIC AND NEONATAL THERAPY

CASE 139

PROBLEM LIST

1. Syphilis Infection
2. Hepatitis B Exposure
3. Hyperbilirubinemia

SOAP NOTE

S: Mother denies history of syphilis infection, reports history of IVDA

O: Jaundiced neonate; Wt 2.885 kg; Cr 1.1; BUN 11; T Bili 12.0; D Bili 0.0; RPR (+), FTA-abs (+); LP (RBC 10, WBC 6, Glu 51, Prot 163, VDRL pending); purulent nasal discharge

A: **Problem 1:** Congenital syphilis infection

Problem 2: Hepatitis B exposure in utero

Problem 3: Hyperbilirubinemia with jaundice

P: **Problem 1: Syphilis Infection**

- Administer aqueous crystalline penicillin G 100,000–150,000 units/kg/day administered as 50,000 units/kg/dose IV q12h for the first 7 days; q8h for 3 additional days (total 10 days therapy) OR procaine penicillin G 50,000 units/kg/dose IM QD × 10 days
- Quantitative nontreponemal test every 2–3 months until nonreactive (follow-up for congenital syphilis)
- Examine CSF every 6 months until cell count normal (follow-up in neurosyphilis)
- Counsel mother regarding therapy for her syphilis infection

Problem 2: Hepatitis B Exposure

- Give hepatitis B immune globulin (HBIG) as soon

as possible after birth (prevention of seropositivity transfer to neonate)
- HBIG 0.5 mL IM within 12 hours of birth
- Three-dose treatment with the hepatitis B virus (HBV) vaccine; begin by at least 1 week of age (for adequate protection)
- HBV vaccine 0.5 mL IM at 0–7 days
- Schedule boosters at 1 and 6 months of age
- Give all IM injections in the anterolateral thigh muscle
- Counsel mother regarding importance of 1 and 6 month boosters as well as importance of other routine immunizations

Problem 3: Hyperbilirubinemia
- Indirect bilirubin concentration not within range considered at risk for kernicterus (>18 mg/dL), but the patient is symptomatic (physiologic jaundice)
- Measure total and direct bilirubin concentrations daily
- Initiate UV light therapy if indirect bilirubin concentrations continue to increase
- Measure total and direct bilirubin concentrations during UV light therapy
- Discontinue therapy when total bilirubin decreases to <12 mg/dL (direct bilirubin should increase as total bilirubin decreases)
- Give additional IV fluids during IV light therapy (to replace insensible (evaporative) water loss through the skin)

ANSWERS
1. c. Transplacental transmission of spirochetes to the fetus in utero
2. b. Purulent nasal discharge
3. d. IVDA
4. c. It has a greater amount of muscle mass in the neonate
5. a. Immature liver conjugation of bilirubin
6. Rationale for using UV light therapy to prevent kernicterus in the neonatal period includes:
   a. The metabolism of bilirubin through the glucuronyl transferase pathway is immature until 1–2 weeks of age.
   b. Unconjugated bilirubin (indirect bilirubin) crosses the blood-brain barrier (increased permeability secondary to developmental issues).
   c. Bilirubin in the brain will cause a yellow staining (kernicterus), which can cause neurologic damage.
   d. UV light therapy metabolizes bilirubin in the skin to harmless metabolites, which are then excreted by the kidney.
7. b. Aspirin
8. c. Allergic reactions
9. b. Increased renal tubular capacity after 7 days of life
10. Counseling topics regarding the use of HBIG and hepatitis B vaccine:

a. The different mechanisms of each form of therapy (i.e., HBIG to prevent seroconversion and the vaccine to provide adequate coverage)
b. Stress the importance of 1- and 6-month booster vaccines for preventing infection in the infant
c. Consent for vaccinations
d. Identification of adverse events (pain at injection site, fever, allergy)
e. Recommendations for treatment of adverse effects (acetaminophen)
11. Risk management steps to reduce medication errors:
   a. Review references (e.g., CDC guidelines for hepatitis B and congenital syphilis) for correct neonatal dosage, contraindications, side effects
   b. Educate mother about medications and importance of vaccinations
   c. Obtain and document informed consent for vaccinations
   d. Monitor for adverse events (allergic reactions)
12. Key points are:
   a. Maternal history in the neonatal period is crucial to ensuring adequate health and well-being throughout life. Maternal prenatal screenings should be a routine part of prenatal care or at delivery (if no prenatal care). Neonates should receive prophylaxis and pharmacotherapy for any congenital infections based on current guidelines. Follow-up along with family counseling is a critical point to ensure prevention of infections and compliance with therapy.
   b. Children are not small adults. The pharmacokinetic principles of absorption, distribution, metabolism, and excretion are different from the adult population and are widely variable during development. Drug dosages and schedules, as well as optimal drug regimens, should be adjusted based on these developmental issues.
   c. Pharmacotherapy in the pediatric and neonatal population should continually be monitored for adverse events, particularly the development of toxicity and allergic reactions.
   d. Compliance issues in pediatric and neonatal therapy are affected not only by the pediatric patient taking the medication, but also by the willingness of the caregiver to give medications and follow-up for routine care and immunizations. Counseling the caregiver on these issues will promote education and compliance with therapeutic regimens.

CASE 142

PROBLEM LIST
1. Nonfunctioning Catheter
2. Change to Peripheral TPN
3. Feeding Intolerance
4. Bloody Nasogastric Aspirates, Guaiac-Positive Stool
5. Hypoalbuminemia
6. Hypermagnesemia
7. Hypertriglyceridemia

SOAP NOTE

S: Nurse reports problems clearing PICC; physician requesting assistance in clearing catheter, beginning peripheral TPN and reinitiating feedings

O: 3.0-kg infant (birth weight 3.4 kg), 6 weeks old, with history of failure to thrive, weight loss, emesis, and diarrhea with feedings; evaluation for gastrointestinal abnormalities/failure to thrive–negative, BP 105/65, HR 145, RR 30, T 37.0°C; (+) BS, bloody appearance of NG tube aspirates, guaiac-positive stool; Na 142; K 4.0; Cl 106; HCO$_3$ 22; BUN 15; SCr 0.6; Glu 88, Alb 1.8; Ca 3.9; PO$_4$ 6.0; Mg 3.0; Trig 250, AST 46; ALT 35; GGT 68; T Bili 1.0; D Bili 0.2; Hgb 13; Hct 37; cultures (stool, blood, urine): negative

A: **Problem 1:** Nonfunctioning catheter probably the result of fibrin deposition

Problem 2: Change to peripheral TPN secondary to nonfunctioning central PICC

Problem 3: Feeding intolerance

Problem 4: Bloody nasogastric aspirates, guaiac-positive stool

Problem 5: Hypoalbuminemia

Problem 6: Hypermagnesemia

Problem 7: Hypertriglyceridemia

P: **Problem 1: Nonfunctioning Catheter**
- Attempt to clear the catheter pharmacologically
- If fibrin clot suspected, instill 10,000 units streptokinase or 2 mg alteplase into catheter
- If precipitates suspected (calcium phosphate binding in the catheter), instill 0.1 N HCl into the catheter
- If saponified material (calcium complexes with fat emulsion) suspected, instill ethanol into the catheter
- Instill selected agent into the lumen of the catheter
- Wait 1–2 hours, then check patency; if occlusion persists, repeat dose and wait 2 more hours
- After waiting period, withdraw selected agent along with additional 5 mL blood (to ensure removal of loosened debris)
- Flush the catheter after removal of selected agent and blood
- If catheter patency cannot be achieved, remove catheter
- Counsel physicians and nurses regarding the FDA warning about urokinase (deviations from the Good Manufacturing Practice, which cannot ensure that the product is free from infectious disease)
- If streptokinase used, ask mother about recent streptococcal infection in herself or her infant to prevent allergic reactions or decreased efficacy

Problem 2: Change to Peripheral TPN
- Limit calcium concentration to 10 mEq/L
- Limit potassium concentration to 40 mEq/L
- Limit dextrose concentration to 10–12.5%
- Continue lipids to prolong survival time of peripheral line
- Consider giving additional calcium orally to provide requirements necessary for adequate bone mineralization
- Consider increasing daily fluid maintenance volume to 120 mL/kg to provide more calories peripherally (an increase of 20 mL/kg will provide CD an additional 7 kcal/kg/day)
- Monitor peripheral line site daily for evidence of infiltration or extravasation
- If optimal caloric intake cannot be provided through peripheral TPN and enteral nutrition for >7–14 days, discuss need for central access to provide nutrient needs and to promote weight gain

Problem 3: Feeding Intolerance
- When initiating enteral feeding again, consider using a specialized elemental infant formula that may be more easily digested and tolerated (Nutramigen, Pregestimil, Alimentum)
- If an elemental formula fails, try a lactose- and sucrose-free formula (Isomil, Prosobee) to assess for carbohydrate intolerance
- Begin with low-volume continuous feedings through NG tube
- Advance volume of feedings gradually as tolerated
- Evaluate daily for intolerance (increased gastric residuals, abdominal distention, vomiting)
- Monitor stool consistency, volume, and frequency
- Monitor daily weights to determine weight gain
- Encourage pacifier use to increase suck-swallow mechanism
- As feedings progress, decrease volume of TPN
- Offer small volumes of formula by bottle
- Increase bottle feedings as tolerated until CD can be maintained and gain weight on bottle feedings alone

Problem 4: Bloody Nasogastric Aspirates, Guaiac-Positive Stool
- Increase ranitidine dosage in TPN to 4 mg/kg/day
- Measure pH of gastric aspirates to determine if ranitidine therapy maintaining pH > 3.5–4
- If ranitidine therapy not increasing pH (i.e., may have developed tolerance), consider the use of other acid suppressive therapy (proton pump inhibitors can be placed through NG tube if compounded in suspension form to protect acid-labile drug while traveling through GI tract)
- Give antacid therapy per NG tube every 1–2 hours

- Monitor appearance of aspirates (evaluating for resolution of bloody appearance)
- Monitor Hct during periods of bloody aspirates (current Hct not consistent with overt GI bleeding)
- Evaluate medication profile for substances that interfere with guaiac testing to evaluate for false-positive stool guaiac (iron in multivitamin preparation)
- If bloody aspirates continue or are voluminous, evaluate for GI bleed

Problem 5: Hypoalbuminemia

- Evaluate for evidence of capillary leak syndrome (stable and does not have evidence of edema consistent with third spacing fluid—a condition that would not require albumin replacement)
- Albumin may be added to TPN solution (compatible with TPN)
- Discuss supplementation to correct albumin deficit with physician since it is controversial, empiric, and expensive
- If supplementation performed, give doses of 0.5–1.0 g/kg/day via TPN until deficit corrected
- Evaluate ways to limit albumin wastage in TPN tubing (i.e., eliminating overfill volume so that entire solution infused)
- If supplementation not performed, do not use albumin as a marker of nutritional gains from TPN (half-life of ≈ 3 weeks)
- Adjust calcium concentration for hypoalbuminemia to avoid providing excessive amounts of calcium (i.e., CD's corrected calcium concentration is WNL–10.7)

Problem 6: Hypermagnesemia

- Decrease magnesium provision in TPN to 2 mEq/L
- Evaluate medication profile for other exogenous sources of magnesium (has been receiving Mylanta, which contains magnesium hydroxide)
- Utilize antacid therapy that does not contain magnesium hydroxide (calcium carbonate a good choice since calcium provisions have been limited in peripheral TPN)
- Do not monitor for changes in magnesium concentrations daily (intracellular cations will take several days for equilibration)

Problem 7: Hypertriglyceridemia

- Visually inspect blood sample for signs of turbidity (turbid blood samples suggest lipemia consistent with intolerance to exogenous lipid products)
- If turbid sample, decrease dose of lipids provided in TPN to 1.5 g/kg/day
- Initiate carnitine therapy at 20 mg/kg/day
- Reevaluate triglyceride concentration in 5–7 days (if < 200, can advance lipids gradually up to 3 g/kg/day)
- If sample is clear, continue lipids and monitor triglyceride concentrations (clear sample may suggest breakdown of endogenous fat stores to provide metabolic needs)
- Continue lipid therapy, even at a reduced dose, while receiving peripheral TPN to promote patency of the peripheral line and to provide a concentrated source of calories

ANSWERS

1. b. Heparin deposition
2. d. Cardiac dysrhythmias
3. Advantages of using lipid emulsion in parenteral nutrition:
   a. Prevention of essential fatty acid deficiency
   b. Provision of a concentrated source of calories
   c. Prolongation of catheter life
4. b. Lipid
5. b. Increasing dextrose concentration
6. Benefits of adding cysteine to CD's TPN:
   a. Enhanced growth
   b. Improved nitrogen retention
   c. Improved calcium and phosphorus stability
   d. Reduced risk for metabolic bone disease and cholestasis
7. c. Multivitamin with iron
8. a. Disaccharidase deficiency
9. d. Bloody aspirates
10. Advantages of using calcium carbonate over Mylanta for antacid therapy in CD:
    a. Elimination of exogenous source of magnesium (pt with hypermagnesemia)
    b. Elimination of additional exogenous source of aluminum (trace elements in TPN contain aluminum contaminant)
    c. Provision of exogenous source of calcium in a patient with high calcium requirements and minimal provision in TPN
11. Mechanism of action of carnitine in the treatment of hypertriglyceridemia is the transport of free fatty acids across the mitochondrial membrane for beta oxidation and energy production (increased fat utilization)
12. d. Provide TPN for 5 days per week
13. a. Low albumin concentration
14. Key points are:
    a. Provide nutrients for basal requirements and growth and development (since CD has only peripheral access at this time, the treatment goal should be to maximize nutrient and caloric provision allowed in a peripheral line and seek other sources of calories and mineral provision outside of TPN, i.e., calcium carbonate therapy).
    b. Use the gastrointestinal tract to provide additional calories with the future goal of weaning the patient completely from TPN.
    c. Provide nutrients in peripheral TPN in a safe and effective manner by limiting dextrose, calcium, and

potassium concentrations, and by maximizing lipid calories and maintenance volume.

d. Continually evaluate patient's response to therapy by monitoring weight gains and losses, tolerance of enteral

feeding, and laboratory measurements, and adjusting nutrient intake according to these factors.

e. Engage the patient's parents and caregivers in all aspects of nutrition management.

SECTION 18 / OB-GYN DISORDERS

CASE 143

PROBLEM LIST

1. Dysmenorrhea
2. *Trichomonas* Vaginitis
3. Bipolar Disorder
4. Contraception
5. Facial Acne

SOAP NOTE

S: "I am having painful pelvic cramping that always occurs a couple of days before my period starts that causes it to hurt when I urinate. I have also noticed a vaginal discharge that is fishy in odor. I would like birth control."

O: History of dysmenorrhea even in anovulatory cycles; normal saline slide: highly motile, pear-shaped, unicellular *Trichomonas vaginalis,* meatal erythema, vaginal malodor, thick gray discharge; euphoria, hyperactivity, and flight of ideas escalating rapidly and lasting a few days to a few months followed by depressive episodes lasting for several weeks; no form of birth control: sexually active with multiple partners; facial skin clear at this time

A: **Problem 1:** Dysmenorrhea: Primary dysmenorrhea occurs in ovulatory cycles and unresponsive to NSAIDs; has had PID twice; therefore, adhesions causing secondary dysmenorrhea probably also present

Problem 2: *Trichomonas* vaginitis: Treatment of both patient and partner required

Problem 3: Bipolar disorder: Depressive episodes triggered by COC use in past

Problem 4: Contraception: Currently receiving no form of birth control; IUD and oral contraceptives have been tried but are not acceptable to SK

Problem 5: Facial acne: Managed with tetracycline

Problem 1: Dysmenorrhea

- Start mefenamic acid 500 mg PO stat, then 250 mg PO q6h PRN
- Laparoscopy to identify presence of adhesions
- May consider removing identified adhesions
- Avoid long-term use of opioids in a bipolar patient (may exacerbate manic episodes)

Problem 2: *Trichomonas* Vaginitis

- Start metronidazole, 2 g PO stat for both patient and partner(s)
- Educate about possibility of disulfiram reaction if taken with alcohol, metallic taste, and brown discoloration of urine with drug
- Assess therapeutic success by checking resolution of symptoms
- Metronidazole, 500 mg PO twice daily for 7 days if therapy fails

Problem 3: Bipolar Disorder

- Continue nortriptyline for depressive symptoms; to prevent a manic episode add lithium, carbamazepine, valproic acid, or gabapentin to stabilize mood
- Avoid COC and other forms of hormonal therapy to avoid aggravation of depression or initiation of depressive episodes

Problem 4: Contraception

- Consider a barrier method, such as a condom with contraceptive foam to protect from pregnancy (if used properly) and help prevent STDs
- Avoid oral contraceptives and other forms of hormonal therapy to avoid aggravation of depressive episodes
- Recommend HIV testing; counsel regarding safe sex

Problem 5: Facial Acne

- Continue tetracycline
- Instruct to take with plenty of fluids
- Avoid sunlight and UV rays

ANSWERS

1. d. Endometriosis
2. d. Malodorous vaginal discharge
3. c. Metronidazole and alcohol-containing products
4. a. Prostaglandin E2
5. d. Clonidine may be used for patients with dysmenorrhea that fail NSAIDs
6. Oral contraceptives alter tryptophan metabolism, resulting in a deficiency in brain serotonin causing OC-related depression.
7. b. NSAIDs
8. b. A few hours prior to menses, 48–72 hours
9. b. Swollen papillae projecting through vaginal secretions
10. Pharmacologic and nonpharmacologic treatment problem(s) present in SK's treatment plan:
    1. Pharmacologic
       a. COC-related depression
       b. Medication side effects
    2. Nonpharmacologic
       a. Counseling on safe sex
       b. Transmission of STDs to others
11. Mechanism of action of the pharmacologic and nonpharmacologic interventions
    a. Nortriptyline–manipulates neurotransmitters in the brain to elevate mood
    b. Gabapentin–exact mechanism unknown; thought to stabilize mood (mania and depressive episodes in a bipolar patient)
    c. Mefenamic acid–blocks action of prostaglandins, resulting in decreased uterine contractions and menstrual blood loss
    d. Tetracycline–antibacterial and anti-inflammatory activity
    e. Metronidazole–inhibits bacterial protein synthesis by binding with 30S and 50S ribosomal subunits
12. Psychosocial factors that may affect SK's adherence to both pharmacologic and nonpharmacologic therapy:
    1. Common emotional disorders presenting in patient with bipolar disorder
       a. Stressful life circumstances may precipitate depression
       b. Depression as a result of dysmenorrhea (a medical illness which may not be managed by NSAIDs)
13. The health care provider's role relative to the proposed psychosocial factors includes:
    a. Individualize a pharmacologic and nonpharmacologic plan
    b. Provide patient education and positive reinforcement
    c. Counsel about medications: with metronidazole complete regimen and avoid all products containing alcohol; antidepressant response usually seen within 4–6 weeks: side effects are seen before benefits
    d. Lifestyle modifications: Counsel on safe sex; stress compliance with contraception to avoid future STDs.
14. Pharmacoeconomic considerations relative to SK's plan of care:
    1. Direct nonmedical
       a. Dysmenorrhea contributes to significant loss of working hours, which in some cases may be severe enough to restrict daily activities.
    2. Direct medical
       a. Clinic personnel
       b. Treatment and complications
15. Key points are:
    a. Dysmenorrhea may be a primary disorder (related to an increase in prostaglandin) or secondary disorder (related to a pelvic pathology) which can have a tremendous impact on a patient's quality of life. Pharmacologic management includes NSAIDs, opioid analgesics, and oral contraceptives. Nonpharmacologic management includes exercise (which may or may not improve pain).
    b. *Trichomonas* vaginitis is a sexually transmitted disease in which both the partner as well as the patient must be treated. Because the patient is sexually active a form of contraception is needed. Although COC may help dysmenorrhea and facial acne, precipitation of depressive episodes by COC warrants the patient to use condoms and spermicides, which may also prevent STDs.

CASE 146

PROBLEM LIST

1. Vulvovaginal Candidiasis with Discharge
2. Pregnant 8 Weeks Gestation
3. Asthma
4. HTN
5. Type 1 DM
6. Epilepsy
7. Impaired Renal Function

SOAP NOTES

S: "I have severe vaginal and vulvar itching, burning, and discharge and I'm 8 weeks pregnant."

O: Erythematous vagina and labia; KOH with pseudohyphae and blastopores (buds); cottage cheese, curd-like discharge, nonmalodorous; 8 weeks gestation; asthma controlled with PRN metaproterenol and prednisone; denies coughing; lungs clear to auscultation; BP 150/100; seizure disorder, maintained on phenytoin: phenytoin level 47.6 (12); FBS 16 mmol/L (290); urine glu 3+ to 4+ HbA$_{1C}$ 8%; BUN 8.9 (25 mg/dL), Cr 123 (1.4 mg/dL), urine protein 1+

A: **Problem 1:** Vaginal itching with discharge: *Candida* vaginitis probably due to pregnancy, uncontrolled DM, and corticosteroid use; requires therapy since symptomatic

Problem 2: Pregnancy: 8 weeks gestation; has several chronic diseases and impaired renal function; requires careful monitoring of drugs and dose adjustments to decrease morbidity and mortality in mother and fetus

Problem 3: Asthma: Inadequate dosing of metaproterenol; QID instead of PRN should decrease corticosteroid use

Problem 4: HTN: Possible complication of long-term uncontrolled type 1 DM; currently taking methyldopa, which is safe in pregnancy

Problem 5: Type 1 DM: Inadequate glucose monitoring, insulin administration, and poor diet

Problem 6: Epilepsy: Adequate seizure control with phenytoin; pregnancy category D

Problem 7: Impaired renal function: Possibly due to poor glucose control and HTN

P: Problem 1: Candidal Infection

- Begin clotrimazole 100 mg suppositories, insert vaginally QHS for 14 days
- Instruct to finish all medications and consider refraining from intercourse during treatment
- Monitor for vulvar burning
- Encourage wearing loose-fitting garments

Problem 2: Pregnancy

- Educate on risks and benefits associated with drug therapy for each disease: risk of drug therapy increasing the chance of birth defects: risk of maternal and fetal morbidity and mortality if diseases are untreated
- Smoking cessation highly recommended
- Consult pharmacist before taking any OTC medications
- Maintain a healthy diet and avoid alcohol and alcohol-containing products
- Begin prenatal care vitamins, schedule visits with OB throughout pregnancy
- Wear a Medic-Alert bracelet noting chronic diseases

Problem 3: Asthma

- Instruct to use metaproterenol 1–2 puffs PO QID and PRN
- Decrease prednisone dose by 5 mg/wk until discontinued to prevent worsening of HTN, DM, infection, or complications with pregnancy
- Counsel on proper use and storage on inhaler; add a spacer if not already using
- Monitor wheezing, SOB, and FEV
- Add topical administration with beclomethasone inhaler if unable to discontinue steroids

Problem 4: HTN

- Increase methyldopa to 250 mg PO TID
- Educate on the importance of adherence and regular BP checks
- Counsel on possible side effects of sedation, N/V, and dry mouth with increased dose
- Methyldopa is cleared renally and accumulation may occur; adjust if necessary

- If HTN not controlled with increased doses of methyldopa (may be given in divided doses up to 4 g/day), consider hydralazine for lowering BP
- Strongly urge to quit smoking and follow prescribed diet

Problem 5: Type 1 DM

- Change insulin regimen to NPH and regular, at a ratio of 2:1 in the morning and 1:1 before the evening meal for "tight" control with sliding scale regular insulin as needed
- Aim of therapy: FBG < 5.55 mmol/L (100 mg/100 mL) and postprandial values, 6.66 mmol/L (120 mg/100 mL), no urine ketones and normal HbA_{1C} (4–6%)
- Frequent blood glucose measurement and dose-appropriate dose adjustments
- Educate on the importance of taking insulin to stabilize blood sugar
- Educate on the signs and symptoms of hypoglycemia (irritability, confusion, sweating) and hyperglycemia (polydipsia, fatigue, polyuria, and blurred vision)
- Stress the importance of maintaining a proper diet

Problem 6: Epilepsy

- Continue phenytoin, 100 mg PO QHS; inadequate seizure control would be dangerous to fetus and CC
- Monitor free and total phenytoin concentrations, PT, PTT, albumin, and for seizure activity; adjust dose accordingly
- Emphasize importance of taking medication and glucose control to avoid seizures
- Educate about risk versus benefit ratio of phenytoin therapy during pregnancy, including birth defects
- Monitor for adverse effects of phenytoin including abnormal bleeding, dizziness, and ataxia
- Supplement with folic acid PO 2.5–5 mg/day

Problem 7: Impaired Renal Function

- Stress importance of glucose control and avoiding diabetic nephropathy
- Monitor BP at each visit; measure urinary protein; employ caution with renally cleared medications and adjust doses for decreased renal function
- Monitor Cr, BUN, and urinalysis
- Avoid the use of nephrotoxic agents if possible
- ACE inhibitors would not be an option due to pregnancy

ANSWERS

1. c. Diabetes mellitus
2. c. Decreased volume of distribution
3. a. Ketoconazole
4. c. EXT–peripheral tingling

5. a. Impaired renal function
6. b. Acute alcohol ingestion
7. Risk factors associated with pregnancy-induced hypertension include DM, HTN, and renal insufficiency
8. b. Phenytoin
9. c. The phenotype of mother and fetus
10. Psychosocial factors affecting pharmacologic and nonpharmacologic therapy include:
    1. Pharmacologic
       a. Candida infections may occur or may fail therapy due to DM as well as impaired renal function
       b. Chronic medications—adherence to complex regimens of insulin at varying times
    2. Nonpharmacologic
       a. Dietary regimens
       b. Caring for three children may add stress
11. Health care provider's role:
    a. Education on disease process and consultation on medications
    b. Stress the importance of taking medication as prescribed
    c. Encourage home blood glucose monitoring
12. b. Monitor BP. Monitor asthma control with peak flow meter.
13. c. Refer to endocrinologist, cardiologist, and high-risk pregnancy provider
14. a. Fetal hydantoin syndrome
15. Pharmacoeconomic considerations
    1. Direct medical
       a. Cost of medications
       b. Cost of glucometer, peak flow meter, strips, and supplies
       c. Office visits for phenytoin levels, prenatal care
    2. Indirect personal
       a. Child care while sick
       b. Decreased productivity
       c. Quality of life
16. Key points are:
    a. Because medication use in pregnancy is a complex issue, effort must be taken to provide the patient, as well as the fetus, with the most safe and effective medication. Mothers should be told that most medications will reach the fetus to some extent.
    b. The importance of patient education to ensure maternal involvement in the decision process regarding medication risk and benefit is imperative.

CASE 147

PROBLEM LIST

1. Infertility
2. "Bumps" Around Rectum
3. History of Hyperthyroidism: Graves' Disease

SOAP NOTES

S: "My husband and I have been trying to conceive but we are not having any luck. Could this be due to my hyperthyroidism? I don't know how significant this is, but I have noticed some bumps around my rectum which have been there for some months."

O: Normal pelvic exam G0P0, LMP 10 days ago; spouse fathered two children in previous marriage; 2–3 small condyloma acuminatum around anus; thyroid function tests: WNL

A: **Problem 1:** Infertility: 32-year-old desiring pregnancy; no apparent anatomical reason for infertility at this time; history of endocrine disorder and infection may contribute to infertility; assessment of ovulatory status necessary prior to therapy with fertility agents

Problem 2: Bumps around the rectum: *Condyloma acuminata,* a sexually transmitted disease (STD), caused by human papillomavirus (HPV)

Problem 3: Hyperthyroidism. Graves' disease in remission; history of hyperthyroidism 4 years ago successfully treated with PTU; following therapy remained euthyroid; thyroid function tests WNL; physical examination unremarkable: no tremors, no myxedema, and mild but stable proptosis; previous Graves' disease may not interfere with conception; reactivation of hyperthyroidism possible

P: **Problem 1: Infertility**

- Treat HPV
- Obtain prolactin and androgen levels
- Instruct to chart basal body temperatures
- Use ovulation kits to determine most fertile time for 2 cycles
- Take daily urine samples until ovulation is detected
- Once ovulation determined, instruct to have intercourse within 12–24 hours
- If ovulation is not detected in the following 2 months and prolactin and androgen levels are WNL, begin clomiphene

Problem 2: Bumps Around the Rectum: *Condyloma acuminata*

- Biopsy to rule out malignancy
- Examine entire anogenital tract due to widespread nature of *Condyloma acuminata*
- Treatment may be applied by patient or physician; instruct to presoak lesion in warm water for 5–10 minutes; with an emery board, rub away loose wart; apply trichloroacetic acid 50% with a cotton applicator once or twice a day for 3 consecutive days and then none applied for 4 consecutive days; repeat until wart is removed (usually within 2–3 months)
- Abstain from sexual activity while being treated; otherwise, activity as tolerated; sex partner should be examined for evidence of warts and treated if needed

Problem 3: History of Hyperthyroidism: Graves' Disease

- Continue to monitor for clinical signs and symptoms of hyperthyroidism
- More frequent monitoring will be required when pregnant

ANSWERS TO QUESTIONS

1. c. Average incubation period usually 10–14 days
2. d. Systolic hypotension
3. a. A TSH level of <0.01 U/ml excludes hyperthyroidism
4. a. PTU is a thioamide that may safely be used by BB if she wishes to become pregnant
5. d. STD
6. b. Basal body temperature
7. b. Burning
8. a. Trichloroacetic acid
9. Mechanism of action of the pharmacologic interventions in this case
   1. Pharmacologic
      a. Trichloracetic acid–chemically destroys genital warts used and prevents reinfection PTU-inhibits both thyroid hormone and extrathyroidal conversion of T3 to T4
   2. Nonpharmacologic
      a. Soak wart in warm water; use emery board to help remove wart.
10. Pharmacoeconomics
    1. Cost of genital wart controlled at home
       a. No therapy has been shown to eradicate genital warts; patient continues to receive medications to manage discomfort and removal of warts
    2. Cost of infertility
       a. Many times the causes of infertility may be unknown and many patients will exhaust all avenues until conception is obtained, which may result in financial, emotional, and physical strain
11. BB may be started on medications that might correct the etiology of her infertility. Medications include:
    Clomiphene to induce ovulation
    Gonadotrophins to manipulate hypothalamic-pituitary failure
    Leuprolide if endometriosis is the cause
12. a. Clomiphene 50 mg PO QD on day 5 of menses; repeat same dose if ovulation occurs without conception
13. Psychosocial factors that may affect SK's adherence to both pharmacologic and nonpharmacologic therapy are:
    1. Chronic medications
       a. Exacerbation of genital warts; unsuccessful conception with fertility medications
    2. Common emotional disorders in patients with infertility problems
       a. Anxiety
       b. Depression
    3. Other barriers
       a. Family dynamics–limited support system
       b. Other stressors in life

c. Limited financial resources–unable to purchase infertility medications

14. Key points are:
    a. There are multiple causes of infertility that may occur in either the male or female reproductive system. A complete physical exam and ROS reveals STD and endocrine conditions, both of which can cause interference with conception. A reproductive and sexual history should also be performed. Diagnostic tests may include a postcoital test (test sperm count) and a hysterosalpingogram (test of tubal patency).
    b. Medications are used based on the specific etiology and include gonadotropin-releasing hormone (GnRH) (leuprolide) and antiestrogens (clomiphene). Procedures include laparoscopy if endometriosis is present.

CASE 148

PROBLEM LIST

1. HSV 2
2. Depression
3. Breast-Feeding Concerns

SOAP NOTES

S: "I am having another really bad herpes outbreak. I am having bad genital pain. I have also been depressed again lately, I just cannot seem to do anything: I don't want to get out of bed in the morning and I am always tired. The only thing worth getting up for is my baby. If it weren't for her nothing would be worth it."

O: HSV-2 with visible vesicles on labia, urethra, and vulva: antibody to HSV–positive; Pap smear: giemsa giant cells; depressive symptoms including decreased mood and appetite and lack of interest; not taking any antidepressants or receiving psychotherapy

A: Problem 1: HSV 2, a STD to which there is no currently available cure; third recurrence in 2 years; may occur at times of stress; depressive episode may have triggered reactivation of the painful vesicles

Problem 2: Depression responded well to amitriptyline but discontinued during pregnancy; now complains of depressive mood, which could be due to the discontinuation of antidepressant, postpartum depression, alcohol use, or previous viral infection

Problem 3: Breast-feeding concerns: Desires to breast-feed her 6-day-old infant; because infant was not offered breast milk during the immediate postpartum period, successful breast-feeding may be reduced; must also consider other factors that may interfere with desire to breast-feed, which include any drug therapy, potential spread of HSV, history of alcohol use, and smoking

Problem 1: HSV-2

- Begin valacyclovir 1000 mg PO QD × 5 days (valacyclovir 1000 mg QD is as effective as acyclovir 500 mg BID for recurrent herpes simplex 2 infections. Valacyclovir has a safety profile similar to acyclovir. *J Antimicrob Chemother* 1999 Oct;44 (4):525–531.)
- Advise to avoid intercourse while genital lesions are visible
- Discuss possible side effects of N/V, headache, and rash with this medication
- For painful lesions take over-the-counter acetaminophen

Problem 2: Depression

- Expresses a high interest in breast-feeding her infant
- Although amitriptyline has been successful in managing depression in the past, the antidepressant is not recommended in nursing mothers
- Start fluoxetine 10 mg PO QD, since has been the most extensively studied antidepressant for use in pregnant and nursing mothers
- Educate about the possible side effects of fluoxetine, which include nausea and vomiting, sleep disturbances, drowsiness, weight loss, and sexual problems
- Instruct to take fluoxetine at bedtime to help lower concentrations in breast milk at feeding times
- Avoid alcohol while on this medication; may potentiate sedation; benefits should be seen in 4–6 weeks; may see some response after 2 weeks
- Follow up with psychotherapy and reassess alcohol consumption in 2 weeks

Problem 3: Breast-Feeding Concerns

- May breast-feed her infant
- Discuss that long-term side effects of fluoxetine on the infant are unknown
- Tobacco use and alcohol use should also be discontinued; discuss options for smoking cessation
- Discuss the advantages of breast-feeding, which include protection from infection, and disadvantages, which include the possible spread of her HSV, avoiding drugs that may pass through the breast milk and cause side effects in the infant
- Must consume foods high in calcium, and continue vitamins since breast milk lacks vitamin D
- Monitor for HSV lesions that may develop on breasts to prevent exposure to infant
- Consult with pharmacist before taking any over-the-counter medications

ANSWERS

1. c. Giemsa is a type of smear that shows multinucleated giant cells, which does not distinguish between varicella-zoster and HSV
2. a. Nonionized drugs
3. c. Prolonged GI transit time in the mother
4. c. Breast milk is equally nutritious as formula supplements and is high in vitamin D
5. c. MW wishes to breast feed
6. a. Pharmacologic treatment problems: MW responded to amitriptyline, a tricyclic antidepressant (TCA); however, she wishes to breast-feed; amitriptyline is secreted in breast milk and not recommended while nursing; fluoxetine is an alternative agent most extensively studied in nursing mothers; weigh risks versus benefits
7. Nonpharmacologic treatment problems include:
   a. Counseling for depression
   b. Smoking and alcohol use
   c. Financial problems–unemployed
   d. Diagnosed with a chronic STD–emotional impact
8. a. Acyclovir 30 mg/kg/day PO in 3 divided doses × 14–21 days
9. c. Alcohol
10. b. Acyclovir
11. Psychosocial factors that may affect MW's adherence to both pharmacologic and nonpharmacologic therapy are:
    1. Issues that patient must address:
       a. Make patient aware that this antidepressant may or may not help with her depression and should be followed up with psychotherapy
       b. Long-term effects with any antidepressant are unknown
    2. Common emotional disorders
       a. Depression
       b. Alcohol and tobacco abuse
       c. Chronic STD and breast feeding concerns
    3. Other barriers
       a. Limited financial resources: unable to purchase medications
       b. Family dynamics: 20-year-old single mom without job
12. May continue relieving stressors with alcohol consumption and cigarette smoking
13. The health care provider's role relative to the proposed psychosocial factors identified:
    a. Individualize a plan for both pharmacologic (compliance) and nonpharmacologic (alcohol and smoking cessation) treatment
    b. Provide patient education and positive reinforcement
    c. Refer to psychotherapist
14. Pharmacoeconomic considerations relative to MW's plan of care include:
    1. Cost of depression
       a. Pharmacotherapy costs of traditional vs alternative care
    2. Cost of HSV care
    3. Indirect personal
       a. Decreased productivity
       b. Quality of life
15. Key points are:
    a. Breast-feeding is a natural, free, convenient way of

providing milk, the only food an infant needs for the first several months of life.

b. Medication use in lactation is a complex issue, and effort must be taken to provide the patient as well as the infant with the most safe and effective medication.

c. Most medications taken by the mother will reach the fetus to some extent.

d. Advantages of breast-feeding include protection against infection, and increased intellectual development in the infant. Advantages for the nursing mother include a

decreased risk of subsequent breast cancer, and facilitation of the return to prepregnancy weight.

e. Patient education is imperative to ensure maternal involvement in the decision process regarding medication risk and benefit.

f. Medications prescribed to nursing mothers should take into account that certain medications can be secreted through the breast milk. Expressing milk several hours prior to dose of medication is one way to prevent exposure to high concentrations of some medications.

SECTION 19 / GERONTOLOGY

CASE 150

PROBLEM LIST

1. Agitation
2. Uncontrolled HTN
3. Parkinson's Disease
4. Constipation

SOAP NOTE

S: Confusion reported by family; drowsy; severe agitation

O: BP 150/94, HR 88, RR 24; confusion, oriented to person only, agitation, bilateral rigidity, slight tremor present, hard stool in rectum; Alk Phos 1.75 (1105)

A: Problem 1: Agitation; currently receiving several CNS depressants

Problem 2: Uncontrolled HTN

Problem 3: Parkinson's disease; signs of adverse drug effects of current therapy

Problem 4: Constipation

P: Problem 1: Agitation

- Work-up for Alzheimer's disease; consider trial of donepezil
- Evaluate continued need for medications with CNS depressant activity, such as thioridazine, alprazolam, flurazepam
- Discontinue thioridazine—no apparent diagnosis and potential to interfere with Parkinson's disease
- Monitor behaviors for patterns and triggers

- Consider low-dose atypical antipsychotic agents for control of agitation
- Discontinue alprazolam and flurazepam (polypharmacy); may cause idiosyncratic reactions in older patients

Problem 2: Uncontrolled HTN

- Schedule follow-up visit for BP check in 7 days
- If BP remains elevated, add an additional antihypertensive agent such as fosinopril 10 mg QD; adjust up to 20 mg PO QD as necessary and tolerated
- Continue potassium supplement for now; monitor serum potassium, especially if fosinopril added
- Monitor BP for target goal of <140/90 mm Hg

Problem 3: Parkinson's Disease

- Taper to discontinue benztropine due to adverse anticholinergic effects
- Monitor response to above and if loses control, add a dopamine agonist such as ropinirole 0.25 mg PO TID
- Consider switching to CR form of levodopa/carbidopa with a 10% to 30% increase in the amount of levodopa

Problem 4: Constipation

- Remove impaction with enema while in emergency department
- Initiate bowel regimen consisting of 70% sorbitol solution 30 mL PO QD; if not effective, add glycerin suppository QD
- Avoid anticholinergic drug therapy
- Maximize fluid intake
- Dietary consult to increase bulk in diet

ANSWERS TO QUESTIONS

1. c. Thioridazine
2. a. Double the dose of levodopa/carbidopa to 25/250 4 tablets PO TID
3. c. Phenolphthalein
4. Management strategies for constipation:
   a. Constipation is defined as no more than two bowel movements per week, or straining upon defecation 25% of the time or more
   b. Assessment issues
      • Adequate fluid: if no, increase to 2–8 8-oz glasses daily if no fluid restrictions
      • Adequate fiber: if no, increase to 2–10 g/day if not contraindicated
      • Recent medication change: if yes, review for constipating medications and change
      • Contributing disease: if yes, rule out or treat GI disorders, metabolic disorders, endocrine disorders, neurologic disorders, immobilizing disorders, respiratory disorders, and muscular disorders
      • Change in activity or exercise level: if yes, increase activity level if possible
      • Bowel program consists of adequate hydration, bulk laxatives, stool softeners, and laxatives as needed
5. d. Problems with balance
6. a. Is not effective in creatinine clearance < 30 mL/min
7. b. Risperidone
8. c. Use 10–30% increase in levodopa dose
9. c. Risperidone
10. Pharmacoeconomic considerations relative to therapy for Parkinson's disease may include:
    a. Generic versus brand name levodopa/carbidopa. Both are effective; this should be joint decision among health care practitioners, patients, and care givers
    b. Sustained-release levodopa/carbidopa products more costly than immediate release; consider costs of mobility
    c. Newer products (dopamine agonists and COMT inhibitors) more costly than older products
    d. Cost of medication and provision of ADLs to a patient with progressive functional decline compared to cost of surgery
11. a. Urinary retention
12. Monitoring parameters for patient SP:
    a. Assessment of Parkinson's disease signs and symptoms—tremor, stiffness, bradykinesia
    b. Medication side effects—nausea, hypotension, dyskinesias, CNS effects (hallucinations, confusion, fatigue, anxiety)
    c. Assessment of hypertension signs and symptoms—blood pressure, pulse
    d. Medication side effects—hypotension, electrolyte imbalances
    e. Behavior monitoring—description, incidence, severity
    f. Medication side effects—anticholinergic effects, EPS, sedation, cardiovascular effects
13. Caregiver issues important to SP's case:
    a. Medication compliance
    b. Monitor for effectiveness and adverse effects from medications
    c. Assist with ADLs such as bathing, grooming, dressing, eating, transferring, toileting
    d. Participate in Parkinson's disease support group
14. Key points are:
    a. Parkinson's disease is a progressive neurologic disorder involving tremor, bradykinesia, muscle rigidity, and postural instability.
    b. Nonpharmacologic therapy consists of physical therapy and occupational therapy to maximize functional abilities.
    c. Drug therapy for Parkinson's disease should maximize functional abilities while minimizing adverse effects.
    d. Drug therapy for Parkinson's disease should be reevaluated and adjusted frequently, based on the functional abilities of the patient.
    e. Constipation can be minimized through consumption of adequate amounts of fluid and fiber, with maximal amount of exercise and by controlling conditions and medications that can contribute to constipation.
    f. Thiazide diuretics, usually first-line therapy for hypertension, are often ineffective in creatinine clearances less that 30 mL/min; alternative agents should be used. Select the agent based on comorbid conditions and patient parameters.

CASE 152

PROBLEM LIST

1. Weight Loss
2. Poorly Controlled Atrial Fibrillation
3. Possible Repeat CVA While Receiving Dipyridamole

SOAP NOTE

S: Often slumps in wheelchair; responds poorly to commands; noted to be lethargic, and sleeping most of the day for the past week; 6-lb weight loss over last 30 days

O: BP 110/70; HR 120; Wt 42.5 kg; Ht 155 cm; irregularly irregular heart rate; dry mucous membranes; poor skin turgor; oriented to person; kyphosis; stool, occult blood: negative; Glu (fasting) 7.8 (140); K 3.3 (3.3); Cr 120 (1.4); digoxin level 3 months prior: 2.3 (1.8); ECG shows atrial fibrillation, ST-T wave changes

A: **Problem 1:** Weight loss secondary to numerous possible causes: failure to thrive post CVA; lethargy and sleeping most of day; furosemide can cause dehydration and glucose intolerance; patient unable to feed herself due to upper body weakness and lethargy.

Problem 2: Poorly controlled atrial fibrillation

Problem 3: Possible repeat CVA while receiving dipyridamole

P: Problem 1: Weight Loss

- Recheck digoxin level
- Discontinue furosemide due to dehydration and reduced fluid intake; no diagnosis for use
- Monitor potassium and discontinue potassium supplement if possible
- Monitor intake and output
- Maximize food and fluid intake; may require assistance
- Evaluate position of patient
- Evaluate feet, use compression stockings and ambulate if possible
- Evaluate for constipation; discontinue psyllium due to poor fluid intake

Problem 2: Poorly Controlled Atrial Fibrillation

- Check echocardiogram to measure atrial chamber size to determine if cardioversion candidate
- Continue digoxin for rate control to decrease occurrence of repeat CVAs; repeat digoxin level and adjust if necessary
- Initiate warfarin therapy; adjust dose to achieve INR between 2 and 3

Problem 3: Possible CVA

- CVA could account for behaviors
- Discontinue dipyridamole due to questionable effectiveness
- Conservative approach is to initiate ASA 325 mg PO QD to prevent additional CVAs; monitor for interaction with warfarin
- Evaluate for ability to cope with cardioversion of atrial fibrillation to prevent further CVA activity

ANSWERS

1. c. Poor skin turgor
2. c. Dipyridamole
3. d. Weight loss
4. Goals of pharmacologic and nonpharmacologic therapy are to remove or limit the obstruction to blood flow, and protect brain cells distal to the obstruction from hypoxic changes via the following:
   a. Antiplatelet therapy with aspirin or ticlopidine
   b. Thrombolytic therapy with streptokinase, anisoylated plasminogen activator complex (APSAC), tissue plasminogen activator (t-PA) single chain (antephase)
   c. Physical therapy and occupational therapy as soon as possible and to the extent required by the specific patient. Assistance with activities of daily living
   d. Carotid endarterectomy (CEA)
5. A decision should be made regarding the issues of DNR (do not resuscitate). Advance directives should be in place for health care decisions regarding how aggressive therapies should be, the use of antibiotic therapy, nutritional support, and general supportive measures.
6. d. 81 mg PO QOD
7. a. Renal function
8. c. Clopidogrel
9. No; mental status has deteriorated to the point where the medications indicated (donepezil and tacrine) are not useful; these agents are indicated for the treatment of mild to moderate dementia
10. Prognosis is poor; comfort measures should be provided
11. Based on the history and presentation, EM's deteriorated mental status is most likely the result of multiple ischemic strokes. Older age may be a contributing factor in that aging is a risk factor for the development of dementia. Medications known to impair cognition such as sedatives and those with anticholinergic effects should be avoided.
12. Psychosocial factors affecting EM's adherence to both pharmacologic and nonpharmacologic therapies include:
    1. Issues patient must address
       a. Willingness to continue with therapy in a terminal situation (failure to thrive)
       b. Refusal of acceptance of nutrition
       c. Participation in rehabilitation therapies
    2. Other barriers
       a. Family participation in therapeutic decisions; additional medications, tube feedings, rehabilitation therapies
       b. Limited financial resources
13. Key points are:
    a. A complete history and physical, including laboratory workup, is necessary to rule out possible causes for the dementia.
    b. Nondrug therapies and social support (patient and family) are necessary.
    c. Drug therapies should address specific problems or symptoms and should be continued as long as effective, then discontinued.
    d. Periodic assessment of the patient's functional status and mental status is necessary to insure appropriate therapeutic interventions.
    e. Patients and families should be encouraged to complete "Advance Directives" to express their choices for care in terminal situations.

CASE 154

PROBLEM LIST

1. Acute Heart Failure
2. Renal Insufficiency
3. Type 1 Diabetes Mellitus

SOAP NOTE

S: 58-year-old male with hypotension following CABG

O: PE: BP 90/50, MAP 63 mm Hg, HR 110 beats/min, PCWP 21 mm Hg, CI 1.2 L/min/m², SVR 2080 dynes/sec/cm⁵, urine output: 20 mL/hr; Cr 150 (1.7); Type 1 DM; home insulin regimen: 26 units of NPH insulin q AM and 12 units of NPH insulin q PM plus 5 units regular insulin 30 minutes before meals; chest x-ray: mild pulmonary edema

A: **Problem 1:** Acute heart failure evolving into cardiogenic shock as evidenced by decreased organ perfusion

Problem 2: Renal insufficiency secondary to decreased perfusion (decreased cardiac output) in addition to baseline diabetic nephropathy

Problem 3: Type 1 diabetes mellitus; at risk for developing diabetic ketoacidosis

P: **Problem 1: Acute Heart Failure**

- Discontinue verapamil, hydrochlorothiazide, and nitrates as they may decrease blood pressure
- Begin inotropic agent: dopamine at 5 μg/kg/min and titrated to response; use lowest effective dose
- Monitor MAP, CI, HR, PCWP, urine output at least every hour
- Goals of therapy: MAP ≥70 mm Hg, CI >2.2 L/min/m², heart rate <120 beats/min, PCWP 16–18 mm Hg; resolution of pulmonary edema, and a urine output ≥0.5 mL/kg/hr

Problem 2: Renal Insufficiency

- Should resolve if adequate cardiac output (renal perfusion) reestablished
- Monitor serum electrolytes, hourly urine output, serum creatinine daily until renal insufficiency resolves
- Patient likely has diabetic nephropathy and therefore renal function may not normalize completely

Problem 3: Type 1 Diabetes Mellitus (DM)

- Monitor blood glucose level every 6 hours; increase frequency if blood glucose levels >11.2 mmol/L (200 mg/dL)
- Begin sliding scale insulin using regular human insulin as follows:
  - Blood glucose <3.4 mmol/L (60 mg/dL) 25 mL 50% dextrose IV push
  - Blood glucose <8.3 mmol/L (150 mg/dL) 0 units SC
  - Blood glucose 8.3–11.1 mmol/L (150–200 mg/dL) 3 units SC
  - Blood glucose 11.1–13.9 mmol/L (200–250 mg/dL) 6 units SC
  - Blood glucose >13.9 mmol/L (250 mg/dL) 10 units SC
- Adjust insulin dose and monitoring frequency to the patient's response
- Monitor for clinical evidence of hypoglycemia: unexplained agitation, tachycardia, diaphoresis, seizures, or CNS depression require assessment of the blood glucose concentration and prompt treatment with 25 mL of 50% dextrose administered IVP if hypoglycemia is present
- Begin NPH/regular insulin regimen once patient tolerates regular ADA diet. Begin with home regimen of 26 units of NPH insulin q AM and 12 units NPH insulin q PM plus 5 units regular insulin before meals. May need to increase doses as HbA$_{1C}$ was elevated on admission.

ANSWERS

1. c. Start dobutamine at 5 μg/kg/min
2. Decreased urine output (less than 0.5 mL/kg/hr) is the only direct evidence of decreased perfusion. Other data suggestive of decreased perfusion are decreased cardiac output, elevated PCWP resulting in pulmonary edema, and decreased blood pressure.
3. a. β$_1$-Agonist
4. d. Increase cardiac output
5. c. Decreased cardiac output
6. The estimation of creatinine clearance using a method such as the Cockroft and Gault equation assumes that creatinine clearance is not changing. In this case, creatinine clearance is decreasing over time as perfusion continues to be impaired. This will result in an overestimation of the calculated creatinine clearance.
7. Decreased renal perfusion as a result of impaired cardiac function. Although patient has underlying diabetic nephropathy which may progress to chronic renal failure, is not a cause of acute renal failure.
8. b. Hyperkalemia

9. d. Diabetic ketoacidosis
10. b. Acute myocardial infarction
11. The use of diuretic agents to increase urine output in acute renal failure patients has not been shown to decrease mortality.
12. a. 500 mL/min
13. d. Serum lipids
14. Intensive insulin therapy has been shown to decrease microvascular complications of diabetes such as retinopathy and neuropathy. Prevention of these complications would significantly maintain a better quality of life. In addition, treatment and complications of retinopathy and neuropathy would be avoided, resulting in less medical costs to the patient.
15. End-of-life issues need to be addressed in life-threatening situations. Ideally, the patient has previously dictated his wishes to family members or the medical team. These decisions involve the use of life-support measures such as mechanical ventilation, resuscitation, medications for hemodynamic support, nutritional support, conditions for withdrawal of life-support. Occasionally, the family is forced to make these decisions on behalf of the patient when the patient cannot speak for himself. These decisions should involve all members of the health care team so that a uniform approach to end-of-life care is achieved.
16. Key points are:
   a. Cardiac events occur frequently in critically ill patients and require numerous pharmacologic treatment strategies, the most important of which is to maximize tissue oxygen supply and minimize tissue oxygen demand.
   b. Decreased organ perfusion may affect the clearance of both renally eliminated drugs and hepatically eliminated drugs.
   c. Optimizing the determinants of oxygen delivery (hemoglobin concentration, oxygen saturation, cardiac output) is critically important to ensuring adequate tissue oxygenation.
   d. Recognition of physiologic triggers, appropriate monitoring, and appropriate therapy is vital for the prevention of diabetic ketoacidosis.

CASE 156

PROBLEM LIST

1. Gastrointestinal Bleeding
2. Sepsis
3. Liver Disease (Cirrhosis)
4. Coagulopathy
5. History of Alcohol Withdrawal
6. Mental Status Changes
7. Chronic Obstructive Pulmonary Disease (COPD)

SOAP NOTE

S: Vomiting bright red blood, abdominal pain; productive cough

O: Icteric sclera, spider angiomas on chest, protuberant abdomen, diffuse abdominal tenderness, hypoactive bowel sounds, abdominal fluid wave present, shifting abdominal dullness present, drowsy; HR 110, T 39.4°C (rectal); Hct 0.30 (30%), Hgb 102 (10.2), Lkcs 17×10^9 (17×10^3), AST 4.5 (270), GGT 60 (60), ALT 3.7 (220), LDH 3.33 (200), Alk Phos 2.0 (118), Alb 20 (2.0), T Bili 94 (5.5), Lkcs differential: 0.79 (79%) polys, 0.14 (14%) bands; INR 2.1; urinalysis: bilirubin positive; paracentesis: cloudy fluid; Lkcs 500/mm^3 with 96% polys; Gram stain reveals many Lkcs and gram-negative rods; FEV$_1$ 65% predicted, FVC 72% predicted; EGD documented esophageal varices, history of prolonged alcohol abuse

A: **Problem 1:** Gastrointestinal bleed secondary to esophageal varicies

Problem 2: Sepsis secondary to subacute bacterial peritonitis; developed while receiving cefotaxime

Problem 3: Liver disease (cirrhosis)

Problem 4: Coagulopathy secondary to liver dysfunction; possible platelet inhibition secondary to aspirin use, vitamin K deficiency, or disseminated intravascular coagulation

Problem 5: History of alcohol withdrawal

Problem 6: Mental status changes secondary to liver dysfunction, sedative administration, or sepsis

Problem 7: COPD secondary to prolonged, heavy cigarette use; PFTs indicate mild obstructive disease; minor symptoms; adequate gas exchange

P: **Problem 1: Gastrointestinal Bleed**
- Discontinue vasopressin 24 hours after bleeding stops; restart if evidence of bleeding
- Continue sucralfate administration until coagulopathy corrected
- Monitor hematocrit every 6 hours until stable, then daily while hospitalized
- Stool guaiac test if bleeding suspected
- Monitor heart rate and blood pressure every 1–2 hours while in ICU, then every 8 hours if stabilized

Problem 2: Sepsis
- Discontinue cefoxitin
- Avoid penicillins secondary to potential allergy
- Start gentamicin 140 mg IV q8h and metronidazole 500 mg IV q8h
- Monitor temperature, blood pressure, heart rate, respiratory rate, urine output every 1–2 hours
- Monitor WBC count and differential, and serum creatinine daily
- Obtain gentamicin peak and trough levels with third dose; adjust peak and trough to achieve levels

of 8–10 mg/L peak and <2 mg/L trough; monitor for resolution or progression of abdominal pain and tenderness

Problem 3: Liver Disease (Cirrhosis)

- Adjust dose of medications that are primarily hepatically eliminated
- Discontinue diazepam
- Educate patient and family on risk of consequences or death related to continued alcohol consumption
- Encourage enrollment into alcohol abuse treatment program
- Institute dietary management including protein intake of 1 g/kg/day, 2000–3000 kcal/day, vitamin and folate supplementation

Problem 4: Coagulopathy

- Give vitamin K 10 mg SC QD × 3 days, then weekly
- Monitor PT, INR, signs of bleeding, hematocrit

Problem 5: History of Alcohol Withdrawal

- Monitor for anxiety, agitation, visual and auditory hallucinations, signs of increased sympathetic tone
- Administer lorazepam 2–4 mg IV as needed for agitation

Problem 6: Change in Mental Status

- Discontinue diazepam as above since hepatically eliminated
- Continue lactulose, titrate to 2–3 bowel movements per day to prevent development of hepatic encephalopathy
- Monitor stool output (daily) and progression or resolution of mental status

Problem 7: History of COPD

- No therapy indicated at this time
- Educate on risks of smoking; encourage enrollment into smoking cessation program
- Consider therapy with nicotine patch or bupropion

ANSWERS

1. Developed peritonitis while receiving cefoxitin, unlikely to respond. Bacterial coverage should include gram-negative aerobes and anaerobes. Single-agent antibiotic therapy option limited by DD's allergy to penicillin drugs.
2. b. Increase bioavailability for high-extraction drugs
3. d. Propranolol
4. Probable disulfiram reaction; inhibition of acetaldehyde dehydrogenase by metronidazole.
5. If emergent decrease in ascitic volume is needed, a paracentesis is performed. For gradual reduction and maintenance therapy, spironolactone is used. Mild diuresis is recommended, since the flux of interstitial fluid to the intravascular space is slow, predisposing the patient to intravascular depletion if rapid diuresis attempted. Spironolactone aids in limiting ascitic volume by inhibiting aldosterone-mediated sodium and water retention. Diuretics may be used in conjunction with spironolactone.

6. $k = \ln(6.5/2.1)/5.5 \text{ hours} = 0.20 \text{ hours}^{-1}$

$$C_{max} = 6.5/e^{-0.20(0.5 \text{ hours})} = 7.2 \text{ mg/L}$$

$$C_{min} = 2.1/e^{0.20(1.5 \text{ hours})}$$

$V = (140 \text{ mg/0.5 hours})1 - e^{-0.20(0.5 \text{ hours})}/$
$0.20 \text{ hours} (7.2 - 1.6e^{-0.20(0.5 \text{ hours})}) = 23 \text{ L}$

$\text{Dosing interval} = (\ln(9/1) / 0.20) + 0.5 \text{ hours}$
$= 11.5 \text{ hours or } 12 \text{ hours.}$

$\text{Rate of infusion} = (23 \text{ L}) (0.20 \text{ hours}^{-1})(9 - 1e^{-0.20(0.5 \text{ hours})}/$
$1 - e^{-0.20(0.5 \text{ hours})} = 392 \text{ mg/hour} \times 0.5 \text{ hour infusion}$
$= 196 \text{ mg or } 200 \text{ mg every } 12 \text{ hours.}$

7. c. Fresh frozen plasma infusion
8. a. *Escherichia coli*
9. c. Increased V
10. Abdominal pain, diffuse abdominal tenderness on exam, Lkcs 17 × 10⁹ (17 × 10³), Lkcs differential: 0.79 (79%) polys, 0.14 (14%) bands; paracentesis: cloudy fluid; Lkcs 500/mm³ with 96% polys; Gram stain reveals many Lkcs and gram-negative rods
11. Cefotetan, cefamandole, cefmetazole, and cefoperazone, which contain a methlytetrathiazole (MTT) side chain, as these may prolong the prothrombin time. (Moxalactam, a noncephalosporin, also contains an MTT side chain and should be avoided.)
12. The goal for this patient is to stop drinking alcohol and smoking cigarettes. Family support is critical to his success. The patient should strongly be encouraged to seek professional treatment for his substance abuse. Financial decisions will be difficult and must involve family since many alcoholics do not hold jobs and lack health insurance. It must be stressed that alcohol has caused most of his health problems and will cause significant morbidity and ultimately early death.
13. b. Cirrhosis, portal hypertension, ascites
14. Alcohol abuse counseling, smoking cessation program, salt restriction to limit ascites formation, 1.0 g/kg/day protein diet to prevent hepatic encephalopathy.
15. d. IM due to coagulopathy
16. Once-daily gentamicin therapy could be used instead of standard dosing. Typically, a dose of 4–7 mg/kg (IBW) every 24 hours. A single trough serum concentration can be monitored every several days, thus decreasing the cost of monitoring. In addition, the once-daily regimen has less risk of renal toxicity compared with standard dosing and thus would avoid costs associated with the treatment of renal insufficiency/failure.
17. Key points are:
   a. Critically ill patients undergo a number of physiologic changes and therapeutic maneuvers that can significantly alter pharmacokinetics and pharmacodynamics within the acute care setting.
   b. The most appropriate route of drug administration

should be individualized for each patient and based on available routes of administration, available dosage forms, the pharmacokinetics and pharmacodynamics of the drug, and the clinical situation.

c. Acute renal failure and hepatic dysfunction are common complications in critically ill patients that can have profound effects on drug product selection and dosing.

d. Successful therapy for substance abuse disorders depends on both pharmacologic and nonpharmacologic treatment strategies.

e. Severe liver dysfunction can cause significant dysfunction in other organ systems and is associated with significant morbidity and mortality.

CASE 158

PROBLEM LIST

1. Allograft Rejection
2. Cyclosporine Toxicity
3. Hypertension
4. Anemia
5. S/P Renal-Pancreatic Transplant

SOAP NOTE

S: Urinating less than normal, confusion, hands shaking more last few days

O: BP 142/96; fine hand tremor present; K 5.0 (5.0), Cr 239 (2.7), Glu 6.1 (111); CBC: Hct 0.3 (30), Hgb 94 (9.4), Lkcs 18 × 10^9 (18 × 10^3), MCV 88 (88); serum amylase: 2.7 μkat/L (162); urine amylase: 1095 μkat/L (65,700); CSA level: 398 (whole blood HPLC); anti-OKT3 antibodies: negative; urinalysis: pH 6.2, specific gravity 1.0, color yellow, appearance cloudy, Lkcs esterase positive, protein negative, glucose negative, ketones negative occult blood negative; CMV blood culture: negative; renal biopsy: 1+ vasculitis, 1+ interstitial changes

A: **Problem 1:** Allograft rejection requiring high-dose steroids

Problem 2: Cyclosporine toxicity with evidence of neurotoxicity, possibly contributing to renal dysfunction; assess diet as contributor to cyclosporine toxicity

Problem 3: Hypertension as preexisting condition; compounded by steroid and cyclosporine therapy, or possibly allograft rejection

Problem 4: Anemia probably due to erythropoietin deficiency associated with chronic renal disease; erythropoietin production should return to normal posttransplant

Problem 5: S/P renal-pancreatic transplant; now with acute allograft rejection

P: Problem 1: Allograft Rejection
- Methylprednisolone 500 mg IV × 3 days
- If no response, start OKT3 5 mg/day × 10 days
- Monitor serum Cr, serum and urine amylase, CD3 cell counts (if on OKT3)
- Decrease cyclosporine dose 50% while on OKT3

Problem 2: Cyclosporine Toxicity
- Hold cyclosporine doses for 2 days; recheck level
- Decrease cyclosporine to 200 mg PO BID
- Monitor mental status, renal function, and cyclosporine levels at least weekly while in hospital, then monthly when stable

Problem 3: Hypertension
- Increase nifedipine XL to 90 mg QD
- Continue clonidine patch for now. Avoid increasing dose as may result in excessive sedation, dry mouth
- Goal blood pressure is ≤ 130/85 mm Hg; monitor daily while in hospital and follow up in clinic following discharge

Problem 4: Anemia
- Obtain serum erythropoietin level to confirm diagnosis
- Monitor renal function; if continues to deteriorate, may start recombinant erythropoietin therapy 2000 units SC 3 times weekly along with ferrous sulfate 325 mg PO QHS as iron stores will become depleted with increased red blood cell production and ultimately decrease erythropoietin response

Problem 5: S/P Renal-Pancreas Transplant
- Continue triple-drug immunosuppressive regimen
- Decrease cyclosporine dose to 200 mg BID due to toxicity; decrease another 50% if OKT3 therapy is started
- Monitor cyclosporine levels every week while in hospital, monthly once stable; goal 50–150 ng/mL whole blood HPLC
- Monitor for drug toxicities

ANSWERS

1. Both acyclovir and ranitidine are > 70% eliminated via the kidneys. CrCl = (140–30)(75)/72(2.7) = 42 mL/min. A 25–50% reduction is required for both drugs. Change to acyclovir 400 mg PO TID and ranitidine 150 mg PO QD. Decrease further if renal function continues to decline.
2. Lifestyle modifications: increase aerobic activity (30–45 min/day), limit sodium intake to ≤ 2.4 g/day or 6 g/day of sodium chloride; limit alcohol intake to 24 oz beer, 10 oz wine, or 2 oz whiskey per day. Counsel on importance of

compliance, rebound hypertension with clonidine withdrawal, and common side effects.

3. c. Headache
4. a. MCV
5. d. 25 hours
6. Erythromycin is a cytochrome P450 enzyme inhibitor and will decrease metabolism of cyclosporine, increasing the risk of toxicity. Inhibition will occur with the first dose of erythromycin. Rifampin is a cytochrome P450 enzyme inducer and will increase the metabolism of cyclosporine, predisposing the patient to allograft rejection. The induction of cyclosporine metabolism will take several days; the effect is not immediate.
7. Beta-blocker therapy should probably be avoided in this patient since this antihypertensive class can decrease insulin release and mask the symptoms of hypoglycemia.
8. b. Cytomegalovirus prophylaxis
9. The health care provider can be key in improving the patient's worries regarding the large expense of medications:
   a. A change of several chronic drugs in this patient's regimen would require less cyclosporine due to cytochrome P450 enzyme inhibition. Such changes include diltiazem or verapamil for nifedipine, ketoconazole for clotrimazole, and cimetidine for ranitidine. Cyclosporine levels must be monitored closely with any of these substitutions. Additionally, most cases of hypertension can be managed with BID dosing. Consider increasing the oral dose of clonidine and discontinuing the clonidine patch. This must be discussed with the patient to assess adherence issues and potentially increased side effects from the oral dosing (increased peak to trough ratio).
   b. Coordinate medication assistance programs through pharmaceutical companies or other social services.
10. d. Skin cancer; postulated to occur as a result of immunosuppression therapy-induced DNA damage, which may be potentiated by ultraviolet light exposure.
11. a. Prednisone
12. PCP prophylaxis with sulfamethoxazole/trimethoprim, calcium, and vitamin D supplementation to prevent osteoporosis. A lipid profile should be checked to assess hyperlipidemia and need for therapy (at increased risk secondary to diabetes).
13. Key points are:
    a. The primary goal of immunosuppressive therapy is to prevent allograft rejection, which remains a major cause of graft loss and morbidity.
    b. The use of immunosuppressive drugs in the prevention of rejection must be balanced against the risks of infection, cardiovascular disease, and malignancy.
    c. Cytomegalovirus is the most important infection in transplant recipients and may predispose allografts to chronic rejection.
    d. Immunosuppressant medications have many toxicities. There are many new chronic medical conditions such as diabetes, hypertension, hyperlipidemia, and osteoporosis that may require treatment following transplantation.
    e. Immunosuppressive medications have narrow therapeutic indices. Patients must be monitored closely for signs and symptoms of efficacy and toxicity.

f. Concomitant therapy with nephrotoxic agents or drugs that interfere with CYP3A4-metabolism should be approached with caution. Increased monitoring is warranted (i.e., SCr, CSA, TAC, or SIR levels).

g. Immunosuppressant agents present a significant economic burden to patients. All immunosuppressive regimens should be evaluated in terms of their pharmacoeconomic benefit.

CASE 159

PROBLEM LIST

1. Septic Shock
2. Acute Respiratory Distress Syndrome (ARDS)
3. Acute Renal Insufficiency
4. Acute Myelocytic Leukemia (AML) with Chemotherapy-Induced Neutropenia and Thrombocytopenia

SOAP NOTE

S: Tired and sore throat for 1 week

O: Mouth ulcerations, diffuse rales throughout both lung fields, liver and spleen enlarged and palpable, no petechiae; BP 80/50, HR 136, RR 40, T 39.4°C (rectal); WBC revealed 43×10^9/L (43×10^3/mL) with 0.4 (40%) blasts, CO_2 12 (12), BUN 21 (60), Cr 185 (2.1), Lkcs 0.2×10^9 (0.2×10^3), Plts 20×10^9 (20×10^3); urinalysis: specific gravity 1.033; (+) granular casts; 0 RBC; 0 Lkcs; Gram stain: no organisms seen; ABG: pH 7.24, pCO_2 25 mm Hg, pO_2 55 mm Hg, 82% hemoglobin saturation on 50% oxygen via face mask; sputum Gram stain: few Lkcs, many gram-negative rods; chest x-ray: diffuse infiltrates throughout both lung fields; bone marrow biopsy—acute myelocytic leukemia (AML)

A: **Problem 1:** Septic shock; multiple risk factors including compromised immune system secondary to AML and neutropenia, pneumonia likely secondary to mechanical ventilation

Problem 2: ARDS secondary to sepsis

Problem 3: Acute renal insufficiency secondary to septic shock; oliguric

Problem 4: AML with chemotherapy-induced neutropenia and thrombocytopenia

P: **Problem 1: Septic Shock**
- Place pulmonary artery catheter for hemodynamic monitoring and therapy guidance
- Treat underlying cause of septic shock, pneumonia with antibiotic therapy immediately; begin empiric

vancomycin 1 g IV QD plus ceftazidime 2 g IV BID
- Maintain blood pressure (systolic ≥ 90 mm Hg) through use of fluids, vasopressors (dopamine, norepinephrine, phenylephrine), or inotropic agents (dobutamine, amrinone, milrinone)
- Monitor blood pressure, PCWP, CO, SVR, resolution of mental status alteration, blood lactate levels, urine output
- Adjust antibiotic therapy according to culture results, if necessary

Problem 2: ARDS
- Intubate for adequate oxygen delivery
- Give fluids to maintain adequate blood pressure; avoid overhydration
- Sedate with lorazepam 2 mg IV q4h plus PRN and/or morphine 2 mg IV q4h plus PRN; adjust according to response; sedation goal: Ramsay score 3
- Administer albuterol for bronchodilation to facilitate lung expansion without increased lung pressures
- Monitor arterial blood gases, PaO_2/FiO_2 ratio, peak inspiratory or plateau pressures (lung)

Problem 3: Acute Renal Insufficiency
- Restore adequate renal perfusion by maintaining adequate blood pressure
- Monitor total fluid intake and urine output, serum potassium, magnesium, and phosphate until renal insufficiency resolves
- Dopamine infusion μg/kg/min or furosemide may be used once intravascular volume repleted; avoid mannitol since it may worsen pulmonary edema

Problem 4: AML/Neutropenia/Thrombocytopenia
- Wait for recovery of bone marrow
- Consider colony stimulating factor therapy if recovery is slow; plan to administer G-CSF 5 μg/kg/day SC until absolute neutrophil count ≥ 10,000/mm³ with next cycle of chemotherapy
- If platelet count decreases below 20,000 or if bleeding occurs administer platelets
- Monitor neutrophil count, platelet count, hematocrit, evidence of bleeding
- Avoid drugs that decrease platelet activity
- Avoid unnecessary invasive procedures

ANSWERS

1. b. IL-1
2. c. Pulmonary capillary wedge pressure: 16 mm Hg
3. a. Stress ulcers–decreased gastrointestinal mucosal blood flow, impaired oxygenation.

Pneumonia–aspiration or invasive tube
Sinusitis (if nasally intubated)
Decreased cardiac output–alter pharmacokinetics of some drugs by decreasing organ perfusion

4. Decreased cardiac output will decrease blood flow to the liver. Expect:
   a. A decrease in clearance of drugs that are highly extracted (dependent of liver blood flow).
   b. A decrease in clearance for drugs that are primarily renally cleared.
5. The Cockroft and Gault equation assumes a steady-state serum creatinine concentration. In a patient with septic shock, the serum creatinine may rise quickly and continue to rise over time. Thus, the calculation of creatinine clearance represents the creatinine clearance at a given time point. With serum creatinine rising, this calculation will overestimate creatinine clearance.
6. a. Mechanical ventilation and coagulopathy
7. d. Pulmonary embolism
8. b. Cost of treating pneumonia
9. d. Bone pain
10. a. Bacterial cell wall synthesis inhibitor; concentration-independent bacterial killing
11. Sucralfate binds phosphate in the gastrointestinal tract and may lead to hypophosphatemia. Adequate phosphate stores needed for muscle cell energy (ATP). Hypophosphatemia may result in decreased respiratory muscle function.
12. d. Increase arterial oxygen content
13. Oliguria, creatinine 185 μmol/L (2.1 mg/dL); BUN 21 mmol/L (60 mg/L); urine specific gravity 1.033, granular casts
14. As with any patient, the pharmacist should be cognizant of the awareness of the patient. Patients who are mechanically ventilated cannot communicate effectively and therefore rely on communication from the health care worker for information regarding their care. The pharmacist should explain to the patient what his/her function is and what changes are being made in his therapy if appropriate. This should also be explained to the family as they are often confused regarding the role of each health care worker involved in the patient's care. The pharmacist should strive to achieve a level of sedation that will keep the patient comfortable but still responsive.
15. Key points are:
   a. Critically ill patients undergo a number of physiologic changes and therapeutic maneuvers that can significantly alter pharmacokinetics and pharmacodynamics within the acute care setting.
   b. Provision of adequate analgesia and sedation is essential in the supportive care of virtually all critically ill patients.
   c. Mechanical ventilation is frequently required in critically ill patients and is associated with numerous complications requiring pharmacologic intervention.
   d. Acute renal failure and hepatic dysfunction are common complications in critically ill patients that can have profound effects on drug product selection and dosing.
   e. Use of prophylactic heparin and stress ulcer prophylaxis (e.g., sucralfate, H_2-antagonists) should be considered in all critically ill patients at risk to develop these complications.

CASE 160

PROBLEM LIST

1. Allograft Rejection
2. Urinary Tract Infection
3. S/P Renal Transplant
4. Hypertension

SOAP NOTE

S: Pain at transplant site, low-grade fever, pain on urination

O: Cushingoid facial feature, pain at allograft site upon palpation; BP 126/86, T 38.5°C; Cr 221 (2.5) [baseline since transplant 123.8 μmol/L (1.4)]; urinalysis: pH 6.2, specific gravity 1.0, color yellow, appearance cloudy, Lkcs esterase positive, protein negative, glucose negative, ketones negative, occult blood negative, bacterial smear positive, many WBC, nitrate positive; urine culture: 100,000 colonies *Escherichia coli;* sensitivity: resistance to ampicillin but sensitive to cefazolin, gentamicin, tobramycin, ceftizoxime, and ciprofloxacin; CMV culture: negative; renal biopsy: 2+ vasculitis, 2+ interstitial rejection; CSA trough level 78 ng/mL

A: **Problem 1:** Allograft rejection requiring rescue therapy; unresponsive to high-dose steroids; adherent with medications

Problem 2: Urinary tract infection requires immediate therapy to minimize risk of urosepsis and further loss of kidney function. Avoid aminoglycoside due to nephrotoxicity

Problem 3: S/P renal transplant—adherent, no signs of drug toxicity

Problem 4: Hypertension well controlled on current regimen; skin irritation from clonidine patch

P: **Problem 1: Allograft Rejection**

- Start OKT3 therapy at 5 mg/day IV for 10 days
- Minimize chills, rigors, fever, gastrointestinal side effects by premedicating with methylprednisolone, diphenhydramine, and acetaminophen
- Monitor CD3 T cell count, goal: undetectable levels; increase OKT3 dose if CD3 T cells remain elevated
- Monitor serum creatinine daily; expect to increase after first few doses and then return to baseline
- Decrease cyclosporine dose by 50% during OKT3 therapy; monitor trough levels

Problem 2: Urinary Tract Infection

- Based on calculated creatinine clearance (41 mL/min), start cefazolin 1 g IV BID
- Monitor serum creatinine and adjust cefazolin dose based on creatinine clearance
- Urinalysis after 3–4 days of therapy; reculture if persistent UTI suspected. (WBC count and temperature may be difficult to interpret with azathioprine and corticosteroids administered)

Problem 3: S/P Renal Transplant

- Resume previous regimen of cyclosporine, azathioprine, and prednisone after OKT3 therapy complete
- Monitor for signs and symptoms of drug toxicity and organ rejection
- Monitor cyclosporine levels every month

Problem 4: Hypertension

- Advise to rotate application site of clonidine patch to avoid skin irritation
- If irritation persists, change to clonidine therapy at 0.2 mg PO BID
- Change nifedipine to sustained-release formulation 30 mg PO QD to increase adherence and decrease potential for adverse effects

ANSWERS

1. Most common: fever, chills, headache, rigors, and hypotension. Others include tremor, seizure, nausea, vomiting, thrombocytopenia, leukopenia, aseptic meningitis, and pulmonary edema (in patients with fluid overload).
2. Inadequate inactivation of CD3 T cells: increase OKT3 dose to 10 mg/day and monitor CD3 T cells.
3. 25% of patients develop antibodies to OKT3. Need to check antibody titer; if ≥ 1:1000, OKT3 therapy will be ineffective.
4. Positive leukocyte esterase, many WBC, many bacteria, nitrate positive.
5. a. Cytomegalovirus infection
6. c. Change from cyclosporine to tacrolimus
7. d. *Pneumocystis carinii* pneumonia prophylaxis
8. Both cyclosporine and corticosteroid use may increase blood pressure.
9. OKT3 binds to T cells, resulting in opsonization and removal by the reticuloendothelial system. Additionally, it disrupts the function of T lymphocytes by removing CD3 molecules from the surface of the T cell.
10. a. 100 mg
11. d. Ganciclovir IV
12. c. T-helper and cytotoxic T-cell hypersensitivity
13. Factors affecting the pharmacoeconomic evaluation of rejection therapies include cost of the medication and administration, response rate, acute and long-term side effects, incidence of infectious complications, cost of complication treatment, necessity for adjunctive drug therapy to decrease infusion-related side effects, potential for resistance development and thus lack of response (OKT3).

14. b. Depression
15. Key points are:
    a. The primary goal of immunosuppressive therapy is to prevent allograft rejection, which remains a major cause of graft loss and morbidity.
    b. Cytomegalovirus is the most important infection in transplant recipients and may predispose allografts to chronic rejection.
    c. Immunosuppressant medications have many toxicities. There are many new chronic medical conditions such as diabetes, hypertension, hyperlipidemia, and osteoporosis that may require treatment following transplantation.
    d. The use of immunosuppressive drugs in the prevention of rejection must be balanced against the risks of infection, cardiovascular disease, and malignancy.